Practice Considerations for Adult-Gerontological Acute Care Nurse Practitioners
2nd Edition
Volume I

Thomas W. Barkley, Jr., PhD, ACNP-BC, FAANP
Professor
Director of Nurse Practitioner Programs
California State University, Los Angeles
School of Nursing
and
President, Barkley & Associates
Los Angeles, California

Charlene M. Myers, DNP, ACNP-BC, CNS
Associate Clinical Professor
Adult Acute Care Nurse Practitioner Program Coordinator
University of South Alabama
College of Nursing
Mobile, Alabama

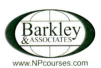

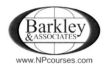
www.NPcourses.com

P.O. Box 69901
West Hollywood, CA 90069

PRACTICE CONSIDERATIONS FOR ADULT-GERONTOLOGY
ACUTE CARE NURSE PRACTITIONERS 2nd EDITION   ISBN 978-0-9864021-4-2
Copyright ©2015 by Barkley & Associates

All rights reserved. No part of this publication may be reproduced or transmitted in any form or by any means, electronic or mechanical, including photocopying, recording, or any information storage and retrieval system, without permission from the publisher. Permissions may be sought directly from Barkley & Associates by the following: phone: 1.866.938.5557 or 1.323.656.1606; fax: 1. 323.656.1620; e-mail: Contact_Us@npcourses.com.

Notice

Knowledge and best practices are subject to change, as new research and further experience expand knowledge. Changes in practice, treatment, and drug therapy may be warranted or appropriate. It is recommended that readers verify the most up-to-date information regarding procedures featured or check the manufacturers of administered products, so as to verify the recommended dose, formula, methods of administration, and contradindications. It is the duty of practitioners, relying on their experience and knowledge of the patient's circumstances, to determine dosages and the best treatment for each patient, while taking all safety precautions. To the fullest extend of the law, neither the Publisher nor the Editors and Authors assume any liability for any injury and/or damage to persons or property arising out of or related to any use of the content in this book.

The Publisher

International Standard Book Number: 978-0-9864021-4-2

Pharmacology Editor: Robert Fellin
Managing Editor: Taylor Spining
Project Manager: Charlie Wang
Staff Coordinator: Chris Cude
Cover Design: Andres Morgan

Preface

Practice Considerations for Adult Gerontology Acute Care Nurse Practitioners 2nd edition is a comprehensive textbook for advanced practice nurses. The text is organized in a systematic fashion, addressing over 350 of the most common conditions experienced by adult patients in acute care. Using an easy-to-read outline format, coverage of each condition includes defining terms, incidence/predisposing factors, subjective and physical examination findings, diagnostic tests, and management strategies.

The text has been written to provide the practitioner with a thorough overview of evidence-based practice guidelines. In this light, the text builds on previous knowledge of anatomy, physiology, and pathophysiology concepts that have not been separately emphasized. Although many practitioners may be highly specialized, this text was designed as a useful tool for the entire scope of acute care nursing practice, including settings such as clinics, emergency departments, medical/surgical departments in hospitals, as well as critical care units. Although this text was developed based on research and expertise, we also feel strongly that collaborative practice with other experts and clinicians is essential to successfully meeting patient goals.

Thomas W. Barkley, Jr.

Charlene M. Myers

Acknowledgments

We gratefully acknowledge the previous authors of the first and second editions of *Practice Guidelines for Acute Care Nurse Practitioners* whose knowledge and dedication provided the foundation for the expansion of this textbook. We would additionally like to thank the outstanding contributors and reviewers of this text. Without the expertise of these scholars, this work would not have been possible.

We also thank the following people at Barkley and Associates:

Pharmacology Editor: Robert Fellin
Managing Editor: Taylor Spining
Project Manager: Charlie Wang
Staff Coordinator: Chris Cude
Cover Design: Andres Morgan

whose combined efforts have produced what we believe is a
state-of-the art, evidence-based, excellent resource for the profession.

Thomas W. Barkley, Jr.

Charlene M. Myers

Distinguished Contributors

Bimbola F. Akintade, PhD, ACNP-BC, MBA, MHA
Assistant Professor
Organizational Systems and Adult Health
Specialty Director
Adult Gerontology Acute Care Nurse Practitioner/Clinical Nurse Specialist Program
University of Maryland
Baltimore, Maryland
23. Measures of Oxygenation and Ventilation, 31. Pneumothorax, 86. Managing the Surgical Patient

Kimberly Alva, MSN, ACNP-BC, CCRN
Acute Care Nurse Practitioner
Neurosurgical Intensive Care Unit
Cedars Sinai Medical Center
Los Angeles, California
4. Neurologic Trauma

Susan J. Appel, PhD, ACNP-BC, FNP-BC, CCRN, FAHA
Professor
The University of Alabama
Capstone College of Nursing
Tuscaloosa, Alabama
47. Diabetes Mellitus, 48. Diabetes-Related Emergencies

Amita Avadhani, DNP, DCC, ACNP-BC, ANP-BC, APN, CCRN
Assistant Professor
Track Coordinator
Adult Gerontology Acute Critical Care Nurse Practitioner Program
Rutgers School of Nursing
Rutgers Biomedical and Health Sciences University
Newark, New Jersey
Critical Care Nurse Practitioner-Adult ICU
Saint Peters University Hospital
New Brunswick, New Jersey
22. Diagnostic Concepts of Oxygenation and Ventilation, 35. Mechanical Ventilatory Support

Thomas W. Barkley, Jr., PhD, ACNP-BC, FAANP
Professor
Director of Nurse Practitioner Programs
California State University, Los Angeles
School of Nursing
President, Barkley & Associates
Los Angeles, California
3. Peripheral Neuropathies, 11. Cardiovascular Assessment, 12. Hypertension, 13. Coronary Artery Disease and Hyperlipidemia, 14. Angina and Myocardial Infarction, 15. Adjunct Equipment/Devices, 16. Peripheral Vascular Disease, 17. Inflammatory Cardiac Diseases, 18. Heart Failure, 19. Valvular Disease, 20. Cardiomyopathy, 21. Arrhythmias, 24. The Chest X-Ray, 25. Pulmonary Function Testing, 26. Obstructive (Ventilatory) Lung Diseases, 27. Restrictive (Inflammatory) Lung Diseases, 28. Pulmonary Hypertension and Pulmonary Vascular Disorders, 29. Chest Wall and Secondary Pleural Disorders, 30. Respiratory Failure, 31. Pneumothorax, 32. Lower Respiratory Tract Pathogens,

33. Obstructive Sleep Apnea, 34. Oxygen Supplementation, 35. Mechanical Ventilatory Support, 47. Diabetes Mellitus, 48. Diabetes-Related Emergencies, 49. Thyroid Disease, 50. Cushing's Syndrome, 51. Primary Adrenocortical Insufficiency (Addison Disease) and Adrenal Crisis, 52. Pheochromocytoma, 53. Syndrome of Inappropriate Antidiuretic Hormone, 54. Diabetes Insipidus, 67. HIV/AIDS and Opportunistic Infections Among Older Adults, 68. Autoimmune Diseases, 69. Integumentary Disorders, 70. Ectopic Pregnancy and STIs, 71. Eye, Ear, Nose, and Throat Disorders, 72. Headache, 73. Fever, 74. Pain, 76. Management of the Patient in Shock, 77. Nutritional Considerations, 78. Fluid, Electrolyte, and Acid-Base Imbalances, 79. Poisoning and Drug Toxicities, 80. Wound Management, 81. Infections, 82. Trauma Considerations, 83. Solid Organ Transplantation, 84. Burns, 85. Hospital Admission Considerations, 86. Managing the Surgical Patient, 87. Guidelines for Health Promotion and Screening, 89. Immunization Recommendations

Catherine Blache, MSN, RN, CCRC
Owner/Director of Research
Precision Clinical Research, LLC
Mobile, Alabama
80. Wound Management, 84. Burns

Bob Blessing, DNP, ACNP-BC
Consulting Associate Professor
Duke University
School of Nursing
Durham, North Carolina
Lead Nurse Practitioner
Neuroscience Critical Care Unit
Duke University Health System
Durham, North Carolina
3. Peripheral Neuropathies, 76. Management of the Patient in Shock

Kelly Blessing, MSN, FNP-BC
Neurology Provider
Duke University Health System
Durham, North Carolina
Family Nurse Practitioner
Cerebrovascular Center
Duke University Health System
Durham, North Carolina
3. Peripheral Neuropathies

Lorris J. Bouzigard, DNP, ACNP-BC, ANP-C, DCC
Acute Care Nurse Practitioner
Internal Medicine Clinic
Louisiana Heart Hospital Medical Group
Lacombe, Louisiana
Adjunct Clinical Instructor
University of South Alabama
Mobile, Alabama
73. Fever

Travis Bradley, MSN, ACNP-BC, CEN
Acute Care Nurse Practitioner
Neuro-Surgical Intensive Care Unit
Cedars-Sinai Medical Center
Los Angeles, California
1. Cerebrovascular Accidents: Brain Attack, 2. Structural Abnormalities

Steven W. Branham, PhD, RN, ACNP-BC, FNP-BC, FAANP, CCRN
Assistant Professor
Acute Care Nurse Practitioner Program
Texas Tech University
College of Nursing
Lubbock, Texas
43. Acute Kidney Injury and Chronic Kidney Disease

Barbara Ann Shelton Broome, PhD, RN, CNS, FAAN
Dean
Kent State University
College of Nursing
Kent, Ohio
88. Major Causes of Mortality in the United States

Fredrick Carlston, MSN, ACNP-BC
Acute Care Nurse Practitioner
Cardiovascular Medicine
Keck Hospital of USC
Los Angeles, California
Acute Care Nurse Practitioner
Cardiology Nuclear Medicine
Cedars-Sinai Medical Center
Los Angeles, California
21. Arrhythmias

Jennifer Coates, MSN, ACNP-BC, MBA, ACNPC
Assistant Clinical Professor
Adult Gerontology Acute Care Nurse Practitioner Program
Drexel University
College of Nursing & Health Professions
Philadelphia, Pennsylvania
29. Chest Wall and Secondary Pleural Disorders, 33. Obstructive Sleep Apnea

Marla Couture, MSN, ACNP-BC, CCRN
Clinical Instructor
Acute Care Department
The University of Alabama at Birmingham
School of Nursing
Birmingham, Alabama
46. Nephrolithiasis

R. Michael Culpepper, MD
Professor
Chief Division of Nephrology
University of South Alabama
College of Medicine
Mobile, Alabama
78. Fluid, Electrolyte, and Acid-Base Imbalances

Rita A. Dello Stritto, PhD, ACNP-BC, CNS, ENP
Associate Professor
Texas Woman's University
Nelda C. Stark College of Nursing
Houston, Texas
49. Thyroid Disease, 50. Cushing's Syndrome, 51. Primary Adrenocortical Insufficiency (Addison Disease) and Adrenal Crisis, 54. Diabetes Insipidus

Lisa Evans, DNP, ACNP-BC
Hospitalist Nurse Practitioner
Director of Skilled Nursing Facility Services
Pulmonary Consultants & Primary Care Physicians
Orange, CA
Lecturer
Adult Gerontology Acute Care Nurse Practitioner Program
California State University, Los Angeles
Los Angeles, California
61. Anemias, 62. Sickle Cell Disease/Crisis, 63. Coagulopathies

Robert Fellin, PharmD, BCPS
Pharmacist
Cedars-Sinai Medical Center
Los Angeles, California
Faculty
Barkley & Associates
Los Angeles, California
9. Parkinson's Disease, 12. Hypertension, 18. Heart Failure, 19. Valvular Disease, 21. Arrhythmias

Alison Forbes, MSN, ACNP-BC, CCRN
Acute Care Nurse Practitioner
Division of Neurocritical Care, Department of Surgery
Harbor UCLA Medical Center
Torrance, California
Lecturer
Adult Gerontology Acute Care Nurse Practitioner Program
California State University, Los Angeles
Los Angeles, California
81. Infections, 82. Trauma Considerations

Catherine L. Fung, MSN, ACNP-BC
General Surgery Acute Care Nurse Practitioner
Division of Upper GI and General Surgery
Keck Hospital of USC
Los Angeles, California
40. Anatomic Intestinal Disorders

Donna Gullette, PhD, ACNP-BC, APRN
Professor
Director of Master of Nursing Science Programs
Associate Dean for Practice
University of Arkansas for Medical Sciences
College of Nursing
Little Rock, Arkansas
69. Integumentary Disorders, 72. Headache

Haley Hoy, PhD, ACNP-BC
Interim Associate Dean, Graduate Programs
University of Alabama Huntsville
Huntsville, Alabama
Acute Care Nurse Practitioner
Lung Transplantation
Vanderbilt Medical Center
Nashville, Tennessee
25. Pulmonary Function Testing, 28. Pulmonary Hypertension and Pulmonary Vascular Disorders

Alicia Huckstadt, PhD, APRN, FNP-BC, GNP-BC, FAANP
Professor
Director of Graduate Programs
Wichita State University
School of Nursing
Wichita, Kansas
36. Peptic Ulcer Disease, 89. Immunization Recommendations

Lisa A. Johnson, DrNP, CRNP, ACNP-BC
Assistant Professor
Director, AGACNP Program
De Sales University
Department of Nursing and Health
Center Valley, Pennsylvania
39. Inflammatory Gastrointestinal Disorders, 68. Autoimmune Diseases

Joan E. King, PhD, ACNP-BC, ANP-BC, FAANP
Professor
Adult-Gerontology Acute Care Nurse Practitioner Program Director
Vanderbilt University
School of Nursing
Nashville, Tennessee
11. Cardiovascular Assessment, 13. Coronary Artery Disease and Hyperlipidemia, 14. Angina and Myocardial Infarction, 18. Heart Failure

Honore Kotler, MSN, ACNP-BC
Lead Acute Care Nurse Practitioner
Comprehensive Transplant Center
Cedars Sinai Medical Center
Los Angeles, California
83. Solid Organ Transplantation

Victoria Ku, MSN, ACNP-BC, CCRN
Acute Care Nurse Practitioner
Thoracic Surgery
Keck Hospital of USC,
Los Angeles, California
Clinical Instructor
West Coast University
Ontario, California
24. The Chest X-Ray

Judi Kuric, DNP, ACNP-BC, CNRN
Assistant Professor
University of Southern Indiana
College of Nursing and Health Professions
Evansville, Indiana
Acute Care Nurse Practitioner
Neurosurgical Private Practice
Louisville, Kentucky
5. Central Nervous System Disorders, 8. Multiple Sclerosis, 9. Parkinson's Disease, 10. Amyotrophic Lateral Sclerosis, 85. Hospital Admissions Considerations

Patrick A. Laird, DNP, ACNP-BC, APRN
Assistant Professor of Clinical Nursing
Adult-Gerontology Acute Care Nurse Practitioner Program Director
The University of Texas Health Science Center at Houston
School of Nursing
Houston, Texas
6. Seizure Disorders

Monique Lambert, DNP, ACNP-BC
Director of the Advanced Practice Institute
RUSH University Medical Center
Chicago, Illinois
52. Pheochromocytoma, 53. Syndrome of Inappropriate Antidiuretic Hormone

Paula McCauley, DNP, ACNP-BC, APRN, CNE
Assistant Clinical Professor
Associate Dean for Academic Affairs
University of Connecticut
School of Nursing
Storrs, Connecticut
Acute Care Program Coordinator
University of Connecticut
School of Nursing
Storrs, Connecticut
77. Nutritional Considerations

Sheila Melander, PhD, ACNP-BC, FCCM, FAANP
Professor
University of Kentucky
College of Nursing
Lexington, Kentucky
15. Adjunct Equipment/Devices, 17. Inflammatory Cardiac Diseases, 20. Cardiomyopathy

Helen Miley, PhD, ACNP-BC. AGACNP-BC
Clinical Associate Professor
Specialty Director
Adult Geriatric Acute Care Nurse Practitioner Program
Rutgers, The State University of New Jersey
Newark, New Jersey
Adult Geriatric Acute Care Nurse Practitioner
Medical Intensive Care Unit
Robert Wood Johnson University Hospital
New Brunswick, New Jersey
12. Hypertension, 87. Guidelines for Health Promotion and Screening

David A. Miller, MD, FCCP
Associate Professor
Family Nurse Practitioner Program
Texas A&M University-Corpus Christi
College of Nursing and Health Sciences
Corpus Christi, Texas
26. Obstructive (Ventilatory) Lung Diseases, 27. Restrictive (Inflammatory) Lung Diseases, 30. Respiratory Failure, 32. Lower Respiratory Tract Pathogens, 67. HIV/AIDS and Opportunistic Infections Among Older Adults, 71. Eye, Ear, Nose, and Throat Disorders

Charlene M. Myers, DNP, ACNP-BC, CNS
Associate Clinical Professor
Adult Acute Care Nurse Practitioner Program Coordinator
University of South Alabama
College of Nursing
Mobile, Alabama
1. Cerebrovascular Accidents: Brain Attack, 2. Structural Abnormalities, 4. Neurologic Trauma, 5. Central Nervous System Disorders, 6. Seizure Disorders, 7. Dementia, 22. Diagnostic Concepts of Oxygenation and Ventilation, 23. Measures of Oxygenation and Ventilation, 25. Pulmonary Function Testing, 29. Chest Wall and Secondary Pleural Disorders, 34. Oxygen Supplementation, 35. Mechanical Ventilatory Support, 36. Peptic Ulcer Disease, 37. Liver Disease, 38. Biliary Dysfunction, 39. Inflammatory Gastrointestinal Disorders, 40. Anatomic Intestinal Disorders, 41. Gastrointestinal Bleeding, 42. Urinary Tract Infections, 43. Acute Kidney Injury and Chronic Kidney Disease, 44. Benign Prostatic Hyperplasia, 45. Renal Artery Stenosis, 46. Nephrolithiasis, 71. Eye, Ear, Nose, and Throat Disorders, 72. Headache, 73. Fever, 74. Pain, 76. Management of the Patient in Shock, 77. Nutritional Considerations, 78. Fluid, Electrolyte, and Acid-Base Imbalances, 80. Wound Management, 86. Managing the Surgical Patient, 87. Guidelines for Health Promotion and Screening, 89. Immunization Recommendations

Marcie Nomura, MSN, ACNP-BC, CCRN
Acute Care Nurse Practitioner
Hepatobiliary Surgery
Cedars-Sinai Medical Center
Comprehensive Transplant Center
Los Angeles, California
74. Pain

Michalyn Pelphrey, MSN, ACNP-BC, CCTC
Acute Care Nurse Practitioner
Liver Transplant
Cedars-Sinai Medical Center
Los Angeles, California
37. Liver Disease, 38. Biliary Dysfunction

Nicole Perez, MSN, ACNP-BC, CCRN
Critical Care Intensivist Nurse Practitioner
Harbor UCLA Medical Center
Torrance, California
Lecturer
Adult Gerontology Acute Care Nurse Practitioner Program
California State University, Los Angeles
Los Angeles, California
41. Gastrointestinal Bleeding

Tobias P. Rebmann, MSN, ACNP-BC, CCRN
Acute Care Nurse Practitioner
Trinity Clinic Cardiothoracic Surgery
Louis and Peaches Owen Heart Hospital
Cardiothoracic Intensive Care Unit
Tyler, Texas
26. Obstructive (Ventilatory) Lung Diseases, 27. Restrictive (Inflammatory) Lung Diseases

Jacqueline Rhoads, PhD, APRN-BC, CNL-BC, PMHNP-BE, FAANP
Professor
Tulane University
School of Tropical Medicine
Center of Applied Environmental Public Health
New Orleans, LA
64. Leukemias

Ivan Robbins, MD
Professor
Director, Pulmonary Vascular Center
Vanderbilt Medical Center
Nashville, Tennessee
28. Pulmonary Hypertension and Pulmonary Vascular Disorders

Jennifer Javier Roberg, MSN, ACNP-BC
Staff Education
Research & Consulting
Kaiser Permanente South Bay
Harbor City, California
44. Benign Prostatic Hyperplasia

Jenna Rush, MSN, ACNP-BC, CCTC
Heart Transplant Coordinator
Cedars-Sinai Medical Center
Comprehensive Transplant Center
Los Angeles, California
65. Lymphoma

Valerie K. Sabol, PhD, ACNP-BC, GNP-BC
Associate Professor
Specialty Director
Adult-Gerontology Acute Care Nurse Practitioner Master's Program
Duke University
School of Nursing
Durham, North Carolina
76. Management of the Patient in Shock

Angela Starkweather, PhD, ACNP-BC, CNRN
Associate Professor and Chair
Department of Adult Health and Nursing Systems
Virginia Commonwealth University
School of Nursing
Richmond, Virginia
7. Dementia, 70. Ectopic Pregnancy and STIs

Michele Talley, MSN, ACNP-BC
Clinical Instructor
Specialty Track Coordinator
Adult-Gerontology Acute Care Nurse Practitioner Program
University of Alabama at Birmingham
School of Nursing
Birmingham, Alabama
42. Urinary Tract Infections, 45. Renal Artery Stenosis

Carol Thompson, PhD, DNP, ACNP-BC, FNP-BC
Professor
University of Kentucky
College of Nursing
Lexington, Kentucky
34. Oxygen Supplementation

Elizabeth A. VandeWaa, PhD
Professor
Adult Health Nursing Department
University of South Alabama
College of Nursing
Mobile, Alabama
79. Poisoning and Drug Toxicities

Paula K. Vuckovich, PhD, PMHCNS-BC
Associate Professor
Psychiatric Mental Health Graduate Option Coordinator
Doctor of Nursing Practice Program Coordinator
California State University, Los Angeles
School of Nursing
Los Angeles, California
75. Psychosocial Problems in Acute Care

Theresa M. Wadas, PhD, DNP, ACNP-BC, FNP-BC, CCRN
Assistant Professor
University of Alabama
Captone College of Nursing
Tuscaloosa, Alabama
16. Peripheral Vascular Disease, 19. Valvular Disease

Colleen R. Walsh, DNP, ACNP-BC, ONC, ONP-C, CS
Contract Assistant Professor of Graduate Nursing
University of Southern Indiana
College of Nursing and Health
Evansville, Indiana
55. Arthritis, 56. Subluxations and Dislocations, 57. Soft Tissue Injury, 58. Fractures, 59. Compartment Syndrome, 60. Back Pain Syndromes, 66. Other Common Cancers

Distinguished Reviewers

Laura Kierol Andrews, PhD, ACNP-BC
Assistant Professor
Yale University
School of Nursing
Orange, Connecticut
Senior Acute Care Nurse Practitioner
Department of Critical Care Medicine
Hospital of Central Connecticut
New Britain, Connecticut

Susan J. Appel, PhD, ACNP-BC, FNP-BC, CCRN, FAHA
Professor
The University of Alabama
Capstone College of Nursing
Tuscaloosa, Alabama

Kelly Arashin, MSN, ACNP-BC
Associate Professor of Graduate Nursing
Armstrong Atlantic State University
School of Nursing
Savannah, Georgia
Acute Care Nurse Practitioner
Critical Care Clinical Nurse Specialist
Hilton Head Hospital
Apollo, Maryland

Melanie Schwartz Binshtok, MS, ACNP-BC, AACC
Adjunct Faculty
Virginia Commonwealth University
School of Nursing
Richmond, Virginia
Inpatient Cardiology Nurse Practitioner
Bon Secours Richmond Health System
Richmond, Virginia

Valeria K. Bisig, MSN, ACNP-BC, FNP-BC
Acute Care Nurse Practitioner
TriHealth Corporate Health
Cincinnati, Ohio

Jennifer M. Blake, MSN, ACNP-BC, CNRN
Neuroscience Nurse Practitioner
Seton Brain and Spine Institute
Austin, Texas

Shari W. Bryant MSN, ACNP-BC, AOCNP
Adjunct Faculty
Acute Care Nurse Practitioner Program
University of Southern Indiana
College of Nursing and Health
Evansville, Indiana
Hospitalist Acute Care Nurse Practitioner
St. Mary's Medical Center
Evansville, Indiana

Megan M. Butts, MSN, ACNP-BC
Neuro Critical Care Nurse Practitioner
Neuroscience Intensive Care Unit
The University of Mississippi Medical Center
Jackson, Mississippi

Sandra K. Callaghan, MSN, NP-C
Family Nurse Practitioner
Specialty in Neurosurgery and Pain Management
Antelope Valley Neuroscience Medical Group
Lancaster, California
Universal Pain Management
CEO, Callaghan, Inc.
Palmdale, California

Jaime Cannon, MSN, ACNP- BC
Acute Care Nurse Practitioner
Montgomery Pulmonary Consultants
Montgomery, Alabama

Melanie A. Caustrita, MSN, ACNP-BC
Hospitalist Nurse Practitioner
Miami Valley Hospital
Dayton, Ohio
Locum Tenens Nurse Practitioner
StaffCare, Inc.
Irving, Texas

Grace Courreges, MSN, ACNP-BC
Acute Care Nurse Practitioner
Sierra Medical Center
El Paso, Texas

Patricia Cunningham, DNSc, PMHNP-BC, PMHCNS-BC, FNP-BC
Associate Professor
Coordinator of the Psychiatric Mental Health
Doctor of Nursing Practice Program
University of Tennessee Health Science Center
College of Nursing
Memphis, Tennessee

Caroline Lloyd Doherty, MSN, AGACNP-BC, AACC
Associate Program Director
Adult-Gerontology Acute Care Nurse Practitioner and
Adult-Gerontology Clinical Nurse Specialist Programs
University of Pennsylvania
School of Nursing
Philadelphia, Pennsylvania

Lisa Evans, DNP, ACNP-BC
Hospitalist Nurse Practitioner
Director of Skilled Nursing Facility Services
Pulmonary Consultants & Primary Care Physicians
Orange, California
Lecturer
Adult Gerontology Acute Care Nurse Practitioner Program
California State University, Los Angeles
Los Angeles, California

Mary Franklin, PhD, ACNP-BC
Clinical Assistant Professor
Wayne State University
College of Nursing
Detroit, Michigan

Connie L. Leonard Geimer, MSN, ACNP-BC, CRNP, CCRN
Acute Care Nurse Practitioner
Pegasus Emergency Group
Gadsden Regional Medical Center
Gadsden, Alabama

Donna L. Gerber, PhD, ACNP-BC, AOCN
Acute Care Nurse Practitioner
Department of Sarcoma
University of Texas M.D. Anderson Cancer Center
Houston, Texas

Darla Gowan, DNP, FNP-BC
Assistant Professor
Division of Graduate Studies in Nursing
Family Nurse Practitioner Program
Indiana Wesleyan University
School of Nursing
Marion, Indiana

Laura Griffin, DNP, ACNP-BC, CCRN
Adjunct Professor
Adult-Gerontology Acute Care Nurse Practitioner Program
Texas Woman's University
School of Nursing
Denton, Texas
Chief Nurse Executive/Chief Clinical Officer
Kindred Sugar Land Hospital
Sugar Land, Texas
Acute Care Nurse Practitioner
Houston Methodist Sugar Land Hospital
Sugarland, Texas

Tonja M. Hartjes, DNP, ACNP-BC, CCRN, CSC
Clinical Associate Professor
Adult-Gerontology Acute Care Nurse Practitioner Program
University of Florida
College of Nursing
Gainesville, Florida

Constance W. Hartman, MSN, ACNP-BC, CCRN
Pulmonary and Sleep Nurse Practitioner
Central Ohio Pulmonary Disease, Inc
Columbus, Ohio

Melissa Hill, MSN, ACNP-BC, APRN, CNRN, CCRN, SCRN
Clinical Instructor
Acute Care Nurse Practitioner
Neuroscience Intensive Care Unit
Medical University of South Carolina
Charleston, South Carolina

Susan Hunt, MSN, ACNP-BC
Adjunct Assistant Professor
Adult-Gerontology Acute Care Nurse Practitioner Program Coordinator
Indiana University
School of Nursing
Indianapolis, Indiana

Lindsay Iverson, DNP, ACNP-BC
Assistant Professor
Adult-Gerontology Acute Care Nurse Practitioner Program Coordinator
Creighton University
College of Nursing
Omaha, Nebraska

Carolyn I. Johnson, MSN, ACNP-BC, ARNP-BC
Post-Acute Rehabilitation Nurse Practitioner
Advanced Registered Nurse Practitioner Manor Care Post-Acute Rehabilitation
Waterloo, Iowa

Karin Jonczak, MSN, ACNP-BC, CRNP, CNRN
Neurovascular Nurse Practitioner
Neurovascular Associates of Abington
Neurosciences Institute
Comprehensive Stroke Center
Abington Memorial Hospital
Abington, Pennsylvania

Vanessa M. Kalis, DNP, ACNP-BC, PNP, CNS
Assistant Professor
Director of the Adult-Gerontologic Acute Care
Doctor of Nursing Practice Program
Brandman University
Irvine, California

Kimberly J. Langer, MSN, ACNP-BC
Associate Professor and Program Coordinator
Acute Care Nurse Practitioner Program
Winona State University
Rochester, Minnesota
Mayo Clinic
Division of Blood and Marrow Transplant
Rochester, Minnesota

Beatrice K. Launius, MSN, ACNP-BC, CCRN
Adjunct faculty
Coordinator Adult-Gerontology Acute Care Nurse Practitioner Program
Northwestern State University
Shreveport, Louisiana
Clinical instructor
Chief Nurse Practitioner Division of Trauma and Critical Care Surgery
Louisiana State University Health Sciences Center Shreveport
Shreveport, Louisiana

Gail Ann Lis, DNP, ACNP-BC
Professor
Madonna University
College of Nursing and Health
Livonia, Michigan

Lisa Marchetti, MSN, ACNP-BC
Nurse Practitioner
Surgical Intensive Care Unit
William Beaumont Hospital
Royal Oak, Michigan

Tara McEnany, DNP, ACNP-BC, FNP-BC
Assistant Professor
Allen College
Unity Point Health
Waterloo, Iowa

Taylor A. Mercier, MSN, ACNP-BC, FNP-BC
Acute Care Nurse Practitioner
Emergency Care Specialist
Spectrum Health Butterworth Emergency Department
Grand Rapids, Michigan

Deidre Meyer, MSN, ACNP-BC
Acute Care Nurse Practitioner
ProMedica Physicians Group
The Toledo Hospital
Toledo, Ohio

Rebecca L. Mogensen, MSN, ACNP-BC, APNP
Acute Care Nurse Practitioner
Division of Hospital Medicine
University of Wisconsin Medical Foundation
University of Wisconsin Hospital and Clinics
Madison, Wisconsin

S. Lori Neal, MSN, ACNP-BC, FNP-BC
Trauma Nurse Practitioner
Erlanger Trauma Services
Chattanooga, Tennessee

Jeni Page, MSN, ACNP-BC
Acute Care Nurse Practitioner
Neurosurgery
Swedish Neuroscience Institute
Seattle, Washington

Elizabeth Palermo, MSN, ACNP-BC, ANP-BC
Assistant Professor of Clinical Nursing
Acute Care Nurse Practitioner Program Specialty Director
University of Rochester
School of Nursing
Rochester, New York
Acute Care Nurse Practitioner
Hospital Medicine Division
Strong Memorial Hospital
Rochester, New York

Carmen Paniagua, EdD, ACNP-BC, AGACNP-BC, APNG-BC, FAANP
Clinical Instructor
Department of Emergency Medicine
University of Arkansas for Medical Sciences
College of Medicine
Little Rock, Arkansas
Adult Acute Care Nurse Practitioner and
Adult-Gerontology Acute Care Nurse Practitioner
Gastroenterology Associates of Southeast Arkansas (GASA)
Pine Bluff, Arkansas

Patty Pawlow, MSN, ACNP-BC
Lecturer
Course Director
Adult Gerontology Acute Care Nurse Practitioner Program
University of Pennsylvania
School of Nursing
Philadelphia, Pennsylvania

Leslie Karns Payne, PhD, ACNP-BC, FNP
Assistant Professor
Baylor University Louise Herrington
School of Nursing
Dallas, Texas

Daniel J. Rauh, MSN, AGACNP-BC, CCRN, EMT-P
Emergency Department Nurse Practitioner
Good Samaritan Hospital
Cincinnati, Ohio

Rosalyn R. Reischman, PhD, ACNP-BC
Adult-Gerontology Acute Care Nurse Practitioner
Program Coordinator
University of Florida
College of Nursing
Gainesville, Florida

Patti Renaud, MSN, ACNP-BC
Acute Care Nurse Practitioner
Hepatobiliary and Transplant Surgery
Henry Ford Health System
Detroit, Michigan

Molly K. Rothmeyer, DNP, APRN, FNP-BC, PNP-AC, Fellow NAPNAP
Adjunct Faculty
Graduate Nursing Program
Maryville University
Catherine McAuley School of Nursing
College of Health Professions
St. Louis, Missouri
Adjunct Faculty
Graduate Nursing Program
Brandman University
Marybelle and S. Paul Musco School of Nursing and Health Professions
Irvine, California

Lori Rubio, DNP, ACNP-BC, MBA, HCM
Acute Care Nurse Practitioner
University Medical Center
Ysleta Clinic
El Paso, Texas

Kara Rumley, MSN, ACNP-BC
Vascular Surgery Acute Care Nurse Practitioner
Regional Hemodialysis Access Coordinator
Evansville Surgical Associates
Evansville, Indiana

Alexandra E. Saborio, MSN, ACNP-BC
Acute Care Nurse Practitioner
Inpatient Specialty Program
Cedars-Sinai Medical Center
Los Angeles, California

Kristine Anne Scordo, PhD, ACNP-BC, FAANP
Professor and Director
Adult-Gerontology Acute Care Nurse Practitioner Program
Wright State University
College of Nursing
Dayton, Ohio

Julie Settles, MSN, ACNP-BC, CEN
Clinical Research Scientist
Indianapolis, Indiana

Michelle R. Smith, MSN, AGACNP-BC
Hospitalist Nurse Practitioner
Indiana University Health Ball Memorial Hospital
Hospitalist Department
Muncie, Indiana

Mary Beth Tombes, MSN, ACNP-BC, CCRC
Clinical Research Nurse Practitioner
Virginia Commonwealth University Massey Cancer Center
Richmond, Virginia

Colleen R. Walsh, DNP, ACNP-BC, ONC, ONP-C, CS
Contract Assistant Professor of Graduate Nursing
University of Southern Indiana
College of Nursing and Health
Evansville, Indiana

Marjorie G. Webb, DNP, ACNP-BC
Associate Professor
Interim Department Chair
Community and Professional Studies
Metropolitan State University
School of Nursing, College of Health
Saint Paul, Minnesota

Brett Whaley, MSN, ACNP-BC
Adjunct Professor
Evolution Health Transitional Care and Urgent Care Program Developer, Manager, and Clinician
Texas Woman's University
College of Nursing
Denton, Texas

Julie L. Yerke, MSN, ACNP-BC
Acute Care Nurse Practitioner
Floyd Medical Center
Rome, GA

Sheila Zielinski, DNP, ACNP-BC, FNP-BC, CCRN, CEN
Intensive Care Unit Nurse Practitioner
Indiana University Health Physicians, Pulmonary & Critical Care
Indiana University Health – Methodist
Indianapolis, Indiana

Volume I
Table of Contents

SECTION ONE
Management of Patients with Neurologic Disorders

1 Cerebrovascular Accidents: Brain Attack, 3
TRAVIS BRADLEY AND CHARLENE M. MYERS

Transient Ischemic Attack, 3
Stroke/Brain Attack, 7
Ischemic Stroke, 8
Hemorrhagic Stroke, 13

2 Structural Abnormalities, 21
TRAVIS BRADLEY AND CHARLENE M. MYERS

Aneurysm, 21
Other Abnormalities, 24
Hydrocephalus, 25
Space-Occupying Lesions (Brain Tumors), 26

3 Peripheral Neuropathies, 31
ROBERT BLESSING, KELLY BLESSING, AND THOMAS W. BARKLEY, JR.

Guillain-Barré Syndrome, 31
Myasthenia Gravis, 35

4 Neurologic Trauma, 40
KIMBERLY ALVA AND CHARLENE M. MYERS

Head Trauma/Traumatic Brain Injury, 40
Spinal Cord Trauma, 46

5 Central Nervous System Disorders, 56
JUDI KURIC AND CHARLENE M. MYERS

Meningitis, 56
Cerebral Abscess, 60
Encephalitis, 61
Encephalopathy, 63

6 Seizure Disorders, 65
PATRICK A. LAIRD AND CHARLENE M. MYERS

7 Dementia, 72
ANGELA STARKWEATHER AND CHARLENE M. MYERS

8 Multiple Sclerosis, 79
   JUDI KURIC

9 Parkinson's Disease, 85
   JUDI KURIC AND ROBERT FELLIN

10 Amyotrophic Lateral Sclerosis, 90
   JUDI KURIC

SECTION TWO

Management of Patients with Cardiovascular Disorders

11 Cardiovascular Assessment, 95
   JOAN KING AND THOMAS W. BARKLEY, JR.

12 Hypertension, 100
   THOMAS W. BARKLEY, JR., HELEN MILEY, AND ROBERT FELLIN

13 Coronary Artery Disease and Hyperlipidemia, 111
   JOAN KING AND THOMAS W. BARKLEY, JR.

14 Angina and Myocardial Infarction, 119
   JOAN KING AND THOMAS W. BARKLEY, JR.
   Fibrinolytic/Thrombolytic Therapy, 127
   Percutaneous Transluminal Coronary Angioplasty (PTCA)/Percutaneous Coronary Intervention (PCI), 132
   Coronary Artery Bypass Graft (CABG) Surgery, 134
   Cardiac Tamponade, 135
   Implications for the Elderly, 136

15 Adjunct Equipment/Devices, 139
   SHEILA D. MELANDER AND THOMAS W. BARKLEY, JR.
   Intra-Aortic Balloon Pump (IABP), 139
   Pacemakers, 142
   Automatic Internal Cardioverter/Defibrillator (AICD), 149

16 Peripheral Vascular Disease, 152
   THERESA M. WADAS AND THOMAS W. BARKLEY, JR.
   Peripheral Vascular Disease: Overview, 152
   Specific Disorders, 156
   Venous Disease, 158

17 Inflammatory Cardiac Diseases, 162
   SHEILA MELANDER AND THOMAS W. BARKLEY, JR.
   Pericarditis, 162
   Endocarditis, 163

18 Heart Failure, 168
   JOAN KING, ROBERT FELLIN, AND THOMAS W. BARKLEY, JR.

19 Valvular Disease, 186
   THERESA M. WADAS, ROBERT FELLIN, AND THOMAS W. BARKLEY, JR.

20 Cardiomyopathy, 193
   SHEILA MELANDER AND THOMAS W. BARKLEY, JR.

21 Arrhythmias, *198*
    FREDRICK CARLSTON, ROBERT FELLIN, AND THOMAS W. BARKLEY, JR.

    Common Cardiac Rhythms/Arrhythmias and Treatment, *198*

SECTION THREE

Management of Patients with Pulmonary Disorders

22 Diagnostic Concepts of Oxygenation and Ventilation, *221*
    AMITA AVADHANI AND CHARLENE M. MYERS

    Pulmonary Perfusion, *221*
    Ventilation, *221*
    Alveolar Diffusion, *222*
    Oxygen Transport in the Circulation, *223*
    Ventilator Adjustments, *225*

23 Measures of Oxygenation and Ventilation, *226*
    BIMBOLA AKINTADE AND CHARLENE M. MYERS

    Oxygenation and Ventilation, *226*
    Pulse Oximetry, *228*
    Measurement of Clinical Perfusion, *229*
    Fluid Resuscitation, *231*

24 The Chest X-ray, *234*
    VICTORIA F. KU AND THOMAS W. BARKLEY, JR.

    General Principles, *234*
    Reading a Chest X-ray, *235*
    Specific Disease Entities, *237*

25 Pulmonary Function Testing, *240*
    HALEY M. HOY, THOMAS W. BARKLEY, JR., AND CHARLENE M. MYERS

26 Obstructive (Ventilatory) Lung Diseases, *245*
    THOMAS W. BARKLEY, JR., ROBERT FELLIN, AND TOBIAS P. REBMANN

    Chronic Obstructive Pulmonary Disease (COPD), *245*
    Asthma, *252*
    COPD and Asthma Dual Diagnosis, *254*
    Bronchiectasis, *255*
    Obstructive Airway Lesions, *255*

27 Restrictive (Inflammatory) Lung Diseases, *261*
    THOMAS W. BARKLEY, JR., TOBIAS P. REBMANN, AND DAVID A. MILLER

    Pneumonia, *261*
    Tuberculosis (TB), *264*
    Acute Respiratory Distress Syndrome (ARDS)/Acute Lung Injury (ALI), *266*
    Idiopathic Pulmonary Fibrosis (IPF), *267*
    Sarcoidosis, *269*
    Heart Failure/Cardiogentic Pulmonary Edema, *271*

28 Pulmonary Hypertension and Pulmonary Vascular Disorders, *275*
    HALEY M. HOY AND THOMAS W. BARKLEY, JR.

    Pulmonary Hypertension, *275*
    Pulmonary Vascular Disorders, *277*

29 Chest Wall and Secondary Pleural Disorders, *285*
    JENNIFER COATES, THOMAS W. BARKLEY, JR., AND CHARLENE M. MYERS

    Disorders of the Chest Wall, *285*
    Pleural Disorders, *286*

30 Respiratory Failure, 289
DAVID A. MILLER AND THOMAS W. BARKLEY, JR.

Definitions and Concepts, 289
The Effects of Aging on the Need for Respiratory Assistance, Including Intubation, 290
Ventilatory Failure, 290
Respiratory Failure, 291
Treatment, 291

31 Pneumothorax, 293
BIMBOLA AKINTADE AND THOMAS W. BARKLEY, JR.

32 Lower Respiratory Tract Pathogens, 296
DAVID A. MILLER AND THOMAS W. BARKLEY, JR.

33 Obstructive Sleep Apnea, 305
JENNIFER COATES AND THOMAS W. BARKLEY, JR.

Characteristics of Breathing and Sleep, 305
Obstructive Sleep Apnea (OSA), 305

34 Oxygen Supplementation, 308
CAROL THOMPSON, THOMAS W. BARKLEY, JR., AND CHARLENE M. MYERS

Basic Principles of Oxygen Supplementation, 308
Facilitation of Ventilation, 310
Devices for Oxygen Supplementation, 311

35 Mechanical Ventilatory Support, 314
AMITA AVADHANI, THOMAS W. BARKLEY, JR., AND CHARLENE M. MYERS

Indications for Mechanical Ventilation, 314
General Principles of Ventilation, 315
Variables for Mechanical Ventilators, 315
Modes of Mechanical Ventilation, 317
Special Aspects of Ventilator Management, 317

SECTION FOUR

Management of Patients with Gastrointestinal Disorders

36 Peptic Ulcer Disease, 323
ALICIA HUCKSTADT AND CHARLENE M. MYERS

Peptic Ulcer Disease, 323
Gastroesophageal Reflux Disease (GERD), 330

37 Liver Disease, 336
MICHALYN D. PELPHREY AND CHARLENE M. MYERS

Major Liver Diseases, 336

38 Biliary Dysfunction, 352
MICHALYN D. PELPHREY AND CHARLENE M. MYERS

Cholecystitis, 352
Acute Pancreatitis, 355

39 Inflammatory Gastrointestinal Disorders, 361
LISA A. JOHNSON AND CHARLENE M. MYERS

Diverticulitis, 361
Inflammatory Bowel Disease, 362
Peritonitis, 365
Appendicitis, 368

40 Anatomic Intestinal Disorders, *371*
CATHERINE FUNG AND CHARLENE M. MYERS

Small Bowel Obstruction, *371*
Large Bowel Obstruction, *374*
Mesenteric Ischemia, *375*

41 Gastrointestinal Bleeding, *378*
NICOLE A. PEREZ AND CHARLENE M. MYERS

Esophageal Varices, *378*
Upper Gastrointestinal Bleeding, *380*
Lower Gastrointestinal Bleeding, *382*

SECTION FIVE

Management of Patients with Genitourinary Disorders

42 Urinary Tract Infections, *387*
MICHELE H. TALLEY AND CHARLENE M. MYERS

Urinary Tract Infections, *387*

43 Acute Kidney Injury and Chronic Kidney Disease, *393*
STEVEN W. BRANHAM AND CHARLENE M. MYERS

Primary Kidney Regulation of Physiologic Functions, *393*
Acute Kidney Injury, *393*
Chronic Kidney Disease, *401*
Modification of Drug Dosages, *406*

44 Benign Prostatic Hyperplasia, *409*
JENNIFER J. ROBERG AND CHARLENE M. MYERS

45 Renal Artery Stenosis, *415*
MICHELE H. TALLEY AND CHARLENE M. MYERS

46 Nephrolithiasis, *420*
MARLA COUTURE AND CHARLENE M. MYERS

Renal Calculi-Nephrolithiasis, *420*

APPENDIX

ICD-9 and ICD-10 Codes

SECTION ONE

Management of Patients With Neurologic Disorders

CHAPTER 1

Cerebrovascular Accidents: Brain Attack

TRAVIS BRADLEY • CHARLENE MYERS

TRANSIENT ISCHEMIC ATTACK

I. **Definition**
   A. Classic definition: sudden or rapid onset of neurologic deficit caused by focal ischemia that lasts for a few minutes and resolves completely within 24 hr
   B. It has been found that with more widespread use of modern imaging techniques for the brain, up to one third of patients with symptoms lasting less than 24 hr actually have a small infarct.
   C. Updated definition: a transient episode of neurological dysfunction caused by focal brain, spinal cord, or retinal ischemia, without acute infarction

II. **Incidence/prevalence**
   A. Incidence is 160/100,000; prevalence is 135/100,000

III. **Etiology**
   A. Atherosclerotic disease
      1. Aorta
      2. Carotid arteries
      3. Vertebral arteries
      4. Intracranial atherosclerosis
   B. Cardiac emboli as seen in arrhythmia (atrial fibrillation), myocardial infarction (MI), congestive cardiomyopathy, and valvular disease
   C. Vasculitis conditions such as moyamoya disease, fibromuscular dysplasia, lupus, and others
   D. Hematologic causes
      1. Red blood cell (RBC) disorders
         a. Increased sludging
         b. Decreased cerebral oxygenation such as in severe anemia
         c. Polycythemia, sickle cell anemia
      2. Platelet disorders
         a. Thrombocytosis
         b. Thrombocytopenia
      3. Increased viscosity/hypercoagulable conditions
         a. Antiphospholipid antibody syndrome (e.g., lupus anticoagulant, anticardiolipin antibody)
         b. Oral contraceptive and/or estrogen use
         c. Antithrombin III deficiency
         d. Protein S and C deficiency

e. Tissue-type plasminogen activator (t-PA) and plasminogen deficiencies
f. Patients particularly at risk for a hypercoagulable state:
    i. Older than 45 years
    ii. History of thrombolytic event
    iii. History of spontaneous abortion
    iv. Related autoimmune conditions (e.g., lupus)
    v. Stroke of unknown cause
    vi. Family history of thrombotic events
4. Myeloproliferative disorders, leukemia with white blood cell count greater than 150,000

E. Intracranial causes
1. Brain tumor
2. Focal seizure
3. Hemorrhage
    a. Subdural hematoma (SDH)
    b. Subarachnoid hemorrhage (SAH)
    c. Intracerebral hemorrhage (ICH), which may cause cerebrovascular dysfunction due to leakage of blood outside the normal vessels

F. Subclavian steal syndrome
1. Localized stenosis or occlusion of a subclavian artery proximal to the source of the vertebral artery, so that blood is stolen from that artery
2. Blood pressure (BP) is significantly lower in the affected arm than in the opposite arm.

G. Others
1. Transient hypotension
2. Osteophytes that cause compression of neck vessels
3. Cocaine abuse
4. Hypoglycemia
5. Migraines

IV. Risk factors

A. A transient ischemic attack (TIA) is an important predictor of stroke.
1. The 90-day risk of stroke after a TIA is as high as 17%
2. The greatest risk is within the first week
3. Approximately one third of stroke patients have a history of TIA

B. Hypertension

C. Cardiac disease, such as the following:
1. Mitral valve disease
2. Anterior wall MI
3. Congestive myopathy
4. Arrhythmia (e.g., atrial fibrillation)

D. Smoking
E. Obesity
F. Hyperlipidemia
G. Elevated homocysteine levels in the elderly
H. Advanced age
I. Diabetes
J. Alcohol and recreational drug abuse

V. Clinical manifestations

A. Carotid artery syndrome
1. Hemianopia, ipsilateral monocular blindness (amaurosis fugax) described as similar to a shade coming down over one eye
2. Visual field cut
3. Paresthesia/weakness of contralateral arm, leg, and face (may be episodic)
4. Dysarthria, transient aphasia

5. Confusion
6. Gait disturbance
7. Carotid bruit may be present
8. Microemboli, hemorrhage, and exudate may be visualized in the ipsilateral retina

B. Vertebrobasilar artery syndrome
1. Visual bilateral disturbances (blurred vision, diplopia, and complete blindness)
2. Vertigo and ataxia
3. Nausea and/or vomiting
4. Sudden loss of postural tone in all extremities while consciousness remains intact (drop attacks)
5. Dysarthria
6. Facial paresthesia
7. Gait instability

VI. Diagnostics/laboratory findings

A. Laboratory evaluation may include the following:
1. Complete blood count (CBC), platelet count, prothrombin time (PT), partial thromboplastin time (PTT), and international normalized ratio (INR) to detect these conditions:
   a. Anemia
   b. Polycythemia
   c. Leukemia
   d. Thrombocytopenia
   e. Hypercoagulopathy
2. Electrolytes, glucose to detect the following:
   a. Hyponatremia
   b. Hypokalemia
   c. Hypoglycemia
   d. Hyperglycemia
3. Lipid profile
   a. Detects hyperlipidemia
4. In selected patients, antinuclear antibody, Venereal Disease Research Laboratory (VDRL) test, and toxicology screen
5. Sedimentation rate, to detect these conditions:
   a. Vasculitis
   b. Infective endocarditis
   c. Hyperviscosity
   d. Giant cell arteritis
6. Homocysteine level
   a. An amino acid
   b. Elevated plasma level associated with increased risk of vascular events
7. Anticardiolipin antibodies (immunoglobulin [Ig]G, IgM, and IgA) and assay for lupus anticoagulant for suspected antiphospholipid antibody syndromes
8. Assays for antithrombin III, proteins S and C, plasminogen, and t-PA

B. Computed tomographic (CT) scan of the head
1. May reveal "silent" ischemia or ischemic images, as well as hemorrhage or infarct and SDH

C. Magnetic resonance imaging (MRI), particularly diffusion-weighted imaging, and perfusion-weighted imaging
1. More sensitive than CT scan to early pathologic changes of ischemic infarction because of its excellent detection of brain edema
2. MRI is also preferred for the detection of lacunar or vertebrobasilar TIAs, or when vascular territory is not well defined.

3. Up to one third of patients with TIAs have an infarct in the territory relevant to their symptoms
D. Duplex ultrasonography
   1. 85% sensitivity and 90% specificity
   2. Useful in identifying hemodynamically significant carotid stenosis
E. CT angiography (CTA)
   1. Evaluation of neck and brain vessels
   2. Requires use of contrast material
      a. Normal renal function
      b. Adequate intravenous access
F. Magnetic resonance angiography (MRA)
   1. Alternative to ultrasound or CT studies
   2. No contrast medium is needed
   3. Can be obtained at the same time as an MRI scan
   4. Good means for assessment of extracranial and intracranial vessels
G. Echocardiography and a 24-hr Holter monitor are used to evaluate for a cardiac source of emboli.
H. Transesophageal echocardiography (TEE) to evaluate the aortic arch, left atrium, and for patent foramen ovale
I. Cerebral angiography for patients whose symptoms suggest involvement of the carotid circulation and who are candidates for carotid endarterectomy (CEA)
J. Chest x-ray for enlarged heart
K. Blood cultures to monitor for infective endocarditis
L. Temporal artery biopsy to detect giant cell arteritis
M. Cardiac enzymes to detect an acute MI
N. Electroencephalography indicated in patients suspected of having a seizure disorder associated with stroke, as well as an underlying toxic-metabolic disorder that may cause seizure activity

VII. Management
A. Address the following underlying risk factors:
   1. Hypertension
   2. Diabetes mellitus (DM)
   3. Obesity
   4. Hyperlipidemia
   5. Smoking
B. Carotid TIAs
   1. Greater than 70%–80% obstruction: intervention is indicated for those who are a good surgical risk
   2. Controversy exists about patients who have 50%–69% obstruction but are symptomatic; should be evaluated on a case-by-case basis by a vascular specialist.
   3. Less than 50% obstruction: surgery is not indicated
   4. Carotid angioplasty and stenting (CAS) is an alternative to CEA
   5. Several recent trials such as the Stenting and Angioplasty with Protection in Patients with High Risk for Endarterectomy (SAPPHIRE) and the Carotid Revascularization Endarterectomy versus Stent Trial (CREST) reveal that CAS is safe and effective.
      a. Determination of CAS versus CEA is largely based on availability of trained personal and institutional expertise
C. Anticoagulation if caused by a cardioembolic event from atrial fibrillation or paroxysmal atrial fibrillation
   1. May prevent recurrent cardioembolic events
   2. Traditional treatment has been a bridging of heparin to warfarin (Coumadin). Although with newer-generation anticoagulants, the heparin bridge may not be necessary.

3. Begin with heparin, 12 units/kg/hr
4. Target PTT should be 1.5–2.5 times patient's baseline value
5. Follow with warfarin, 5–10 mg PO (orally), which is indicated for the following:
   a. TIA caused by embolism arising from a mural thrombus after an MI
   b. TIA caused by embolus in patients with mitral stenosis or prosthetic heart valves
   c. Recurrent TIAs despite platelet antiaggregant agents
   d. INR of 2–3 is considered therapeutic
D. Common antiplatelet therapy
   1. Aspirin (acetylsalicylic acid) decreases incidence of subsequent stroke by 15%–30% in male patients with TIAs; dose of 81–325 mg/day is as effective as higher doses and causes fewer adverse effects
   2. Clopidogrel (Plavix)
      a. Indicated for secondary prevention of ischemic stroke, MI, and other vascular events in patients who cannot tolerate aspirin, or in patients who were taking aspirin at the time of the event
      b. Dosage is 75 mg/day PO
      c. May cause thrombotic thrombocytopenia purpura during the first 2 weeks of treatment
   3. Aspirin, 25 mg/extended-release dipyridamole, 200 mg (Aggrenox)
      a. Both drugs suppress platelet aggregation but do so through different mechanisms
      b. Combination treatment is more effective than either drug alone
      c. Recommended dose is one capsule PO twice a day
      d. Significantly more expensive than aspirin therapy
      e. Main side effect is headache

STROKE/BRAIN ATTACK

I. **Definition**
   A. Rapid onset of a neurologic deficit involving ischemia to a certain vascular territory and lasting longer than 24 hr
   B. A stroke in evolution is an enlarging infarction manifested by neurologic defects that increase over 24–48 hr
   C. Because of advances in early recognition and treatment, stroke dropped from being the third leading cause of death to the fourth. It remains the leading cause of disability.
   D. Stroke can be classified as ischemic and hemorrhagic
   E. Eighty percent of strokes are caused by blood clots that produce ischemic areas in the brain; remaining 20% of strokes are caused by ICH

II. **Etiology and risk factors**
   A. Same as for TIA
   B. Cocaine-related stroke is increasingly common
   C. Women who use oral contraceptives and who smoke are at high risk
   D. Hyperlipidemia raises the risk of ischemic stroke
   E. Low cholesterol increases the risk of hemorrhagic stroke

III. **Public education**
   A. Need to increase public awareness of the warning signs of stroke to facilitate early treatment
   B. Five "suddens" of stroke:
      1. Sudden weakness
      2. Sudden speech difficulty
      3. Sudden visual loss
      4. Sudden dizziness
      5. Sudden severe headache
   C. Need to call 9-1-1 and/or active emergency medical systems (EMS) to expedite best chance of meeting treatment window limits

D. Should be treated like a heart attack; "brain attack" may become new nomenclature
IV. **Prehospital stroke management**
   A. Implementation strategies for emergency medical services within stroke systems of care policy statement:
      1. Dispatched to highest level of care available in the shortest possible time
      2. Time between call and dispatch of response team less than 90 seconds
      3. EMS response time less than 8 min
      4. On-scene time less than 15 min barring extenuating circumstances
      5. Travel time equivalent to trauma or acute MI calls
V. **Stroke systems of care**
   A. Goals of creating stroke systems of care include stroke prevention, community stroke education, optimal use of EMS, effective acute and subacute stroke management, rehabilitation, and performance review of stroke care delivery.
   B. Hospitals with the capacity and commitment to deliver acute stroke care in the emergency department and stroke unit are essential to effective stroke care.
   C. Transporting patients to stroke centers optimizes their chance of timely therapy and decreases the morbidity and mortality associated with stroke.
VI. **Primary stroke center**
   A. Established in 2004 by The Joint Commission (TJC); currently more than 800 primary stroke centers exist
   B. Have dedicated and organized stroke resources that lead to increased rates of intravenous t-PA administration, increased lipid profile testing, improved deep vein thrombosis prophylaxis, and better clinical outcomes
VII. **Comprehensive stroke center**
   A. Criteria established in 2011 by the American Stroke Association
   B. Ability to offer 24/7 state-of-the-art care on the full spectrum of cerebrovascular disease
   C. Neurocritical care units and interventional radiology for cerebral interventions essential
   D. Can be part of a "hub and spoke" model of care to maximize stroke care
   E. Even patients with a large infarct, but outside intervention window, should be admitted to a neurocritical care unit for complication management.

ISCHEMIC STROKE

I. **Etiology**
   A. Caused by a thrombus that occludes a blood vessel in the head or neck (30%)
      1. Progression of symptoms over hours to days, or can be sudden
      2. Patients often have a history of TIA
      3. Predisposing factors:
         a. Atherosclerosis
         b. Hypertension (HTN)
         c. DM
         d. Hyperlipidemia
         e. Vasculitis
         f. Hypotension
         g. Smoking
         h. Connective tissue disorders
         i. Trauma to the head and neck
   B. Caused by embolism (25%)
      1. Very rapid onset
      2. History of TIA
      3. Predisposing factors:
         a. Atrial fibrillation
         b. Mitral stenosis and regurgitation

CHAPTER I   Cerebrovascular Accidents: Brain Attack

      c. Endocarditis
      d. Mitral valve prolapse

II. Clinical manifestations (depending on the cerebral vessel involved)
  A. Middle cerebral artery
    1. Hemiplegia (involves upper extremity and face more often than lower extremity)
    2. Hemianesthesia
    3. Hemianopia (blindness of half the field of vision)
    4. Eyes may deviate to the side of the lesion
    5. Aphasia if dominant hemisphere is involved
    6. Neglect syndrome
    7. Occlusions of various branches of the middle cerebral artery may cause different findings (involvement of the anterior division may cause expressive aphasia, and involvement of the posterior branch may produce receptive aphasia).
  B. Anterior cerebral artery
    1. Hemiplegia (lower extremity more often than upper extremity)
    2. Primitive reflexes
    3. Confusion
    4. Abulia
    5. Bilateral anterior infarction may cause behavioral changes and disturbance in memory.
  C. Vertebral and basilar arteries
    1. Decreased level of consciousness (LOC)
    2. Vertigo
    3. Dysphagia
    4. Diplopia
    5. Ipsilateral cranial nerve findings
    6. Contralateral (or bilateral) sensory and motor deficits
  D. Deep penetrating branches of major cerebral arteries (lacunar infarction)
    1. Most common: less than 5 mm in diameter
    2. Associated with poorly controlled HTN or diabetes
    3. Contralateral pure motor or sensory deficits
    4. Ipsilateral ataxia with crural (pertaining to the leg or thigh) paresis
    5. Dysarthria with clumsiness of the hand

III. Diagnostics/laboratory findings
  A. CT scan of the head without contrast should be done initially
    1. Preferable to MRI in the acute stage to rule out cerebral hemorrhage as MRI is usually not as readily available, especially for patients who present with stroke symptoms and are on anticoagulation therapy; also will rule out abscess, tumor, and SDH
    2. Appears as an area of decreased density
    3. Lacunar infarcts appear as small, punched-out, hypodense areas.
    4. Initial CT scan may be negative, and the infarct may not be visible for up to 24 hr
  B. Chest radiography
    1. May reveal cardiomegaly or valvular calcification
    2. Neoplasm may suggest metastasis rather than stroke as the cause of neurologic deficits
    3. Dilated aorta may reveal aortic dissection.
  C. CBC, sedimentation rate, blood glucose, VDRL, lipid profile, INR, PTT prior to anticoagulation, blood urea nitrogen/serum creatinine (Cr) to evaluate renal function before contrast media may be given, homocysteine level, drug screen, and blood alcohol level
  D. Electrocardiogram (ECG) (if unrevealing, may place patient on cardiac monitor/Holter monitor)
  E. Blood cultures if endocarditis is suspected
  F. Echocardiography with bubble study
  G. TEE to detect dysfunction of left atrium (thrombus)

H. Carotid duplex ultrasonography
I. MRI/MRA: Diffusion-weighted MRI is more sensitive than conventional MRI in detecting cerebral ischemia.
J. CTA
   1. Can provide information regarding vascular anatomy with three-dimensional reconstruction (requires the use of contact dye)
   2. May allow for rapid evaluation and diagnosis in hospitals without MRI capability
   3. Can be used to image the carotid arteries instead of duplex ultrasonography, and will show internal carotid artery structure
   4. CT perfusion can also be performed as part of the CTA, which can provide evidence of salvageable tissue (penumbra) or an already completed infarct, and may affect the treatment plan.
K. Cerebral angiography continues to be the gold standard for complete evaluation of intracranial and extracranial vessels
L. Lumbar puncture (LP)
   1. Not always necessary but may be helpful if the cause of stroke is uncertain
   2. Obtain a CT scan first to rule out cerebral hemorrhage or any expanding mass that could lead to herniation if LP is performed

IV. **Management**
   A. Correct treatment depends on a correct diagnosis of stroke type; therefore, it is imperative that diagnostic tests be completed quickly. A report from the National Institute of Neurological Disorders and Stroke advocates the following goals, which are based on time of arrival:
      1. Perform an initial emergency department evaluation within 10 min
      2. Notify the stroke team or neurologist within 15 min
      3. Start a CT scan within 25 min
      4. Obtain a CT scan interpretation within 45 min
      5. Administer thrombolytics, if appropriate, within 60 min
      6. Transfer the patient to an inpatient bed within 3 hr
   B. BP control
      1. Acute lowering of systemic BP is not recommended because it may lead to further damage in the ischemic penumbra, in which autoregulation may be defective, and may clinically worsen the stroke.
      2. Most patients with acute cerebral infarction have an elevated BP, which usually returns to baseline within 48 hr without any special treatment.
      3. BP control may be warranted, however, in the following conditions:
         a. Systolic BP (SBP) exceeds 220 mmHg, and diastolic BP (DBP) exceeds 120 mmHg (malignant hypertension)
         b. Hypertensive encephalopathy is present
         c. Vital organs are compromised
         d. Aortic dissection
         e. Symptomatic cardiac disease
         f. Patient is receiving t-PA therapy
            i. Some experts recommend decreasing BP in those who are receiving intravenous heparin therapy as well, although this is not universally accepted.
         g. In patients who are candidates for t-PA, BP should be lowered to SBP less than 185 and DBP less than 110 prior to t-PA administration. After t-PA administration, SBP should be maintained less than 180 and DBP less than 105.
      4. When indicated, BP should be lowered by approximately 15% and closely watched for neurological deterioration related to decreased perfusion.

5. The current 2013 Stroke Guidelines recommend the use of either labe IV push over 1–2 min, can repeat once; or nicardipine, intravenous drip 2.5–15 mg/hr for BP management.
6. An alternative is esmolol (Brevibloc), 2.5 grams/250 ml NS or 2 grams/10 continuous infusion titrated to desired BP; maximum dose should not excee 300 mcg/kg/min.

C. Anticoagulation
   1. Intravenous heparin has historically been used as a treatment for acute stroke. However, it does not reduce the severity of a stroke that has occurred and is no longer routinely recommended. The decision to even consider the use of heparin in the acute management of stroke should be determined by a neurology expert.
   2. It may be used in patients with stroke in evolution and in hypercoagulable states, or in patients with very high-risk or recurrent emboli.
   3. Heparin may increase the risk of transformation from ischemic stroke to hemorrhagic stroke and, therefore, is not recommended for massive stroke.
   4. No loading dose of heparin is recommended as the potential risk of hemorrhagic transformation is high. A maintenance infusion of 12 units/kg/hr (max 1000 units/hr) can be started. PTT should be 1.5–2.5 patient's baseline value.
   5. Heparin followed by warfarin (5–10 mg/day PO) is indicated as secondary prevention in suspected cerebral embolism resulting from the following:
      a. Mural thrombus
      b. Mitral stenosis
      c. Atrial fibrillation
      d. Mechanical heart valves
   6. Several newer anticoagulants are now on the market and targeted at stroke prevention for patients with atrial fibrillation or paroxysmal atrial fibrillation.
      a. Dabigatran (Pradaxa) is a direct thrombin inhibitor. Originally used to prevent thromboembolic events after orthopedic procedures, the randomized evaluation of long-term anticoagulation therapy (RE-LY) study demonstrated that dabigatran had benefit compared with warfarin for prevention of stroke in patients with atrial fibrillation.
         i. Food and Drug Administration approved in 2010 at 150 mg BID, or 75 mg BID in renally-impaired patients
      b. Apixaban (Eliquis) is a factor Xa inhibitor also recently approved for stroke prevention in patients with atrial fibrillation. Standard dose is 5 mg BID or 2.5 mg BID for patients greater than 80 years of age, body weight 60 kg or less, or Cr greater than 1.5 mg/dl.
      c. Rivaroxaban (Xarolto) is a factor Xa inhibitor approved for stroke prevention in patients with atrial fibrillation. Standard dose is 20 mg daily with evening meal for patients with creatinine clearance greater than 50 ml/min, or 15 mg daily with evening meal for patients with creatinine clearance 15–50 ml/min. Avoid use when CrCl less than 15 mL/min.
      d. Because of the mechanism of action of the above three drugs, no routine lab draws of PTT or INR are necessary for ongoing treatment and may facilitate better patient compliance.
      e. If acute hemorrhage develops, holding anticoagulants or use of activated charcoal may reverse bleeding. Empiric fresh frozen plasma, factor VII, or factor IX complex may be attempted in emergency situations.
      f. The decision to use one of the newer anticoagulants should be determined after a thorough discussion between the neurologist, cardiologist, patient, and/or family has occurred. The risks and benefits should be carefully examined.

7. CT scan may be necessary after 48 hr to determine whether any hemorrhaging has occurred.
8. Anticoagulation is contraindicated if CT scan or LP suggests cerebral hemorrhage, tumor, abscess, SDH, or epidural hematoma.
9. Use cautiously in patients with a history of GI bleeding, bleeding tendencies, severe HTN, or a large cerebral infarct
10. May be used after a completed stroke if embolization is determined to be the cause

D. Antiplatelet therapy may be used for non-cardioembolic stroke patients not due to vertebral or carotid dissection.
1. Aspirin, 81–325 mg/day PO
   a. Continues to be the least expensive and most widely used antiplatelet medication
2. Clopidogrel (Plavix), 75 mg PO daily
3. Aggrenox (aspirin, 25 mg immediate release, and dipyridamole, 200 mg extended release), 1 tablet BID (1 in the morning and 1 at night)
   a. Approved for stroke prevention
   b. Study has shown that this combination may reduce stroke by 22% compared with aspirin therapy alone

E. Mannitol and/or hypertonic saline can be used for cerebral edema that may occur on the second or third day.
   a. Mannitol (0.25–1 gram/kg IV every 4–6 hr) may help decrease elevated intracranial pressure (ICP) by overall osmotic diuresis. Side effects can include acute kidney injury. Serum osmolality should be monitored.
   b. Hypertonic saline (23.4%) can be administered as an intravenous push through a central line in the event of an acute decompensation. Standard dose is 30 ml IV administered over greater than 30 min; subsequent doses dependent on ICP
   c. Hypertonic saline (3%) can be administered as an intravenous drip to maintain a higher sodium level at the discretion of the intensivist. Standard dose is initial bolus of 250–300 ml IV over 60 min, followed by continuous infusion titrated to treatment goals including 145–155 mEq/L and serum osmolality 310–320 mOsm/L. Recommend checking sodium levels every 6 hr and adjusting drip PRN.

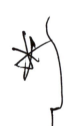

F. Corticosteroids are used to reduce vasogenic cerebral edema related to tumor burden but are not recommended for cytotoxic edema from strokes. Hypertonic solutions are used to reduce cytotoxic edema associated with cerebral infarct.
G. t-PA is now being used, if appropriate conditions are met, as thrombolytic therapy for acute stroke when the patient is brought in within 3–4.5 hr after the stroke. The traditional window of 3 hr has been expanded to 4.5 hr with certain criteria listed below. Such conditions include the following:
1. Availability of a physician with appropriate expertise to diagnose the stroke
2. 24-hr availability of CT scanning to assess for hemorrhage
3. Capability of facility to manage intracranial hemorrhage or transfer to higher level of care
4. Patients must seek help early and have a well-defined onset of symptoms.
   a. Commonly called "last known well time"
5. Patient's condition must be carefully examined for contraindications, such as the following:
   a. Previous and/or current hemorrhage
   b. Previous stroke or head trauma within 3 months
   c. Major surgery within 14 days
   d. Urinary or GI hemorrhage within 24 days
   e. Seizure at stroke onset
   f. Arterial puncture at noncompressible site within 7 days
   g. Elevated PTT and PT (longer than 15 seconds)

CHAPTER 1 Cerebrovascular Accidents: Brain Attack

        h. Oral anticoagulants or heparin with elevated PTT within 48 hr
        i. Serum glucose level less than 50 or greater than 400 mg/dl
        j. SBP greater than 185 mmHg or DBP greater than 110 mmHg
        k. Active internal bleeding within 22 days
    6. Additional criteria for patients within the 3- to 4.5-hr window
        a. Inclusion:
            i. Ischemic stroke causing measurable deficit
            ii. Onset of symptoms within 3–4.5 hr
            iii. Age greater than 18 years
        b. Exclusion:
            i. Age greater than 80 years
            ii. Severe stroke (National Institutes of Health Stroke Scale greater than 25)
            iii. Taking an oral anticoagulant regardless of international normalized ratio
            iv. History of both diabetes and prior ischemic stroke
            v. SBP greater than 185 mmHg or DBP greater than 110 mmHg
    7. Dose: 0.9 mg/kg (maximum dose of 90 mg) given over 60 min, with 10% of the calculated dose given as an initial bolus over one min
        a. Admit to stroke unit
        b. Vital signs and neuro checks every 15 min during and for 2 hr after administration, then every 30 min for 6 hr, then hourly until 24 hr after t-PA onset
  H. Surgery and CEA may be indicated for those with high-grade extracranial carotid artery disease (greater than 70%) if not at high risk
  I. Rehabilitation should take a multidisciplinary approach
  J. Additional treatment options
    1. Mechanical reperfusion
        a. There are numerous devices available that are used to mechanically retrieve a clot from within a cerebral artery.
        b. Examples include the MERCI device, the Solitaire device, the Trevo device, and the Penumbra device
        c. Use is largely determined by the experience and expertise of the user and the institution
    2. Combined intra-arterial (IA) and intravenous thrombolysis
        a. The Interventional Management of Stoke (IMS) study evaluated the use of IA t-PA in patients who received standard intravenous t-PA but displayed little or no improvement by the end of the t-PA administration.
        b. The initial IMS and then IMS trial two showed good rates of recanalization of the occluded artery with comparable safety data to t-PA alone; however, the IMS trial three was stopped early for reported futility. Although the artery was recanalized, it has been reported that overall outcomes were not significantly better. Further study is warranted.

HEMORRHAGIC STROKE

I. **Definition**
  A. Condition resulting from bleeding into the subarachnoid space or brain parenchyma
  B. Accounts for approximately 14% of all cerebral infarctions

II. **Etiology**
  A. SAH
    1. Ruptured saccular aneurysm (85%)
    2. Arteriovenous malformation (AVM) (8%)
    3. Cryptogenic
  B. ICH
    1. Usually associated with HTN

2. Predisposing factors
   a. HTN
   b. Use of anticoagulants or thrombolytics
   c. Use of illicit street drugs (e.g., cocaine)
   d. Heavy use of alcohol
   e. Hematologic disorders

III. **Clinical manifestations**
   A. SAH
      1. Sudden headache of intense severity that radiates into the posterior neck region and is worsened by neck and head movements; often described as a "thunderclap headache" or "worst headache of my life"
      2. Grading scales: standardized way to describe SAH patients among providers
         a. Hunt and Hess classification (clinical assessment)
            i. Grade I: asymptomatic or slight headache
            ii. Grade II: moderate to severe headache, stiff neck, no focal signs other than cranial nerve palsy
            iii. Grade III: drowsy, mild focal deficit, or confusion
            iv. Grade IV: stupor, hemiparesis
            v. Grade V: deep coma, decerebration
         b. Fisher grade (based on CT findings)
            i. Grade I: no blood detected
            ii. Grade II: diffuse or vertical layers less than 1 mm thick
            iii. Grade III: localized clot and/or vertical layer 1 mm or more
            iv. Grade IV: intracerebral or intraventricular clot with diffuse or no SAH
   B. ICH
      1. Elevation in BP, often to very high levels (90% of patients)
      2. Headache (40%)
      3. Vomiting is an important diagnostic sign, particularly if the hemorrhage lies in the cerebral hemisphere (49%).
      4. Sudden onset of neurologic deficits that can rapidly progress to coma or death, depending on area involved (50%)
      5. Basal ganglia hemorrhage
         a. Conjugate deviation of eyes to the side of the lesion
         b. Decreased LOC
         c. Contralateral hemiplegia
         d. Hemisensory disturbance
      6. Thalamic hemorrhage
         a. Downward deviation of the eyes, looking at the nose
         b. Pupils pinpoint with a positive reaction
         c. Coma is common
         d. Flaccid quadriplegia
      7. Cerebellar hemorrhage
         a. Ipsilateral lateral conjugate gaze paresis
         b. Pupils equal, round, reactive to light (PERRL)
         c. Inability to stand or walk
         d. Facial weakness
         e. Ataxia of gait, limbs, or trunk
         f. Vertigo and dysarthria

IV. **Diagnostics/laboratory findings**
   A. SAH
      1. CT scan of the head will assist in differentiating between an ischemic and a hemorrhagic stroke.

a. Sensitivity of CT in the first 3 days after an aneurysmal SAH is very high (close to 100%). After 5–7 days, the rate of a negative CT scan increases, and LP should be considered.
b. Aneurysms less than 3 mm in size are unreliably demonstrated on CTA
c. Depending on site, size, CT scan quality, and whether or not fine cuts were obtained, aneurysm itself may be seen in 50% of cases when contrast material is given.
2. LP if CT scan is unavailable or negative and suspicion is high
   a. Contraindicated in any expanding mass because it may cause herniation
   b. A funduscopic examination must be performed prior to the procedure to rule out papilledema if no CT available
   c. Cerebrospinal fluid (CSF) will be uniformly grossly bloody, although this may not occur if the bleed is small. In a true SAH, the LP reveals 103–106 RBCs/mm
   d. Opening pressure may be elevated
   e. Xanthochromia is present
      i. Yellowish discoloration of CSF produced by blood breakdown products
      ii. Xanthochromia appears no earlier than 2–4 hr after bleeding occurs
      iii. Cerebral angiography
         (a) Used to determine source of bleed, presence of an aneurysm, and best source of treatment (medical or surgical)
         (b) May demonstrate vasospasm
         (c) Should be performed after the patient has been stabilized
3. CTA is beneficial in patients who are too unstable to undergo cerebral angiography or in an emergent setting prior to surgical evacuation of clot.

B. ICH
   1. CT scan without contrast
      a. To confirm a bleed and determine the size and site
      b. May reveal structural abnormalities such as aneurysms, AVMs, or brain tumors that may have caused the bleed, as well as complications such as herniation, intraventricular hemorrhage, or hydrocephalus
   2. Cerebral angiography may be performed
      a. To determine whether the source is an aneurysm or an AVM
      b. Should be considered for all patients without a clear cause of hemorrhage who are surgical candidates, particularly young, normotensive patients who are clinically stable
      c. Timing depends on the patient's clinical state and the neurosurgeon's judgment about the urgency of surgery, if needed
   3. MRI and MRA may be useful for detecting structural abnormalities (i.e., AVMs and aneurysms). Gradient recalled echo MRI may be useful in detecting hemorrhage
   4. CTA may be used to allow noninvasive imaging of large and medium-sized vessels
   5. CBC, platelet count
   6. Electrolytes
   7. ECG
   8. Chest x-ray
   9. Bleeding time
   10. PT/PTT
   11. Liver enzymes
   12. Renal studies
   13. LP is contraindicated: may cause herniation in the presence of a large hematoma

V. **Management**
   A. SAH
      1. Basic ABCs first; many patients may need to be intubated if unable to protect airway

2. External ventricular drain (EVD) placement if hydrocephalus seen on CT scan; relieving the pressure from acute hydrocephalus may dramatically improve a patient's LOC
3. Strict bed rest in a quiet, stress-free environment
4. Cardiac monitoring
5. Treat symptomatically for headache or anxiety (acetaminophen and/or escalating opiates). Avoid use of nonsteroidal anti-inflammatory drugs due to bleeding risk.
6. Have the patient avoid all forms of straining and exertion.
7. Order stool softeners and laxatives (docusate [Colace], 100–200 mg PO/NG twice a day)
8. Seizure prophylaxis
   a. Up to 26% of patients with SAH will experience seizures
   b. Short-term seizure prophylaxis is used to prevent seizures in the acutely ill patient and prevent spikes in BP and possible rebleeding of the aneurysm.
   c. Commonly used medications include:
      i. Phenytoin sodium (Dilantin), 100 mg IV every 8 hr, titrate to blood level 10–20 mcg/ml for 7 days
      ii. Levetiracetam (Keppra), 500 mg IV or PO twice a day for 7 days
         (a) Alternative to phenytoin; there is limited literature to support use for this indication and is not approved as monotherapy for seizures
   d. If the patient has a seizure during the acute phase, consider continuing antiepileptic therapy for a longer duration.
9. Acute hypertension can contribute to aneurysm re-rupture and should be aggressively managed.
   a. Maintain SBP less than 160 mmHg
   b. Consider intravenous titratable nicardipine drip or
   c. Labetalol, 10 mg intravenous push
   d. Hydralazine, 10–20 mg IV push if patient has bradycardia
10. Cerebral edema can be reduced with mannitol and/or hypertonic saline solutions.
    a. Mannitol, 0.25–1 gram/kg IV every 4–6 hr
    b. Saline, 3% solution, loading dose of 250–300 ml IV over 60 minutes, followed by continuous infusion titrated to treatment goals, including 145–155 mEq/L and serum osmolality of 310–320 mOsm/L
    c. Saline, 23.4% solution, 30 ml IV administered over 30 min or longer, subsequent doses dependent on ICP
11. Surgical clipping or endovascular coiling should be performed as early as possible. Interventional choice of aneurysm obliteration is dependent on the size and location of the aneurysm, the patient's age and clinical condition, and the neurosurgeon's experience.
12. Coil embolization and/or stent placement for ruptured aneurysm: performed by trained neurovascular surgeon or neuroradiologist.
    a. Nonsurgical procedure involving the threading of tiny coils through a microcatheter into the aneurysm
    b. May be used when bleeding is in a difficult-to-reach area of the brain
13. Cerebral vasospasms
    a. Vasospasms occur in approximately 30% of patients. It is most frequent between days 7 and 10 after aneurysm rupture and usually resolves after 21 days. It may be associated with the presence of a thick clot in the subarachnoid space.
    b. Symptoms, which include confusion, decreased LOC, localizing neurological deficits, headache, and increased ICP, may or may not be present. Cerebral infarction can occur with severe vasospasm

CHAPTER I   Cerebrovascular Accidents: Brain Attack

- c. Calcium channel blockers (nimodipine) may be used to treat cerebral blood vessel spasm after SAH from ruptured aneurysms (60 mg PO/NGT every 4 hr for 3 weeks). Recent studies demonstrate improved neurological outcomes by processes other than preventing large vessel narrowing.
- d. If symptomatic vasospasm occurs, the patient is usually treated with IVF loading. Traditional "triple H" therapy has been modified to euvolemia maintenance and induced hypertension.
    - i. Aim for a hematocrit of approximately 30% (although optimal hemoglobin levels are still to be determined)
    - ii. Monitor cardiac output and central venous pressure if necessary
    - iii. The goal is to optimize the low shear rate viscosity of the whole blood and to ensure cerebral perfusion pressure (CPP) that is adequate to restore regional cerebral blood flow in perfusion areas beyond the vasospastic vessels
- e. Treatment is less risky if the aneurysm has been clipped
- f. Balloon angioplasty or IA vasodilators may be used for vasospasms resistant to the preceding treatments
- g. Daily transcranial Doppler ultrasounds should be performed to monitor for vasospasm

14. Rebleeding
    - a. Rebleeding is unpredictable but often occurs between days 2 and 19 after initial rupture and is thought to originate from fibrinolysis of the clot at the site of the ruptured aneurysm.
    - b. Forty percent of patients rebleed, and approximately half of these rebleeds are fatal; therefore, efforts to seal off an aneurysm should be made as soon as possible.
    - c. Neurologic deterioration is generally abrupt
    - d. A repeat CT scan, and occasionally a repeat LP, is needed to confirm rebleeding
    - e. The use of antifibrinolytic agents (aminocaproic acid, tranexamic acid) to prevent rebleeding and decrease mortality in patients with subarachnoid hemorrhage is controversial. Use of these agents has been associated with an increase in cerebral ischemia and no significant decrease has been noted in mortality rate or in degree of disability among survivors.
    - f. For patients with an unavoidable delay in obliteration of aneurysm, a significant risk of rebleeding, and no compelling medical contraindications, short term (less than 72 hr) therapy with tranexamic acid or aminocaproic acid is reasonable to reduce the risk of every aneurysm rebleeding.

15. Cerebral salt wasting
    - a. Hyponatremia develops after aneurysmal SAH
    - b. Excessive secretion of natriuretic peptides that causes hyponatremia from excessive natriuresis and volume contraction
    - c. Crystalloid fluid replacement to maintain euvolemia
    - d. Three percent saline solution to correct hyponatremia
    - e. Consider fludrocortisone to aid in correction of hypovolemia and hyponatremia and to maintain euvolemia

16. Fever
    - a. Most common medical complication in aneurysmal SAH
    - b. The presence of fever that is noninfectious (central) has been associated with severity of injury, amount of hemorrhage, and development of vasospasm
    - c. May be a marker of a systemic inflammatory state
    - d. Fever often associated with worse cognitive outcomes
    - e. Aggressive fever management is recommended

B. ICH

1. Initial management should be directed toward the basic airway, breathing, and circulation and toward focal neurologic deficits.
2. Intubation is indicated for insufficient ventilation, for hypoxia (partial pressure of oxygen [P_{O_2}] less than 60 mmHg or partial pressure of carbon dioxide [P_{CO_2}] greater than 50 mmHg), and for obvious risk of aspiration.
3. Oxygen should be administered to all patients with possible ICH
4. Control severe HTN
   a. Should be achieved through short-acting agents like nicardipine that are titratable
   b. The goal is to decrease the risk of ongoing bleeding from ruptured small arteries and arterioles.
   c. Overaggressive treatment of HTN may decrease CPP and, therefore, worsen brain injury, particularly in the setting of increased intracranial pressure.
   d. However, recent studies demonstrate that SBP kept above 140–150 mmHg was associated with more than double the risk of subsequent death or dependency.
   e. Further study is still warranted, but current evidence suggests that acute lowering of SBP to 140 mmHg is probably safe.
   f. Patients should be carefully monitored during the BP lowering phase, and if neurological exam deteriorates, consider increasing the BP goal to improve cerebral perfusion
5. CPP (Mean arterial pressure[MAP]-ICP) should be kept at 50–70 mmHg
6. Some suggested medications for elevated BP include the following:
   a. Labetalol (Trandate), 5–10 mg IV push
   b. Nicardipene (Cardene), intravenous titratable drip, 2.5–15 mg/hr
   c. Esmolol (Brevibloc), maintenance, 50–300 mcg/kg/min
7. If BP falls to less than 90 mmHg, pressors should be given (dopamine, 2–20 mcg/kg/min; phenylephrine, 0.5–5 mcg/kg/min (50–400 mcg/min); epinephrine, 0.01–0.2 mcg/kg/min (1–10 mcg/min); or norepinephrine [Levophed], 0.01–0.5 mcg/kg/min (1–40 mcg/min).
8. Maintain ICP at less than 20 mmHg and CPP at greater than 50–70 mmHg
   a. Mannitol for cerebral edema (0.25–1 gram/kg of a 20% solution) given intravenously every 4–6 hr
      i. Because of its rebound phenomenon, mannitol is recommended for 5 days or less
      ii. Serum osmolality should be measured BID for those receiving osmotherapy and should be kept at no greater than 320 mOsm/L. Watch renal function carefully and fluid balance status.
   b. Hypertonic saline may also be used to treat cerebral edema
      i. Three percent saline infusions may be started with sodium checks every 6 hr. Administer loading dose of 250–300 ml IV over 60 minutes, followed by continuous infusion titrated to treatment goals. Goal sodium levels of up to 145–155 mEq/L and serum osmolality of 310–320 mOsm/L are at the discretion of the intensivist.
      ii. Twenty-three percent saline may be given in an acutely decompensating patient as an emergency measure to treat elevated ICP. Administer as 30 ml IV over 30 min or longer; subsequent doses dependent on ICP.
   c. Ventricular drain for secondary hydrocephalus
      i. Use should not exceed 7 days because of possible infectious complications
      ii. Intravenous antibiotic prophylaxis may be used if ventricular catheter is non-antibiotic coated
   d. If hyperventilation is used, PCO_2 should be maintained at 30–35 mmHg
   e. Steroids are not recommended
9. Supportive measures

    a. IVFs (normal saline fluid of choice)
        i. Excessive administration can worsen cerebral edema
        ii. Goal is euvolemia.
        iii. Fluid balance is calculated by measuring daily urine production and adding 500 ml for insensible losses plus 300 ml per degree in febrile patients.
    b. Phenytoin (Dilantin), 100 mg every 8 hr, titrate to blood level 10–20 mcg/ml
        i. Levetiracetam (Keppra), 500 mg IV/PO twice a day, as an alternative to phenytoin
    c. Nutritional support
    d. Maintain body temperature with acetaminophen (Tylenol), 650 mg for temperature greater than 101.3°F (38.5°C)
    e. Physical therapy
    f. Skin care/turning
10. Surgery
    a. Indicated for patients with cerebellar hemorrhage greater than 3 cm in diameter
    b. Indicated for those with surgically accessible cerebral hematoma generally extending to within one cm of the cortical surface
    c. Patients with a hemorrhage greater than 1 cm from the cortical surface or with a GCS score of 8 or less tended to do worse with surgical removal as compared with medical management.
    d. Must take into account age and overall prognosis when considering a surgical intervention

BIBLIOGRAPHY

Adams, H. P., Jr. (2009). Secondary prevention of atherothrombotic events after ischemic stroke. *Mayo Clinic Proceedings, 84*(1), 43–51.

Bederson, J. B., Connolly, E. S., Batjer, H. H., Dacey, R. G., Dion, J. E., Diringer, M. N., ... Rosenwasser, R. H. (2009). Guidelines for the management of aneurysmal subarachnoid hemorrhage: A statement for healthcare professionals from a special writing group of the Stroke Council, American Heart Association. *Stroke, 40*(3), 994–1025.

Broderick, J. P. (2004). William M. Feinberg lecture: Stroke therapy in the year 2025: Burden, breakthrough, and barriers to progress. *Stroke, 35*(1), 205–211.

Connolly, E. S., Rabinstein, A. A., Carhuapoma, J. R., Derdeyn, C. P., Dion, J., Higashida, R. T., ... Vespa, P. (2012). Guidelines for the management of aneurysmal subarachnoid hemorrhage: A guideline for healthcare professionals from the American Heart Association/American Stroke Association. *Stroke, 43*(6), 1711–1737.

Diringer, M. N., Scalfani, M. T., Zazulia, A. R., Videen, T. O., & Dhar, R. (2011). Cerebral hemodynamic and metabolic effects of equi-osmolar doses mannitol and 23.4% saline in patients with edema following large ischemic stroke. *Neurocritical Care, 14*(1), 11–17.

Easton, J. D., Saver, J. L., Albers, G. W., Alberts, M. J., Chaturvedi, S., Feldmann, E., ... Sacco, R. L. (2009). AHA/ASA scientific statement: Definition and evaluation of transient ischemic attack. *Stroke, 40*, 2276–2293.

Elliott, J., & Smith, M. (2010). The acute management of intracerebral hemorrhage: A clinical review. *Anesthesia & Analgesia, 110*(5), 1419–1427.

Ferrero, E., Ferri, M., Viazzo, A., Gaggiano, A., Ferrero, M., Maggio, D., ... Nessi, F. (2010). Early carotid surgery in patients after acute ischemic stroke: Is it safe? A retrospective analysis in a single center between early and delayed/deferred carotid surgery on 285 patients. *Annals of Vascular Surgery, 24*(7), 890–899.

Ferri, F. F. (2010). *Practical guide to the care of the medical patient* (8th ed.). St. Louis, MO: Mosby.

Frontera, J. A., Fernandez, A., Schmidt, J. M., Claassen, J., Wartenberg, K. E., Badjatia, N., ... Mayer, S. A. (2009). Defining vasospasm after subarachnoid hemorrhage. What is the most clinically relevant definition? *Stroke, 40*, 1963–1968.

Furie, K. L., Kasner, S. E., Adams, R. J., Albers, G. W., Bush, R. L., Fagan, S. C., . . . Wentworth, D. (2011). Guidelines for the prevention of stroke in patients with stroke or transient ischemic attack: A guideline for healthcare professionals from the American Heart Association/American Stroke Association. *Stroke, 42*(1), 227–276.

Harrigan, M. R., Rajneesh, K. F., Ardelt, A. A., & Fisher III, W. S. (2010). Short-term antifibrinolytic therapy before early aneurysm treatment in subarachnoid hemorrhage: Effects on rehemorrhage, cerebral ischemia, and hydrocephalus. *Neurosurgery, 67*(4), 935–940.

Jamieson, D. G. (2009). Diagnosis of ischemic stroke. *The American Journal of Medicine, 122*(4), S14–S20.

Jauch, E. C., Saver, J. L., Adams, H. P., Jr., Bruno, A., Connors, J. J., Demaerschalk, B. M., . . . Yonas, H. (2012). Guidelines for the early management of patients with acute ischemic stroke: A guideline for healthcare professionals from the American Heart Association/American Stroke Association. *Stroke, 44*(3), 870–947.

Kwon, W. K., Park, D. H., Park, K. J., Kang, S. H., Lee. J. H., Cho, T. H., & Chung, Y. G. (2014). Prognostic factors of clinical outcome after neuronavigation-assisted hematoma drainage in patients with spontaneous intracerebral hemorrhage. *Clinical Neurology and Neurosurgery, 123*, 83–89.

Lansberg, M. G., O'Donnell, M. J., Khatri, P., Lang, E. S., Nguyen-Huynh, M. N., Schwartz, N. E., . . . Aki, E. A. (2012). Antithrombotic and thrombolytic therapy for ischemic stroke. *Chest, 141*(2 Suppl), e601S–e636S.

Lu, A. Y., Ansari, S. A., Nyström, K. V., Damisah, E. C., Amin, H. P., Matouk, C. C., ... Bulsara, K. R. (2014). Intra-arterial treatment of acute ischemic stroke: The continued evolution. *Current Treatment Options in Cardiovascular Medicine, 16*(2), 1–10.

Manno, E. M. (2010). Update on intracerebral hemorrhage. *Critical Care Neurology, 18*(3), 598–610.

Martinez-Vila, E., & Sieira, P. I. (2010). Current status and perspectives of neuroprotection in ischemic stroke treatment. *Cerebrovascular Diseases, 11*(1), 60–70.

Mlynash, M., Olivot, J. M., Tong, D. C., Lansberg, M. G., Eyngorn, I., Kemp, S., ... Albers, G. W. (2009). Yield of combined perfusion and diffusion MR imaging in hemispheric TIA. *Neurology, 72*(13), 1127–1133.

Morgenstern, L. B., Hemphill, J. C., III, Anderson, C., Becker, K., Broderick, J. P., Connolly, E. S., Jr., . . . Tamargo, R. J. (2010). Guidelines for the management of spontaneous intracerebral hemorrhage: A guideline for healthcare professionals from the American Heart Association/American Stroke Association. *Stroke, 41*(9), 2108–2129.

National Institute of Neurological Disorders and Stroke (NINDS). (2004). *Stroke: Hope through research. (NIH Publication No. 99-2222).* Retrieved from http://www.ninds.nih.gov/disorders/stroke/detail_stroke.htm

Overview of hemorrhagic stroke. (2014). In R. S. Porter & J. L. Kaplan (Eds.), *The Merck Manual Home Health Handbook.* Retrieved from http://www.merckmanuals.com/home/brain_spinal_cord_and_nerve_disorders/stroke_cva/overview_of_hemorrhagic_stroke.html

Papadakis, M. A., & McPhee, S. J., (Eds.) (2014). *Current medical diagnosis and treatment* (53rd ed.). New York, NY: McGraw Hill Education.

Seevinck, P. R., Deddens, L. H., & Dijkhuizen, R. M. (2010). Magnetic resonance imaging of brain angiogenesis after stroke. *Angiogenesis, 13,* 101–111.

Vijayaraghavan, K., & Deedwania, P. (2011). Renin-angiotensin-aldosterone blockade for cardiovascular disease prevention. *Cardiology Clinics, 29*(1), 137–156.

CHAPTER 2

Structural Abnormalities

TRAVIS BRADLEY • CHARLENE M. MYERS

ANEURYSM

I. **Definition**
   A. Abnormal dilatation of an arterial wall in which the intima bulges outward
   B. Usually caused by abnormal weakening
   C. Usually occurs with a sudden increase in systolic blood pressure that is caused by events such as straining or sexual intercourse, which may precipitate a rupture

II. **Types**
   A. Berry (saccular)—congenital aneurysm of a cerebral vessel
      1. Tends to occur at arterial bifurcations
      2. More common in adults
      3. Frequently multiple
      4. Usually asymptomatic
      5. May be associated with polycystic kidney disease or coarctation of the aorta
   B. Fusiform—aneurysm that is tapered at both ends and spindle shaped; all walls of the blood vessel dilate more or less equally, creating tubular swelling
      1. More common in the vertebrobasilar system
   C. Mycotic—caused by or infected by microorganisms (bacterial)
   D. Traumatic

III. **Location**
   A. Most intracranial aneurysms, 85%–95%, are located in the carotid system.
      1. 30% occur in the anterior communicating artery
      2. 25% occur in the posterior communicating artery
      3. 20% occur in the middle cerebral artery
   B. Some intracranial aneurysms, 5%–15%, occur in the posterior circulation.
      1. 10% occur in the basilar artery
      2. 5% occur in the vertebral artery
   C. Multiple intracranial aneurysms, usually two or three in number, are found in 20%–30% of patients.
   D. Rupture results in the following:

1. Subarachnoid hemorrhage (SAH)—most common (see Cerebrovascular Accidents: Brain Attack)
2. Intraventricular hemorrhage—13%–28%
3. Intracerebral hemorrhage—less common (see Cerebrovascular Accidents: Brain Attack)
4. Subdural hematoma—rare (see Neurologic Trauma)

IV. Risk factors

A. Evidence supports the association of intracranial aneurysm with heritable connective tissue disorders (e.g., polycystic kidney disease, Ehlers–Danlos syndrome type IV, neurofibromatosis type I, Marfan syndrome) and their familial occurrence.
B. Some of the patients with aneurysmal SAH, 7%–20%, have a first- or second-degree relative with a confirmed intracranial aneurysm.
C. Cigarette smoking is an environmental factor.
   1. The risk of an aneurysmal SAH is approximately three to ten times higher among smokers.
   2. Risk increases with the number of cigarettes smoked.
   3. Smoking decreases the effectiveness of α1-antitrypsin, the main inhibitor of proteolytic enzymes (protease), such as elastase; the imbalance between protease in smokers may result in the degradation of a variety of connective tissues including the arterial wall.
D. Risk is higher among women than among men older than 50 years.
   1. Suggests a role for hormonal factors
   2. Premenopausal women have a low risk of aneurysmal SAH.
   3. Postmenopausal women have a relatively high risk.
   4. Postmenopausal women receiving hormone replacement therapy have an intermediate risk.
E. A moderate to high level of alcohol consumption is an independent risk factor for aneurysmal SAH. Recent heavy use of alcohol, in particular, appears to increase the risk of SAH.
F. Aneurysm size of 7 mm or greater has a higher risk of rupture.
G. Incidence:
   1. Overall estimates in the United States are 14.5 aneurysmal SAH per 100,000 adults.
   2. Incidence increases with age; the typical age at onset is greater than 50 years. It is rare in children.
   3. Women have a 1.24 times greater risk than men.
   4. African Americans and Hispanics have higher incidence than Caucasians.

V. Signs/symptoms

A. Most aneurysms are asymptomatic until they rupture, at which time, SAH results (see signs and symptoms of SAH in Cerebrovascular Accidents: Brain Attack).
B. Some focal neurologic deficits may be related to compression of adjacent structures.
C. Small amounts of blood from the aneurysm ("warning leaks") may precede the major hemorrhage by a few hours or days. These may cause the patient to have headaches, nausea, and neck stiffness.
   1. Often referred to as a "sentinel" headache
D. Ophthalmologic examination may reveal unilateral or bilateral subhyaloid hemorrhages in approximately one fourth of patients with aneurysmal SAH. These hemorrhages are venous in origin, are located between the retina and the vitreous membrane, and are convex at the bottom and flat on the top.
E. Some aneurysms have a mass effect, causing the patient to become symptomatic. These aneurysms are generally large or giant (25 mm or larger).
   1. The most common symptom of mass effect is headache.
   2. The most common sign is palsy of cranial nerve III (pupils).

CHAPTER 2   Structural Abnormalities

3. Brain stem dysfunction, visual field defects, trigeminal neuralgia, cavernous sinus syndrome, seizures, and hypothalamic–pituitary dysfunction may also occur, depending on the location of the aneurysm.
4. These aneurysms carry a high risk of rupture (approximately 6% per year).

VI. **Laboratory/diagnostics**
  A. A computed tomography (CT) scan or a magnetic resonance angiography can be performed to obtain a baseline value for ventricular size and to rule out infarct/hemorrhage. These studies are noninvasive and carry a lower complication rate than is associated with conventional catheter angiography.
    1. CT scans are sensitive in detecting acute hemorrhage, and they show the presence of SAH in almost 100% of patients who undergo scanning within the first 24 hr after hemorrhage.
    2. The sensitivity of CT scanning decreases sharply after 5–7 days because blood is cleared rapidly from the subarachnoid space.
    3. CT scans are also useful in detecting any associated intracranial hemorrhage or hydrocephalus, and the distribution of blood may offer important clues about the location of the ruptured aneurysm.
  B. Cerebral angiography can be ordered to discern the size, shape, location, and number of aneurysms, as well as the occurrence of arterial spasm. The risk of permanent neurologic complications is lower than previously recognized, and cerebral angiography has a high level of diagnostic accuracy. Angiography provides superior spatial resolution and lacks the flow-related artifacts that may affect magnetic resonance angiography.
  C. Magnetic resonance imaging (MRI) angiography does not require contrast material and can be used to detect intracranial aneurysms as small as 2–3 mm in diameter.
  D. Standard MRI is the best method for detecting the presence of a thrombus within the aneurysmal sac.
  E. CT angiography with a 64-slice scanner is an accurate tool for detecting and characterizing aneurysms and can aid in the decision to clip or coil an aneurysm. Helical CT angiography has the ability to demonstrate the relation of the aneurysm to bony structures of the skull base; it can be performed safely in patients who have been treated with ferromagnetic clips, which are a contraindication to MRI angiography.
  F. Lumbar puncture: If the CT scan is negative but a strong clinical suspicion of SAH persists, then a lumbar puncture should be performed. Herniation may occur if intracranial pressure is increased (see Cerebrovascular Accidents: Brain Attack).
  G. Elevations in white blood cell count and sedimentation rate are indicators of a ruptured aneurysm.

VII. **Management**
  A. Surgery
    1. Choosing surgery for patients with an unruptured intracranial aneurysm involves weighing the risk of intracranial rupture against the risks associated with brain surgery.
    2. Size, location, and previous SAH are the most important features for predicting aneurysmal rupture.
       a. As noted in the Cooperative Study of Intracranial Aneurysms and Subarachnoid Hemorrhage, which involved 6,038 ruptured aneurysms, the critical size for rupture is 7–10 mm. Many studies support the critical size as larger than 10 mm.
       b. Major compressive symptoms (e.g., headache and neurologic signs and symptoms) should lead to consideration of surgery.
       c. Coexisting medical problems or factors that favor the need for surgery must be considered (e.g., hypertension and poorly controlled hypertension) to prevent the risk of bleeding.
    3. Early (within 72 hr of the bleed) surgery is desirable for eliminating the risk of rebleed and for allowing aggressive treatment for vasospasm, should it occur.

4. Late: after 7 days post bleed
5. Methods
    a. Clipping
    b. Wrapping
    c. Embolization
    d. Endovascular treatment: Soft metallic coils are inserted within the lumen of the aneurysm. The goal is complete obliteration of the aneurysmal sac.
B. Medical management if surgery is not feasible, as outlined for SAH in Cerebrovascular Accidents: Brain Attack, is continued for approximately 6 weeks.

VIII. **Possible complications**
A. Vasospasm
1. It occurs several days to 3–4 weeks after treatment.
2. Calcium channel blockers (nimodipine, 60 mg every 4 hr for 21 days) have been shown to improve outcomes.
3. Intravascular volume expansion, induced hypertension, or transluminal balloon angioplasty of involved cranial vessels may also be used after the aneurysm has been obliterated.
B. Rebleeding
1. It is greatest within 2–24 hr of the first hemorrhage.
2. Approximately 20% of patients will have further bleeding within 2 weeks, and 40% within 6 months.
3. Prevent hypertensive episodes (see Cerebrovascular Accidents: Brain Attack)
4. Antifibrinolytic agents: Aminocaproic acid or tranexamic acid, used during the first 2 weeks after hemorrhage, has been shown to reduce the risk of rebleeding.
    a. Short-term therapy (less than 72 hr) indicated for patients with unavoidable delay in obliteration of aneurysm, significant risk of rebleeding, and no significant medical contraindications to reduce risk of early aneurysm bleeding
    b. The use of antifibrinolytic agents (e.g., aminocaproic acid, tranexamic acid) to prevent rebleeding and decrease mortality in patients with subarachnoid hemorrhage is controversial. It has been associated with an increase in cerebral ischemia and no significant decrease has been noted in mortality rate or in degree of disability among survivors.
C. Hydrocephalus (see Communicating Hydrocephalus)
1. Caused by interference in the flow of cerebrospinal fluid (CSF)
2. Acute hydrocephalus occurs in 15%–87% of patients with aneurysmal SAH.
3. Chronic hydrocephalus requiring shunt placement occurs in 8.9%–48% of patients with aneurysmal SAH.
4. Acute hydrocephalus is usually managed by the placement of an external ventricular drain or lumbar drain.
D. Seizures
E. Increased intracranial pressure

OTHER ABNORMALITIES

I. **Arteriovenous malformations (AVMs)**
A. AVMs are the condition of dilated arteries and veins with dysplastic vessels, no capillary bed, and no intervening neural parenchyma.
B. In adults, AVMs are medium to high pressure and high flow.
C. AVMs usually present with hemorrhage.
D. AVMs are congenital lesions with a lifelong risk of bleeding of approximately 2%–4% per year.
E. Treatment options are as follows: embolization, stereotactic radiosurgery, and/or surgical excision.

CHAPTER 2 Structural Abnormalities

II. **Dural arteriovenous fistula**
   A. It is different from an AVM, more of a direct fistula.
   B. It is an arteriovenous shunt contained within the leaflets of the dura matter exclusively supplied by the branches of the carotid or vertebral arteries before they penetrate the dura.
   C. Evidence suggests these are not congenital but acquired lesions, usually resulting from collateral revascularization after thrombosis of a venous sinus.
   D. It usually presents with tinnitus, headache, or visual changes.
   E. Treatment options are as follows: embolization, stereotactic radiosurgery, and/or surgical excision

III. **Chiari malformation**
   A. It is a heterogeneous group of conditions with a common factor of CSF flow disruption through the foramen magnum; some are congenital, and some are acquired.
   B. There are four types, although types 1 and 2 most common
   C. Cerebellar tonsillar herniation is the most common type
   D. Surgery is usually the treatment of choice

HYDROCEPHALUS

I. **Definition**
   A. Hydrocephalus is a condition in which an excessive amount of CSF accumulates within the cerebral ventricles.
      1. The human brain makes approximately 500 ml of CSF per day, most of which is generated by the choroid plexus within the ventricular system.
         a. CSF circulates around the brain and spinal cord and is reabsorbed in the venous system.
   B. Hydrocephalus is a common neurosurgical problem that leads to changes in cerebral blood flow caused by displacement, deformation, stretching, or decrease in the caliber of cerebral vessels.
      1. Change in the vessels causes a change in vascular resistance and cerebral perfusion pressure, which is important for cerebral microcirculation.
   C. Normal pressure hydrocephalus is an unusual cause of dementia.
      1. Although the cause is often idiopathic, it may occur as a late complication of intracerebral infection, Alzheimer's disease, or SAH. CSF opening pressure is usually 5–18 mmHg (70–245 mm H_2O).
      2. The syndrome develops subacutely for a few weeks; in some patients, no predisposing reason is identified.

II. **Etiology**
   A. Oversecretion/overproduction of CSF
   B. Obstruction of CSF (lesions or tumors)
   C. Impaired absorption
   D. Normal pressure hydrocephalus may follow head injury, SAH, or meningoencephalitis.

III. **Classification**
   A. Communicating
      1. Ventricles are patent; obstruction occurs beyond the fourth ventricle.
      2. Caused by impaired absorption or overproduction
      3. Usually occurs 4–20 days after aneurysmal rupture, although it may occur at any time
   B. Noncommunicating
      1. Obstruction occurs within or next to the ventricular system, preventing CSF made in the lateral and third ventricles from circulating normally; thus, this fluid no longer communicates with the subarachnoid space.
      2. It is related to lesions or tumors

IV. **Signs/symptoms (adults)**
   A. Acute hydrocephalus

1. Papilledema
2. Headache
3. Nausea and vomiting
4. Gait change
5. Upgaze
   B. Normopressure hydrocephalus
      1. Classic triad
         a. Dementia
         b. Gait disturbance
         c. Urinary incontinence
V. **Management**
   A. Acute: external ventricular drain
   B. Chronic: ventricular shunt
   C. Endoscopic third ventriculostomy (Mixter surgery) has been used in noncommunicating hydrocephalus to enable the surgeon to control the condition without the need for ventricular shunting and without long-term complications associated with shunts.
      1. The advantage of endoscopic surgery is that, when feasible, it can be performed with minimal disruption of neural tissue, thus frequently allowing patients to become mobilized rapidly, resulting in shorter hospitalizations and reduced costs.

SPACE-OCCUPYING LESIONS (BRAIN TUMORS)

I. **Definition**
   A. Brain tumors consist of primary neoplasms (originating in the brain) or secondary neoplasms (originating from sites other than the brain, such as the lung, the breast, the genitourinary tract, and the gastrointestinal tract) located within the intracranial vault.
   B. Glioblastoma multiforme is the most common primary tumor, followed by meningioma and astrocytoma.
   C. The cause is unknown; however, genes and viruses may be associated with these lesions.
II. **Types and characteristics**

Table 2.1	Primary intracranial tumors	
Tumor	**Clinical Features**	**Treatment and Prognosis**
Glioblastoma multiforme	Commonly nonspecific, and complaints of increased intracranial pressure. As the tumor grows, focal deficits develop.	Course is rapidly progressive, with poor prognosis. Total surgical removal is usually not possible and response to radiation therapy is poor.
Astrocytoma	A glioma whose presentation is similar to that of glioblastoma multiforme, but its course is more protracted, often extending for several years. Cerebellar astrocytoma, especially in children, may have a more benign course.	Prognosis is variable. By the time of diagnosis, total excision is usually impossible; tumor often is not radiosensitive. In cerebellar astrocytoma, total surgical removal is often possible.
Medulloblastoma	A glioma is seen most frequently in children. Generally arises from roof of fourth ventricle and leads to increased intracranial pressure accompanied by brain stem and cerebellar signs. May seed subarachnoid space.	Treatment consists of surgery combined with radiation therapy and chemotherapy.

Table 2.1	Primary intracranial tumors	
Tumor	**Clinical Features**	**Treatment and Prognosis**
Ependymoma	A glioma arising from the ependyma of a ventricle, especially the fourth ventricle; leads to early signs of increased intracranial pressure. Arises also from central canal of spinal cord.	Tumor is not radiosensitive and is best treated surgically, if possible.
	A slow-growing glioma. Usually arises in cerebral hemisphere in adults. Calcification may be visible on skull x-ray.	Treatment is surgical and is usually successful.
Brain stem glioma	Occurs during childhood with cranial nerve palsies and then with long-tract signs in the limbs. Signs of increased intracranial pressure occur late.	Tumor is inoperable; treatment is by irradiation and with a shunt for increased intracranial pressure.
Cerebellar hemangioblastoma	Presents with disequilibrium, ataxia of trunk or limbs, and signs of increased intracranial pressure; sometimes familial. May be associated with retinal and spinal vascular lesions, polycythemia, and hypernephromas.	Treatment is surgical.
Pineal tumor	Manifests with increased intracranial pressure; sometimes associated with impaired upward gaze (Parinaud's syndrome) and other deficits indicative of midbrain lesion.	Ventricular decompression by shunting is followed by surgical approach to tumor; irradiation is indicated if tumor is malignant. Prognosis depends on histopathologic findings and extent of tumor.
	Originates from remnants of the Rathke pouch above the sella, depressing the optic chiasm. May occur at any age but usually in childhood, with endocrine dysfunction and bitemporal field deficits.	Treatment is surgical, but total removal may not be possible.
Acoustic neuroma	Ipsilateral hearing loss is the most common initial symptom. Subsequent symptoms may include tinnitus, headache, vertigo, facial weakness or numbness, and long-tract signs (may be familial and bilateral when related to neurofibromatosis). Most sensitive screening tests are MRI and brain stem auditory evoked potential.	Treatment is excision by translabyrinthine surgery, craniectomy, or a combined approach. Outcome is usually good.
Meningioma	Originates from the dura mater or arachnoid; compresses, rather than invades, adjacent neural structures. Increasingly common with advancing age. Tumor size varies greatly. Symptoms vary with tumor site (e.g., unilateral exophthalmos [sphenoidal ridge], anosmia, and optic nerve compression [olfactory groove]). Tumor is usually benign and is readily detected by CT scan; may lead to calcification and bone erosion visible on plain x-rays of skull.	Treatment is surgical. Tumor may recur if removal is incomplete. If removal is incomplete, patients may undergo radiation to decrease the risk of recurrence.
Primary cerebral lymphoma	Associated with AIDS and other immunodeficient states. Presentation may occur with focal deficits or with disturbances of cognition and consciousness. May be indistinguishable from cerebral toxoplasmosis.	Treatment is by whole brain irradiation; chemotherapy may have an adjunctive role. Prognosis depends on CD4 count at diagnosis.

III. **Signs/symptoms**
   A. Vary—depending on the type, location, and growth of the tumor; most symptoms do not develop until the tumor is well advanced
   B. Progressive neurological deficit, 68%, usually motor deficit
   C. Headache, 54%
   D. Seizures, 26%
   E. Other signs and symptoms can include:
      1. Hydrocephalus
      2. Dysphagia
      3. Confusion
      4. Lethargy
      5. Vision changes
      6. Endocrine disturbances

IV. **Laboratory/diagnostics**
   A. MRI is the procedure of choice for imaging all types of brain tumors because of its high sensitivity, capacity to delineate small tumors in sites near bone, sensitivity to tissue edema, and inherent multiplanar capability that allows an accurate localization of tumors and the identification of their relation to normal structures.
   B. CT scan may be useful for screening patients with known cancers elsewhere in the body and patients with atypical headache. Contrast medium may be needed. If CT scan is negative but suspicion is strong, an MRI should be performed. CT scan is effective for following the progression of a diagnosed tumor.
   C. Cerebral angiography can facilitate the assessment of the vascularity of lesions and/or their proximity to blood vessels.
   D. Electroencephalography can detect the presence and location of seizure activity.
   E. Open brain biopsy (craniotomy) or CT- or MRI-directed stereotactic needle biopsy provides a definitive diagnosis.
   F. Metastatic workup is necessary.
      1. Chest x-ray
      2. Mammogram
      3. Bone scan
      4. Prostate examination
      5. Chest/abdominal/pelvic CT

V. **Management**
   A. Referral to oncologist, as pharmacologic therapy is determined by the hematologist or oncologist
   B. Chemotherapy, depending on the type and stage of tumor
      1. Carmustine (BCNU), lomustine (CCNU), cisplatin, and procarbazine are the agents most commonly used for malignant glioma in adults.
   C. Radiation therapy, depending on the type of tumor
      1. Malignant gliomas are not radiosensitive; however, radiation increases the survival rate in affected patients.
   D. Corticosteroids
      1. Dexamethasone (Decadron)
         a. Preferred over methylprednisolone
         b. Standard dose at initiation of therapy is 4–10 mg IV/PO four times a day.
         c. Monitor for adverse effects
         d. Taper slowly, and discontinue if possible
         e. Patients with incompletely treated tumors may not tolerate the decrease in dosage (e.g., they continue to show neurologic deterioration/cerebral edema) and, therefore, may require long-term steroid usage during their last months of life.

  f. Prescribe a concurrent H_2 blocker to prevent gastric irritability associated with steroid use: ranitidine (Zantac), 150 mg PO BID; or famotidine (Pepcid), 20 mg PO BID.
  g. Watch for hyperglycemia-related to steroid use
 2. Methylprednisolone (Solu-Medrol), 120–200 mg IV in 4–6 divided doses (although optimal dosing not well defined) to reduce tumor-associated edema
E. For patients with severe cerebral edema, or in situations where intracranial pressure becomes life threatening, an osmotic diuretic may be necessary. Mannitol (Osmitrol) in the usual dose of 0.25−2 grams/kg of a 20% solution IV for 3–5 minutes can reduce intracranial pressure.
F. In patients with recurrent seizures caused by tumor location and/or edema, anticonvulsants may be necessary.
 1. The agent of choice for many practitioners is phenytoin (Dilantin), 1 gram IV or PO as a loading dose, followed by 300 mg/day in divided doses as a maintenance dose.
 2. Levetiracetam (Keppra) may also be used, with a starting dose of 500 mg IV or PO BID.
G. Brachytherapy (the stereotactic implantation of interstitial radionuclide sources [wafer]) may have a positive effect on survival in patients with glioblastoma.
H. The modified linear accelerator used with stereotactic guidance, the gamma knife, and the proton beam are other noninvasive stereotactic radiosurgical methods that have produced some successful results.
I. If obstructive hydrocephalus is present, surgical shunting can produce dramatic benefit.

BIBLIOGRAPHY

Aminoff, M. J., & Kerchner, G. A. (2014). Nervous system disorders. In. M. A. Papadakis & S. J. McPhee (Eds.), *Current Medical Diagnosis & Treatment* (53rd ed., p. 954). New York, NY: McGraw-Hill Education.

Armstrong, T. S. (2009). *Head's up on the treatment of malignant glioma patients. Oncology Nursing Forum, 36*(5), E232-E240. doi:10.1188/09.ONF.E232-E240

Bederson, J. B., Sander Connoly, E., Hunt Batjer, H., Dacey, R. G., Dion, J. E., Diringer, M. N., . . . Rosenwasser, R. H.(2009). Guidelines for the management of aneurysmal subarachnoid hemorrhage. A statement for healthcare professionals from a special writing group of the Stroke Council, American Heart Association. *Stroke*. Advance online publication. doi:10.1161/STROKEAHA.108.191395

Connolly, E. S., Rabinstein, A. A., Carhuapoma, J. R., Derdeyn, C. P., Dion, J., Higashida, R. T., . . . Hoh, B. L. (2012). Guidelines for the management of aneurysmal subarachnoid hemorrhage: A guideline for healthcare professionals from the American Heart Association/American Stroke Association. *Stroke, 43*(6), 1711-1737. doi:10.1161/STR.0b013e3182587839

Dea, N., Borduas, M., Brendan, K., Fortin, D., Mathieu, D. (2010). Safety and efficacy of gamma knife surgery for brain metastases in eloquent locations. *Journal of Neurosurgery, 113*, 79-83. doi:10.3171/2010.8.GKS10957

Ferri, F. F. (2011). *Practical guide to the care of the medical patient* (8th ed.). St. Louis, MO: Mosby/Elsevier.

Gagliano, N., Costa, F., Cossetti, C., Pettinari, L., Bassi, R., Chiriva-Internati, M., . . . Pluchino, S. (2009). Glioma-astrocyte interaction modifies the astrocyte phenotype in a co-culture experiment model. *Onocology Reports, 22*, 1349-1356. doi: 10.3892/or_00000574

Gallagher, R., Osmotherly, P., Chiarelli, P. (2014). Idiopathinc normal pressure hydrocephalus, what is the physiotherapist's role in assessment for surgery? *Physical Therapy Reviews, 19*(4), 245-251.

Greenberg, M. (2010). *Handbook of neurosurgery* (7th ed.). New York, NY: Thieme.

Hickey, J. V. (2011). *Clinical practice of neurological and neurosurgical nursing* (2nd ed.). Philadelphia, PA: Lippincott Williams & Wilkins.

Jauch, E. C., Saver, J. L., Adams, H. P., Jr., Bruno, A., Connors, J. J., Demaerschalk, B. M., . . . Yonas, H. (2013). Guidelines for the early management of patients with acute ischemic stroke: A guideline for healthcare professionals from the American Heart Association/American Stroke Association. *Stroke, 44,* 870-947. doi:10.1161/STR.0b013e318284056a

Kernan, W. N., Ovbiagele, B., Black, H. R., Bravata, D. M., Fang, M. C., Fisher, M., . . . Wilson, J. A. (2014). Guidelines for the prevention of stroke in patients with stroke and transient ischemic attack: A guideline for healthcare professionals from the American Heart Association/American Stroke Association. *Stroke, 45,* 2160-2236. doi:10.1161/STR.0000000000000024

Kondziella, D., & Waldemar, G. (2013). *Neurology at the bedside.* New York, NY: Springer Publishing.

Longo, D., Fauci, A., Kasper, D., & Hauser, S. (2011). *Harrison's principles of internal medicine: Volumes 1 and 2* (18th ed.). New York, NY: McGraw-Hill Education.

Lynn-McHale Wiegand, D. J. (2011). *AACN procedure manual for critical care* (6th ed.). Philadelphia, PA: Elsevier/Saunders.

McPhee, S. J., Papadakis, M. A., & Tierney, L. M. (Eds.). (2014). *Current medical diagnosis and treatment* (53rd ed.). New York, NY: McGraw-Hill/Appleton & Lange.

Proust, F., Matinaud, O., Gérardin, E., Derrey, S., Levèque, S., Bioux, S., . . . Fréger, P. (2009). Quality of life and brain damage after microsurgical clip occlusion or endovascular coil embolization for ruptured anterior communicating artery aneurysms: Neuropsychological assessment. *Journal of Neurosurgery, 110,* 19-29. doi:10.3171/2008.3.17432

Tisell, M., Tullberg, M., Hellström, P., Edsbagge, M., Högfeldt, M., Wikkelso, C. (2011). Shunt surgery in patients with hydrocephalus and white matter changes. *Journal of Neurosurgery, 114*(5), 1432-1438. doi:10.3171/2010.11.JNS10967

Wyckoff, M., Houghton, D., & LePage, C. (2009). *Critical care: Concepts, role, and practice for the acute care nurse practitioner.* New York, NY: Springer Publishing.

Zaidi, H., Del Guerra, A. (2011). An outlook on future design of hybrid PET/MRI systems. *Medical Physics, 38*(10), 5667-5689. doi:10.1118/1.3633909

CHAPTER 3

Peripheral Neuropathies

ROBERT BLESSING • KELLY BLESSING • THOMAS W. BARKLEY, JR.

GUILLAIN–BARRÉ SYNDROME

I. **Definition**
   A. Guillain–Barré syndrome (GBS) is an acute, usually rapidly progressive, form of inflammatory demyelinating radiculoneuropathy; typically motor greater than sensory.
   B. Characterized by a monophasic course of muscular weakness, mild distal sensory loss, and autonomic dysfunction, with the majority of patients reporting an antecedent infection
      1. The maximum deficit is usually attained by week 4.
   C. Most frequently acquired demyelinating neuropathy

II. **Etiology**
   A. Unknown, although an autoimmune basis is probable
   B. Majority of cases are triggered by an antecedent infection, suggesting a response involving antibodies cross-reacting with both humoral and cellular immunity with peripheral nerve gangliosides
   C. Frequent antecedent infections include the following: upper respiratory infections, *Campylobacter jejuni* enteritis, cytomegalovirus infection, Epstein Barr virus infection, hepatitis infection, HIV, and mycoplasma infection
   D. Immunological response may vary between subtypes.
      1. In cases of *C. jejuni* exposure, ganglioside antibodies, such as GM1, lead to the formation of membrane-attacking complexes damaging axons and disturbing nerve conduction in muscles.
      2. In cases of acute inflammatory demyelinating polyneuropathy, the most common subtype of GBS, T cells initiate complement and macrophage activity, leading to myelin destruction.

III. **Significance**
   A. Incidence/prevalence in the United States
      1. 1.3–3 cases/100,000 annually
      2. Nonseasonal, nonepidemic in nature
      3. Incidence increases with age
         a. 0.8 cases/100,000 at age 18
         b. 3.2 cases/100,000 at age 60

B. Systems affected: nervous, endocrine/metabolic
C. Predominant age/sex
1. All ages
2. Men affected more frequently (1.25:1)
3. Bimodal peaks of occurrence in the 15- to 35-year-old group and the 50- to 75-year-old group

IV. **Signs/symptoms**
A. May differ somewhat between subtypes of the disease
B. Usually symmetric, rapidly progressive distal muscle weakness and paresthesia, beginning in the legs and ascending rapidly to the arms, face, and oropharynx
1. Progression to total motor paralysis can ensue, leading to death from respiratory failure; therefore, this condition is considered a medical emergency.
C. Demyelinating neuropathy occurs in most patients, but approximately 5% of cases present with a primary axonopathy. This subtype, called the Miller Fisher variant, may present with descending paralysis and often involves eye muscles on presentation.
1. The Miller Fisher variant may also include a triad of symptoms, including ophthalmoplegia, ataxia, and areflexia.
D. Deep tendon reflexes are often significantly reduced or absent on presentation, although this may take days to develop.
E. Weakness is more prominent than sensory signs and symptoms and may be more prominent proximally.
F. Sensory involvement can present early, but usually without the objective signs of sensory dysfunction (e.g., stocking distribution sensory loss).
1. Patient may have hyperesthesia, which may make the touch of a hand or a bed sheet very painful
2. Perception of joint position, vibration, and temperature may diminish
G. Bulbar involvement: bilateral facial and oropharyngeal paresis
H. Difficulty swallowing (may have cranial nerve involvement)
I. Urinary retention
J. Respiratory paralysis (involvement of intercostal muscles)
K. Autonomic dysfunction often presents as a hyper-sympathetic state with unexplained tachycardia, but may include bradycardia, blood pressure fluctuations, inappropriate antidiuretic hormone secretion, cardiac arrhythmias, and pupillary changes.
L. Most patients will have a good outcome without sequelae after appropriate treatment and management, but approximately 5% will die from complications.

V. **Laboratory/diagnostics**
A. Cerebrospinal fluid
1. Albuminocytologic dissociation or elevation in cerebrospinal fluid protein (especially immunoglobulin [Ig]G) without pleocytosis (lack of nucleated cells)
2. Normal values may be seen on presentation.
3. Elevation may not occur until the second week of illness.
4. Protein elevation may be very high (greater than 1000 mg/dl) but may not be elevated until symptoms have been present greater than 1 week.
B. Complete blood count: Early leukocytosis may be seen with a left shift that resolves during the course of illness.
C. If diagnosis is strongly suspected, a repeat lumbar puncture may be indicated.

VI. **Pathological findings**
A. Segmental demyelination of peripheral nerves and axonal degeneration
B. Inflammatory lesion: lymphocyte and macrophage invasion of myelin sheath
C. Presence of antibodies depending on subtypes (i.e., GM1 or anti-GQ1b)

CHAPTER 3   Peripheral Neuropathies

D. Special tests: motor and sensory nerve conduction studies and needle electromyography, which reveals slowed conduction velocities and prolonged motor, sensory, and F-wave latencies or absent F-waves; decreased nerve conduction related to demyelination

VII. **Management**
  A. There is no known cure for Guillain–Barré syndrome. However, there are therapies that lessen the severity and accelerate recovery in many patients.
  B. Refer to neurology—treatment is usually determined by a specialist, rather than general practitioner. Most therapies outside of intravenous immunoglobulin (IVIG) and plasmapheresis are not FDA-labeled.
  C. Severe acute polyneuropathy is a medical emergency. Initiate therapy as soon as possible following diagnosis. Delayed therapy, even 2 weeks after first motor symptoms, may prove to be ineffective.
  D. Admit to the intensive care unit for constant monitoring and vigorous support of vital functions
  E. Measure vital capacity and arterial blood gases
     1. Intubation with mechanical ventilation may be indicated for the following: vital capacity less than 12–15 ml/kg, partial pressure of oxygen in arterial blood (PaO_2) less than 70, negative inspiratory force weaker than negative 20 cm H2O or rapidly worsening, difficulty clearing secretions, and/or concerns of aspiration
  F. Anticipate respiratory support by mechanical ventilation.
  G. Monitor patients with autonomic dysfunction (bradyarrhythmias, tachyarrhythmias, orthostatic hypotension, systemic hypertension, and hypotension) PRN, as dysautonomia is a leading cause of mortality in patients with GBS.
  H. Immunomodulating treatment with IVIG and plasmapheresis are both considered first-line therapy and deemed equivalent in efficacy.
     1. Combination of therapies does not offer additional benefit.
     2. Corticosteroids are not indicated for patients with GBS.
        a. IVIG
           i. Has been used traditionally as an alternative to plasmapheresis (0.4 grams/kg/day IV for 5 consecutive days)
           ii. The major component is the IgG molecule and is derived from healthy donated blood-neutralizing pathogenic antibodies and limiting activation of the complement system.
           iii. Recommended within 2 weeks (possibly 4 weeks) of symptom onset
           iv. Decision to use this over plasmapheresis is usually determined by available resources and comorbidities increasing potential complications such as heart disease, renal insufficiency, and IgA deficiency
        b. Plasmapheresis
           i. Recommended as first-line treatment, especially for patients with severe symptoms such as impaired independent walking or ventilator dependency
           ii. Mechanically removes antibodies and activated complements from the blood
           iii. The routine frequency is five times (approximately 50 ml/kg) every other day for acute severe cases.
           iv. Shorter courses of therapy have been reported for less severe cases or chronic conditions.
           v. Although data are limited, plasmapheresis may reduce time on ventilator.
           vi. The decision to use this over IVIG is usually determined by available resources and comorbidities increasing potential complications such as labile blood pressure, unstable angina, septicemia, and venous access difficulties.
        c. Other potential agents
           i. Interferons

- (a) Inhibitory glycoproteins that act as cellular immunomodulators that may inhibit antigen presentation and tumor necrosis factor secretion
- (b) May decrease T-cell proliferation, increase anti-inflammatory cytokine production, and modulate macrophage activity
- I. Prevention of thromboembolic events
  1. Thromboembolic events are a leading cause of mortality in patients with GBS.
  2. Heparin (5,000 units SQ every 8 hr) or low-molecular weight heparin along with sequential compression devices is indicated.
  3. Therapeutic anticoagulation may be considered in patients without contraindications and determined by risk factors other than those derived from GBS.
- J. Pain management
  1. Pain may be significant in GBS, especially during the reinnervation phase.
  2. Suitable analgesics range from nonsteroidal anti-inflammatory agents to opioids.
  3. Neuropathic pain medications may be beneficial (e.g., gabapentin and pregabalin)
- K. Stress ulcer prevention, especially in those receiving ventilatory support
  1. Ranitidine, 150 mg PO/NG every 12 hrs or 50 mg IV every 8 hrs
  2. Famotidine, 20 mg PO/NG/IV every 12 hrs
  3. Cimetidine, 300 mg PO/NG/IV every 6 hrs or 37.5–50 mg/hr via continuous infusion
- L. Encourage fluid intake to maintain adequate urine output
- M. Monitor serum electrolytes
- N. Maintain skin integrity, protect skin from trauma and pressure, reposition frequently
- O. Apply moist heat to relieve pain and to permit early physical therapy
- P. Range of motion
  1. Perform passive range-of-motion exercises immediately
  2. Perform active range-of-motion exercises when acute symptoms subside
  3. Prevention of joint contractures is very important
- Q. Nutrition management
  1. Assess pharyngeal function
  2. If patient has difficulty swallowing, initiate enteric or parental nutrition.
- R. Emotional support and social counseling
- S. Interdisciplinary care team is necessary to provide the complex care needed for patients and families

VIII. Follow-up
- A. Patient will require physical rehabilitation to regain strength
- B. Subsequent development of chronic course: chronic inflammatory demyelinating polyradiculoneuropathy
  1. Chronic inflammatory demyelinating polyradiculoneuropathy has an insidious onset after GBS and may continue for years.
  2. Plasmapheresis benefits one third of patients, as do immunosuppressive agents (azathioprine).

IX. Expected course and prognosis
- A. Weakness and paralysis progress during a 2-week period, stabilize, and then gradually improve. Improvement for a period of months is common.
- B. 10%–23% of patients require ventilatory support
- C. 7%–22% of patients are left with mild disability, mild weakness, or reflex loss
- D. Approximately 10% of patients—those with a more prolonged course—may have severe residual defects.
- E. Axonal regeneration requires 6–18 months
- F. Mortality occurs at a rate of approximately 5%

MYASTHENIA GRAVIS

I. **Definition**
   A. Disorder of the neuromuscular junction resulting in a pure motor syndrome; characterized by weakness that may fluctuate most notably after prolonged muscle use, particularly of the extraocular, pharyngeal, facial, cervical, proximal limb, and respiratory musculature
   B. Caused by an autoimmune attack on the acetylcholine receptor (AChR) complex at the postsynaptic membrane of the neuromuscular junction, resulting in AChR dysfunction and jeopardizing normal muscular transmission
   C. Onset may be sudden or severe (myasthenic crisis) but typically is mild and intermittent for many years.

II. **Significance**
   A. The reported prevalence is 14–20 cases per 100,000 population with 10–20 new cases per million.
   B. Predominant age is 20–40 years, but it can occur at any age (1–80 years). The incidence in women peaks in the third decade, in men in the fifth and sixth decades.
      1. Bimodal distribution
      2. May be under recognized in elderly patients
   C. Female-to-male ratio of 2:1 in early adulthood, but it becomes more equally distributed later in life

III. **Signs/symptoms**
   A. Ptosis—ocular muscles are affected initially in 40% of patients and eventually in 80%
   B. Diplopia
   C. Facial weakness
   D. Fatigue from chewing
   E. Bulbar muscle weakness resulting in dysphagia and dysarthria
   F. Dysphonia
   G. Neck weakness
   H. Fatigue after exercise
   I. Proximal limb weakness with upper limbs more noticeable than lower
   J. Respiratory weakness
   K. Generalized weakness
   L. Sensory modalities and deep tendon reflexes remain normal
   M. Severe generalized quadriparesis may develop, especially in relapse

IV. **Myasthenic crisis**
   A. Myasthenia crisis, defined by respiratory failure, is an emergency that occurs in up to 20% of MG patients and requires mechanical ventilation.
   B. It weakens oropharyngeal and laryngeal muscles, causing airway obstruction.
   C. It affects 10%–15% of patients with the greatest risk within 2–3 years of diagnosis.
   D. Increasing muscle weakness and diplopia may be seen prior to onset of crisis.
   E. Patients with muscle-specific kinase (MuSK) antibody-positive are more likely to have crisis.
   F. Common precipitating factors include:
      1. Infections
      2. Stress (trauma and surgery)
      3. Rapid introduction, escalation, or tapering of steroids
      4. Withdrawal of cholinesterase inhibitors
      5. Exposure to drugs
         a. Neuromuscular blocking agents
         b. Antibiotics including macrolides, aminoglycosides, and fluoroquinolones
         c. Cardiovascular agents, including β-blockers, calcium channel blockers, procainamide, and quinidine

d. Quinine
e. Magnesium
f. Iodinated contrast agents
g. Botulinum toxin
h. Chemotherapeutic agents such as cisplatin

V. **Laboratory/diagnostics**
   A. Strategy for diagnostic testing based on clinical, serological, and electrodiagnostic findings and may include edrophonium testing
   B. Antibody testing: AChR and MuSK
      1. AChR is positive in 80%–85% of generalized myasthenia patients.
      2. MuSK antibodies are present in nearly half of those negative for AChR.
      3. Seronegative (approximately 10%) may have antibody-clustered AChRs.
   C. Electrodiagnostics
      1. Repetitive nerve stimulation: A decremental response occurs after maximal voluntary contraction; this is seen more frequently in the proximal, cervical, or facial muscles and is considered positive if motor response declines more than 10%.
      2. Single-fiber electromyography: highly sensitive but less specific, technically difficult to perform, and limited availability
         a. Single-fiber electromyography assesses temporal variability between two muscle fibers within the same motor unit (jitter). MG is a condition in which jitters are increased.
   D. Edrophonium (Tensilon) test: short duration (less than 5 minutes); used in MG for differentiating between myasthenic and cholinergic crises
      1. Requires objective improvement in a testable muscle
      2. Administer 2 mg IV as a test dose, while monitoring electrocardiogram for changes in heart rate or rhythm (cholinergic side effects may include increased salivation, sweating, flushing urgency, and periorbital fasciculations)
      3. After observing for approximately two minutes, additional dosing may be required up to a total of 10 mg.
      4. In MG, a sudden, brief improvement in muscle function occurs, whereas those in cholinergic crises worsen
      5. Dangerous cardiorespiratory depression may occur, and atropine and equipment to maintain respiration must be available during the test.
   E. MRI or CT scan of the anterior mediastinum may document an associated thymoma.
   F. Laboratory data that may be present with MG:
      1. Thyroid function test: Patients with MG have a greater incidence of thyroid disease.
      2. Vitamin B12 levels may be low because of associated pernicious anemia.
      3. Antinuclear antibodies, antithyroid antibodies, and rheumatoid arthritis factor are often present.
      4. Lumbar puncture is typically normal

VI. **Management**
   A. Typically outpatient, but focus will be on inpatient management
   B. Inpatient care includes symptomatic and immunosuppression management of MG as well as myasthenic crisis.
   C. General measures: management is difficult and should be carried out by a neurologist who specializes in neuromuscular disease
   D. Symptomatic management
      1. Cholinesterase inhibitors: pyridostigmine bromide (Mestinon)
         a. First-line therapy for general management
         b. Slows down degradation, thereby increasing availability of acetylcholine at the neuromuscular junction
         c. Dosing: tailored to individual requirements throughout the day

CHAPTER **3** Peripheral Neuropathies

> > > i. 30–60 mg PO every 4–6 hr initially, with a maximum daily dose of 360 mg
> > > ii. Average daily dose: 600 mg/day
> > > iii. Mild MG: 60–360 mg/day
> > > iv. Severe MG: maximum daily dose as high as 1500 mg
> > d. Onset of effect is 30 minutes, duration 4 hr
> > e. Longer-acting preparation is available for patients on stable dosing.
> > f. Monitor patient for cholinergic adverse effects, such as nausea, vomiting, diarrhea, increased salivation, bronchial secretions, and cramps. These adverse effects can be controlled with propantheline (15 mg may be given 15–30 minutes prior to administration of pyridostigmine).
> 2. Drugs to try to avoid in patients with MG include:
> > a. Ketolides
> > b. Aminoglycosides
> > c. Polypeptides (when not used topically)
> > d. Glycopeptides
> > e. Lincosamide
> > f. Class 1 antiarrhythmics
E. Immunomodulating therapy: necessary for patients with MG and may require lifelong therapy (IVIG and plasmapheresis for rapid immunomodulating therapies, see myasthenic crisis)
> 1. Prednisone
> > a. Should be administered to those who have responded poorly to anticholinesterase drugs and, if indicated, have already undergone thymectomy
> > b. Dose is determined on an individual basis
> > c. High initial dose can gradually be tapered to a lower maintenance dose
> > d. Continue to taper very slowly, attempting to establish the minimum dosage necessary to maintain remission
> 2. Azathioprine
> > a. Widely used as a nonsteroidal immunosuppressant and can be used as monotherapy
> > b. Dose is started at 50 mg/day, titrated up to 2–3 mg/kg PO per day if well tolerated
> > c. May cause macrocytosis and lymphopenia (drug should not be discontinued for this effect)
> > d. If remission not achieved, refer to specialist for other immune modulating therapies (e.g., methotrexate, cyclosporin, mycophenolate, or tacrolimus)
F. Management of impending myasthenic crisis
> 1. Airway and ventilatory management
> > a. Patients with bulbar weakness, declining vital capacity (less than 20 ml/kg), maximal inspiratory force of negative 30 cm H_2O, or weak or ineffective cough that increases work of breathing, should be admitted to an intensive care unit to monitor for possible intubation and mechanical ventilation.
> > b. Vital capacity may not be reliable in patients having difficulty maintaining a seal around a spirometer mouthpiece.
> 2. Rapid immunomodulating therapies (IVIG and plasmapheresis are equivocal in efficacy in myasthenic crisis)
> > a. IVIG
> > > i. Therapy that has been used traditionally as an alternative to plasmapheresis
> > > ii. Dosing: 1 gram/kg/day IV for 2 days or 400 mg/kg/day IV for 5 days, for a total of 1–2 grams/kg IV for 2–5 days
> > > iii. Major component is IgG molecule and is derived from healthy donated blood-neutralizing pathogenic antibodies and limiting activation of the complement system

              iv. Decision to use over plasmapheresis usually determined by available resources and comorbidities increasing potential complications, such as heart disease, renal insufficiency, and IgA deficiency
         b. Plasmapheresis
              i. Mechanically removes antibodies and activated complements from the blood
              ii. Routine frequency is five times (approximately 50 ml/kg) every other day for acute severe cases.
              iii. Shorter courses of therapy have been reported for less severe cases or chronic conditions.
              iv. Decision to use over IVIG usually determined by available resourcets and comorbidities increasing potential complications such as labile blood pressure, unstable angina, septicemia, venous access difficulties

VII. **Associated conditions**
    A. Thymoma (present in 10%–15% of patients with MG)
       1. CT scan is indicated to assess for presence
       2. Thymectomy may result in long-term improvement in patients with suspected thymoma
       3. Thymectomy is generally delayed if patient is in acute respiratory failure
    B. Thymic hyperplasia
    C. Thyrotoxicosis
    D. Other autoimmune disease

BIBLIOGRAPHY

Barth, D., Nabavi Nouri, M., Ng, E., Nwe, P., & Bril, V. (2011). Comparison of IVIG and PLEX in patients with myasthenia gravis. *Neurology, 76*, 2017–2023.

Cavaicante, P., Bernasconi, P., & Mantegazza, R. (2012). Autoimmune mechanisms in myasthenia gravis. *Current Opinion in Neurology, 25*(5), 621–629.

Chhibber, V., & Weinstein, R. (2012). Evidence-based review of therapeutic plasma exchange in neurological disorders. *Seminars in Dialysis, 25*, 132–139.

Jacob, S., Stuart, V., Lashley, D., & Hilton-Jones, D. (2009). Myasthenia gravis and other neuromuscular junction disorders. *Practical Neurology, 20*, 364–371.

Huan, M., & Smith, A.G. (2012). Weakness (Guillain-Barré syndrome). In K. L. Roos (ed.), *Emergency Neurology* (211-234). New York, NY: Springer Science and Business Media.

Hui, D. (2011) *Approach to Internal Medicine: A Resource Book for Clinical Practice* (3rd ed.). New York, NY: Springer Science and Business Media.

Kieseier, B. C., Lehmann, H. C., & Meyer, G. (2012). Autoimmune diseases of the peripheral nervous system. *Autoimmunity Reviews, 11*, 191–195.

Maggi, L., & Manteegazza, R. (2011). Treatment of myasthenia gravis, focus on pyridostigmine. *Clinical Drug Investigation, 13*(10), 691–701.

Myasthenia Gravis Association. *Myasthenia Gravis Medication List*. Retrieved from http://mgakc.org/wp-content/uploads/2011/07/MGA-Medication-List-12-1-12.pdf

Patwa, H. S., Chaudhry, V., Katzberg, H., Rae-Grant, A. D., & So, Y. T. (2012). Evidenced-based guideline: Intravenous immunoglobulin in the treatment of neuromuscular disorders: Report of the therapeutics and technology assessment subcommittee of the American Academy of Neurology. *Neurology, 78*, 1009–1015.

Spillane, J., Higham, E., & Kullmann, D. (2012). Easily missed? Myasthenia gravis. *BMJ, 345*. doi:10.1136/bmj.e8497

Vincent, J. L., Abraham, E., Moore, F. A., Kochanek, P. M., & Fink, M. P. (2011). *Textbook of critical care* (6th ed.). Philadelphia, PA: Elsevier Saunders.

Xiao, J., Simard, A. R., Shi, F., & Hao, J. (2013). New strategies in the management of Guillain–Barre Syndrome. *Clinical Reviews in Allergy and Immunology*.

Yuebing, L. (2013). Myasthenia gravis: Newer therapies offer sustained improvement. *Cleveland Clinic Journal of Medicine, 80*(11), 711–721.

CHAPTER 4

Neurologic Trauma

KIMBERLY ALVA • CHARLENE M. MYERS

HEAD TRAUMA/TRAUMATIC BRAIN INJURY

I. **Head trauma accounts for two thirds of all casualties of motor vehicle accidents.**
   A. Head trauma is the leading cause of death in all trauma cases.
   B. Anatomic structures and physiologic functions of the head provide protection for the brain.
      1. Scalp
      2. Skull
      3. Cerebral meninges (pia mater, arachnoid, and dura mater)
      4. Cerebrospinal fluid (CSF)
   C. The brain is dependent on glucose (25%) and oxygen (20%) for functioning.

II. **Mechanism of injury**
   A. Acceleration/deceleration
   B. Deformation
   C. Blunt trauma
   D. Penetrating injury
      1. High-velocity object
      2. Low-velocity object
   E. Coup-contrecoup injuries: brain tissue injury directly at the site of impact (coup) and at the pole opposite of the site of impact (contrecoup) that may be caused by movement of cranial contents within the skull

III. **Categories of injury**
   A. Primary head injury
      1. Scalp laceration
         a. The most common head injury
         b. May result in profuse bleeding caused by the great vascular supply to the scalp (monitor for signs and symptoms of hypovolemia, such as increased heart rate and decreased blood pressure)
         c. Apply direct pressure to control bleeding (first assess for skull fracture)
         d. Suture/staple laceration after thorough examination and cleansing
            i. Lidocaine 1% with epinephrine should be used on scalp lacerations to help control bleeding.

CHAPTER **4** Neurologic Trauma

      ii. Do not use lidocaine with epinephrine on lacerations located on the nose or ears.
2. Skull fracture
   a. Simple: no displacement of bone
      i. Observe for scalp laceration; protect the cervical spine
      ii. May indicate underlying brain injury
   b. Depressed: bone fragment depressing the thickness of the skull
      i. Patients often have a scalp laceration
      ii. Patient may be asymptomatic or may have an altered level of consciousness
      iii. Surgery is often required to elevate and debride the wound.
      iv. Prophylactic broad-spectrum antibiotics should be initiated
      v. Tetanus toxoid, if indicated
      vi. Institute seizure precautions
   c. Basilar: fracture in the floor of the skull
      i. Raccoon eyes—periorbital ecchymosis
      ii. Battle sign—mastoid ecchymosis
      iii. Otorrhea and/or rhinorrhea (positive Dextrostix test result, halo or target sign, and salty taste in mouth); do not obstruct the flow
      iv. Prophylactic antibiotic coverage
      v. Oral intubation and oral gastric tube are indicated in place of nasal intubation and nasogastric tube
3. Brain injury
   a. Concussion: transient, reversible alteration in brain functioning
      i. Brief loss of consciousness and amnesia of events
      ii. Lethargy, headache, nausea, and dizziness
      iii. Do not give opioids or other sedating medications. Evaluate for changes in the level of consciousness.
      iv. May need to admit to hospital if unconsciousness lasts longer than 2 minutes
   b. Contusion: bruising to the surface of the brain with varying degrees of edema; contrecoup injury
      i. Most commonly seen in the frontal or temporal regions; the skull is rough and jagged, and the brain may be damaged as it moves across underlying structures
      ii. Variable levels of consciousness and amnesia
      iii. Nausea, vomiting, and/or dizziness
      iv. Visual disturbances
      v. Institute seizure precautions
      vi. Brain stem contusion: posturing, variable temperature, and variable vital signs
B. Hematoma
   1. Epidural hematoma (EDH): most commonly seen in the temporal/parietal region; associated with skull fracture resulting in arterial injury, causing bleeding into the epidural space between the skull and the dura mater
      a. Brief loss of consciousness
      b. "Lucid interval"
      c. Deterioration—may be rapid
         i. Obtundation
         ii. Contralateral hemiparesis
         iii. Ipsilateral pupil dilatation
      d. Evaluation and treatment
         i. Obtain CT scan (noncontrast)
         ii. Medical therapy based on Brain Trauma Foundation (BTF) if EDH is less than 15 mm thick, has a midline shift less than 5 mm, and the patient has a Glasgow coma score (GCS) greater than 8; serial CT scans and close neurological assessments

iii. Surgical intervention if an EDH is greater than 30 cm; should be evacuated regardless of GCS
2. Subdural hematoma: most commonly caused by tearing of bridging veins, causing bleeding between the dura mater and the brain tissue
   a. Most frequently seen type of intracranial bleeding
   b. Acute: develops over minutes to hours
      i. Drowsiness, agitation, and confusion
      ii. Headache
      iii. Unilateral or bilateral pupil dilatation
      iv. Late hemiparesis
      v. Obtain CT scan (noncontrast)
      vi. If subdural hematoma meets surgical criteria, surgery is indicated immediately (surgical indications: greater than 10 mm thickness with greater than 5 mm midline shift regardless of GCS, or in a patient with deteriorating GCS less than 9 despite the size of the hematoma).
   c. Chronic: develops over days or weeks, generally occurs in elderly patients
      i. Headache
      ii. Memory loss
      iii. Personality changes
      iv. Incontinence
      v. Ataxia
      vi. Obtain CT scan (noncontrast)
      vii. Surgery is usually required (burr holes or craniotomy), but close monitoring may be sufficient if the hematoma is small.
C. Infection
   1. Meningitis
   2. Brain abscess
D. Cerebral edema/elevated intracranial pressure (ICP)/herniation
   1. Clinical manifestations
      a. Decrease in the level of consciousness
      b. Herniation—indicated by pupillary dilation; "blown pupil"
      c. Cushing triad—present in combination in only about one third of patients, indicates increasing ICP and impending cerebral herniation
         i. Hypertension: Widening pulse pressure (systolic blood pressure will increase in attempts to maintain a constant cerebral perfusion pressure [CPP]); CPP = mean arterial pressure (MAP) - ICP
         ii. Decreased respiratory rate
         iii. Bradycardia
E. Neurologic examination
   1. AVPU (A—awake; V—responds to verbal stimuli; P—responds to painful stimuli; U—unresponsive)
   2. GCS (range: 3–15) used to assess the level of consciousness; a score of 8 or below is considered comatose
   3. Posturing
      a. Decorticate: flexion of arms, wrists, fingers; adduction of arm against thorax; extension, internal rotation, and/or plantar flexion with lower extremities
      b. Decerebrate: stiff extension, adduction, and internal rotation of upper extremities (palms pronated); stiff extension and plantar flexion of lower extremities (clenched teeth and hyperextended back, more of the brain stem is involved)
F. Electrolyte disturbances in brain injury
   1. Hyponatremia—most common electrolyte disturbance in brain injury
      a. Syndrome of inappropriate antidiuretic hormone

CHAPTER 4   Neurologic Trauma

      b. Cerebral salt wasting (CSW): The differentiation of CSW from the syndrome of inappropriate antidiuretic hormone is imperative as the treatment differs significantly.
  2. Hypernatremia
      a. Diabetes insipidus: increased urinary output with specific gravity of 1.005 or less; may cause severe hypernatremia if left untreated
         i. Often seen in herniation syndromes
      b. Use of osmotic (mannitol) and thiazide diuretics

IV. **Management of traumatic brain injury**
  A. Consult a neurosurgeon
  B. Limit secondary injury
  C. Prevent hypotension and hypoxemia
    1. Both may increase morbidity and mortality from traumatic brain injury
    2. According to BTF guidelines, resuscitation should be aimed at maintaining a systolic blood pressure greater than 90 mmHg and a partial pressure of arterial oxygen (PaO_2) greater than 60 mmHg.
    3. The administration of blood is another way to improve tissue perfusion to the brain by optimizing the oxygen-carrying capacity of intravascular fluid. The goal is to maintain hematocrit at 30%–33%.
  D. Treating cerebral edema/elevated ICP/herniation
    1. Hyperventilation/hyperoxia
      a. Hyperventilation ($PaCO_2$ [partial pressure of carbon dioxide in arterial blood], 25–30 mmHg) has been used for decades to cause cerebral vasoconstriction and thereby lower ICP. Cerebral vasoconstriction caused by hyperventilation has also been known to cause cerebral ischemia.
      b. Experts now recommend that hyperventilation should not be used routinely, especially during the first 24 hr after injury, unless ICP is severely high or the patient requires suctioning.
         i. BTF guidelines specifically recommend that hyperventilation should be undertaken to bring $PaCO_2$ to less than 35 mmHg only if a measured increase in ICP is reported, or if increased ICP is suspected because of physical signs, while intracranial hypertension is refractory to other interventions.
         ii. Other methods known to control ICP (e.g., elevating the head of the bed, sedation, paralysis, mannitol, CSF drainage) should be instituted first.
  E. Sedation and analgesia
    1. Opioid sedatives help lower ICP by reducing metabolic demand and relieving anxiety and pain.
    2. Short-acting opioids are the best choices
      a. IV fentanyl (2 mcg/kg test dose; 2–5 mcg/kg/hr continuous infusion) or sufentanil (Sufenta) (10–30 mcg test dose; 0.05–2 mcg/kg/hr continuous infusion)
         i. Fentanyl and sufentanil have the potential to slightly raise ICP
         ii. Morphine may be used in this setting, but is longer acting.
      b. These may be supplemented with propofol (Diprivan) (0.5 mg/kg test dose; 20–75 mcg/kg/min continuous infusion [not to exceed 5 mg/kg/hr]) or benzodiazepines, such as diazepam (Valium [2.5–10 mg]) or lorazepam (Ativan [0.5–2 mg]), if the patient remains agitated or ICP remains elevated.
    3. Neuromuscular blocking agents—use removes the ability to perform a neurological assessment; should only be given after consultation with the neurologist or neurosurgeon
      a. Vecuronium (Norcuron) or cisatracurium (Nimbex)
         i. Dosage should be individualized and a peripheral nerve stimulator or train-of-four (TOF) monitor should be used to measure neuromuscular function during administration.

ii. Cisatracurium, 0.1–0.2 mg/kg bolus, followed by 1–10 mcg/kg/min continuous infusion; titrate to TOF
    b. Can be used to help lower ICP in patients in whom confusion, posturing, or severe agitation is interfering with treatment or diagnostic testing
    c. Patient must be sedated and intubated with an adequate set rate on the ventilator
    d. Paralytic agents also may be needed to help oxygenate and ventilate the patient
F. Steroids
   1. Corticosteroids in multiple studies, including the CRASH trial, have shown to increase morbidity and mortality.
      a. The BTF highly recommends that steroids not be used in traumatic brain injury.
G. Hyperosmolar therapy
   1. Mannitol—drug of choice in an emergency situation when brain herniation is pending
      a. Creates an osmotic gradient across the blood-brain barrier that pulls water from the central nervous system into the intravascular space
      b. May enhance cerebral oxygen delivery via decreased blood viscosity, increased CPP, or both
      c. May also provide some cytoprotective effects through oxygen-free radical scavenging
      d. Administer as a bolus (0.25–1 grams/kg) or continuous infusion
      e. Results are quick, occurring usually within 10–20 min, and can last up to 6 hr
      f. May need to avoid use in patients with renal failure
      g. Monitor serum osmolarity. Maintain serum osmolarity less than 320 mOsm
      h. Monitor electrolytes, especially serum sodium
      i. Monitor blood pressure closely
         i. Hypotension is an adverse effect that results from dehydration caused by diuresis.
         ii. The goal is to attain beneficial effects without inducing dehydration.
      j. Volume replacement may be necessary to keep the patient euvolemic and to prevent hypotension (e.g., replace urinary with isotonic crystalloids).
      k. An indwelling urinary catheter should be in place and urine output recorded each hour.
   2. Hypertonic saline (3% or 23% NaCl)
      a. The effect is on the osmotic mobilization of fluid across the blood-brain barrier, similar to mannitol
      b. May exacerbate pulmonary edema in patients with cardiac or pulmonary issues
      c. May be given as a bolus or a continuous infusion
H. ICP monitoring
   1. ICP monitoring is appropriate for the following:
      a. Comatose patients (GCS score of 3–8) with an abnormal CT scan
      b. Comatose patients with a normal CT scan and two of the following:
         i. Older than 40 years of age
         ii. Unilateral or bilateral motor posturing
         iii. Hypotension
   2. ICP monitoring is not routinely appropriate for patients with mild or moderate head injury.
   3. Ventricular catheter allows the practitioner to measure ICP and to drain CSF
   4. If the ICP is greater than 20–25 mmHg for greater than 5 minutes, treatment should be initiated to lower ICP.
   5. Monitoring of ICP allows the practitioner to calculate CPP (CPP = MAP − ICP)
   6. Ideally, CPP should be maintained at a minimum of 60 mmHg.
I. Seizure prophylaxis in traumatic brain injury

1. It is recommended that anticonvulsants such as phenytoin (Dilantin) may be used to prevent early posttraumatic seizures in those at high risk after a head injury.
    a. IV loading dose of 15–20 mg/kg, followed by maintenance dose 5 mg/kg/day
2. Levetiracetam (Keppra) is used for prophylaxis of both early and late seizures after trauma
    a. Easier to use and better side effect profile compared to phenytoin; however, further research is needed to ascertain that levetiracetam may be an acceptable alternative to phenytoin
    b. Treatment protocols range from 7–30 days; may be administered in daily doses of 1000 mg, 2000 mg, and 3000 mg, given as twice-daily dosing
3. Prophylactic use is not recommended for preventing late posttraumatic seizures.
4. Prophylactic seizure treatment is not suggested to be used longer than 7 days.

J. DVT/VTE prophylaxis
   1. Use graduated compression stockings or intermittent pneumatic compression (IPC) stockings until patients are ambulatory
   2. Low molecular weight heparin (LMWH) or unfractionated heparin (UFH) should be used in combination with mechanical prophylaxis.
       a. Note an increased risk for expansion of intracranial hemorrhage
   3. There is insufficient evidence for precise recommendations concerning the preferred agent, dose or timing of pharmacologic prophylaxis for DVT.

K. Neurological assessment and management of traumatic brain injury (TBI) patient
   1. It is an ongoing process
   2. GCS score may be necessary every 30–60 minutes for the first 24 hr
       a. Note whether the patient is receiving sedation and/or paralytics; cannot assess GCS while on paralytics
   3. Pupil size and reaction
   4. Vital signs
   5. All patients with head injury are presumed to have a cervical spine injury until proven otherwise. Once the patient's condition has stabilized, a cervical spine series should be ordered.
   6. Avoid any condition (e.g., fever, pain, and shivering) that increases metabolic rate and therefore increases the demand for O_2 and glucose.

L. Hypothermia
   1. Possibly improves clinical outcomes by controlling ICP
       a. Lowering the temperature to 89.6°F–91.4°F
       b. There is no evidence that hypothermia improves mortality. Some studies have shown improved GCS. Currently, it is not recommended by national guidelines but may be used in practice.

M. Decompressive craniectomy
   1. Surgical intervention where part of the skull is removed (placed in the abdomen, stored, or discarded) to allow swelling of the brain
   2. Used in patients with increased ICP refractory to treatment
       a. It is considered for those who have failed to respond to conservative therapy.
       b. Studies have shown that ICP normalizes after a craniectomy.

N. Brain oxygenation monitoring
   1. Prevention of secondary brain injury relies on providing adequate oxygen and metabolic substrate to the brain.
   2. Brain tissue oxygen monitoring allows the clinician to gauge the adequacy of oxygen delivery to the brain.
   3. Different ways to monitor:
       a. Jugular venous oxygen saturation ($SjvO_2$) provides global O_2 saturation within the brain; normal value is 55%–70%.

b. Brain tissue oxygen monitoring (PbrO$_2$): Levels lower than 15 mmHg during the resuscitation phase of TBI predict poor outcome.

V. **Brain death**
   A. A condition where the patient has sustained irreversible cessation of all functions of the entire brain, including the brainstem
   B. The Uniform Determination of Death Act has been adopted by most states to assist in determining death in all situations.
   C. A patient cannot be declared brain dead as a result of the following conditions:
      1. Hypothermic (temperature less than 32°C)
      2. Drug intoxication or poisoning
      3. Severe electrolyte, acid base, or endocrine disturbance
   D. Examination to determine brain death
      1. No spontaneous movement
      2. Absence of brain stem reflexes
         a. Fixed and dilated pupils
         b. No corneal reflexes
         c. Absent doll's eyes
         d. Absent gag reflex
         e. Absent vestibular response to caloric stimulation
      3. Absence of breathing drive (apnea)—must perform apnea test
      4. Must have absence of all of the above before making consideration of brain death
   E. Ancillary tests for brain death
      1. Electroencephalography
      2. Cerebral angiography
      3. Transcranial doppler
      4. Cerebral blood flow study
      5. CT angiogram of brain

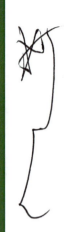

SPINAL CORD TRAUMA

I. **Mechanisms of injury**
   A. Motor vehicle accidents account for the largest number of spinal cord injuries (SCIs) (40%)
   B. Falls or falling objects (10%–20%)
   C. Acts of violence (15%)
   D. Sports-related injuries (13%)
   E. Penetrating wounds (12%)

II. **Spinal cord injuries**
   A. Rapid acceleration/deceleration
      1. Hyperextension
         a. Usually occurs as the result of a fall onto the face, forehead, or chin
         b. Rear-end collisions may result in rupture of the anterior longitudinal ligament
         c. Hyperextension may cause the cord to stretch, resulting in central cord syndrome (see Section IX. Spinal cord lesions [syndromes], C)
      2. Hyperflexion: greatest stress occurs at C5-C6, causing bilateral facet dislocations
      3. Vertical column loading (compression)
         a. Occurs in diving accidents or falls, when the patient lands on the feet or buttocks
         b. Vertebral body is compressed and/or shattered, resulting in a "burst" fracture, and bone fragments may become embedded in the cord.
         c. Injuries commonly occur at the level of C1 with diving accidents
      4. Whiplash: sudden hyperextension of the spine that stretches the ligaments as a result of the force of the lower body moving forward and the backward and downward movement of the head
   B. Distraction injuries: result from hanging

CHAPTER **4** Neurologic Trauma

C. Penetrating trauma
  1. Gunshot wound
  2. Stab wound
  3. Bony fragments
D. Hematoma
E. Pathologic fractures: occur in patients with osteoporosis or metastatic disease

III. **Epidemiology**
  A. Incidence
    1. Sixty percent of SCIs involve the cervical spine
    2. Approximately 8,000 SCIs occur each year, or 32.1 per million
    3. Approximately 40% of patients with SCI die before they reach the hospital or during the initial resuscitation phase.
    4. Average hospital costs: $80,200 for quadriplegics and $72,000 for paraplegics
    5. Average lifetime care costs of a young adult with an SCI exceed $1 million

IV. **Age**
  A. More common in young men (82%)
  B. More common in younger persons (80% younger than 40 years, and 50% between 15 and 25 years of age)

V. **Anatomy and physiology**
  A. 33 vertebrae
    1. Cervical spine (C1-C7)
      a. Highly flexible in nature, small in diameter
      b. Therefore, many fractures occur
    2. Thoracic spine (T1-T12)
      a. Articulates with the ribs
      b. Less common site for fracture because of its stability
    3. Lumbar spine (L1-L5)
      a. Highly mobile, yet large in diameter
      b. Requires a greater amount of force to fracture
    4. Sacral spine (S1-S5)
    5. Coccygeal vertebrae (3–5 coccyges)
  B. Spinal cord
    1. Gray matter
    2. White layer
    3. Meningeal layer (pia mater, arachnoid, and dura mater)

VI. **Assessment**
  A. History
    1. Mechanism of injury, such as the following:
      a. Speed of impact
      b. Blunt versus penetrating forces
      c. Flexion, extension, rotation, or distraction to the spine
      d. Height of fall
      e. Use of restraints or deployed airbag
      f. Extent of vehicular damage
      g. Position of patient in vehicle
    2. Patient complaints, such as the following:
      a. Back pain
      b. Neck pain
      c. Numbness
      d. Paresthesia
    3. Motor/sensory response
    4. Prehospital treatment

B. Physical assessment
  1. Problems with airway, breathing, and circulation and life-threatening injuries are treated first
  2. Pulmonary complications account for most of the early deaths that occur after acute traumatic quadriplegia
  3. Assess respiratory ability
     a. Chest excursion
     b. Use of intercostal muscles or diaphragm
     c. Cervical cord injury above C3 results in respiratory arrest
     d. C5-C6 injuries spare the diaphragm, and diaphragmatic breathing occurs
     e. T1-L2 lesions cause loss of intercostal muscle use
  4. Intubation if necessary
     a. Jaw thrust maneuver
     b. Apnea
     c. Breathing difficulty
     d. Diaphragmatic fatigue
  5. Arterial blood gases should be monitored closely
  6. Monitor for pneumonia, pulmonary edema, and pulmonary emboli
C. Motor assessment
  1. Inability to perform the functions listed here indicates that the lesion is above the level indicated
     a. Deltoids (C4): apply pressure to shoulders and ask patient to shrug shoulders
     b. Biceps (C5): have patient flex arm (gravity), then apply pressure by trying to straighten the arm. Tell patient not to let you straighten it (resistance)
     c. Wrist (C6): have patient hyperextend the wrist (gravity) and apply pressure by trying to straighten the wrist; tell the patient not to let you push down (resistance)
     d. Triceps (C7): have patient extend arm (gravity) and try to pull arm up to the flexed position; tell patient not to let you bend arm (resistance)
     e. Intrinsic (C8): have patient abduct (fan) fingers and try to push them together
     f. Hip flexion: have patient bend knee and apply pressure to determine resistance (L2-L4)
     g. Knee extension: while hip is flexed and knee bent, have patient try to extend the knee (L2-L4)
  2. Grade strength using the following scale:
     a. 5: normal movement against gravity and full resistance
     b. 4: full range of motion against moderate resistance and gravity
     c. 3: full range of motion against gravity, not against resistance
     d. 2: extremity can move, but not against gravity (can roll but not lift)
     e. 1: muscle contracts, but extremity cannot move
     f. 0: no visible or palpable muscle contraction or movement of extremity (flaccid)
  3. All motor groups must be comprehensively assessed
  4. Complete lesion
     a. Patient lacks sensory function, proprioception, and voluntary motor activity below the level of spinal cord damage
     b. Worse prognosis for recovering neurologic function
  5. Incomplete lesion
     a. Parts of the spinal cord at the level of the lesion are intact.
     b. Sacral sparing occurs
     c. Note sensory perception and voluntary contraction of the anus around the examiner's finger
D. Sensory function
  1. Begin at the area of no feeling and proceed to the area of feeling

2. Assess response to pain
    a. Great toe: L4
    b. Back of leg: S1-S3
    c. Perianal area: S4-S5
    d. Umbilicus: T10
    e. Nipple line: T4
    f. Ring and little fingers: C8
    g. Middle finger: C7
    h. Thumb: C6
    i. Top of shoulder: C4
3. If the patient is unable to feel pain, the lesion is at or above the spinal nerve level indicated

E. Evaluate the patient's back
   1. Perform a well-coordinated log-roll maneuver
   2. Maintain in-line spinal stabilization
   3. Gently palpate spine for pain, tenderness, or gaps between spinous processes
   4. Observe for entrance/exit wounds, impaled objects, and other signs of injury

VII. **Key signs of various levels of injury**
   A. C2-C3
      1. Respiratory paralysis (breathing center-C3)
      2. Flaccid paralysis
      3. Areflexia (deep tendon reflexes [DTRs])
      4. Loss of sensation below the mandible
   B. C5-C6
      1. Diaphragmatic breathing
      2. Paralysis of intercostal and abdominal muscles
      3. Quadriplegia
      4. Anesthesia below the clavicle and the ulnar half of the arms
      5. Areflexia (with possible exception of the biceps reflex)
      6. Fecal and urinary retention
      7. Priapism (spontaneous erection)
   C. T12-L1
      1. Paraplegia
      2. Anesthesia in the legs
      3. Areflexia in the legs
      4. Fecal and urinary retention
      5. Priapism (spontaneous erection)
   D. L1-L5
      1. Flaccid paralysis to partial flaccid paralysis
      2. Abdominal and cremasteric reflexes present
      3. Ankle and plantar reflexes absent

VIII. **Multisystem impact of SCIs**
   A. Cardiovascular
      1. Hypotension
         a. Caused by loss of sympathetic tone in patients with high thoracic or cervical injury with pooling of blood into the periphery
         b. If associated with a neurologic deficit, normal or decreased heart rate, and warm, vasodilated extremities, spinal shock is suspected.
         c. For initial fluid resuscitation, use 2–3 L of Lactated Ringer's solution. (Do not overload. Possible loss of cardiac contractility puts the patient at risk for congestive heart failure and pulmonary edema.)
         d. Rule out hypovolemia as a cause of hypotension

e. Vasopressors (dopamine) and hemodynamic monitoring may be indicated if patient is unresponsive to intravenous fluids
2. Bradycardia
   a. Caused by sympathetic blockade and may lead to arrhythmia (junctional or ventricular escape)
   b. Be alert for conditions that promote bradycardia in patients with SCIs: hypoxia, hypothermia, and vagal stimulation
   c. Be sure the patient is well oxygenated
   d. Maintain body temperature at greater than 96.8°F
   e. Administer atropine for symptomatic bradycardia (decreased level of consciousness, urinary output, and blood pressure)
3. Vasovagal reflex
   a. Induced by straining, coughing, or bearing down
   b. Frequently induced by suctioning, which leads to hypoxia, and by vagal stimulation (bradycardia—cardiac arrest)
   c. Oxygenate and hyperventilate with 100% O_2 prior to suctioning
   d. Limit suctioning to 10 seconds
   e. Monitor cardiac rate and rhythm
4. Poikilothermy
   a. Patient's temperature is dependent on the temperature of the environment; this association is the result of interruption of the sympathetic pathways to the temperature-regulating centers in the hypothalamus
   b. Maintain temperature of the environment
5. Venous thrombosis
   a. A venous stasis in the legs and pelvis resulting from decreased blood flow and flaccid paralysis
   b. Administer deep venous thrombosis prophylaxis (low-dose heparin, 5,000 units subcutaneously BID, or low molecular weight heparin [Lovenox], 30–40 mg subcutaneously BID); use antiembolic stockings, range of motion, and vena cava filters
   c. Measure thighs and calves for swelling from deep venous thrombosis
6. Orthostatic hypotension
   a. Occurs when patients move from supine to sitting position; it is related to venous pooling in the legs and abdomen caused by loss of skeletal muscle pump and impaired sympathetic nervous system control
   b. Use thigh-high stockings and abdominal binders to promote venous return
   c. Raise the head of the bed gradually, and monitor blood pressure closely

B. Gastrointestinal
1. Abdominal injuries resulting from trauma
   a. Difficult to diagnose in SCI because abdominal pain and muscular rigidity—telltale signs of internal bleeding—are absent if the patient has sensory and motor deficits.
   b. Assess patient for abdominal distention; monitor hematocrit and hemoglobin and blood volume
   c. Perform diagnostic peritoneal lavage
2. Curling's ulcer
   a. Patients with central nervous system injury may have this type of stress ulcer as a result of vagally stimulated gastric production and/or release of adrenocorticotropic hormone.
   b. Assess gastric pH, and administer H_2 antagonists (ranitidine, 150 mg PO quarterly for 12 hr) for prevention and treatment
   c. Warm and cold water lavage may be used to treat bleeding
   d. Monitor patient for coagulation defects

e. Gastrectomy may be necessary in severe cases
3. Gastric atony and ileus
   a. Related to loss of central control
   b. Leads to severe gastric distention that in turn can lead to respiratory compromise, vomiting, and aspiration
   c. Place a nasogastric tube to lower wall suction, note amount and quality of aspirate
4. Loss of bowel function
   a. Patient cannot sense when the bowel is full or cannot perform the Valsalva maneuver to aid in evacuation
   b. May lead to obstruction or autonomic dysreflexia
   c. Initiate a bowel program—suppository same time every day, AM or PM

C. Genitourinary
   1. Autonomic dysreflexia
      a. Distended bladder is the most common cause, although it can result from any noxious stimuli (e.g., distended bowel, wrinkled sheets, pressure ulcers, constrictive clothing, constrictive devices such as foot splints, and shoes that are tied too tightly).
      b. Hypertensive crisis that may result from a noxious stimulus in injuries above T6—the sympathetic outflow level
      c. SCI may result in denervation of the bladder, which may become overdistended.
      d. Noxious stimulus below the level of injury triggers the sympathetic nervous system, causing massive release of catecholamines.
      e. Result of catecholamine release is vasoconstriction
      f. Vasodilatation occurs above the site of injury—red, flushed, warm skin, as well as headache, vasocongestion, and diaphoresis.
      g. Piloerection occurs below the level of injury
      h. Place a urinary catheter to monitor urinary output and to decompress the bladder
      i. Do not drain bladder rapidly if cardiovascular system suggests autonomic dysreflexia (no more than 600 ml at a time)
   2. Urinary tract infection
      a. May result from urinary retention or catheterization
      b. Intermittent catheterization is recommended
      c. Early detection is essential to prevent sepsis or prolonged spinal shock.

D. Musculoskeletal
   1. Impaired skin integrity related to abnormal nerve supply and poor circulation
   2. Paralysis
      a. Muscle atony and wasting
      b. Contractures
      c. Perform passive range of motion and positioning, and use hand splints and boots to prevent foot drop

E. Psychological devastation
   1. Effects on the patient
      a. Disturbance of self-concept
      b. Ineffective coping
      c. Feelings of powerlessness
      d. Denial, anger, and depression
   2. Practitioner's response
      a. Be honest with a positive attitude
      b. Include patient in his or her care
      c. Set limits of behavior, and be consistent with care
      d. Take an interdisciplinary approach, including the following:
         i. Social services
         ii. Psychiatry

iii. Physical therapy
iv. Occupational therapy
v. Pastoral care

IX. **Spinal cord lesions (syndromes)**
   A. Anterior cord syndrome
      1. Probably the most devastating of the syndromes
      2. Disruption of blood flow through the anterior spinal artery
      3. Flexion injuries
      4. Weakness or paralysis with loss of sense of pain and temperature
      5. Proprioception intact
   B. Posterior cord syndrome
      1. Rare injury resulting from disruption of the posterior column
      2. Decrease in touch proprioception and vibration
   C. Central cord syndrome
      1. Hyperextension injuries with stretching of the cord and subsequent hemorrhaging in the center of the cord
      2. Greater motor loss and sensation in the upper extremities than in the lower extremities because the upper extremities are controlled by the central portion of the cord
   D. Brown-Séquard syndrome
      1. Stab wounds, gunshot wounds, fractures of the vertebral process, and spinal cord tumors
      2. One side of the spinal cord is damaged
      3. Ipsilateral motor loss and contralateral loss of pain and temperature sensation
      4. Extremities that can move have no feeling, and those that have feeling cannot move

X. **Laboratory/diagnostics**
   A. Cervical vertebrae
      1. Cross-table lateral position first; all seven vertebrae must be seen; to do so, the following may be required:
         a. Firmly pulling the patient's shoulders down
         b. Lateral swimmer's view
      2. Obtain anteroposterior x-ray if lateral x-ray is abnormal
      3. Obtain open-mouth odontoid x-ray for conscious patient for visualization of C2
      4. Failure to obtain basic radiographic studies is the primary reason for missed diagnosis of cervical spine injury.
   B. Thoracic vertebrae
      1. Perform lateral and anteroposterior x-rays
      2. View all 12 vertebrae
   C. Lumbar vertebrae
      1. Perform lateral and anteroposterior views
      2. View all five lumbar vertebrae
   D. CT may be helpful for clear identification of normal cervical spine anatomy or the presence of bony fragments.
   E. Films in flexion/extension position or oblique films at times for further delineation of suspected fractures
   F. Myelogram detects compression of the cord by herniated disks, bone fragments, or foreign matter, which requires surgical intervention.
   G. MRI can provide further information regarding cord impingement, hematomas, and infarcts. Cord contusion or hemorrhage cannot be visualized by any other technique.

XI. **Management**
   A. Consult neurosurgeon
   B. Airway maintenance
      1. Perform nasotracheal intubation or cricothyrotomy, if necessary
      2. Do not hyperextend or rotate the neck

3. Administer oxygen
C. Immobilization
   1. Use protective devices (e.g., cervical collar and spine board)
   2. Do not remove device until x-rays have been obtained and cleared
   3. Perform log roll only (will require more than two people)
D. Intravascular fluids (limit to appropriate levels)
   1. Distinguish neurogenic shock (warm, dry extremities; bradycardia) from hypovolemic shock (cool, clammy skin; tachycardia)
E. Monitor blood pressure very closely because perfusion to the spinal cord is crucial
   1. Hypotension must be avoided to prevent ischemia caused by decreased blood flow and perfusion to the spinal cord, which may produce neuronal injury and neurologic deficit.
   2. Attempts should be made to maintain MAP at 85–90 mmHg
F. Bladder catheterization
G. Nasogastric intubation
H. Corticosteroids (controversial)
   1. It may be useful in the early treatment (within the first 8 hr) of patients with acute, nonpenetrating SCI to reduce swelling.
      a. Reduce damage to cellular membranes that contributes to neuronal death after injury
      b. Reduce inflammation near the injury
      c. Suppress activation of immune cells that appear to contribute to neuronal damage
   2. Improvement is noted 6 weeks to 6 months after injury
   3. Monitor patient for elevation in blood glucose levels
   4. Monitor patient for other adverse effects, such as the following:
      a. Immunosuppression
      b. Fluid and electrolyte disturbances
      c. Adrenocortical insufficiency
      d. Impaired wound healing
      e. Gastrointestinal disturbances
I. Preliminary clinical trials of another agent, GM-1 ganglioside
   1. Although evidence does not support a significant clinical benefit, may potentially be useful in acute SCI for preventing secondary damage caused by the following:
      a. Oxidative free radicals
      b. Calcium-mediated damage
      c. Proteases
      d. Cytoskeletal dysfunction
      e. Excitotoxicity
      f. Immune reactions
      g. Apoptosis
      h. Necrosis
   2. Studies suggest that it may also improve neurologic recovery from SCI during rehabilitation.
J. Antibiotics for penetrating injuries
K. Maintain room temperature; avoid poikilothermy
L. Provide meticulous skin care: order rotating bed for respiratory therapy (postural drainage) and skin therapy
M. Prepare for insertion of skeletal tongs and traction (Stryker frame, kinetic bed, or halo vest) used to assist in restoration of the spine to a normal position (reduction)
   1. At least 10 lb of weight is initially applied.
   2. Weight is applied on the basis of 5 lb per interspace (i.e., a C5-C6 injury would require 25–30 lb of traction).
   3. Muscle relaxants are helpful
   4. Lateral x-rays are taken to assess vertebral alignment as weights are applied.

5. Too much weight can pull the spine apart, resulting in distraction injury
6. If paralytics are needed, weight may have to be reduced.
N. Fixation: involves stabilizing vertebral fracture with wires, plates, and other types of hardware
O. Fusion: involves attaching injured vertebrae to uninjured vertebrae with bone grafts and steel rods
P. Surgery may be indicated to remove bony fragments or to drain hematomas that compress the cord
Q. Rehabilitation begins upon admission; follow an interdisciplinary approach
R. Electrical stimulation devices or neural prostheses were recently approved by the FDA but are still experimental. These can be implanted in the body to allow some hand movement and bladder/bowel control; some may also assist with breathing.

BIBLIOGRAPHY

Adams, J. P., Bell, D., & McKinlay, J. (Eds.). (2010). *Neurocritical care: A guide to practical management*. London, UK: Springer-Verlag London Limited.

Aarabi, B., & Yukuwa, Y. (2011). Emergency room evaluation of the spinal injury patient including assessment of spinal shock. *Spine and Spinal Cord Trauma: Evidence-Based Management*.

Aries, M. J., Czosnyka, M., Budohoski, K. P., Steiner, L. A., Lavinio, A., Kolias, A. G., ... Smielewski, P. (2012). Continuous determination of optimal cerebral perfusion pressure in traumatic brain injury. *Critical Care Medicine, 40*(8), 2456–2463.

Brain Trauma Foundation. (2007). Guidelines for the management of severe traumatic brain injury (3rd ed.), *Journal of Neurotrauma, 24*(Suppl 1), S1–S106.

Burns, S. (2014). *AACN Essentials of Critical Care Nursing* (3rd ed.). New York, NY: McGraw-Hill.

Fehlings, M. G., Rabin, D., Sears, W., Cadotte, D. W., & Aarabi, B. (2010). Current practice in the timing of surgical intervention in spinal cord injury. *Spine, 35*(21S), S166–S173.

Ferri, F. F. (2014). *Practical guide to the care of the medical patient* (9th ed.). St. Louis, MO: Mosby.

Greenberg, M. S. (2010). *Handbook of neurosurgery* (7th ed.). New York, NY: Thieme.

Gupta, R., Bathen, M. E., Smith, J. S., Levi, A. D., Bhatia, N. N., & Steward, O. (2010). Advances in the management of spinal cord injury. *Journal of the American Academy of Orthopaedic Surgeons, 18*(4), 210–222.

Haddad, S. H., & Arabi, Y. M. (2012). Critical care management of severe traumatic brain injury in adults. *Scand J Trauma Resusc Emerg Med, 20*(12). Retrieved from http://www.ncbi.nlm.nih.gov/pmc/articles/PMC3298793/

Hartings, J. A., Vidgeon, S., Strong, A. J., Zacko, C., Vagal, A., Andaluz, N., ... Bullock, M. R. (2014). Surgical management of traumatic brain injury: A comparative-effectiveness study of 2 centers. *Journal of Neurosurgery, 120*(2), 434–446.

Hickey, J. V. (2011). *The clinical practice of neurological & neurosurgical nursing* (6th ed). Philadelphia, PA: Lippincott Williams & Wilkins.

Krassioukov, A., Eng, J. J., Claxton, G., Sakakibara, B. M., & Shum, S. (2010). Neurogenic bowel management after spinal cord injury: A systematic review of the evidence. *Spinal Cord, 48*, 718–733.

Mulligan, R. P., Friedman, J. A., Mahabir, R. C. (2010). A nationwide review of the associations among cervical spine injuries, head injuries, and facial features. *Journal of Trauma-Injury Infection & Critical Care, 68*(3), 587–592.

Oddo, M., Levine, J. M., Frangos, S., Carrera, E., Maloney-Wilensky, E., Pascual, J. L., ... LeRoux, P. D. (2009). Effect of mannitol and hypertonic saline on cerebral oxygenation in patients with severe traumatic brain injury and refractory intracranial hypertension. *J Neurol Neurosurg Psychiatry, 80*, 916–920.

Olson, D. A. (2013). In S. A. Berman (Ed.), *Head injury*. Retrieved from http://emedicine.medscape.com/article/1163653-overview

Papadakis, M. A., McPhee, S. J., & Rabow, M. W. (2013). *Current medical diagnosis and treatment* (53rd ed.). New York, NY: McGraw Hill/Appleton & Lange.

Park, S., Roederer, A., Mani, R., Schmitt, S., LeRoux, P. D., Ungar, L. H., . . . Kasner, S. E. (2011). *Neurocritical Care, 15*(3), 469–476.

Paul, P. & Williams, B. (2009). *Brunner & Suddarth's textbook of Canadian medical-surgical nursing*. Philadelphia, PA: Lippincott Williams & Wilkins.

Rabchevsky, A. G., & Kitzman, P. H. (2011). Latest approaches for the treatment of spasticity and autonomic dysreflexia in chronic spinal cord injury. *Neurotherapeutics, 8*(2), 274–282.

Rangel-Castilla, L., Lara, L. R., Gopinath, S., Swank, P. R., Valadka, A., & Robertson, C. (2010). Cerebral hemodynamic effects of acute hyperoxia and hyperventilation after severe traumatic brain injury. *Journal of Neurotrauma, 27*(10), 1853–1863.

Roy, R. R., Harkema, S. J., & Edgerton, V. R. (2012). Basic concepts of activity-based interventions for improved recovery of motor function after spinal cord injury. *Archives of Physical Medicine and Rehabilitation, 93*(9), 1487–1497.

Skandsen, T., Kvistad, K. A., Solheim, O., Strand, I. H., Folvik, M., & Vik, A. (2010). Prevalence and impact of diffuse axonal injury in patients with moderate and severe head injury: A cohort study of early magnetic resonance imaging findings and 1-year outcome. *Journal of Neurosurgery, 113*(3), 556–563.

Spiotta, A. M., Stiefel, M. F., Gracias, V. H., Garuffe, A. M., Kofke, W. A., Maloney-Wilensky, E., . . . Le Roux, P. D. (2010). *Journal of Neurosurgery, 113*(3), 571–580.

Stein, M. B., & McAllister, T. W. (2009). Exploring the convergence of posttraumatic stress disorder and mild traumatic brain injury. *The American Journal of Psychiatry, 166*(7).

Urbano, L. A., & Oddo, M. (2012). Therapeutic hypothermia for traumatic brain injury. *Current Neurology and Neuroscience Reports, 12*(5), 580–591.

Walker, J. (2009). Spinal cord injuries: Acute care management and rehabilitation. *Nursing Standard, 23*(42), 47–56.

Wyckoff, M., Houghton, D., & LePage, C. (Eds.). (2009). *Critical Care: Concepts, Role, and Practice for the Acute Care Nurse Practitioner*. New York, NY: Springer.

CHAPTER 5

Central Nervous System Disorders

JUDI KURIC • CHARLENE M. MYERS

MENINGITIS

I. **Definition**
   A. Inflammation of the arachnoid, dura mater, and/or pia mater of the brain or spinal cord (also known as the meninges), which is caused by viral, bacterial, or fungal infections
II. **Etiology/predisposing factors**
   A. Predisposing factors for the development of meningitis include sinusitis, otitis media, mastoiditis, pneumonia, trauma, and congenital malformations.
   B. Bacterial meningitis
      1. Profound and life threatening; may be fatal within hours
      2. Bacteria that are present in the meninges attract inflammatory cells and cytokines, causing a breach in the blood brain barrier, which allows white blood cells (WBCs), fluids, and other infection-fighting particles to enter the meninges.
      3. Neutrophils gather in the area and begin making exudates within the subarachnoid space.
      4. Exudates cause the cerebrospinal fluid (CSF) to thicken and decrease the flow of CSF through the brain and the spinal cord.
         a. *Streptococcus pneumoniae* (pneumococcal meningitis)
            i. Most common and most serious bacterial meningitis that may cause neurologic damage ranging from deafness to severe brain damage
            ii. Occurs frequently in infants (younger than 2 years), adults with weakened immune systems, and the elderly
            iii. Rates in children younger than 2 years have decreased since the pneumococcal 7-valent conjugate vaccine (Prevnar) has been available.
         b. *Neisseria meningitidis* (meningococcal meningitis)
            i. May occur in schools, colleges, and other group settings
            ii. Spreads through contact with drainage of the nasopharynx or with blood
            iii. High-risk groups include infants younger than 1 year, people with suppressed immune systems, travelers to foreign countries where the disease is endemic, and college students (freshman in particular) who reside in dormitories.
         c. *Haemophilus influenzae*

i. At one time, this was the most common cause of acute bacterial meningitis.
ii. *H. influenzae B* (Hib) vaccine has greatly reduced the number of cases in the United States.
iii. Children most at risk are those in daycare and children who do not have access to the vaccine.
   d. *Escherichia coli* and *Enterobacter*, *Klebsiella*, and *Proteus*
      i. May occur in infants, the elderly, and immunosuppressed patients
   e. Atypical bacterial meningitides (less common)
      i. *Listeria monocytogenes*
      ii. Staphylococci (*Staphylococcus aureus* and *Staphylococcus epidermidis*)
      iii. *Mycobacterium tuberculosis*
      iv. Streptococci
   f. Meningitis may follow an upper respiratory tract infection or head trauma.
C. Aseptic or viral meningitis
   1. Pia and arachnoid space are filled with lymphocytes but not with exudate forms.
   2. Much more benign and self-limited than bacterial meningitis
   3. Most viral meningitis occurs in late summer and early fall.
   4. Transmission usually occurs via cough, saliva, and fecal matter of an infected person.
   5. Caused by viruses
      a. Enterovirus (most common)
      b. Arbovirus
      c. Mumps
      d. Varicella zoster
      e. Herpes simplex types 1 and 2
      f. Measles
      g. Rubella
      h. Cytomegalovirus
      i. Influenza
      j. Epstein-Barr virus
      k. Human immunodeficiency virus (HIV)
   6. Fungal
      a. Most common in immunocompromised (particularly in patients with AIDS through inhalation and bloodstream spread)
      b. *Candida albicans*
      c. *Coccidioides immitis*
      d. *Cryptococcus neoformans* (most common fungal meningitis; found in bird droppings)
      e. *Histoplasma capsulatum*
      f. *Aspergillus*
D. Syphilis
III. **Clinical manifestations**
   A. Severe headache
   B. Stiff neck (nuchal rigidity) related to meningeal irritation (meningismus)
   C. Photophobia, may have diplopia
   D. Fever of 101°F–103°F (38°C–40°C); toxic appearance
   E. Altered mental status
   F. Cranial nerve palsy
   G. Seizures
   H. Chills, myalgias
   I. Kernig's sign
      1. Flex the patient's leg at the knee, then at the hip, to a 90° angle, and then extend the knee

2. In a patient with meningitis, this maneuver will trigger pain and spasms of the hamstring muscles caused by inflammation of the meninges and spinal nerve roots.
- J. Brudzinski's sign
  1. Flex the patient's head and neck to the chest
  2. The legs will flex at the hips and at the knees in response to this movement.
- K. Nausea and vomiting
- L. Purpura or petechiae may be seen with meningococcal meningitis.
  1. Located on the trunk, lower extremities, mucous membranes, conjunctiva
  2. Patients with rapidly evolving rash, indicative of poor outcome, require emergent care
- M. Vertigo
- N. Exaggerated deep tendon reflexes

IV. **Laboratory findings/diagnostics**
- A. Lumbar puncture (LP) should be performed as soon as a diagnosis is suspected.
  1. CT scan of the head should be completed prior to the LP in patients with altered level of consciousness, papilledema, neurologic deficits, new-onset seizures, immunocompromised state, or history of central nervous system (CNS) disease
- B. LP in bacterial meningitis (see table 5.1)
  1. Appearance of CSF: cloudy
  2. Opening pressure: elevated (greater than 180 mm H_2O)
  3. Cells: increased WBCs (100–5,000/mm; most are polymorphonuclear cells)
  4. Total protein: increased (100–500 mg/dl [normal, 15–45 mg/dl])
  5. Glucose: decreased (5–40 mg/dl or 0.3 times blood glucose level [normal 45–80 mg/dl or 0.6 times blood glucose level])
  6. Culture: bacteria present on Gram stain and culture
- C. LP in viral meningitis
  1. Appearance of CSF: clear, occasionally cloudy
  2. Opening pressure: usually normal (less than 180 mm H_2O)
  3. Cells: increased WBCs (50–1,000/mm; most are mononuclear cells)
  4. Total protein: normal or slightly increased (less than 200 mg/dl)
  5. Glucose: normal (greater than 45 mg/dl)
  6. Culture: no bacteria present; demonstration of virus requires special technique

Table 5.1	Comparison of cerebrospinal fluid in bacterial versus viral meningitis	
	Bacterial	**Viral**
Appearance	Cloudy	Clear (occasionally cloudy)
Opening pressure	Elevated (greater than 180 mm H_2O)	Normal (less than 200 mm H_2O)
Cells	Increased white blood cells (100–5,000 mm) Most are polymorphonuclear	Increased white blood cells (50–1,000 mm) Most are mononuclear
Total protein	Increased (100–500 mg/dl)	Normal or slightly increased (less than 200 mg/dl)
Glucose	Decreased (5–40 mg/dl or 0.3 times blood glucose level)	Normal (greater than 45 mg/dl)
Culture	Bacteria present on Gram stain	No bacteria present

CHAPTER 5   Central Nervous System Disorders

D. CT scan of the head is indicated in patients with focal neurologic signs or diminished level of consciousness.
E. In patients who have signs, symptoms, and CSF findings typical of bacterial meningitis but in whom no organisms are found, follow-up CT scans should be obtained, even if clinical improvement occurs, because such patients may have a brain abscess and may require neurosurgical intervention.
F. An additional maneuver in assessing for meningitis is to elicit jolt accentuation of the patient's headache by asking the patient to turn his or her head horizontally at a frequency of two to three rotations per second.
    1. Worsening of a baseline headache is a positive sign.
    2. Include examination of the cranial nerves, motor and sensory systems, and reflexes, as well as testing for Babinski's reflex
G. Assess the ears, sinuses, and respiratory system.
H. Obtain blood and sputum cultures, nasopharyngeal specimen.
I. Obtain complete blood count (CBC), electrolytes, coagulation profiles, and liver/renal panel.
J. Chest, skull, and sinus films or chest CT scan may be necessary to facilitate detection of primary infection
K. Serology (antigen tests)
    1. Latex agglutination tests
        a. Can detect antigens of encapsulated organisms such as *S. pneumoniae*, *H. influenzae*, *N. meningitidis*, and *C. neoformans*
        b. Rarely used, beneficial in patients who have been pretreated with antibiotics and who have a negative Gram stain and CSF
    2. Polymerase chain reaction testing of CSF
        a. Has been employed to detect bacteria (*S. pneumoniae*, *H. influenzae*, *N. meningitidis*, *M. tuberculosis*, *Borrelia burgdorferi*, and *Tropheryma whippelii*) and viruses (herpes simplex, varicella-zoster, cytomegalovirus, Epstein-Barr virus, and enterovirus) in patients with meningitis
        b. Test results are rapid and are obtained within hours.
    3. Enzyme linked immunosorbent assay (ELISA)
        a. Detects immunoglobulin (Ig)M early in the infection and IgG as the disease progresses
    4. HIV/AIDS testing

V. **Management**
A. Consult infectious disease specialist, particularly for cases in which the preferred therapy cannot be used or when the pathogens/organism is resistant to usual therapy
B. Antibiotics must be initiated immediately in those suspected to have meningitis. See table 5.2 for empiric treatment.
C. Meningococcal meningitis: patients 18–60 years of age with penicillin-susceptible infection: aqueous penicillin G (4 million units IV every 4 hr); continue until 5–7 days after the patient becomes afebrile
    1. If penicillin-intermediate sensitivity: ceftriaxone, 2 grams IV every 12 hr, or cefotaxime, 2 grams IV every 4–6 hr
D. *H. influenzae* meningitis that is β-lactamase negative: ampicillin, 2 grams IV every 4 hr
    1. If β-lactamase positive: third-generation cephalosporin (ceftriaxone [Rocephin], 2 grams IV every 12 hr or cefotaxime, 2 grams IV every 4 hr)
E. Aseptic meningitis: supportive therapy
    1. Treat the severely ill empirically with antibiotics.
F. Tuberculosis: isoniazid (INH), 5 mg/kg/day (maximum, 300 mg/day) plus pyridoxine, 50 mg PO daily; rifampin (RIF), 600 mg IV/PO daily; pyrazinamide (PZA), 15–30 mg/kg once daily (maximum, 2000 mg/day); ethambutol (EMB), 15–25 mg/kg once daily (maximum, 1600 mg/day)

Table 5.2	Empiric Treatment for Suspected Meningitis	
	Common Pathogens	**Drugs of First Choices**
2–50 years	*N. meningitidis, S. pneumoniae, H. influenzae*	Vancomycin weight based dose to achieve vancomycin trough level of 15–20 mg/L PLUS Ceftriaxone 2 grams IV every 12 hr or Cefotaxime 2 grams IV every 4–6 hr
Older than 50 years	*S. pneumoniae, N. meningitidis, H. influenzae, L. monocytogenes*, aerobic gram-negative bacilli	Vancomycin weight based dose to achieve Vancomycin trough level of 15–20 mg/L PLUS Ampicillin 2 grams IV every 4 hr PLUS Ceftriaxone 2 grams IV every 12 hr or cefotaxime 2 grams IV every 4–6 hr
Neurosurgery or Head Trauma	*S. aureus, Enterobacteriaceae*, Resistant gram negative bacilli, *S. pneumoniae*	Cefepime 2 grams IV every 8 hr PLUS Vancomycin weight based dose to achieve vancomycin trough level of 15–20 mg/L

aIn those allergic to penicillin and third-generation cephalosporin, consult with infectious disease specialist or pharmacist for alternative therapy.

- G. If *S. Pneumonia* is suspected, add dexamethasone, 0.15 mg/kg IV every 6 hr for 2–4 days
    1. Should be administered prior to, or with, first antibiotic dose, not after regimen has already been started.
- H. Anticonvulsants (lorazepam or diazepam) for acute seizure control
- I. Acetaminophen, 325–1000 mg every 4 hr PRN for pain/fever (not to exceed 3000 mg/24 hr)
- J. Intravenous hydration with lactated Ringer's solution or normal saline; avoid hypotonic solutions and dextrose 5% in water

CEREBRAL ABSCESS

I. **Definition/etiology**
   - A. Infected space-occupying lesion containing pus, cells, and other materials in the brain
   - B. Usually due to bacterial or fungal infection from a different primary source, generally in or near the brain
        1. Otitis media
        2. Mastoid infection
        3. Sinusitis
        4. Oral surgery (rare)
   - C. Other sources for abscess
        1. Lung infection/empyema
        2. Skin infection
        3. Bacterial endocarditis
        4. Bronchiectasis
        5. Congenital heart disease
        6. Penetrating trauma, skull fracture, intracranial procedures

II. **Clinical manifestations (symptoms depend on location in the brain)**
   - A. General: ill appearance, lethargic
   - B. Elevated body temperature may or may not be present
   - C. Signs of increased intracranial pressure: nausea, vomiting, altered level of consciousness, focal neurologic deficit
   - D. Neurologic: speech and visual disturbances, hemiparesis, seizures, headache
   - E. Patients go through two phases of symptoms with cerebral abscess

1. Stage I: initial formation of abscess
   a. Headache, chills, fever, malaise
   b. Confusion, drowsiness, speech disorder
2. Stage II: due to expanding cerebral mass
   a. Vague signs and symptoms of brain tumor: recurrent headache of increased severity, confusion, drowsy, stupor, flulike symptoms

III. **Diagnosis/treatment**
   A. Laboratory studies
      1. Elevated WBC count, elevated sedimentation rate
      2. LP (need CT prior to procedure)—elevated opening pressure, mild increase in protein level
      3. CT scan of the head—identify space-occupying lesion with contrast enhancement
         a. Multiple lesions possible
      4. Magnetic resonance imaging (MRI) of the head: similar to CT; more information on necrosis versus edema
   B. Treatment: identification of pathogen and primary infection source are key to successful treatment; long-term (6–12 weeks) antibiotic treatment is given
   C. Surgical removal and debridement is considered in abscesses that are greater than 2.5 cm and easily accessible.
   D. Outcome is directly related to neurologic status of patient at the time of diagnosis

ENCEPHALITIS

I. **Definition**
   A. Acute inflammation of the brain caused by virus, bacteria, fungus, or parasite; viral encephalitis is most common

II. **Etiology**
   A. Herpes simplex virus (HSV) encephalitis
      1. Most common cause of acute sporadic viral encephalitis in the United States
   B. Mumps, measles, varicella-zoster virus
   C. Possible influenza
   D. Tick infestation
      1. Lyme disease
      2. Rocky Mountain spotted fever
      3. Eastern equine encephalitis
      4. Japanese encephalitis (1 year after travel to Asia)
      5. La Crosse encephalitis
      6. St. Louis encephalitis (3,000 cases/year)
      7. Western equine encephalitis
      8. West Nile virus
         a. Transmission of West Nile virus
            i. Mosquitoes become infected when they feed on infected birds.
            ii. The mosquito circulates the virus in the blood for several days.
            iii. During this time, the mosquito can infect humans and other animals by biting to take blood.
            iv. The virus is injected into the human or animal, where it multiplies and may cause illness.
   E. Toxoplasmosis
      1. Commonly seen in patients with AIDS
   F. Enteroviruses, polioviruses
   G. Rabies
   H. Cytomegalovirus (CMV), HIV, rubella virus

III. **Signs and symptoms (vary based on organism and area involved)**
   A. General: anxious, lethargic, possibly comatose
   B. Vital signs: unstable if advanced CNS infection, fever
   C. Eyes: nystagmus, ocular paralysis, photophobia
   D. Gastrointestinal: nausea/vomiting
   E. Musculoskeletal: nuchal rigidity
   F. Neurologic: severe headache, altered level of consciousness, ataxia, dysphagia, hemiparesis, stupor progressing to coma, confusion, olfactory or gustatory hallucinations, seizures, aphasia, cranial nerve deficit, Babinski reflex

IV. **Diagnostic testing**
   A. Standard laboratory tests
      1. Complete blood count
      2. Chemistry
      3. Liver function tests
      4. Culture of body fluids: blood, urine, stool, nasopharynx, sputum
   B. LP
      1. Elevated WBC count
      2. Red blood cell count normal (elevated with HSV)
      3. Protein: normal or slightly elevated
      4. Glucose: normal or slightly elevated
   C. Possible open brain biopsy to identify treatable causes

V. **Specific diagnostic testing**
   A. Electroencephalogram (EEG): abnormal with slowing or epileptiform activity; temporal lobe abnormalities suggest HSV infection
   B. Measurement of IgM antibody in serum and CSF
      1. Collect within 8 days; use the IgM antibody capture enzyme-linked immunosorbent assay (MAC-ELISA)
   C. IgM does not cross the blood-brain barrier; if it is present in the CSF, a CNS infection (likely, encephalitis) is suggested.

VI. **Imaging diagnostics**
   A. CT scan
   B. MRI
   C. Brain scan
   D. Usually normal initially; later, nonspecific abnormalities are identified
   E. If temporal lobe disease exists, a diagnosis of HSV infection is suggested.

VII. **Treatment for encephalitis**
   A. Admit to the intensive care unit; most treatment is supportive
   B. Intravenous fluids
   C. Respiratory support
   D. Circulatory support
   E. Prevention of secondary infection
   F. Anticonvulsants (lorazepam or diazepam for acute seizure treatment)
   G. Monitor for cerebral edema.
   H. Monitor for syndrome of inappropriate antidiuretic hormone secretion.

VIII. **Specific treatments**
   A. Consult an infectious disease specialist
   B. Acyclovir, 10 mg/kg IV every 8 hr for adults, is used for herpes simplex virus—administer as early as possible, adjust dose for renal impairment
      1. Acyclovir should be initiated in all patients with suspected encephalitis, pending results of diagnostic studies

C. Other empirical antimicrobial agents should be initiated on basis of specific epidemiologic or clinical factors, including appropriate therapy for presumed bacterial meningitis, if clinically indicated
D. No specific antiviral therapy is available for other causes.
E. Supportive care

IX. **Reporting encephalitis**
A. The Centers for Disease Control and Prevention has devised standards for reporting cases of encephalitis in humans, mosquitoes, and birds.
B. Each state has specific guidelines regarding human, mosquito, and bird notification.
C. Guidelines are available for handling dead birds and mosquitoes at www.cdc.com.

ENCEPHALOPATHY

I. **Definition**
A. Dysfunction of the brain caused by a disease or disease process

II. **Etiology**
A. Hepatic
B. Hypertensive
C. Metabolic (lactic acidosis, metabolic acidosis)
D. Electrolytes (hyponatremia, hypoglycemia, hypercalcemia)
E. Uremic
F. Anoxic-ischemic
G. Hypercapnic
H. Endocrine (hyperparathyroidism, Cushing's disease)
I. AIDS
J. Thiamine deficiency (Wernicke disease)

III. **Clinical manifestations**
A. Depends on cause and may include the following:
   1. Headache
   2. Inattentiveness, impaired judgment
   3. Motor incoordination
   4. Drowsiness
   5. Confusion
   6. Stupor
   7. Coma
   8. Altered mental status or personality changes

IV. **Diagnosis**
A. Depends on clinical event
   1. Physical presentation
   2. Serum laboratory analysis (ammonia)
   3. CSF analysis
   4. EEG activity
   5. MRI

V. **Management**
A. ABCs of emergency care (airway, breathing, and circulation)
B. Correction of underlying cause
   1. Specific treatment determined by underlying cause (i.e., hepatic = lactulose, anoxia = oxygen, hypoperfusion of CNS = vasopressors)
C. Prevention of irreversible neurologic injury
D. Anticonvulsant therapy for seizures (lorazepam or diazepam for treatment of acute seizures), if clinically indicated

BIBLIOGRAPHY

Bader, M. K., & Littlejohn, L. R. (2010). *AANN core curriculum for neuroscience nursing* (5th ed.). Glenview, IL: American Association of Neuroscience Nurses.

Bamberger, D. (2010). Diagnosis, Initial Management, and Prevention of Meningitis. *Am Fam Physician, 82*(12), 1491–1498.

Centers for Disease Control. (2010). *St. Louis encephalitis*. Retrieved from http://www.cdc.gov/sle/

Centers for Disease Control. (2010). *Eastern equine encephalitis*. Retrieved from http://www.cdc.gov/EasternEquineEncephalitis/

Centers for Disease Control. (2013). *Japanese encephalitis*. Retrieved from http://www.cdc.gov/japaneseencephalitis/

Centers for Disease Control. (2013). *West Nile virus: information for health care providers.* Retrieved from http://www.cdc.gov/westnile/healthCareProviders/

Ferri, F. F. (2010). *Practical guide to the care of the medical patient* (8th ed.). St. Louis, MO: Mosby.

Hasbun, R., & Bronze, M. S. (2014). *Meningitis*. Retrieved from http://emedicine.medscape.com/article/232915-overview

Ibrahim, S. I., Cheang, P. P., & Nunez, D. A. (2010). Incidence of meningitis secondary to suppurative otitis media in adults. *Journal of Laryngology and Otology, 124*(11), 1158–1161.

Longo, D., Fauci, A., Kapser, D., & Hauser, S. (2011). *Harrison's principles of internal medicine* (18th ed.). New York, NY: McGraw Hill/Appleton & Lange.

Molyneux, E., Nizami, S. Q., Saha, S., Huu, K. T., Azam, M., Bhutta, Z. A., . . . Qazi, S. A. (2011). 5 versus 10 days of treatment with ceftriaxone for bacterial meningitis in children: A double-blind randomised equivalence study. *Lancet, 377*(9780), 1837–1845.

Papadakis, M. A., McPhee, S. J., & Tierney, L. M. (Eds.). (2013). *Current medical diagnosis and treatment* (52nd ed.). New York, NY: McGraw Hill/Appleton & Lange.

Thigpen, M. C., Whitney, C. G., Messonnier, N. E., Zell, E. R., Lynfield, R., Hadler, J. L., . . . Schuchat, A. (2011). Bacterial meningitis in the United States, 1998–2007. *New England Journal of Medicine, 364*(21), 2016–2025.

Thwaites, G. E. (2012). The mangement of suspected encephalitis. *British Medical Journal, 344*, e3489. doi: 10.1136/bmj.e3489

Waghdhare, S., Kalantri, A., Joshi, R., & Kalantri, S. (2010). Accuracy of physical signs for detecting meningitis: A hospital-based diagnostic accuracy study. *Clinical Neurology and Neurosurgery, 112*(9), 752–757.

CHAPTER 6

Seizure Disorders

PATRICK A. LAIRD • CHARLENE M. MYERS

I. **Definition**
   A. Seizure disorders are transient disturbances of the cerebral function caused by an abnormal paroxysmal neuronal discharge within the brain; epilepsy is the term used to describe recurrent, unprovoked seizures

II. **Etiology**
   A. Cause may be unknown
   B. Metabolic disorders
      1. Acidosis
      2. Electrolyte imbalance (e.g., hyponatremia, hypocalcemia)
      3. Hypoglycemia
      4. Hypoxia
      5. Alcohol or barbiturate withdrawal are the most common causes of new-onset seizures in adults
   C. Central nervous system (CNS) infection
   D. Head trauma
   E. Tumors and other space-occupying lesions
   F. Vascular disease (common with advancing age and the most common cause of onset of seizure disorder at age 60 or older)
   G. Degenerative disorders, such as Alzheimer's disease in later life
   H. The most common cause of seizures is noncompliance with a drug regimen on the part of a patient in whom epilepsy has been diagnosed.

III. **Clinical manifestations**
   A. Focal seizures: cortical discharges localized within one cerebral hemisphere
      1. Focal seizures without dyscognitive features
         a. Consciousness is preserved; rarely lasts longer than 1 minute
         b. Jacksonian march movements: convulsive jerking or paresthesias/tingling that spreads to different parts of the limb or body
         c. Todd's paralysis: localized paresis in the involved region lasting minutes to hours

d. Sensory symptoms
   i. Flashing lights
   ii. Simple hallucinations
   iii. Alterations in taste
   iv. Olfactory changes (intense smells)
   v. Paresthesias
   vi. Buzzing
e. Autonomic symptoms
   i. Abnormal epigastric symptoms
   ii. Pallor
   iii. Sweating
   iv. Flushing
   v. Pupillary dilatation
   vi. Piloerection
f. Speech arrest or vocalization
g. Nausea
h. May have an aura: subjective events not directly observable
i. Psychic symptoms
   i. Déjà vu
   ii. Dreamy states
   iii. Fear
   iv. Distortion of time perception
2. Focal seizures with dyscognitive features
   a. Most common seizure in epileptics
      i. Any simple partial seizure onset followed by impairment of consciousness
   b. Automatisms may occur
      i. Lip smacking
      ii. Chewing
      iii. Swallowing
      iv. Sucking
      v. Picking at clothes
   c. May begin with a stare at the time consciousness is impaired
   d. Frequently begin with an aura
B. Generalized seizures—originates in all areas of cortex simultaneously
   1. Typical absence seizures
      a. Sudden loss of consciousness (5–30 seconds), with eyes fluttering or muscles spasms occurring at a rate of 3 per second; begins and ends so quickly that it may not be apparent
      b. Common in children (ages 6–14 years)
      c. Occasionally accompanied by mild clonic, tonic, or atonic components
      d. Autonomic components (enuresis)
      e. Can accompany automatisms
      f. If the seizure occurs during conversation, the patient may miss a few words or may break off for a few seconds.
      g. Frequently occur several times a day, often when the patient is sitting quietly; infrequent during exercise
   2. Atypical absence seizures
      a. Alteration in consciousness typically longer
      b. Often accompanied by obvious motor signs
      c. May be associated with structural abnormalities of the brain
      d. Less responsive to anticonvulsants

3. Generalized tonic-clonic seizures: Neuronal discharge spreads throughout the entire cerebral cortex.
   a. Often begins abruptly followed by an outcry (caused by air being forced out of the lungs due to generalized muscle tonicity)
   b. Loss of consciousness and falling
   c. Respiration is arrested.
   d. Tonic (muscle rigidity) then clonic (synchronous muscle jerks) contractions of the muscles of the extremities, trunk, and head
   e. Commonly with urinary incontinence
   f. Usually lasts 2–5 minutes
   g. May be preceded by a prodromal mood change and followed by a postictal state
      i. Deep sleep
      ii. Headache
      iii. Muscle soreness
      iv. Amnesia of events
      v. Nausea
      vi. Confusion
      vii. Combination of any of the above
C. Status epilepticus: a series of seizures lasting longer than 5 minutes with the patient never returning to baseline between seizures
   1. Aggressive treatment is required for a patient with continuing seizures lasting 5–10 minutes or seizures without intervening consciousness.
   2. Status epilepticus is a medical emergency requiring immediate treatment.
   3. The longer the seizure activity lasts, the more difficult it is to control the seizure.

IV. **Diagnosis**
   A. Obtain a thorough history from the patient, the family, and/or the observers of the event
   B. Twenty-four-hour continuous EEG is an important test for supporting the diagnosis of epilepsy, differentiating between types of seizures, and providing a guide to prognosis.
      1. Focal abnormalities indicate partial seizures
      2. Generalized abnormalities indicate primary generalized seizures
      3. A normal EEG does not rule out a seizure
   C. CT scan or MRI of the head—performed for all new-onset seizures, especially after age 30, because of the possibility of an underlying neoplasm
      1. MRI preferred over CT scan to identify specific lesions in non-emergent cases
   D. Lumbar puncture (if indicated) is performed to assess for an infectious process after CT scan or MRI has been used to rule out expanding mass that may increase intracranial pressure (ICP).
   E. Twenty-four-hour EEG to document seizure activity
   F. Blood analysis
      1. Complete blood count
      2. Glucose, liver, and renal function tests
      3. Venereal Disease Research Laboratory test
      4. Electrolytes
      5. Magnesium
      6. Calcium
      7. Antinuclear antibody
      8. Erythrocyte sedimentation rate
      9. Arterial blood gases
   G. Urinalysis, drug screen
   H. Serum prolactin rises two to three times above normal for 10–60 minutes after occurrence of 80% of tonic-clonic or complex partial seizures

V. Management

A. Initial management is supportive
B. Most seizures are self-limiting
  1. Maintain open airway
  2. Place patient in left lateral decubitus position
  3. Protect the patient from injury
  4. Administer oxygen if the patient is cyanotic
  5. Do not force airways or objects (e.g., tongue blade) between the teeth until the muscles have relaxed because this may cause the tongue to occlude the airway or teeth to break off and cause a partial obstruction
  6. Start with intravenous (IV) normal saline
  7. Perform ECG, and monitor respiration and blood pressure
C. For status epilepticus:
  1. Benzodiazepines are first-line treatment, as these are able to rapidly control seizures
  2. Lorazepam (Ativan), 0.1 mg/kg (4–8 mg with a maximum dose of 10 mg) at 2 mg/minute; IV diazepam (Valium), 0.1 mg/kg at 5 mg/minute (maximum, 20 mg); or midazolam (Versed), 0.1–0.3 mg/kg IV for a maximal dose of 10 mg (if IV lorazepam is not available)
  3. If IV access is not available, nurse practitioner may prescribe midazolam 10 mg IM in patients greater than 40 kg or 5 mg IM for body weight between 13 and 40 kg
  4. Monitor for respiratory depression after medications are given; intubation may become necessary
  5. Increase normal saline if the patient becomes hypotensive
  6. Phenytoin (Dilantin) should be administered simultaneously with lorazepam or diazepam and saline at 50 mg/minute until a loading dose of 20 mg/kg is reached
     a. Fosphenytoin (Cerebyx) does not irritate the veins and can be given with all common IV solutions; it may be administered more quickly than phenytoin (150 mg/minute vs. 50 mg/minute) without risk of cardiovascular collapse
        i. It is also more expensive
  7. If the above measures to abort status epilepticus are unsuccessful, intubate and administer phenobarbital (Luminal), 100 mg/minute IV to a maximum of 20 mg/kg.
  8. If still unsuccessful after 60 minutes, consider general anesthesia with propofol (Diprivan), loading dose of 3–5 mg/kg, followed by an infusion of 30–100 mcg/kg/min.
D. Clinical pharmacology of the antiepileptic drugs (AEDs) (Table 6.1)
E. Drugs for specific types of seizures (Table 6.2)
F. Titrate dosages to achieve adequate serum levels. If a first drug partially controls seizures at a maximal therapeutic level, add a second drug to achieve therapeutic levels. Evaluation of serum phenytoin may require additional correction based on serum albumin level and/or current renal function; consult pharmacist for appropriate correction of phenytoin levels to avoid unnecessary dosage adjustments.
G. If the patient is seizure-free, monitor the patient, not the levels.
H. One should never abruptly withdraw an anticonvulsant from a patient; these drugs should be tapered.
I. Vagus nerve stimulation is used in conjunction with medications by patients with severe, uncontrolled seizures. Stimulation is typically applied for 30 seconds every 5 minutes. When the vagus is stimulated, resultant impulses in some way interrupt or prevent abnormal neuronal firing.

Table 6.1 Clinical pharmacology of antiepileptic drugs

Drug	Product name	Dosing schedule	Daily maintenance dosage in adults, mg	Target serum level, mcg/ml	Induces hepatic drug metabolism
Traditional antiepileptic drugs					
Carbamazepine	Tegretol	3 times daily	600–1800	4–12	Yes
	Epitol	3 times daily			
	Tegretol-XR	2 times daily			
	Carbatrol	2 times daily			
	Equetro	2 times daily			
Ethosuximide	Zarontin (generic)	1–2 times daily	750	40–100	No
Phenobarbital		1–2 times daily	60–120	15–45	Yes
Phenytoin	Dilantin-125	2–3 times daily	200–300	10–20	Yes
	Dilantin Infatab	2–3 times daily			
	Phenytek	1 time daily			
	Dilantin (ER capsules)	1 time daily			
Primidone	Mysoline	3–4 times daily	500–750	5–15[d]	Yes
Valproic acid	Depakene	3–4 times daily	750–3000	40–100	No
	Depakote	3–4 times daily			
	Depakote ER	2 times daily			
	Stavzor	2–3 times daily			
Additional antieplileptic drugs					
Gabapentin	Neurontin	3 times daily	1200–3600	ND	No
Lacosamide	Vimpat	2 times daily	200–400	ND	No
Lamotrigine	Lamictal, Lamictal ODT	2 times daily	400[bc]	ND	No
	Lamictal XR	1 time daily			
Levetiracetam	Keppra	2 times daily	2000–3000	ND	No
Oxcarbazepine[a]	Trileptal	2 times daily	900–2400	3–40	No
Pregabalin	Lyrica	2–3 times daily	150–600	ND	No
Rufinamide	Banzel	2 times daily	3200	ND	Yes[e]
Tiagabine	Gabitril	2–4 times daily	16–32	ND	No

Note: To avoid serious adverse effects, all anticonvulsant medications must be tapered up or down while drug levels and other pertinent diagnostic test results (laboratory and radiologic) are monitored. Patients should be maintained at the lowest effective dose. ND = not determined; ER = extended release; XR = extended release; ODT = orally disintegrating tablet. Adapted with permission from "Drugs for Epilepsy," by R.A. Lehne, 2013, *Pharmacology for Nursing Care, 8th Edition*, p. 232. Copyright 2013 by WB Saunders.

[a]Oxcarbazepine does not induce enzymes that metabolize antiepileptic drugs, but it does induce enzymes that metabolize other types of drugs. [b]Dosages must be decreased in patients taking valproic acid. [c]Dosages must be increased in patients taking drugs that induce hepatic drug–metabolizing enzymes. [d]Target serum levels are 5 to 15 mcg/ml for primidone itself and 15 to 40 mcg/ml for phenobarbital derived from primidone. [e]Rufinamide produces mild induction of CYP3A4.

Table 6.2	Drugs for specific types of seizures	
Seizure Type	**Traditional AEDs**	**Newer AEDs**
Focal Seizures With and without dyscognitive features	Carbamazepine Phenytoin Valproic Acid Phenobarbital Primidone	Ezogabine Oxcarbazepine Gabapentin Lacosamide Lamotrigine Levetiracetam Pregabalin Topiramate Tiagabine Vigbatrin Zonisamide
Generalized **Tonic-clonic**	Carbamazepine Phenytoin Valproic Acid Phenobarbital Primidone	Lamotrigine Levetiracetam Topiramate
Absence **Typical and atypical**	Ethosuximide Valproic Acid	Lamotrigine
Myoclonic	Valproic Acid	Lamotrigine Levetiracetam Topiramate

Note. To avoid serious adverse effects, all anticonvulsant medications must be tapered up and down while drug levels and other pertinent diagnostic test results (laboratory and radiologic) are carefully monitored. Patients should be maintained at the lowest effective dose. AED=anti-epileptic drug. Adapted from "Drugs for Epilepsy," by Richard A. Lehne, 2013, *Pharmacology for Nursing Care, 8th Edition*, p. 228. Copyright 2013 by WB Saunders, with permission.

BIBLIOGRAPHY

Aminoff, M. J., & Kerchner, G. A. (2014). Nervous system disorders. In M. A. Papadakis, S. J. McPhee, M. W. Rabow, & T. G. Berger (Eds.), *CURRENT Medical Diagnosis & Treatment 2014*. New York, NY: McGraw-Hill.

Bothamley, J., & Boyle, M. (2009). *Medical conditions affecting pregnancy and childbirth*. Oxford: Radcliffe Pub.

Engel, J. (2013). *Seizures and epilepsy*. Oxford, UK: Oxford University Press.

Foreman, B., & Hirsch, L. J. (2012). Epilepsy emergencies: Diagnosis and management. *Neurologic Clinics, 30*(1), 11–41.

French, J. A., & Pedley, T. A. (2009). Initial management of epilepsy. *New England Journal of Medicine, 359*(2), 166–176.

Holtkamp, M., & Meierkord, H. (2011). Nonconvulsive status epilepticus: A diagnostic and therapeutic challenge in the intensive care setting. *Therapeutic Advances in Neurological Disorders, 4,* 169–181.

Kwan, P., Schachter, S. C., & Brodie, M. J. (2011). Current concepts: Drug-resistant epilepsy. *New England Journal of Medicine, 365*(10): 919–926.

Lee, K. (Ed.). (2012). *The NeuroICU book*. New York, NY: McGraw-Hill.

Lehne, R. A. (2013). *Pharmacology for nursing care* (8th ed.). St. Louis, MO: WB Saunders.

Lowenstein, D. H. (2012). Seizures and epilepsy. In A. S. Fauci, E. Braunwald, D. L. Kasper, S. L. Hauser, D. L. Longo, J. L. Jameson, et al. (Eds.), *Harrison's principles of internal medicine* (18th ed.). New York, NY: McGraw Hill.

Loscalzo, J. (Ed.). (2012). *Harrison's principles of internal medicine* (18th ed., pp. 3251–3270). New York, NY: McGraw-Hill.

Marik, P. E., & Varon, J. (2004). The management of status epilepticus. *Chest, 126*(2), 582–591.

Marx, J. A., Hockberger, R. S., & Walls, R. M. (2014). *Rosen's emergency medicine: Concepts and clinical practice* (8th ed., expert consult premium edition). Philadelphia, PA: Elsevier.

Shorvon, S., Guerrini, R., Cook, M., & Lhatoo, S. (2012). *Oxford textbook of epilepsy and epileptic seizures.* Oxford, UK: Oxford University Press.

Silbergleit, R., Durkalski, V., Lowenstein, D., Conwit, R., Pancioli, A., Palesch, Y., & Barsan, W. (2012). Intramuscular versus intravenous therapy for prehospital status epilepticus. *New England Journal of Medicine, 366*(7), 591–600.

CHAPTER 7

Dementia

ANGELA STARKWEATHER • CHARLENE M. MYERS

I. **Definition**
   A. Dementia is a broad (global) acquired impairment of intellectual function (cognition) that is usually progressive and interferes with normal social and occupational activities.
   B. The key features of dementia consist of an intact arousal state and impairment of memory, intellect, and personality.
   C. The disorder is characterized by one or more of the following:
      1. General decrease in level of cognition
      2. Behavioral disturbance
      3. Interference with daily function and independence
   D. It causes loss of mental functions such as thinking, memory, and reasoning.
   E. It is not a disease but rather a group of symptoms caused by various diseases.
   F. Refer to Psychosocial Problems in Acute Care chapter for ways to differentiate dementia from delirium.

II. **Etiology**
   A. As many as 50 known causes of dementia
   B. Develops when parts of the brain that are involved with learning, memory, and decision making are affected by various infections or diseases
   C. Alzheimer's-type dementia (AD)
      1. AD is the most common form of dementia in the elderly.
      2. It accounts for 60%–80% of dementia cases.
      3. Neuronal damage in AD is irreversible; therefore, the disease cannot be cured.
      4. The histopathology of AD is characterized by neuritic plaques, neurofibrillary tangles, and degeneration of cholinergic neurons in the hippocampus and cerebral cortex.
      5. β-amyloid is present in high levels in AD; this may contribute to neuronal injury
      6. AD results in cerebral atrophy
   D. Diseases that cause degeneration or loss of nerve cells in the brain
      1. Alzheimer's disease
      2. Parkinson's disease
      3. Huntington's disease

E. Vascular
   1. Multi-infarct dementia
   2. Stroke
   3. Arteritis (15%–20%)
F. Infectious
   1. HIV
   2. Syphilis
   3. Meningitis
   4. Encephalitis
   5. Abscess
   6. Creutzfeldt-Jakob disease
G. Postencephalitic syndrome, central nervous system anoxia (drug overdose, cardiac arrest)
H. Nutritional deficiencies
   1. Vitamin B12 deficiency
   2. Folate deficiency
   3. Other vitamin deficiencies
I. Toxic reactions
   1. Chronic alcoholism
   2. Drug toxicity
J. Subdural hematoma
K. Hydrocephalus
L. Chronic seizures
M. Illness other than in the brain
   1. Kidney
   2. Liver
   3. Congestive heart failure
   4. Hypercapnia
   5. Hypoxemia
   6. Rhythm disturbance
   7. Acute myocardial infarction
   8. Hypothyroidism/hyperthyroidism
N. Hearing loss
O. Blindness
P. Lewy body dementia
Q. Electrolyte imbalance

III. **Signs/symptoms**
A. Onset may be slow, continuing over a period of months or years
B. Confusion and memory deficits (usually short term in nature: asking the same question, repeatedly forgetting that the question was already answered)
C. Misplacing things: putting an iron in the refrigerator
D. Problems with language: forgetting simple words or using wrong words
E. Impaired abstract reasoning: unable to balance a checkbook because of forgetfulness about what the numbers are and what to do with them
F. Higher cognitive functions may be impaired.
   1. Aphasia: language difficulties that may be cognitive or receptive
   2. Apraxia: inability to perform previously learned purposeful movements (i.e., previously learned tasks) or to use objects properly
   3. Agnosia: loss of comprehension of auditory, visual, or other sensations, although the sensory sphere is intact; inability to recognize objects, shapes, persons, sounds, smells, and so forth
   4. Impaired executive functioning (abstracting/organizing)

G. Disorientation: patients may become easily lost, even in familiar surroundings, or may wander
H. Patients may have difficulty with learned tasks, such as dressing or cooking.
I. Poor judgment: patients may forget that they are watching a child and may leave the child at home
J. Loss of initiative: becoming passive; not wanting to go places or see other people
K. Emotional problems such as depression, lability, or flattened affect
L. Changes in mood: fast mood swings, calm to tears to anger in minutes
M. Agitation, anxiousness, and sleeplessness
N. Drastic personality changes: irritable, suspicious (paranoid ideation), and fearful
O. Patients often lose insight into their deficits
P. Difficulty recognizing family and friends
Q. Severe symptoms include the following:
   1. Loss of speech
   2. Loss of appetite
   3. Weight loss
   4. Loss of bowel and bladder control
   5. Total dependence on caregiver
R. Clouding of consciousness and orientation does not occur until the terminal stages.

IV. **Laboratory/diagnostics**
   A. History
      1. Preferably with family members available to give adequate history of cognitive and behavior changes
      2. Often, the spouse or other informant brings the problem to the practitioner's attention.
      3. Self-reported memory loss does not usually correlate with dementia.
   B. Physical examination
      1. Neurologic examination
      2. Cognitive testing
         a. Attempt the Folstein Mini-Mental State Examination to screen for dementia
            i. The maximum score is 30
            ii. A score of 23 or less indicates cognitive impairment
            iii. LOCAM-LT—mnemonic for Folstein components
               (a) Level of consciousness
               (b) Orientation
               (c) Concentration/calculation
               (d) Attention
               (e) Memory
               (f) Language
               (g) Thought process
         b. Document the progression of disease over time by repeating testing at 3- to 6-month intervals
      3. Examination should include observations of memory, thinking, concentration, attention, judgment, insight, and behavior
      4. Mini-cognitive test: recall of three unrelated words, clock-drawing task
   C. Screening laboratory examination
      1. Glucose
      2. Electrolytes
      3. Magnesium
      4. Calcium
      5. Liver tests
      6. BUN/creatinine
      7. Thyroid function tests

CHAPTER 7 Dementia

      8. Vitamin B12 level, folate
      9. Venereal Disease Research Laboratory test
    10. HIV (selected patients)
    11. Complete blood count with differential, clotting studies
    12. Arterial blood gases
    13. Cultures: blood, urine, and sputum
    14. Serum levels of ingested drugs
    15. Illicit drugs and alcohol levels in selected patients
    16. Albumin
D. Other tests, depending on patient history and findings of physical examination
    1. CT of the head/MRI
       a. Note: for tumor, subdural hematoma, infarction, hemorrhage, hydrocephalus, and atrophy
    2. PET scan—may be useful in differentiating dementia types or pathologic processes in which clinical symptoms are similar
    3. Lumbar puncture—to rule out neurosyphilis, chronic meningitis, and normal pressure hydrocephalus
    4. Electroencephalography
    5. Chest X-ray—to rule out congestive heart failure, chronic lung disease, pulmonary embolus, and infection
    6. Electrocardiogram
E. Identification of treatable causes is very important.
    1. Drug induced
    2. Depression
    3. Hypothyroidism/hyperthyroidism
    4. Hypoglycemia
    5. Vitamin B12 or folate deficiency
    6. Subdural hematoma
    7. Liver failure
    8. Normal pressure hydrocephalus
    9. Stroke
    10. CNS infection
    11. Generalized infection
    12. Cerebral neoplasm
    13. Renal failure
    14. Alcohol abuse
    15. Hypoxia
    16. Hypercalcemia
    17. Vasculitis
    18. Cardiopulmonary disorder
    19. Anemia
F. Diagnostic and Statistical Manual of Mental Disorders (5th ed.; DSM-V; American Psychiatric Association; 2013) criteria for dementia
    1. Memory impairment
    2. At least two of the following:
       a. Aphasia
       b. Apraxia
       c. Agnosia
       d. Disturbances in executive functioning
    3. Disturbance in one or two of the above significantly interferes with work, social activities, or relationships.
    4. Disturbance does not occur exclusively during delirium.

V. Management

A. Supportive care: consult social services or other resources for transitioning between acute and home or skilled nursing care
B. Treat underlying precipitating illnesses
C. Attempt to withdraw, reduce, or stop all nonessential medications
D. Maintain nutrition: dietary consult
E. Avoid restraints, except for safety
F. Speech therapy/physical therapy
G. Address safety issues: coordinate appropriate safety measures with the patient's caregiver to prevent injury from falls, wandering, cooking, driving, and so forth
H. Because a cholinergic deficiency is present in Alzheimer's disease, cholinesterase inhibitors modestly improve cognition, behavior, and function, and they slightly delay disease progression.
I. In patients with Alzheimer's-related dementia, the clinical benefit of pharmacologic therapy is often modest and temporary.
J. Treatment for mild to moderate Alzheimer's-type dementia includes the following:
   1. Donepezil (Aricept), 5 mg PO once daily at bedtime; titrate to 10 mg orally once daily at 4–6 weeks; if suboptimal clinical response, may increase to maximum dose of 23 mg PO once daily at 3 months
      a. Well tolerated with convenient dosing; drug of choice
      b. It may cause syncope, bradycardia, and arteriovenous (AV) block; provide caregiver education and obtain baseline electrocardiogram before starting therapy
      c. Monitor for AV block, syncope, bradycardia and seizures
      d. Nausea and weight loss may occur
   2. Rivastigmine (Exelon): initial dose, 1.5 mg PO BID; maximum dose, 6 mg BID
      a. It should be administered with food to enhance absorption
      b. Similar to other cholinesterase inhibitors, it can cause peripheral cholinergic adverse effects
      c. Monitor for hypotension, syncope
      d. Significant weight loss (7% of initial weight) occurs in 19%–26% of patients
      e. Rivastigmine transdermal patch daily: start with 4.6 mg once a day for 4 weeks, then 9.5 mg once a day for 4 weeks, then maximum of 13.3 mg once a day
   3. Galantamine hydrobromide (Razadyne): Begin at 4 mg PO BID for a minimum of 4 weeks, after which the dosage may be increased to 8 mg BID. Four weeks later, the dosage may be increased again to 12 mg BID. Maximum dose is 24 mg/day; however, for patients with moderate renal or hepatic impairment, the maximum dose is 16 mg daily.
      a. In those with severe renal and hepatic impairment, this drug should be avoided. Caution should be used in patients with cardiac conduction defects.
      b. Monitor for sinus bradycardia, AV block, and syncope
K. Treatment for moderate to severe dementia includes the following:
   1. N-methyl-d-aspartate receptor antagonist
      a. Memantine (Namenda)
         i. Used to prevent the progression of Alzheimer's disease
         ii. Blocks pathologic stimulation of N-methyl-d-aspartate receptors and protects against further damage in patients with vascular dementia
         iii. Initiate with 7 mg PO once daily; titrate in 7-mg increments at intervals of least 1 week as tolerated to a target dose of 28 mg once daily; MAX, 28 mg/day
            (a) Low creatinine clearance (CrCl): reduce dosage to 14 mg PO once daily
         iv. May demonstrate greater efficacy when paired with cholinesterase inhibitors such as donepezil
         v. Monitor closely at initiation of therapy for Stevens-Johnson syndrome

L. Medications that affect serotonin have been useful in controlling aggression and agitation; use remains controversial.
   1. Atypical antipsychotics are the preferred treatment for dementia-related aggression and agitation in elderly patients.
      a. Examples
         i. Olanzapine (Zyprexa): initiate with 2.5 mg PO daily; titrate up to 5 mg BID MAX
         ii. Quetiapine (Seroquel): initiate with 25 mg PO at bedtime; titrate up to 75 mg BID MAX
         iii. Risperidone (Risperdal): initiate with 0.25–1 mg PO daily; dosage may be adjusted, not to exceed 1.5–2 mg daily
         iv. Ziprasidone (Geodon): initiate with 10 mg IM every 2 hr or 20 mg IM every 4 hr; switch to PO when possible
      b. Used for short periods and in low doses
      c. May produce considerable side effects, such as tardive dyskinesia and/or extrapyramidal and anticholinergic symptoms
   2. Studies show typical antipsychotics do not provide much benefit to dementia patients, except haloperidol (Haldol) in treating aggression
      a. Administer 0.5–10 mg IV/IM or PO initially, and observe patient for 20–30 minutes
         i. If the patient's condition remains unmanageable and the patient has had no adverse reactions to haloperidol, double the dose and continue to monitor
   3. Lithium (do not start lithium at a facility that cannot monitor levels; rarely used due to narrow therapeutic index)
   4. Buspirone (not used frequently due to delayed onset of action)
M. Benzodiazepines often preferred when controlling agitation and aggression
   1. Clonazepam (Klonopin): initiate 0.25 mg PO BID; increase by 0.125–0.25 mg BID every three days; target dose is 1 mg daily, 4 mg daily MAX
      a. Use cautiously; may cause paradoxical agitation or increase risk of falls or injury
   2. Lorazepam (Ativan), 1 mg IV every hour, may also be administered if needed
N. Emotional lability has been decreased by either of the following medication in some cases:
   1. Imipramine (Impril), 25–50 mg PO at bedtime; if tolerated, may increase to maximum 100 mg daily
      a. Tricyclic antidepressants such as imipramine usually avoided due to anticholinergic effects
   2. Sertraline (Zoloft): initiate at 25 mg PO daily; after one week, increase to 50 mg based on response and tolerance; 200 mg daily MAX
   3. Citalopram (Celexa): initiate at 20 mg PO daily; maximum dosage, due to risk of QT prolongation
O. Depression responds to the usual doses of tricyclic antidepressants, as well as to selective serotonin reuptake inhibitors, which have fewer anticholinergic adverse effects.
P. Other possible treatments under investigation but currently not supported by results of clinical trials include the following:
   1. Vitamin E and selegiline (Carbex) because of their antioxidant properties; use with caution in heart failure as high-dose therapy may be associated with increased mortality; currently not recommended as evidence to support vitamin E is mixed
   2. Nonsteroidal anti-inflammatory drugs because of properties in lowering plaque-producing amyloidogenic proteins; caution advised as these agents may raise rate of cardiovascular events; risks currently outweigh potential benefits
   3. Ginkgo biloba; investigated on grounds of increased cholinergic transmission; evidence is inconsistent at this time
   4. Antibiotics to treat chlamydia pneumonia, on grounds of association between *Chlamydia pneumoniae* and vascular dementia

5. In vitro studies have shown that rifampin and tetracyclines interfere with accumulation of β-amyloid peptide.
6. Statins may reduce amyloid peptides due to association between cholesterol in the brain and amyloid processing.

BIBLIOGRAPHY

American Psychological Association. (2013). *Diagnostic and statistical manual of mental disorders* (5th ed.). Washington, DC: APA Press.

Birks, J. & Evans, J.G. (2009) Gingko balboa for cognitive impairment and dementia. *Cochrane Database of Systematic Reviews,* (1). doi: 10.1002/14651858.CD003120.pub3.

Gaugler, J. E., Kane, R. L., Johnson, J. A., & Sarour, K. (2013). Sensitivity and specificity of diagnostic accuracy in Alzheimer's disease: A synthesis of existing evidence. *American Journal of Alzheimers Disease and Other Dementias, 28*(4), 337–347.

Harris, J. (2013). Cognitive approaches to early Alzheimer's disease diagnosis. *Medical Clinics of North America, 97*(3), 425–438.

Harrison-Dening, K. (2013). Dementia: Diagnosis and early interventions. *British Journal of Neuroscience Nursing, 9*(3), 131–137.

Landreville, P., Voyer, P., & Carmichael, P. (2013). Relationship between delirium and behavioral symptoms of dementia. *International Psychogeriatrics, 25*(4), 635–643.

McGuinness, B., O'Hare, J., Craig, D., Bullock, R., Malouf, R., & Passmore, P. (2010). Statins for the treatment of dementia. *Cochrane Database of Systematic Reviews,* (8). doi:10.1002/14651858.CD007514.pub2.

Papadakis, M., & McPhee, S. (2013). *Current medical diagnosis & treatment* (52nd ed., pp. 1005–1010). New York, NY: McGraw-Hill.

Schwarz, S., Froelich, L., & Burns, A. (2012). Pharmacological treatment of dementia. *Current Opinion in Psychiatry, 25*(6), 542–550.

Teipel, S. J., Grothe, M., Lista, S., Toschi, N., Garaci, F. G., & Hampel, H. (2013). Relevance of magnetic resonance imaging for early detection and diagnosis of Azheimer disease. *Medical Clinics of North America, 97*(3), 399–424.

van de Glind, E., Van Enst, W. A., Van Muster, B. C., Olde-Rikkert, M. G. M., Scheltens, P. . . . Hooft, L.(2013). Pharmacological treatment of dementia: A scoping review of systematic reviews. *Dementia and Geriatric Cognitive Disorders, 36*(¾), 211–228.

Yamamoto, H., Watanabe, T., Miyazaki, A., Katagiri, T., Idei, T. . . . Kamajima, K. (2005). High prevalance of *Chlamydia pneumoniae* antibodies and increased high-sensitive C-reactive protein in patients with vascular dementia. *Journal of the American Geriatrics Society, 53(4),* 583–589. doi: 10.1111/j.1532-5415.2005.53204.x

CHAPTER 8

Multiple Sclerosis

JUDI KURIC

I. **Definition**
   A. Demyelinating disease of the central nervous system
   B. An acquired, immune-mediated disease
   C. Neurological symptoms can be caused by isolated inflammation, demyelination, and axonal damage leading to nerve conduction delays, alterations, or complete blocks.
   D. Characterized by relapses (attacks or exacerbations) and remissions (recovery or improvements)

II. **Etiology/predisposing factors**
   A. Increased prevalence in populations living a greater distance from the equator
   B. Women have a 2–3 times higher incidence than men
   C. Onset of disease is earlier in women than men.
   D. Caucasians have highest risk
      1. African Americans have half the occurrence rate as Caucasians in the same geographic region.
      2. Northern Europeans, especially Scandinavians, are more likely to develop multiple sclerosis (MS).
   E. Risk in non-Caucasians can increase with movement from a low-risk to high-risk geographic region
   F. Seventy to 80% of persons with MS have onset in their 20s-40s.
   G. Approximately 10%–20% of MS patients have an afflicted family member.
   H. Patients with MS have a 5- to 7-year shorter life expectancy.
   I. No clear etiology but thought to have a multifactorial cause
      1. Viral infection is a precursor to exacerbation
      2. No identified link to several proposed viruses
         a. Measles
         b. Distemper
         c. Herpes
         d. Chlamydia
         e. Epstein-Barr

f. Retrovirus
3. No specific genetic association

III. Clinical manifestations
A. Classification of disease
1. Relapsing-remitting (RR-MS)
    a. Clear and defined episodes of relapses and recovery
        i. Recovery can be full or there can be some residual deficit.
    b. There is no clinical progression between the relapse episodes.
    c. Usual initial presentaetion of 85%–90% with MS
2. Secondary progressive (SP-MS)
    a. Usually initiates with RR-MS, followed by deterioration or progression of the disease
    b. Clinical progression noted between relapsing episodes
    c. Patients usually do not return to baseline after relapsing episode.
3. Primary progressive (PP-MS)
    a. Continued disease progression from the initial neurologic episode
    b. Some plateaus and minor temporary improvements
    c. Most commonly occurs in patients with onset after 40 years of age
    d. Occurs in about 10%–15% of MS patients
4. Progressive relapsing (PR-MS)
    a. Progressive disease from the onset with clear relapses after onset
    b. Recovery from the relapses may be full or partial.
    c. Continued progression of the disease between relapses
    d. Neurological status does not return to baseline after the relapse
    e. Occurs in about 5% of MS patients
5. Malignant MS
    a. Very rapid onset and progressive deterioration
    b. Significant disability and death with short period of time
6. Benign MS
    a. No deterioration after 10 years following onset of disease
    b. Unable to predict, identified only in historical review of the patient's disease process
B. Subjective neurological symptom that lasts at least 24 hr, resulting in increased disability
1. Motor weakness, spasticity, or stiffness
2. Sensory alterations of numbness, burning, tingling, tightness, and pain
3. Brain stem symptoms of double vision, dysarthria, dysphasia, dysphagia, and vertigo
4. Visual deficits: field defect, decreased acuity, impaired color perception, and pain with eye movement
5. Cerebellar symptoms: gait ataxia, intention tremor, and uncoordinated movements
6. Cognitive dysfunction: short-term memory, slowed processing, and difficulty with higher level problem solving
7. Fatigue: overall fatigue and limb fatigue
    a. Present in 90% of patients
8. Sleep disorders
9. Bladder, bowel, and sexual dysfunction
    a. Bladder urgency, frequency, and incontinence
    b. Frequent UTIs
    c. Constipation
    d. Erectile dysfunction
10. Seizure
11. Tonic spasms
C. Objective examination findings
1. Sensory track disturbances, present in 20%–50% of patients

CHAPTER **8**   Multiple Sclerosis

   a. Decreased vibratory sense
   b. Decreased position sense
   c. Decreased pinprick perception
   d. Decreased temperature sensation
  2. Reflex alterations
   a. Abnormal deep tendon reflexes
   b. Positive Babinski sign
   c. Positive Hoffman sign
   d. Spastic limb weakness
  3. Brain stem alterations
   a. Nystagmus
   b. Hearing loss
   c. Tinnitus
  4. Cerebellar
   a. Ataxia
   b. Tremor
   c. Lack of coordination
  5. Visual facial
   a. Optic neuritis (initial symptom in 25% of patients)
   b. Optic disk pallor
   c. Pupil defect
   d. Visual field defect
   e. Trigeminal neuralgia
  6. Frontal lobe
   a. Cognitive dysfunction
   b. Emotional lability or disinhibition
IV. **Laboratory findings/diagnostics**
 A. Complete neurological exam with noted deficits
 B. MRI
  1. Demonstrates white mater lesions in brain
  2. Demonstrates lesions in spinal cord
  3. Demonstrates T2-weighted lesions in periventricular white matter of brain and spinal cord
  4. Gadolinium enhancement on T1 imaging
  5. Hypodensities (black holes) on T1 imaging
  6. Cerebral atrophy
 C. Cerebrospinal fluid (CSF) analysis
  1. Consistent with MS if there is elevated IgG and oligoclonal bands in CSF, but not serum
   a. Bands present in about 70% of MS-positive patients
   b. Presence indicates MS; absence does not rule out the disease
 D. Evoked potentials
  1. Evidence of slowed conduction or prolonged evoked response
  2. Used less frequently; not conclusive, supports other diagnostics
 E. McDonald Diagnostic Criteria (2010)
  1. Applied after clinical evaluation of the patient
  2. A new T2 and /or gadolinium-enhancing lesion on follow-up MRI, with reference to a baseline scan regardless of the timing of the baseline MRI
  3. Simultaneous presence of asymptomatic gadolinium-enhancing and nonenhancing lesions at any time
 F. No better explanation for these neurologic events
  1. Specific MRI findings, abnormal CSF findings, and abnormal evoked potentials
  2. One of three outcomes: MS, possible MS, or not MS

V. Management
A. Referral to neurology
B. Mild acute exacerbations that do not produce functional decline may not require treatment.
C. Acute intervention for relapse
   1. Glucocorticoids, oral or intravenous
      a. High dose (500–1000 mg/day), usually with IV methylprednisolone; duration is dependent on clinical response
   2. Thought to promote early recovery from exacerbation but does not have any long-term effect
   3. Short-term pulse therapy preferred to prevent long-term steroid effects
D. Disease modification medications
   1. Reduces relapse, delays disability, and reduces MRI lesion burden (volume)
   2. Initiate early once diagnosis is established
      a. Immunomodulators
         i. Fingolimod (Gilenya)
            (a) Relapsing forms
            (b) Dose: 0.5 mg orally once daily
            (c) Observe for 6 hr after first dose for bradycardia
            (d) Adverse effects: first dose bradycardia, atrioventricular block, infection, macular edema, cough, headache, diarrhea, elevation of liver enzymes, increased blood pressure
         ii. Interferon beta-1b
            (a) Betaseron or Extavia
               1. Relapsing form
               2. 0.0625 mg SQ every other day; increase every 2 weeks by 0.0625 mg to recommended dosage of 0.25 mg SQ every other day
               3. Depression/suicidality
               4. Injection site necrosis
               5. Lymphopenia
         iii. Interferon beta-1a
            (a) Avonex
               1. Relapsing form
               2. 30 mcg IM once weekly or 7.5 mg IM each week until 30 mcg once weekly is reached
               3. Influenza-like symptoms
               4. Fatigue
               5. Myalgia
               6. Depression
            (b) Rebif
               1. Relapsing form
               2. Titration to 22 mcg dose: 4.4 mcg SQ 3 times a week for weeks 1 and 2; increase to 11 mcg SQ 3 times a week for weeks 3 and 4, then 22 mcg SQ 3 times a week
               3. Titration to 44 mcg dose: 8.8 mcg SQ 3 times a week for weeks 1 and 2; increase to 22 mcg SQ 3 times a week for weeks 3 and 4, then 44 mcg SQ 3 times a week
               4. Influenza-like symptoms (slightly less than Avonex)
               5. Fatigue
               6. Leukopenia
         iv. Glatiramer acetate (Copaxone)
            (a) RR-MS form

- (b) 20 mg SQ daily or 40 mg SQ 3 times a week at least 48 hr apart on the same 3 days each week
- (c) Injection site reaction
- (d) Flushing
- (e) Nausea
  - v. Natalizumab (Tysabri)
    - (a) Restricted use; relapsing form that is intolerant to other agents; only available through TOUCH® Prescribing Program to prescribers, infusion centers, and pharmacies associated with infusion centers
      1. Only prescribed to patients who are enrolled/meet all of the requirements; contact 1–800–456–2255 for details/enrollment
    - (b) 300 mg IV infused over 1 hr; given in 4 week intervals
    - (c) Infusion reaction (potential anaphylaxis)
    - (d) Fatigue
    - (e) Black box warning: natalizumab increases the risk of progressive multifocal leukoencephalopathy (PML), an opportunistic viral infection of the brain that usually leads to death or severe disability
- b. Immunosuppressant agents
  - i. Mitoxantrone (Novantrone)
    - (a) Secondary progressive, progressive relapsing, or worsening relapsing-remitting
    - (b) 12 mg/m^2 IV every 3 months
    - (c) Should not be administered to patients who have received a cumulative dose of 140 mg/m^2 or greater
    - (d) Cardiotoxicity: left ventricular ejection fraction and electrocardiogram evaluation are required prior to administration of each dose; if signs/symptoms of congestive heart failure develop, do not exceed maximum allowable lifetime cumulative dose
    - (e) Adverse effects: alopecia, diarrhea, nausea, vomiting
    - (f) Black box warning: increases risk of developing secondary acute myeloid leukemia
  - ii. Off-label immunosuppressants
    - (a) Methotrexate
    - (b) Cyclophosphamide
    - (c) Mycophenolate mofetil
- E. Symptom management for common complications
  1. Spasticity
  2. Fatigue
  3. Mood disorders
  4. Immobility
  5. Seizures
  6. Incontinence
  7. Cognitive effects
  8. Gait disturbances
  9. Sexual dysfunction

BIBLIOGRAPHY

Bader, M. K., & Littlejohn, L. R. (2010). *AANN core curriculum for neuroscience nursing* (5th ed.). Glenview, IL: AANN.

Langer-Gould, A., Brara, S., Beaber, B., & Zhang, J. (2013). Incidence of multiple sclerosis in multiple racial and ethnic groups. *Neurology, 80*(19), 1734–1739. doi:10.1212/WNL.0b013e3182918cc2

Luzio, C., & Keegan, B. (2014, January 29). *Multiple sclerosis*. Retrieved from http://emedicine.medscape.com/article/1146199-overview

Maloni, H. (2013). Multiple sclerosis: Managing patients in primary care. *Nurse Practitioner, 38*(4), 24–36.

Perrin Ross, A., Halper, J., & Harris, C. J. (2012). Assessing relapses and response to relapse treatment in patients with multiple sclerosis. *International Journal of MS Care, 14*(3), 148–159.

Polman, C., Reingold, S., Banwell, B., Clanet, M., Cohen, J., Filippi, M., . . . Wolinski, J. (2011). Diagnostic criteria for multiple sclerosis: 2010 revisions to the McDonald criteria. *Annuals of Neurology, 69*(2), 292–302. doi:10.1002/ana.22366

Rice, C. M. (2014). Disease modification in multiple sclerosis: An update. *Practical Neurology, 14*(1). doi:10.1136/practneurol-2013–000601

Rice, C., Cottrell, D., Wilkins, A., & Scolding, N. (2013). Primary progressive multiple sclerosis: Progress and challenges. *Journal of Neurology, Neurosurgery, and Psychiatry, 84*(10), 1100–1106.

Ross, A., & Thrower, B. W. (2010). Recent developments in the early diagnosis and management of multiple sclerosis. *Journal of Neuroscience Nursing, 42*(6), 342–353.

Rovira, A., Auger, C., & Alonzo, J. (2013). Magnetic resonance monitoring for lesion evolution in multiple sclerosis. *Therapeutic Advances in Neurological Disorders, 6*(5), 298–310. doi:10.1177/1756285613484079

Ruto, C. (2013). Special needs populations: Care of patients with multiple sclerosis. *AORN Journal, 98*(3), 281–293. doi:10.1016/j.aorn.2013.07.002

CHAPTER 9

Parkinson's Disease

JUDI KURIC • ROBERT FELLIN

I. **Definition**
   A. A neurodegenerative disorder caused by the depletion of dopamine-producing cells in the midbrain (substantia nigra)
   B. Cardinal symptoms of resting tremor, rigidity, and slowness of movement
II. **Etiology/predisposing factors**
   A. Approximately 60,000 new cases diagnosed annually in the United States
   B. Average age of onset is 60 years
   C. Incidence is slightly higher among men than women
   D. Caucasians have a slightly higher prevalence
   E. No single cause has been identified
   F. Environmental and genetic factors suggested as causative factors
      1. Multiple gene mutations have been identified, including the PARK1 gene, which is identified in Italian and Greek families.
      2. Occupational exposure to heavy metals, such as copper and manganese, has been associated with an increased risk.
III. **Clinical manifestations**
   A. Classic triad
      1. Resting tremor, most commonly of the arm and leg
      2. Rigidity: arms, legs, and neck stiffness with restricted range of motion
      3. Bradykinesia: slow movements in a deliberate manner
   B. Additional motor symptoms
      1. Postural instability: slumped posture and loss of posture reflexes
      2. Pull test: patient steps backwards to recover from a slight tug from behind
      3. Falls develop late in the disease process as a result of instability, gait problems, and diminished reflexes.
   C. Gait—classic attributes
      1. Diminished arm swing
      2. Shuffling steps; related to short, restricted steps
      3. Bent forward posture: fast, short steps; tendency for forward acceleration

4. "Frozen" gait: patient gets stuck or frozen while ambulating
D. Neuropsychiatric manifestations
   1. Depression
   2. Dementia
   3. Anxiety
   4. Psychosis
   5. Apathy
   6. Sleep disturbances
   7. Disinhibition
E. Autonomic dysfunction (medications used to treat Parkinson's disease [PD] also have autonomic side effects)
   1. Urinary incontinence
   2. Sexual dysfunction
   3. Constipation
   4. Orthostatic hypotension
   5. Impaired thermoregulation
   6. Sensory abnormalities (pain and paresthesia)
F. Craniofacial abnormalities
   1. Masked face: expressionless, fixed, and immobile face; staring eyes with mouth slightly open
   2. Dysphagia
   3. Involuntary closure of the eye lid
   4. Impaired sense of smell
   5. Excessive drooling
   6. Dysarthria

IV. **Laboratory findings/diagnostics**
A. History and physical exam are the basis for diagnosis
   1. Physical exam findings of tremor, rigidity, impaired balance, and gait alterations are the central findings that suggest PD.
B. CT scan and MRI are usually normal in PD but may be useful in assessing a differential diagnosis
C. Positron emission tomography scans are used primarily in research and are not specific for diagnosis
D. Clinical ratings scales, such as the Unified Parkinson's Disease Rating Scale, provide a standard evaluation and measure of the disease and its progression.

V. **Treatment (see Table 9.1)**
A. Referral to neurologist
B. Pharmacological intervention provides symptom relief and can improve functioning
   1. Carbidopa-levodopa combination (Sinemet) is the standard treatment
   2. Dopamine agonists (ropinirole and pramipexole) may reduce the risk of developing motor complications and alleviate symptoms
   3. Anticholinergics (trihexyphenidyl and benztropine mesylate) are helpful in treating tremors, but may cause confusion; use cautiously
   4. Amantadine (Symmetrel) is used early in the disease, helpful with dyskinesias
   5. MAO-B inhibitors (rasagiline and selegiline) may be helpful in the treatment of motor symptoms
C. "On-off" phenomena described when the medication is working, then stops working. This is characterized by motor function fluctuations. The addition of catechol-O-methyltransferase prevents the breakdown of dopamine and helps with these phenomena.
D. Neuroprotective agents have been investigated to prevent degeneration of neurons. The findings have been conflicting and more research is progressing in this area.

Table 9.1 Pharmacologic Agents for Parkinson's Disease

Agent	Initial Dosage	Adverse Effects	Comments
Dopaminergic Agents			
Carbidopa/levodopa (Sinemet): 10 mg/100 mg, 25 mg/100 mg, 25 mg/250 mg Sinemet CR: 25 mg/100 mg, 50 mg/200 mg	IR: 25/100 PO TID CR: 50/200 PO BID	GI upset, arrhythmias, dyskinesias, on-off and wearing-off phenomena, confusion, dizziness, headache, hallucinations	• Most effective drug for the symptomatic treatment of PD • Use with COMT/MAO-B inhibitors prolongs duration of effect • Sinemet is available as immediate release and sustained release
Dopamine Agonists			
Bromocriptine (Parlodel)	1.25 mg PO BID	Nausea, vomiting, postural hypotension, dyskinesias, confusion, impulse control disorders, sleepiness	• Can be used as monotherapy (mild disease) or in combination with levodopa/carbidopa • Reduce the frequency of "off periods" and may allow reduction of levodopa/carbidopa dose Pramipexole: • Requires slow titration • Adjust dose for renal dysfunction Ropinirole: • Many drug-drug interactions • Contraindicated in patients with a history of psychotic illness or recent MI or active peptic ulceration
Pramipexole (Mirapex, Mirapex ER)	IR: 0.125 mg PO TID ER: 0.375 mg PO daily		
Ropinirole (Requip, Requip XL)	IR: 0.25 mg PO TID Requip XL: 2 mg PO daily		
Monoamine Oxidase Inhibitors			
Rasagiline (Azilect)	0.5–1 mg PO daily	Orthostatic hypotension, rash, weight loss, GI upset, arthralgia, ataxia, dyskinesia, headache	• Adjunct therapy only • Provides modest improvements in motor function • Rasagiline is more potent than selegiline. • May cause serotonin syndrome: avoid TCADs, SSRIs Selegiline: • BBW: increases the risk of suicidal thinking and behavior in children, adolescents, and young adults • Many drug interactions: avoid meperidine, tramadol, methadone, propoxyphene, cyclobenzaprine, OTCs
Selegiline (Eldepryl)	5 mg PO BID		

Table 9.1 Pharmacologic Agents for Parkinson's Disease

Agent	Initial Dosage	Adverse Effects	Comments
COMT Inhibitors			
Entacapone (Comtan)	200 mg PO with each dose of levodopa/carbidopa	Diarrhea, abdominal pain, orthostatic hypotension, sleep disturbances, orange discoloration of the urine	• Adjunct therapy with levodopa/carbidopa only • Extends the effects of levodopa and alleviates "wearing off" phenomenon • Reduce dose of levodopa by 30% upon initiation of treatment. Entacapone: • Available as combination product with carbidopa/levodopa = Stalevo Tolcapone: • Liver toxicity, requires signed patient consent, monitor LFT's • BBW: risk of potentially fatal, acute fulminant liver failure
Tolcapone (Tasmar)	100 mg PO TID with each dose of levodopa/carbidopa		
Anticholinergic Agents			
Benztropine (Cogentin)	0.5–1 mg PO every bedtime	Sedation, nausea, constipation, dry mouth, blurred vision, drowsiness, dizziness, tachycardia, hypotension, nervousness, urinary retention	• May improve tremor and rigidity; have little effect on bradykinesia • Increase dose gradually until benefit occurs • Taper dose when withdrawing therapy • Use of anticholinergic agents is limited due to the development of intolerable side effects, necessitating dosage reduction or drug discontinuation
Biperiden (Akineton)	2 mg PO TID		
Trihexyphenidyl (Artane)	1 mg PO daily		
Miscellaneous			
Amantadine (Symmetrel)	100 mg PO BID	Restlessness, depression, irritability, insomnia, agitation, excitement, hallucinations, confusion, headache, heart failure, postural hypotension, urinary retention, anorexia, nausea, constipation, dry mouth	• Less efficacious than levodopa • Provides modest symptomatic benefit for tremor as well as rigidity and bradykinesia • Benefit is limited as duration of efficacy may last only few weeks • Reduce dose for renal impairment • May cause livedo reticularis

Note. IR = immediate release; CR = controlled release; ER = extended release; BBW = black box warning.

E. Deep brain stimulation surgery has replaced ablative procedures (e.g., pallidotomy and thalamotomy)
   1. Mechanism is unknown; the outcome of deep brain stimulation surgery enables near normal motor function. Patient selection and screening are essential for the positive outcomes of this treatment.
   2. Consult neurology/neurosurgery for evaluation
F. Adequate nutrition
G. Exercise
   1. Physical and occupational therapy may improve mobility, stiffness, balance, and gait
H. Management of neuropsychiatric comorbidities

BIBLIOGRAPHY

Bader, M. K., & Littlejohn, L. (2010). *AANN core curriculum for neuroscience nursing* (5th ed.). Glenview, IL: AANN.

Exercise and physical therapy. Retrieved from http://pdcenter.neurology.ucsf.edu/patients-guide/exercise-and-physical-therapy

Hickey, J. (Ed.). (2013). *The clinical practice of neurological and neurosurgical nursing* (7th ed.). Baltimore, MD: Lippincott.

Longo, D., Fauci, A., Kasper, D., Hauser, S., Jameson, J., & Loscalzo, J. (Eds.). (2012). *Harrison's manual of medicine* (18th ed.). New York, NY: McGraw-Hill.

Oertel, W., Berardelli, A., Bloem, B., Bonuccelli, U., Burn, D., Deuschl, G., . . . Trenkwalder, C. (2011). Late (complicated) Parkinson's disease. In N. Gilhus, M. Barnes, & M. Brainin (Eds.), *European handbook of neurological management* (2nd ed., Vol. 1, pp. 237–267). Oxford, UK.

Oertel, W., Berardelli, A., Bloem, B., Bonuccelli, U., Burn, D., Deuschl, G., . . . Trenkwalder, C. (2011). Early (uncomplicated) Parkinson's disease. In N. Gilhus, M. Barnes, & M. Brainin (Eds.), *European handbook of neurological management* (2nd ed., Vol. 1, pp. 217–236). Oxford, UK.

Papadakis, M. A., McPhee, S. J., & Tierney, L. M. (Eds.). (2013). *Current medical diagnosis and treatment* (52nd ed.) New York, NY: McGraw Hill/Appleton & Lange.

CHAPTER 10

Amyotrophic Lateral Sclerosis

JUDI KURIC

I. **Definition**
   A. Disease of the motor neurons causing asymmetric weakness
   B. Symptom presentation largely occurs with weakness in the upper or lower extremity
   C. Symptoms less likely to present with dysarthria and dysphagia or respiratory weakness

II. **Etiology/predisposing factors**
   A. Mean age of disease onset is 50 years
   B. Men are slightly more likely to develop amyotrophic lateral sclerosis (ALS) than women, although the numbers equalize when women approach menopause.
   C. Familial ALS is an inherited autosomal dominant trait that accounts for 5%–10% of cases.
   D. Remainder of causes unknown

III. **Clinical manifestations**
   A. Classification of disease—El Escorial criteria
      1. Classified by the presence of upper motor neuron (UMN) and lower motor neuron (LMN) symptoms in regions—brain stem, cervical, thoracic, and lumbosacral
      2. Categories
         a. Possible—UMN and LMN signs in one region
         b. Probable—UMN and LMN signs in two regions
         c. Probable lab supported—UMN signs in one or more regions and electromyogram (EMG) positive denervation in two or more limbs
         d. Definite—UMN and LMN signs in bulbar region plus two spinal regions
   B. Progressive weakness over weeks to months
   C. Sensation intact in all areas
   D. Muscle atrophy
   E. Small muscle fasciculations
   F. Abnormal reflexes (hyperreflexia)
   G. Spasticity

IV. **Laboratory findings/diagnostics**
   A. Serum CK may be slightly elevated
   B. EMG—denervation
   C. Muscle biopsy
      1. Small regions grouped with atrophic muscle fibers
   D. MRI—no abnormality that can explain UMN alterations

V. Management
A. Supportive treatment and consult to palliative care—average survival is 2–5 years after diagnosis
1. Immobility
2. Altered respiratory function may be managed with non-invasive ventilation, suction, etc.
3. Dysphagia and poor nutrition may be managed with altering food consistency, nutritional supplements, etc.
4. Pain–refer patient to pain management specialist
5. Anxiety (refer to Psychosocial Problems in Acute Care chapter for anti-anxiety agents)
6. Communication deficits
7. Medication: riluzole (Rilutek), 50 mg PO every 12 hr has been shown to extend survival rate by months but is not curative. Recommended by the American Association of Neuroscience Nursing to be offered to slow disease progression in patients with ALS

BIBLIOGRAPHY

Bader, M. K., & Littlejohn, L. (2010). *AANN core curriculum for neuroscience nursing* (5th ed.). Glenview, IL: AANN.

Gordon, P., Cheng, B., Katz, I., Mitsumoto, H., & Rowland, L. (2009). Clinical features that distinguish PLS, upper motor neuron-dominant ALS, and typical ALS. *Neurology, 72*(22), 1948–1952.

Hickey, J. (2013). *The clinical practice of neurological and neurosurgical nursing* (7th ed.). Baltimore, MD: Lippincott.

Longo, D., Fauci, A., Kasper, D., Hauser, S., Jameson, J., & Loscalzo, J. (Eds.). (2012). *Harrison's manual of medicine* (18th ed.). New York, NY: McGraw-Hill.

McClellan, F., Washington, M., Ruff, R., & Selkirk, S. (2013). Early and innovative symptomatic care to improve quality of life of ALS patients at Cleveland VA ALS Center. *Journal of Rehabilitation Research and Development, 50*(4), vii–xvi.

Miller, R., Jackson, C., Kasarskis, E., England, J., Forshew, D., Johnston, W., . . . Woolley, S. (2009). Practice parameter update: The care of the patient with amyotrophic lateral sclerosis: Drug, nutritional, and respiratory therapies (an evidence-based review). *Neurology, 73*(15), 1218–1226.

Miller, R., Jackson, C., Kasarskis, E., England, J., Forshew, D., Johnston, W., . . . Woolley, S. (2009). Practice parameter update: The care of the patient with amyotrophic lateral sclerosis: Multi-disciplinary care, symptom management, and cognitive/behavioral impairment. *Neurology, 73*(15), 1227–1233.

Papadakis, M., McPhee, S., & Tierney, L.(Eds.). (2013). *Current medical diagnosis and treatment* (52nd ed.). New York, NY: McGraw Hill/Appleton & Lange.

Sreedharan, J. H. (2013). Amyotrophic lateral sclerosis: Problems and prospects. *Annals of Neurology, 74*(3), 309–316.

Van den Berg, J. P., Kalmijn, S., Lindeman, E., Veldink, J. H., de Visser, M., Van der Graaff, M. M., . . . Van den Berg, L. H. (2005). Multidisciplinary ALS care improves quality of life in patients with ALS. *Neurology, 65*(8), 1264–1267.

SECTION TWO
Management of Patients With Cardiovascular Disorders

CHAPTER 11

Cardiovascular Assessment

JOAN KING • THOMAS W. BARKLEY, JR.

I. **Cardiac cycle review**
   A. Systole
      1. Atrioventricular (AV) valves (tricuspid and mitral valves) close
      2. Semilunar valves (aortic and pulmonic valves) open
   B. Diastole
      1. Aortic/pulmonic valves close
      2. Tricuspid and mitral valves open
      3. Rapid ventricular filling (75% filling of the ventricles)
      4. Atrial contraction (atrial kick) (25% filling of the ventricles)
II. **Auscultatory areas of the precordium—characterized by location at which valvular activity is heard best**
   A. Aortic—second right intercostal space (ICS) at the right sternal border (S2 heart sound louder than S1)
   B. Pulmonic—second left ICS at the left sternal border (S2 louder than S1)
   C. Erb's point—third ICS at the left sternal border
   D. Tricuspid—left lower sternal border at the fifth ICS (closure of AV valves)
   E. Mitral—fifth ICS midclavicular line (S1 louder than S2)
III. **S1 heart sound**
   A. Denotes closure of the mitral and tricuspid (AV) valves
   B. Occurs almost simultaneously with apical and carotid impulses
   C. Coincides with the R wave on ECG
   D. More easily heard than S2 at the apex
IV. **S2 heart sound**
   A. Denotes closure of the aortic and pulmonic (semilunar) valves
   B. Occurs at the onset of diastole (note that diastole is between S2 and S1)
   C. Heard louder than S1 at the base of the heart
V. **Split S2 heart sound**
   A. Transient split occurs on inspiration because of late closure of the pulmonic valve and early closure of aortic valve.

B. Late closure of the pulmonic valve is associated with increase in venous return to the right ventricle with inspiration.
C. Early closure of the aortic valve is associated with a decrease in venous return to the left ventricle related to an increase in pulmonary capacity during inspiration.
D. Heard best in the pulmonic auscultatory area
E. S2 returns to a single sound during expiration.
F. If the patient holds his or her breath, the sounds will disappear.
G. Normal physiological finding in children and young adults
H. May occur approximately every fourth heartbeat

VI. **S3 heart sound**
A. Referred to as a ventricular gallop
B. Caused by passive filling of blood into a noncompliant left ventricle
C. Heard early in diastole (0.12–0.16 seconds after S2) at the left lower sternal border (apex)
D. Heard best with the bell of the stethoscope
E. Occurs with such conditions as heart failure and cardiomyopathy when fluid overload is present
F. Normal sound associated with pregnancy (i.e., hyperdynamic state of increased volume)
G. Sounds like the word "Ken-tuc-ky"

VII. **S4 heart sound**
A. Referred to as an atrial or presystolic gallop
B. Produced by blood entering a noncompliant left ventricle during atrial contraction
C. Associated with increased ventricular diastolic pressures
D. Heard late in diastole; immediately before S1
E. Most clearly heard at the left lower sternal border (apex) with the bell of the stethoscope
F. Occurs with such conditions as myocardial infarction, hypertension, left ventricular hypertrophy, and heart failure
G. Sounds like the word "Ten-ne-ssee'"
H. It is not heard if the patient is in atrial fibrillation secondary to a loss of atrial kick.

VIII. **Summation gallop**
A. S3 and S4 heard together
B. Highly suggestive of severe myocardial failure

IX. **Murmurs**
A. "Blowing" or "swooshing" sound that results from turbulent blood flow; identified by the following variables:
 1. Timing—is the murmur systolic or diastolic, pansystolic or holosystolic, pandiastolic or holodiastolic?
 2. Loudness—graded I through VI
  a. Grade I/VI—barely audible
  b. Grade II/VI—clearly audible but faint
  c. Grade III/VI—moderately loud, easily heard
  d. Grade IV/VI—loud, associated with a thrill
  e. Grade V/VI—very loud; heard with one corner of stethoscope off the chest wall
  f. Grade VI/VI—loudest: no stethoscope needed
 3. Pitch—is the pitch high, low, or medium? Is it crescendo, decrescendo, plateau, or crescendo-decrescendo (diamond shaped murmur)?
 4. Quality—is the quality musical, blowing, rumbling, or harsh?
 5. Location—in what area is the murmur best heard?
 6. Radiation—is the murmur heard at other auscultatory areas (e.g., neck, back, left axilla)?
 7. Posture—does the murmur disappear or become louder with changes in posture?
B. Early diastolic murmurs—due to incompetent semilunar valves (e.g., aortic or pulmonic regurgitation)
 1. Decrescendo quality (diminishes in intensity)

2. High pitch (heard best with the diaphragm of the stethoscope)
3. Aortic regurgitation (aortic insufficiency)—sound intensifies if patient sits forward and holds their breath
4. Pulmonic regurgitation—low to medium pitched murmur
C. Diastolic rumbling murmurs—due to mitral stenosis and tricuspid stenosis
  1. Mitral stenosis
     a. Low-pitched; heard best with the bell of the stethoscope
     b. Decrescendo-crescendo quality
     c. Heard best at the apex; better in the left lateral position
     d. Murmur follows an opening snap
     e. Heard early in diastole but extends through diastole as patient's condition worsens
     f. Does not radiate
     g. Associated with rheumatic heart disease, myxomas or congenital malformation
  2. Tricuspid stenosis
     a. Mid-diastolic murmur heard louder with inspiration
     b. Heard best along the left sternal border
D. Midsystolic ejection murmurs—due to obstruction of forward flow through semilunar valves
  1. Aortic stenosis
     a. Harsh crescendo-decrescendo murmur that radiates to the carotids
     b. Heard best with the diaphragm over the aortic area
     c. Associated with aortic valve sclerosis in older adults, rheumatic heart disease, hypertrophic cardiomyopathy
  2. Pulmonic stenosis
     a. Medium-pitched
     b. Crescendo-decrescendo (diamond shaped)
     c. Radiates
E. Pansystolic regurgitant murmurs—due to backward flow
  1. Mitral regurgitation
     a. Holosystolic high pitched blowing sound
     b. Heard best at the apex and radiates to left axilla
     c. Lateral position intensify the sound
     d. Associated with endocarditis, rheumatic heart disease and rupture of the papillary muscles after an acute myocardial infarction
  2. Tricuspid regurgitation
     a. Soft systolic blowing sound
     b. Heard best at the left lower sternal border
     c. Intensifies during inspiration

X. Clicks
A. Midsystolic click
  1. Most common type
  2. Associated with mitral valve prolapse
B. Aortic ejection click
  1. Related to stenosis
  2. Occurs during early systole
  3. Audible at apex and base of the heart
C. Pulmonic ejection click
  1. Occurs during early systole
  2. Audible at the base of the heart only

XI. Friction rub
A. "Scratchy," high-pitched sound
B. Classic sound of pericarditis (inflammation)
C. Usually heard best at the apex with the patient leaning forward

D. Remains audible if the patient holds their breath
XII. **Peripheral pulse amplitude**
　A. Graded on a scale from 0–4
　　1. Bounding: +4
　　2. Full: +3
　　3. Normal: +2
　　4. Diminished: +1
　　5. Absent: 0
XIII. **Electrocardiographic changes associated with electrolyte disturbances**
　A. Hyperkalemia
　　1. Tall, peaked T waves
　　2. Widening of the QRS complex
　　3. Prolongation of the P wave/PR interval
　　4. Increased levels of K+ decrease ventricular depolarization and slow AV conduction.
　B. Hypokalemia
　　1. Premature ventricular contractions (PVC's) both unifocal and multifocal
　　2. U waves which follow the T wave and are of lower amplitude
　　3. Less common changes include bradycardia, atrial flutter, and AV block
　　4. Potentiated effects of digitalis toxicity
　C. Hypercalcemia
　　1. AV blocks, bundle branch block, and bradycardia related to increased contractility of the heart and shortening of the QT interval (period of ventricular repolarization)
　　2. Potentiated effects of digitalis toxicity
　D. Hypocalcemia
　　1. Bradycardia, ventricular ectopy and asystole because low calcium levels decrease contractility
　　2. Decreased cardiac output and hypotension
　　3. Decreased efficacy of digitalis
　E. Hypermagnesemia
　　1. Rarely evident in the acute care setting
　　2. Usually related to renal failure or over-administration of magnesium during replacement therapy
　F. Hypomagnesemia
　　1. Changes similar to those associated with hypokalemia and hypocalcemia
　　　a. Appearances of U wave
　　　b. Prolonged PR/QT intervals
　　　c. Widened QRS complexes
　　　d. Flattened T waves
　　　e. Supraventricular tachycardia (SVT)
　　　f. Ventricular arrhythmia
　　　g. Torsades de pointes
　　2. Note: Hypomagnesemia may cause hypertension and coronary/systemic vasospasm.
　　3. Hypomagnesemia usually must be corrected before replacement therapy for hypokalemia and hypocalcemia can be effective.
XIV. **Cardiovascular changes with the elderly**
　A. Heart valves—become more fibrous and rigid
　B. Conduction—decrease in number of cells in SA node and AV node
　C. Rhythm—decrease in rate both average rate and maximal rate
　　1. Takes longer for heart rate to return to resting rate when stressed
　　2. Tachyarrhythmias are poorly tolerated because of reduced ventricular compliance.

XV. **Assessment of jugular venous distension (as an indication of central venous pressure)**
   A. Patient sitting at 45° angle
   B. Assess for pulsation of the internal jugular vein
   C. Measured in centimeters from the angle of Louis
   D. The angle of Louis is approximately 5 cm right of atrium
   E. Measure vertically in centimeters from the angle of Louis to where height of pulsation is seen
   F. Add measurement to 5 cm for total; 7–9 cm is considered normal
   G. Higher than 9 cm is indication of volume overload

BIBLIOGRAPHY

Bonow, R., & Mann, D. (2012). *Braunwald's Heart Disese: A Textbook of Cardiovascular Medicine* (9th ed.). Philadelphia, PA: Elsevier.

Foreman, M, Milisen, K., & Fulmer, T. (2009). *Critical care nursing of older adults*. New York, NY: Springer Publishing Company.

Hall, J. (2010). *Guyton and Hall textbook of medical physiology* (12th ed.). Philadelphia, PA: W.B. Saunders Elsevier.

Marino, P. (2014). *The ICU book*. Philadelphia, PA: Wolters Kluwer Health/Lippincott, Williams & Wilkins.

Siedel, H, Ball, J., Dains, J., & Flynn, J. (2010). *Mosby's guide to physical examination* (7th ed.). Philadelphia, PA: Mosby Elsevier.

Urden, L. D., Stacy, K., & Lough, M. E. (2013). *Critical care nursing: diagnosis and management* (7th ed.). St. Louis, MO: Mosby.

CHAPTER 12

Hypertension

THOMAS W. BARKLEY, JR. • HELEN MILEY • ROBERT FELLIN

I. **Definition**
   A. Sustained elevation of systolic blood pressure (SBP) of 140 mmHg or above, or diastolic blood pressure (DBP) of 90 mmHg or above on numerous occasions
   B. Includes individuals currently taking antihypertensive pharmacologic agents
   C. Previous expert opinions, such as the JNC 7, identified BP as based on the average of two or more properly measured seated BP readings on each of two or more office visits. (see table 12.1)
   D. In contrast to JNC 7, JNC 8 emphasizes treatment thresholds.

Table 12.1	JNC 7 blood pressure thresholds		
Classifications	**Systolic BP**		**Diastolic BP**
Normal	< 120	and	< 80
Prehypertension	120 to 139	or	80 to 89
Hypertension			
Stage 1	140 to 159	or	90 to 99
Stage 2	≥ 160	or	≥ 100

II. **Incidence/predisposing factors**
   A. Affects 20%–30% of African Americans
   B. Affects 10%–15% of Caucasians in the U.S.
   C. Affects approximately 60 million Americans
   D. Hypertension (HTN) is a leading risk factor for coronary artery disease, stroke, congestive heart failure, renal failure, and retinopathy.

III. **Types and theories**
   A. Primary—referred to as "essential" or "idiopathic"
      1. Cause is unknown
      2. Represents 95% of all cases of HTN
      3. Onset is usually between ages 25 and 55
      4. Exacerbating factors

CHAPTER 12   Hypertension

        a. Obesity
        b. Excessive alcohol consumption (more than two drinks a day)
        c. Cigarette smoking
        d. Use of nonsteroidal anti-inflammatory drugs
     5. Theories of etiology include the following:
        a. Genetic and environmental factors
        b. Elevated intracellular calcium and sodium levels
        c. Sympathetic nervous system hyperactivity
        d. High renin-angiotensin activity causing vascular dysfunction
  B. Secondary—related to other known causes or disease processes
     1. Represents 5% of all cases of HTN
     2. Etiology includes the following:
        a. Estrogen use (via oral contraceptives or hormone replacement therapy)
        b. Renal disease
        c. Pregnancy
        d. Endocrine disorders, such as pheochromocytoma
  C. Isolated systolic HTN—common with aging
     1. Generally defined as a systolic BP greater than 140 and a diastolic BP less than 90
     2. Widening pulse pressure is a good indication and the Framingham point scale is a good predictor.
     3. Poorly understood
     4. May account for 65%–75% of HTN in the elderly
     5. Effectively treated with diuretics and long-acting calcium channel blockers, among others

IV. **Subjective and physical examination findings**
  A. Often none; known as the "silent killer"
  B. Elevated blood pressure (140/90 mmHg or higher)
  C. May complain of classic suboccipital "pulsating" headache, usually in the early morning and resolving throughout the day
  D. May complain of epistaxis, light-headedness, and visual disturbances, among others
  E. S4 heart sound may be present, related to left ventricular hypertrophy
  F. Retinal changes are present with severe, chronic disease.
  G. Rare findings, such as hematuria

V. **Diagnostics/laboratory testing**
  A. Laboratory data are usually unremarkable with uncomplicated disease.
  B. Consider ordering the following:
     1. CBC and electrolytes with hemoglobin levels (establish baseline)
     2. Urinalysis
     3. Blood urea nitrogen and creatinine concentrations
     4. Fasting glucose level
     5. Lipid panel
     6. Electrocardiogram (establish baseline, and rule out arrhythmias)
     7. Chest X-ray (rule out cardiomegaly, for example)
     8. Echocardiogram (if left ventricular, hypertrophy is suspected)
     9. Angiotensin-converting enzyme (ACE) inhibitor (Captopril) stimulation test (if indicated, to rule out renovascular HTN)
    10. Overnight 1-mg dexamethasone suppression test (if indicated, to rule out Cushing's syndrome)
    11. Aldosterone level (if indicated, to rule out aldosteronism)
    12. Plasma catecholamine level (if indicated, to rule out pheochromocytoma)

Table 12.2	JNC 8 Hypertension Treatment Recommendations	
	Population	**Goal BP**
Recommendation 1	Adults ≥ 60 years of age	SBP < 150 mmHg or DBP < 90 mmHg (Grade A)
Recommendation 2	Adults < 60 years of age	DBP < 90 mmHg (Grade A)
Recommendation 3	Adults < 60 years of age	SBP < 140 mmHg (Grade E)
Recommendation 4	Adults ≥ 18 with CKD	SBP < 140 mmHg or DBP < 90 mmHg (Grade E)
Recommendation 5	Adults ≥ 18 with DM	SBP < 140 mmHg or DBP < 90 mmHg (Grade E)
Recommendation 6	Non-African-American	Thiazide type diuretic CCB ACEI ARB (Grade B)
Recommendation 7	African-American	Thiazide diuretics CCB (Grade B) (Grade C for patients with DM)
Recommendation 8	Adults over 18 Adults with CKD	ACEI ARB (Grade B) Regardless of race or other medical conditions
Treatment Goal		
Recommendation 9	• Treatment goal for initial treatment is 1 month • Increase dose or add second drug • Continue to assess monthly until goal is reached • Do not use and ACEI and ARB together • Refer to hypertensive specialist if 3 or more drugs are needed	

Note. JNC = Joint National Committee; BP = blood pressure; SBP = systolic blood pressure; DBP = diastolic blood pressure; CKD = chronic kidney disease; DM = diabetes mellitus; CCB = calcium channel blockers; ACEI = Angiotensin converting enzyme inhibitor; ARB = angiotensin receptor blocker. Grade A = strong recommendation; Grade B = moderate recommendation; Grade C = weak recommendation; Grade E = expert opinion but insufficient evidence for recommendation.

Table 12.3	Blood pressure classification and treatment recommendations for adults age 18 and older	
Category	**Systolic, mmHg**	**Diastolic, mmHg**
Normal for patients ≥ 60	< 150	< 90
Normal for patients < 60	< 140	< 90

VI. Goal of treatment based on JNC 8 (see table 12.2)
VII. Classification for initial hypertensive measurements (see table 12.3)
VIII. Management
    A. Principle—in sequential order
        1. Analyze baseline studies
        2. See algorithm for the treatment of HTN (Figure 12.1)
        3. Use nonpharmacologic strategies
        4. Employ pharmacologic measures
    B. Nonpharmacologic strategies
        1. Restriction of dietary sodium (no more than 100 mmol per day—2.4 grams sodium or 6 grams salt)
        2. Weight loss, if overweight

3. Adopt a DASH (Dietary Approaches to Stop Hypertension) diet (rich in fruits, vegetables, and low-fat dairy products, with reduced saturated and total fat)
4. Exercise (aerobic exercise 30–40 min each day on most days of the week)
5. Stress management planning
6. Reduction or elimination of alcohol consumption (fewer than two drinks daily for men, or one drink daily for women and lighter-weight persons)
7. Smoking cessation
8. Maintenance of adequate potassium, calcium, and magnesium intake

C. Pharmacologic measures (refer to Table 12.4 for specific drug names and dosages)
 1. Based on degree of blood pressure elevation and/or the presence of end-organ damage, cardiovascular disease, or other risk factors

Table 12.4	Common Oral Hypertensive Agents	
	Agent	**Usual Dose/Frequency**
Diuretics: **Thiazide**	chlorothiazide (Diuril) chlorthalidone (Hygroton) hydrochlorothiazide indapamide (Lozol) metolazone (Zaroxolyn)	250–500 mg BID 12.5–25 mg daily 12.5–50 mg daily 1.25–2.5 mg daily 2.5–10 mg daily or BID
Loop	bumetanide (Bumex) ethacrynic acid (Edecrin) furosemide (Lasix) torsemide (Demadex)	0.5–2 mg daily or BID 25–100 mg daily 10–40 mg daily 5–10 mg daily
Potassium sparing	eplerenone (Inspra) spironolactone (Aldactone)	50–100 mg daily 25–50 mg daily
Arterial Vasodilators	hydralazine (Apresoline) minoxidil (Loniten)	10–100 mg BID or four times a day 5–100 mg daily or BID
Direct Renin Inhibitor	aliskiren (Tekturna)	150–300 mg daily
β-adrenergic Blocking Agents	acebutolol (Sectral) atenolol (Tenormin) betaxolol (Kerlone) bisoprolol (Zebeta) carvedilol (Coreg) labetalol (Normodyne) metoprolol (Lopressor) nadolol (Corgard) pindolol (Visken) propranolol (Inderal) timolol (Blocadren)	25–100 mg daily 25–100 mg daily 5–20 mg daily 2.5–10 mg daily 12.5–50 mg BID 200–800 mg BID 50–100 mg daily or BID 40–120 mg daily 10–40 mg BID 10–120 mg BID 20–40 mg BID
ACE Inhibitors	benazepril (Lotensin) captopril (Capoten) enalapril (Vasotec) fosinopril (Monopril) lisinopril (Zestril) moexipril (Univasc) perindopril (Aceon) quinapril (Accupril) ramipril (Altace) trandolapril (Mavik)	10–40 mg daily 12.5–100 mg BID or TID 5–40 mg daily or BID 10–40 mg daily 5–40 mg daily 7.5–30 mg daily 4–8 mg daily 10–80 mg daily 2.5–20 mg daily 1–4 mg daily

Table 12.4	Common Oral Hypertensive Agents	
	Agent	**Usual Dose/Frequency**
Angiotensin II Receptor Antagonists	candesartan (Atacand) eprosartan mesylate (Teveten) irbesartan (Avapro) losartan (Cozaar) olmesartan (Benicar) telmisartan (Micardis) valsartan (Diovan)	8–32 mg daily 400–800 mg daily or BID 75–300 mg daily 25–100 mg daily 20–40 daily 20–80 mg daily 40–320 mg daily or BID
Calcium Channel Blocking Agents	verapamil IR verapamil (Calan SR)	80–320 mg twice or TID 120–240 mg daily or BID
	diltiazem IR diltiazem (Dilacor XR)	45–270 mg BID 180–360 mg daily
	amlodipine (Norvasc) felodipine (Plendil) isradipine (Dynacirc) nicardipine (Cardene SR) nifedipine (Adalat CC) nisoldipine (Sular)	2.5–10 mg daily 2.5–20 mg daily 2.5–10 mg BID 60–120 mg BID 30–90 mg daily 10–40 mg daily
Peripheral α_1-Antagonists	prazosin (Minipress) terazosin (Hytrin) doxazosin (Cardura)	1–10 mg BID 1–10 mg daily or BID 1–16 mg daily
Central α_2-Agonists	clonidine (Catapres) methyldopa (Aldomet)	0.1–0.6 mg BID 250–500 mg TID

2. Goal of therapy—to prescribe the least number of medications possible at the lowest dosage to attain acceptable blood pressure, thereby decreasing cardiovascular and renal morbidity and mortality
3. Thiazide diuretics, first-line drug of choice for hypertension:
    a. Increase excretion of sodium and water
    b. Reduce morbidity and mortality
    c. Screen for sulfa allergy before administering
    d. May cause hypokalemia, hypomagnesemia, hyperglycemia, hyponatremia, hypercalcemia, etc.
4. ACE inhibitors:
    a. Cause vasodilation and block sodium and water retention
    b. Do not initiate if potassium is greater than 5.5 mEq/L
    c. Contraindicated in pregnancy
    d. Do not use in combination with ARB
    e. May cause cough, rash, taste disturbances, hyperkalemia, renal impairment, etc.
5. Angiotensin II-receptor blockers; reserved for patients intolerant to ACE inhibitors:
    a. Cause vasodilation and block sodium and water retention
    b. Do not initiate if potassium is greater than 5.5 mEq/L
    c. Contraindicated in pregnancy
    d. Do not use in combination with ACE inhibitor
    e. May cause cough, hyperkalemia, headache, taste disturbances, renal impairment, etc.
6. Calcium channel blocking agents:
    a. Monitor heart rate, especially when administering verapamil and diltiazem
    b. May be used for angina, arrhythmias, and migraines
    c. May cause headache, flushing, bradycardia, etc.
7. Beta-blocking agents:

a. Directly relax the heart
b. May also be used for angina and arrhythmias
c. Monitor heart rate and avoid use in patients with asthma/COPD
d. Not first-line therapy
e. May cause dizziness, bradycardia, heart block, fatigue, insomnia, nausea, etc.
8. Peripheral alpha-1 antagonists:
   a. Cause vasodilation
   b. Take first dose at bedtime
   c. Primarily used as adjunct therapy
   d. May be used for benign prostatic hyperplasia
   e. May cause first-dose syncope, dry mouth, orthostasis, dizziness, headache, nausea, etc.
9. Central alpha-2 agonists:
   a. Prevent vasoconstriction, cause vasodilation, and slow the heart rate
   b. Methyldopa is the drug of choice in pregnancy, clonidine is available as a transdermal patch
   c. Do not discontinue use abruptly, as it may cause withdrawals and rebound hypertension
   d. Primarily used as adjunct therapy
   e. May cause dry mouth, sedation, depression, headache, bradycardia, etc.
10. Arterial vasodilators:
    a. Directly relax the vascular smooth muscle resulting in arterial vasodilation
    b. Reduce frequency in renal dysfunction
    c. May cause reflex tachycardia
    d. Used primarily as adjunct therapy and is available intravenously
    e. May cause nausea, flushing, dizziness, orthostatic hypotension, etc.
11. Direct renin inhibitors:
    a. Inhibits renin, which decreases plasma renin activity (PRA) and inhibits the conversion of angiotensinogen I to angiotensin I
    b. Does not offer advantage over any other available regimens and is expensive
    c. Teratogenic, avoid use in pregnancy
    d. May cause diarrhea, dizziness, headache, hyperkalemia, etc.
12. Adrenergic antagonists:
    a. Depletes catecholamine stores to decrease blood pressure; depression of sympathetic nerve function
    b. Reserpine reserved for third-line therapy and is contraindicated in renal failure
    c. Guanethidine dose should be adjusted for patients with renal failure
    d. Rarely used due to significant adverse effects, such as drowsiness, nasal stuffiness, depression, and atrial fibrillation/arrhythmia
13. Special considerations
    a. Neither age nor gender usually affects agent responsiveness.
    b. Thiazide-type diuretics are usually recommended for first-line treatment.
    c. Beta blockers, ACE inhibitors, adrenergic receptor blockers, and calcium channel blockers are also useful alone or in combination therapy.
14. Refer to examples of commonly prescribed preparations in table 12.4
15. Follow guidelines regarding blood pressure measurement, primary prevention, goals of therapy, and treatment and adherence in the JNC 8 (Eighth Report of the Joint National Committee on Prevention, Detection, Evaluation, and Treatment of High Blood Pressure) Guide to Prevention and Treatment of Hypertension Recommendations (Table 12.2).
16. Refer often to the algorithm for treatment of HTN (see Figure 12.1)
17. Consider drug interactions with antihypertensive therapy (Table 12.6)

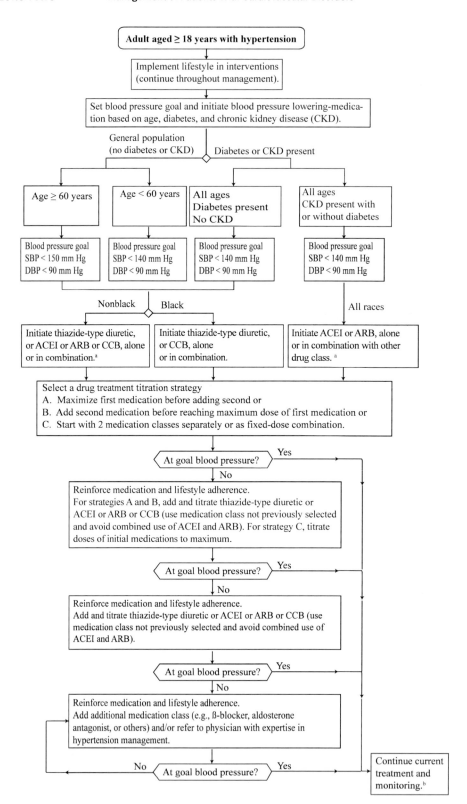

Figure 12.1. 2014 Hypertension Guideline Management Algorithm. SBP = systolic blood pressure; DBP = diastolic blood pressure; ACEI = angiotensin-converting enzyme; ARB = angiotensin receptor blocker; CCB = calcium channel blocker. Adapted with permission from "2014 Evidence-Based Guideline for the Management of High Blood Pressure in Adults," by P. A. James, S. Oparil, B. L. Cater, W. C. Cushman, C. D. Hummelfarb, J. Handler . . . E. Ortiz, 2014, *The Journal of the American Medical Association, 311*(5). Copyright 2014 by the American Medical Association.

[a]ACEIs and ARBs should not be used in combination.

[b]If blood pressure fails to be maintained at goal, reenter the algorithm where appropriate based on the current individual therapeutic plan.

Table 12.5	Prevention and treatment of hypertension recommendations

Blood pressure measurement	• Patient should do the following:
	  • Be seated with feet flat on floor, back and arm supported, and arm at heart level
	  • Rest for 5 minutes before measurement
	  • Wear short sleeves
	  • Not drink coffee or smoke cigarettes 30 min before having blood pressure taken
	  • Go to the bathroom before the reading; having a full bladder can change your blood pressure reading
	• Clinician should do the following:
	  • Use a cuff of appropriate size for the patient; the (cuff) bladder should encircle at least 80% of the upper arm
	  • Use calibrated or mercury manometer

Primary prevention	• Quit smoking to reduce cardiovascular risk • Maintain a healthy weight; lose weight if needed • Restrict sodium intake to no more than 100 mmol/day • Limit alcohol intake to no more than 1–2 drinks per day • Be active; get at least 30–45 minutes of aerobic activity on most days • Maintain adequate potassium intake of about 90 mmol per day • Maintain adequate intakes of calcium and magnesium for general health
Goal	• Set a clear goal of therapy based on patient's risk. Control blood pressure to the levels below: • Less than 140/90 mmHg for patients
Treatment	• Begin with lifestyle modifications for all patients • Be supportive! • Add pharmacologic therapy if blood pressure remains uncontrolled/ out of goal • Start with a thiazidetype diuretic, but also consider ACE inhibitor, angiotensinreceptor blocker, calcium channel blocker, or combination • If no response, try a drug from another class or add a second drug from a different class.
Adherence	• Encourage lifestyle modifications. Be supportive! • Educate the patient and family about the disease. Involve them in measurement and treatment • Maintain communication with patient • Empathy promotes adherence, trust, and motivation • Keep care inexpensive and simple • Consider cultural beliefs, practices, and individual attitudes when treating

Note. Adapted from "The seventh report of the Joint National Committee on prevention, detection, evaluation, and treatment of high blood pressure," by the National Institutes of Health National Heart, Lung, and Blood Institute, NIH Publication No. 04-5230, 2004.

Table 12.6 Select drug interactions with antihypertensive therapy

Drug class	Increase efficacy	Decrease efficacy	Effect on other drugs
Diuretics	• Diuretics that act at different sites in the nephron (e.g., furosemide + thiazides)	• Resin-binding agents • NSAIDs • Steroids	• Diuretics raise serum lithium levels. • Potassium-sparing agents may exacerbate hyperkalemia caused by ACE inhibitors.
β-blockers	• Cimetidine (hepatically metabolized β-blockers) • Quinidine (hepatically metabolized β-blockers) • Food (hepatically metabolized β-blockers)	• NSAIDs • Withdrawal of clonidine • Agents that induce hepatic enzymes, including rifampin and phenobarbital	• Propranolol hydrochloride induces hepatic enzymes to promote clearance of drugs with similar metabolic pathways. • β-blockers may mask and prolong insulin-induced hypoglycemia. • Heart block may occur with nondihydropyridine calcium antagonists. • Sympathomimetics cause unopposed α-adrenoceptor-mediated vasoconstriction. • β-blockers enhance angina-inducing potential of cocaine.
ACE inhibitors	• Chlorpromazine or clozapine	• NSAIDs • Antacids • Food decreases absorption (moexipril)	• ACE inhibitors may raise serum lithium levels. • ACE inhibitors may exacerbate effect of potassium-hyperkalemic sparing diuretics.
α-blockers Central α₂-agonists and peripheral neuronal blockers		• Tricyclic antidepressants (and probably phenothiazines) • Monoamine oxidase inhibitors • Sympathomimetics or phenothiazines antagonize guanethidine monosulfate or guanadrel sulfate • Iron salts may reduce methyldopa absorption	• Prazosin may decrease clearance of verapamil hydrochloride. • Methyldopa may increase serum lithium levels. • Severity of clonidine hydrochloride withdrawal may be increased by β-blockers. • Many agents used in anesthesia are potentiated by clonidine hydrochloride.
Calcium antagonists	• Grapefruit juice (some dihydropyridines) • Cimetidine or ranitidine (hepatically metabolized calcium antagonists)	• Agents that induce hepatic enzymes, including rifampin and phenobarbital	• Cyclosporine levels increase[a] with iltiazem hydrochloride, verapamil hydrochloride, mibefradil dihydrochloride, or nicardipine hydrochloride (but not with felodipine, isadipine, or nifedipine). • Nondihydropyridines increase levels of other drugs metabolized by the same hepatic enzyme system, including digoxin, quinidine, sulfonylureas, and theophylline. • Verapamil hydrochloride may lower serum lithium levels.

Note. NSAIDs = nonsteroidal anti-inflammatory drugs; ACE = angiotensin-converting enzyme. Adapted from "The sixth report of the Joint National Comittee on prevention, detection, evaluation, and treatment of high blood pressure," by the National Institutes of Health National Heart, Lung, and Blood Institute, NIH Publication No. 98-4080, 1997.

[a]This is a clinically and economically beneficial drug-drug interaction because it retards the progression of accelerated atherosclerosis in heart transplant recipients and reduces the required daily dose of cyclosporine.

CHAPTER 12   Hypertension

IX. **Hypertensive urgencies and emergencies**
   A. Hypertensive urgencies
      1. Characterized by severe elevations in blood pressure of 180/110 mmHg or higher without progressive target organ dysfunction
      2. Majority of patients present as noncompliant or inadequately treated hypertensive individuals, often with little or no evidence of target organ damage
      3. Parenteral therapy is rarely required for such asymptomatic patients
      4. May or may not be associated with severe headache, shortness of breath, epistaxis, or severe anxiety
      5. Oral therapy may include the following:
         a. Clonidine (Catapres)
            i. Alpha-adrenergic stimulant
            ii. Dosage is 0.2 mg PO, then 0.1 mg every hour until BP is controlled or total of 0.8 mg is given
            iii. Patient may experience sedation
            iv. Rebound HTN is possible if drug is discontinued after chronic use
         b. Captopril (Capoten)
            i. ACE inhibitor
            ii. Dosage is 12.5–25 mg PO
   B. Hypertensive emergencies
      1. Situations associated with severe elevations in blood pressure of 180/120 mmHg or higher. May occur at a lower blood pressure if complicated by evidence of impending or progressive target organ dysfunction
      2. Examples:
         a. Hypertensive encephalopathy
         b. Intracerebral hemorrhage
         c. Acute myocardial infarction
         d. Acute left ventricular failure with pulmonary edema
         e. Unstable angina pectoris
         f. Dissecting aortic aneurysm or eclampsia
      3. Require immediate blood pressure reduction to prevent or limit target organ damage
      4. Acute management possibilities for hypertensive emergencies
         a. Critical care unit nursing care and an arterial line are indicated
         b. Blood pressure should be lowered to 160–180 mmHg systolic or to less than 105 mmHg diastolic (no more than 25% within minutes to 1–2 hr), and then gradually lowered over several days with oral therapy to prevent additional complications such as coronary, cerebral, or renal ischemia.
         c. Nicardipine: first drug of choice
            i. Dosage is 2.5–15 mg/hr IV
         d. Sodium nitroprusside (Nipride): second drug of choice
            i. Dosage is 0.25–10 mcg/kg/min IV
            ii. May cause rapid, profound hypotension
            iii. Do not give for longer than 72 hr because of the risk of cyanide poisoning
         e. Nitroglycerin: used especially in patients with ischemia
            i. Dosage is 5–200 mcg/min IV
         f. Esmolol hydrochloride (Brevibloc)
            i. Dosage is 500 mcg/kg IV given over 1 min; maintenance dosage is 50–300 mcg/kg/min
               (a) No bolus unless heart rate is above 100
         g. Labetalol hydrochloride (Normodyne, Trandate)
            i. Used especially with hypertension associated with pregnancy
            ii. Start with 10–20 mg, then

iii. 20–80 mg IV bolus over 10 min, or continuous infusion of 0.5–2 mg/min
h. Hydralazine (Apresoline)
   i. Dosage is 5–20 mg IV and may be repeated in 20 min
   ii. Contraindicated in patients with coronary artery disease and aortic dissection
i. Fenoldopam (Corlopam)
   i. Dosage is 0.03–0.1 mcg/kg/min IV; increase or decrease by 0.05–0.1 mcg/kg/min no sooner than every 15 min
      (a) Administer for up to 48 hr
   ii. May cause reflex tachycardia, hypotension, and increased intraocular pressure

BIBLIOGRAPHY

Barkley, T. W., Jr. (2014). *Acute care nurse practitioner certification review manual.* West Hollywood, CA: Barkley & Associates.

Czernichow, S., Zanchetti, A., Turnbull, F., Barzi, F., Ninomiya, T., Kengne, A. P., . . . Bruce, N. (2011). The effects of blood pressure reduction and of different blood pressure-lowering regiments on major cardiovascular events according to baseline blood pressure: Meta-analysis of randomized trials. *Journal of Hypertension, 29*(1), 4–16.

Ferri, F. F. (2011). *Ferri's clinical advisor: Instant diagnosis and treatment* (8th ed.). Philadelphia, PA: Elsevier.

Haro, J. D., Bleda, S., Florez, A., Varela, C., Esparza, L., & Acin, F. (2010). Ms481 long-term pleiotropic effect of statins upon nitric oxide and C-reactive protein levels in patients with peripheral arterial disease. *Atherosclerosis Supplements, 11*(2), 206–207.

Himmelfarb, J., & Sayegh, M. H. (2010). *Chronic kidney disease, dialysis, and transplantation companion to Brenner & Rector's the kidney* (3rd ed.). Philadelphia: Saunders/Elsevier.

Hudnut, F. (2013). Comment on "Beyond medications and diet: Alternative approaches to lowering blood pressure: A scientific statement from the American Heart Association". *Hypertension, 63*(1), e3.

James, A., Oparil, S., Carter, B., Cushman, W. C., Dennison-Himmelfarb, C., Handler, J., . . . Ortiz, E. (2014). 2014 evidence-based guideline for the management of high blood pressure in adults report from the panel members appointed to the Eighth Joint National Committee (JNC 8). *Journal of the American Medical Association, 311*(5), 507–20.

Kaplan, N. M., & Weber, M. A. (2010). *Hypertension essentials* (2nd ed.). Sudbury, MA: Physicians' Press.

Kaplan, N. M., Aronson, M. D., Bakris, G. L., & Forman, J. P. (2013). Perioperative management of hypertension. *UptoDate.* Waltham, MA: UpToDate. Retrieved from http://www.uptodate.com/contents/perioperative-management-of-hypertension

Mancia, G., Fagard, R., Narkiewicz, K., Redon, J., Zanchetti, A., Bohm, M., . . . Wood, D. A. (2013). 2013 ESH/ESC guidelines for the management of arterial hypertension: The task force for the management of arterial hypertension of the European Society of Hypertension (ESH) and of the European Society of Cardiology (ESC). *European Heart Journal, 34*(28), 2159–2219.

McPhee, S. J., Papadakis, M. A., & Tierney, L. M. (Eds.). (2014). *Current medical diagnosis and treatment* (46th ed.). New York, NY: McGraw Hill/Appleton & Lange.

Ogihara, T., Saruta, T., Raguki, H., Matsuoka, H., Shimamoto, K., Shimada, K., . . . Valsartain in Elderly Isolated Systolic Hypertension Study Group. (2010). Target blood pressure for treatment of isolated systolic hypertension in the elderly: Valsartan in elderly isolated systolic hypertension study. *Hypertension, 56*(2), 196–202.

Phillips, R. A. (2012). Controversies in blood pressure goal guidelines and masked hypertension. *Annals of the New York Academy of Sciences, 1254*(1), 115–122.

Strom, B. L. (2013). *Sodium intake in populations: Assessment of evidence.* Washington DC: National Academies Press.

Thelan, L. A., Urden, L. D., & Lough, M. E. (2009). *Critical care nursing: Diagnosis and management* (5th ed.). St. Louis, MO: Mosby.

CHAPTER 13

Coronary Artery Disease and Hyperlipidemia

JOAN KING • THOMAS W. BARKLEY, JR.

I. **Definition of Coronary Artery Disease (CAD)**
   A. Partial or complete blockage or narrowing of the coronary arteries, usually as the result of atherosclerosis; coronary vasospasm is also a cause
II. **Incidence/predisposing factors/risk factors**
   A. Heart disease continues to be the leading cause of death for men and women in the U.S.
   B. Coronary heart disease costs the United States $108.9 billion each year.
   C. Responsible for approximately 646,000 emergency department visits each year
   D. Accounts for 4.4 million cardiac procedures annually and 6.4 million hospital discharges
   E. Non-modifiable risk factors
      1. Age: increasing age increases risk
      2. Gender: men are six to eight times more likely to have CAD than premenopausal women; the incidence in postmenopausal women who are unprotected by estrogen is approximately equal to the incidence in men
      3. Race: white men die more frequently from CAD than do men of other ethnic backgrounds; women of other ethnic backgrounds die from CAD slightly more frequently than Caucasian women
      4. Heredity: family history of CAD increases risk
   F. Modifiable risk factors
      1. Smoking
         a. Increases in low-density lipoproteins (LDLs) and decreases in high-density lipoproteins (HDLs)
         b. Smokers have a two to six times greater risk of death from CAD than do nonsmokers
      2. Hypertension—risk of CAD is three times greater when BP exceeds 160/95 mmHg
      3. Diabetes: CHD risk equivalent—uncontrolled diabetes increases risk
      4. Obesity (visceral body fat) (BMI greater than 30) and/or sedentary lifestyle
      5. Increased stress and type A personality
      6. Use of oral contraceptives (especially if the woman is older than 35 years of age)
      7. Hyperlipidemia

a. Elevations in triglyceride level, LDLs, and very low density lipoproteins (VLDLs) are associated with increased risk of CAD
b. Low HDL levels are also associated with increased risk

III. **Laboratory/diagnostic testing**
A. A1c is closely tied with elevated triglycerides (TG)
B. For patients with suspected CAD who present with intermittent chest pain, do the following:
1. 12-lead ECG
2. See Angina and Myocardial Infarction chapter—management of angina/acute MI
3. Stress testing (exercise stress test or thallium/Lexiscan stress test)
4. Hemoglobin A1c as a corollary of triglycerides
C. 12-lead ECG/stress testing
1. Controversy exists regarding screening of asymptomatic patients in terms of resting ECG or stress testing and calcium scoring.
2. Studies have not shown significant differences between asymptomatic individuals with and without CAD.
D. Patients should be screened for hypertension every time they seek any health care.
E. Pulse pressure (systolic pressure minus the diastolic pressure)
1. Studies have correlated an increase in pulse pressure with higher mortality.
2. Recent studies have suggested that the higher the pulse pressure, the greater the risk for CAD.
F. Cholesterol screening that uses a fasting lipoprotein profile (total cholesterol, LDL, HDL, and TG levels) should be employed for all adults beginning at age 20 and at least every 5 years thereafter in accordance with the National Cholesterol Education Program.
G. Plasma lipoprotein testing after a 9- to 12-hour fast
1. Total cholesterol
   a. Desirable: less than 200 mg/dl
   b. Borderline high: 200–239 mg/dl
   c. High: 240 mg/dl or greater
2. VLDLs contain mostly triglycerides and 10%–15% of total serum cholesterol
   a. Normal triglyceride level: less than 150 mg/dl
   b. Borderline high: 150–199 mg/dl
   c. High: 200–499 mg/dl
   d. Very high: 500 mg/dl or greater
3. LDLs contain 60%–70% of total serum cholesterol in combination with HDLs; level is inversely correlated with HDL levels. Primary target of therapy is as follows:
   a. Optimal: less than 100 mg/dl
   b. Near optimal/above optimal: 100–129 mg/dl
   c. Borderline high: 130–159 mg/dl
   d. High: 160–189 mg/dl
   e. Very high: 190 mg/dl or greater
4. HDLs contain 20%–30% of total cholesterol; level is inversely correlated with LDL levels and directly correlated with risk of coronary disease
   a. Low: less than 40 mg/dl
   b. High: 60 mg/dl or greater
5. Historically, goals for patients with diabetes or documented coronary artery disease:
   a. LDL less than 70
   b. HDL greater than 40
   c. TG less than 150

IV. **Lifestyle changes to modify risk factors**
A. Initiate therapeutic lifestyle changes (TLCs) if LDL is above optimal goal
1. TLC diet
   a. Saturated fat less than 5%–6% of calories

CHAPTER 13   Coronary Artery Disease and Hyperlipidemia

      b. Cholesterol less than 200 mg/day
      c. Consider increased viscous (soluble) fiber (10–25 grams/day) and plant stanols/sterols (2 grams/day) as therapeutic options to enhance LDL lowering.
    2. Weight management
    3. Increased physical activity
  B. Smoking cessation
  C. Control of hypertension—see Hypertension chapter
  D. Control of diabetes, including metabolic syndrome—see Diabetes Mellitus chapter
  E. Stress management
  F. Discontinuance of oral contraceptives for women at risk for CAD who are older than age 35; consider other means of contraception
  G. Estrogen therapy may play a role in limiting CAD; however, estrogen therapy is not recommended as a prevention method for postmenopausal women.
  H. Control of cholesterol through modifiable means or via pharmacologic therapy—see section hereafter

V. Management of high blood cholesterol in adults
  A. Acquire a fasting lipoprotein profile after a 9- to 12-hour fast
  B. Identify total cholesterol, TGs, and LDL and HDL parameters
  C. Identify the presence of clinical atherosclerotic disease that confers high risk for coronary heart disease (CHD) events (CHD risk equivalent):
    1. Clinical CHD
    2. Symptomatic carotid artery disease
    3. Peripheral arterial disease
    4. Abdominal aortic aneurysm
    5. Diabetes
  D. Determine the presence of major risk factors (other than LDL) that modify LDL goals:
    1. Cigarette smoking
    2. Hypertension (BP 140/90 mmHg or higher, or patient is on antihypertensive medication)
    3. Low HDL (less than 40 mg/dl). Note: HDL of 60 mg/dl or greater counts as a "negative" risk factor; thus, its presence removes one risk factor from the total count.
    4. Family history of premature CHD (CHD in male first-degree relative younger than age 55; CHD in female first-degree relative younger than age 65)
    5. Age (men age 45 or older; women age 55 or older)
    6. Note: in the Adult Treatment Panel (ATP) III national guidelines, diabetes is regarded as a CHD risk equivalent
  E. The latest American College of Cardiology and the American Heart Association (ACC/AHA) guidelines recommend using the new Pooled Cohort Risk Assessment Equations developed by the Risk Assessment Work Group to estimate the 10-year atherosclerotic cardiovascular disease (ASCVD) risk (defined as first occurrence nonfatal and fatal MI, and nonfatal and fatal stroke) for the identification of candidates for statin therapy.
    1. The estimated risk of ASCVD is based on:
      a. Age
      b. Sex
      c. Race
      d. Total cholesterol
      e. HDL cholesterol
      f. Systolic blood pressure
      g. Diabetic status
      h. Smoking status

2. To estimate more closely the total burden of ASCVD, the current guideline recommends a comprehensive assessment of the estimated 10-year risk for an ASCVD event that includes both CHD and stroke. This is in contrast to the use of an estimated 10-year risk for hard CHD (defined as nonfatal MI and CHD death).
3. To support the implementation of these guidelines, the new Pooled Cohort Equations CV Risk Calculator and Prevention Guideline Tools (web-based) are available at http://my.americanheart.org/cvriskcalculator and http://www.cardiosource.org/science-and-quality/practice-guidelines-and-quality-standards/2013-prevention-guideline-tools.aspx. In addition, links to download apps for mobile-based devices are also available.

F. Identify individuals who may benefit from statin therapy:
1. Individuals with clinical evidence of ASCVD
2. Individuals with elevated LDL-C of 190 mg/dl or higher
3. Diabetics between ages of 40–75 with LDL-C between 70–189 mg/dl but without clinical evidence of ASCVD
4. Individuals without ASCVD or diabetes with LDL-C between 70–189 mg/dl but with an estimated 10-year risk ASCVD of 7.5% or higher

G. Initiate TLC (everyone)
1. Heart healthy lifestyle habits are the foundation of ASCVD prevention. Recalculate estimated 10-year ASCVD risk every 4–6 years for individuals with all of the following criteria:
    a. Age 40–75 years
    b. Not receiving cholesterol-lowering drugs
    c. Without clinical ASCVD or DM
    d. With LDL-C 70–189 mg/dl

H. Initiate drug therapy (adults greater than 21) (see Tables 13.1 & 13.2)
1. High-intensity statin therapy should be initiated/continued as first-line therapy in women and men ≤ 75 years of age who have clinical ASCVD, unless contraindicated.
    a. Moderate-intensity statin therapy should be used when high-intensity statin therapy is contraindicated/statin-associated adverse effects are present.
    b. Individuals with clinical ASCVD who are 75 years of age or older, it is reasonable to evaluate the potential for ASCVD risk-reduction benefits and for adverse effects, drug-drug interactions, and to consider patient preferences when initiating a moderate or high-intensity statin.
2. Adults 21 years of age or older with primary LDL-C of 190 mg/dl or greater should be treated with statin therapy (10-year ASCVD risk estimation not required). Use high-intensity statin therapy unless contraindicated.
    a. Individuals unable to tolerate high-intensity statin therapy, use the maximum tolerated statin.
    b. Reasonable to intensify statin therapy to achieve at least a 50% LDL-C reduction

Table 13.1	Indications for statin therapy	
High-Intensity Statin Therapy	**Moderate-Intensity Statin Therapy**	**Low-Intensity Statin Therapy**
Daily dose lowers LDL-C on average, by greater than 50%	Daily dose lowers LDL-C on average, by approximately 30 to less than 50%	Daily dose lowers LDL-C on average, by less than 30%
atorvastatin 40–80 mg rosuvastatin 20–40 mg	atorvastatin 10–20 mg rosuvastatin 5–10 mg simvastatin 20–40 mg pravastatin 40–80 mg lovastatin 40 mg fluvastatin 80 mg pitavastatin 2–4 mg	simvastatin 10 mg pravastatin 10–20 mg lovastatin 20 mg fluvastatin 20–40 mg pitavastatin 1 mg

CHAPTER 13 Coronary Artery Disease and Hyperlipidemia

Table 13.2	Commonly used medications			
Agents	**Usual Dose**	**Lipid/lipoprotein Effects**	**Common Adverse Effects**	**Comments**
HMG-CoA reductase inhibitors (statins)				
atorvastatin (Lipitor) fluvastatin (Lescol) lovastatin (Pravachol) pitavastatin (Livalo) pravastatin (Pravachol) rosuvastatin (Crestor) simvastatin (Zocor)	See table 13.1	Decreases LDL Modestly decreases TG	Myopathy/myositis, hepatic dysfunction, N/V/D, abdominal pain, HA, insomnia, rhabdomyolysis, diabetes	Many drug-drug interactions Monitor LFT's Consider decreasing when 2 consecutive LDL-C less than 40 mg/dL
Bile Acid Sequestrants				
cholestyramine (Questran)	4 grams PO BID to QID	Modestly decrease LDL Increases TG	Constipation, dyspepsia, bloating, stomach cramps, abdominal distension, obstruction	Several drug-drug interactions Used as adjunct therapy Contraindicated when TG greater than 300 mg/dL Malabsorption of vitamins A, D, E, & K
colesevelam (Welchol)	875 mg PO BID or 3750 mg PO daily with a meal			
colestipol (Colestid)	2–16 grams PO daily or in divided doses			
Fibrates				
gemfibrozil (Lopid)	600 mg PO BID with/before meals	Decreases TG Slightly decreases LDL Possibly increases HDL	Mild abdominal bloating, N/V/D, gallstones, altered taste, rash	Several drug-drug interactions Contraindicated severe hepatic/renal impairment Concurrent use with statins = increased risk of myositis, rhabdomyolysis and hepatotoxicity Monitor LFT's
fenofibrate (Tricor)	48–145 mg PO daily with or without food			
fenofibric Acid (Trilipix)	45–135 mg PO daily with or without food			
Cholesterol Absorption Inhibitor				
ezetimibe (Zetia)	10 mg PO daily	Decreases LDL	Diarrhea, abdominal pain, fatigue, arthralgia	Primary role will be *in combination* with a statin in patients unable to achieve/sustain target LDL levels with statin alone or in patients with contraindication/intolerance to statins Outcome data ??

Agents	Table 13.2	Commonly used medications		
	Usual Dose	Lipid/lipoprotein Effects	Common Adverse Effects	Comments
Niacin				
immediate-release	500–2000 mg grams PO 2–3 times daily MAX 6 grams/day	Decreases LDL Decreases TG Increases HDL	Flushing, pruritus, hyperglycemia, hyperuricemia, ulcers, HA, dizziness, nausea, hepatotoxicity	Take aspirin 30 minutes before dose to reduce flushing Monitor LFT's Combination therapy with statins or in patients intolerant of statins
extended-release	500–2000 mg PO QHS MAX 2 grams/day			

Note. HMG-CoA = 3-hydroxy-3-methylglutaryl-coenzyme A; LDL = low-density lipoprotein; TG = triglycerides; N/V/D = nausea/vomiting/diarrhea; HA = headache; LFT = liver function tests; PO = per os; BID = two times a day

      c. After the maximum intensity of statin therapy has been achieved, addition of a non-statin drug may be considered to further lower LDL-C.
3. Moderate-intensity statin therapy should be initiated or continued for adults 40–75 years of age with DM.
    a. High-intensity statin therapy is reasonable for adults 40–75 years of age with DM with a 7.5% or higher estimated 10-year ASCVD risk unless contraindicated.
    b. Adults with DM, who are less than 40 or greater than 75 years of age, it is reasonable to evaluate the potential for ASCVD benefits and for adverse effects, for drug-drug interactions, and to consider patient preferences when deciding to initiate, continue, or intensify statin therapy.
4. The Pooled Cohort Equations should be used to estimate 10-year ASCVD risk for individuals with LDL-C 70–189 mg/dl without clinical ASCVD to guide initiation of stain therapy for the primary prevention of ASCVD.
    a. Adults 40–75 years of age with LDL-C 70–189 mg/dl without clinical ASCVD or diabetes and an estimated 10-year ASCVD risk 7.5% or higher should be treated with moderate to high-intensity statin therapy.
    b. Reasonable to offer treatment with a moderate-intensity statin to adults 40–75 years of age, with LDL-C 70–189 mg/dl, without clinical ASCVD or diabetes and an estimate 10-year ASCVD risk of 5%–7.5%
I. Identify metabolic syndrome, and treat if present after 3 months of TLC.
    1. Clinical identifications of metabolic syndrome is defined by any three of the following five criteria:
        a. Abdominal obesity: A simple measure of waist circumference is recommended to identify the body weight component of metabolic syndrome.
            i. In men, greater than or equal to 101.6 cm (40 inches)
                (a) Some men with marginally increased waist sizes (e.g., 37–39 inches) may have a strong genetic predisposition to insulin resistance and therefore, may develop multiple metabolic risk factors.
                (b) These patients should benefit from TLC similar to those men with waist sizes greater than 40 inches.
            ii. In women, larger than 88.9 cm (35 inches)
        b. Triglycerides: defining level, 150 mg/dl or above or on drug treatment for elevated triglycerides
        c. HDL: defining levels

CHAPTER 13   Coronary Artery Disease and Hyperlipidemia

        i. Men: less than 40 mg/dl
        ii. Women: less than 50 mg/dl
    d. BP: defining levels
        i. 130 mmHg or greater systolic or
        ii. 85 mmHg or greater diastolic or
        iii. On antihypertensive drug treatment in patient with a history of hypertension
    e. Fasting glucose: defining level, hemoglobin A1c, or on drug treatment for elevated glucose
        i. 100 mg/dl or greater
  2. Treatment of metabolic syndrome; lifestyle interventions and pharmacotherapy, if necessary, should be used to achieve hemoglobin A1c less than 7.
    a. Treat underlying causes (overweight/obesity and physical inactivity):
        i. Intensify weight management
        ii. Increase physical activity
    b. Treat lipid and nonlipid risk factors if they persist despite these lifestyle therapies
        i. Treat hypertension
        ii. Use aspirin for patients with CHD to reduce prothrombotic states
        iii. Treat elevated triglycerides and/or low HDL (as shown below)
J. Treat elevated triglycerides
  1. Treatments for triglycerides of 150 mg/dl or greater:
    a. Primary aim is to reach LDL goal
    b. Intensify weight management
    c. Increase physical activity
    d. Intensify/optimize treatment of DM
    e. Restriction/avoidance of alcohol
    f. If triglyceride level is 200 mg/dl or greater after LDL goal is reached, set a secondary goal for non-HDL cholesterol (total cholesterol minus HDL cholesterol) that is 30 mg/dl higher than the LDL goal.
        i. CHD and CHD risk equivalent (10-year risk for CHD greater than 20%)
            (a) LDL goal: less than 100 mg/dl
            (b) Non-HDL goal: less than 130 mg/dl
        ii. Multiple (two or more) risk factors and 10-year risk of 20% or less
            (a) LDL goal: less than 130 mg/dl
            (b) Non-HDL goal: less than 160 mg/dl
        iii. Zero or one risk factor
            (a) LDL goal: less than 160 mg/dl
            (b) Non-HDL goal: less than 190 mg/dl
    g. If triglyceride level is 200–499 mg/dl after LDL goal is reached, despite aforementioned measures, consider adding a drug if needed to reach non-HDL goal.
        i. Intensify therapy with LDL-lowering drug, OR
        ii. Add nicotinic acid or fibrate to further lower VLDL level
        iii. Because of the increased risk of myositis, rhabdomyolysis and hepatotoxicity, use caution when adding a fibrate with a statin.
    h. If triglyceride level is 500 mg/dl or greater, first lower triglycerides to prevent pancreatitis
        i. Very low-fat diet (15% or less of calories from fat)
        ii. Weight management and physical activity
        iii. Treatment of primary hypertriglyceridemia: fibrates, niacin, or omega-3 fatty acids (see above for risks associated with fibrates and statins)
            (a) Patients not on a statin: gemfibrozil (Lopid) or fenofibrate (Tricor) are the agents of choice
        iv. When triglycerides are less than 500 mg/dl, turn to LDL-lowering therapy.

K. Treat low-HDL cholesterol level (less than 40 mg/dl) if present
   1. First, reach LDL goals, then
   2. Intensify weight management and increase physical activity
L. Treat triglyceride levels:
   1. If triglyceride level is 200–499 mg/dl, achieve non-HDL goal
   2. If triglyceride level is less than 200 mg/dl (isolated low HDL) in CHD or CHD equivalent, consider nicotinic acid or fibrate
M. Complications of CAD—see specific complications
N. Angina—see Angina and Myocardial Infarction chapter
O. Myocardial infarction—see Angina and Myocardial Infarction chapter
P. Congestive heart failure—see Heart Failure chapter
Q. Peripheral vascular disease—see Peripheral Vascular Disease chapter
R. Hypertension—see Hypertension chapter

BIBLIOGRAPHY

Baron, R. (2012). In S. J. McPhee, M. A. Papadakis, M. & Rabow, M. (Eds.), *Current medical diagnosis and treatment* (51st ed.). New York, NY: McGraw Hill.

Berglund, L., Brunzell, J. D., Goldberg, A. C., Goldberg, I. J., Sacks, F., Murad, M. H., & Stalenhoef, A. F. H. (2012). Evaluation and treatment of hypertriglyceridemia: An Endocrine Society clinical practice guideline. *The Journal of Clinical Endocrinology & Metabolism, 97*(9), 2969–2989.

Boumaiza, I., Omezzine, A., Romdhane, M., Rejeb, J., Rebhi, L., Bouacida, L., . . . Bouslama, A (2014). Metabolic syndrome according to three definitions in Hamman-Sousse Sahloul Heart Study: A city based Tunisian study. *Advances in Epidemiology.* Retrieved from http://www.hindawi.com/journals/aep/2014/891297/

Bueche, J.L. (2010). Special topics in adult nutrition: chronic disease nutritional assessment. In J. Sharlin, & S. Edelstein (Eds.), *Essentials of Life Cycle Nutrition* (197–217). Sudbury, MA: Jones & Bartlett Publishers.

Foss-Freitas, M.C., Gomes, P.M., Andrade, R.G.G., Figueiredo, R.C., Pace, A.E., Dal Fabbro, A.L., . . . Foss, M.C. (2013). Prevalance of the metabolic syndrome using two proposed definitons in a Japanese-Brazilians community. *Diabetology & Metabolic Syndrome, 4*(38). doi:10.1186/1758–5996–4–38

Foster, J., & Prevost, S. (Eds). (2012). *Advanced practice nursing of adults in acute care.* Philadelphia, PA: F. A. Davis Company.

Gerstein, H.C., & Punthakee, Z. (2011). Dysglycemia and the risk of cardiovascular events. In S. Yusuf., J. Cairns, J. Camm, E.L. Fallen, & B.J. Gersh (eds.), *Evidence-Based Cardiology* (3rd ed.). Hoboken, NJ: John Wiley and Sons.

Godara, H., Hirbe, A., Nassif, M., Otepka, H., & Rosenstock, A. (Eds.). (2014). *The Washington manual of medical therapeutics* (34th ed.). Philadelphia, PA: Wolters Kluwer/Lippincott Williams & Wilkins.

Griffin, B., Callahan, T., & Memon, V. (Eds.). (2013). *Manual of cardiovascular medicine* (4th ed.). Philadelphia, PA: Wolters Kluwer/Lippincott Williams & Wilkins.

Gunder, L., & Martin, S. (2011). *Essentials of Medical Genetics for Health Professionals.* Sudbury, MA: Jones and Bartlett Publishers.

Ramos, L. M. (2014). Cardiac diagnostic testing: What bedside nurses need to know. *Critical Care Nurse, 34*(3), 16–26.

Stone, N., Robinson, A., Lichtenstein, C., Merz, N. B., Blum, C., Eckel, R.., . . . Wilson, P. (2013). ACC/AHA Guideline on the treatment of blood cholesterol to reduce atherosclerotic cardiovascular risks in adults: A report of the American College of Cardiology/American Heart Association Task Force on Practice Guidelines. Retrieved on December 15, 2013 from http://circ.ahajouurnals.org

CHAPTER 14

Angina and Myocardial Infarction

JOAN KING • THOMAS W. BARKLEY, JR.

I. **Definition/etiology**
   A. Angina means "squeezing and choking of the chest" related to ischemia
   B. Myocardial infarction (MI) is necrosis of myocardial tissue
   C. Pathology—supply/demand mismatch: the demand for myocardial oxygen is greater than the ability of the coronary arteries to supply oxygen

II. **Incidence/predisposing factors/general comments**
   A. Incidence
      1. Heart disease is the leading cause of death in the United States.
      2. One of every six deaths in the United States is caused by coronary heart disease.
      3. Approximately 10 million people in the United States have angina.
      4. Approximately 635,000 Americans will have a new MI each year, and 280,000 will have a recurrent attack.
      5. Each year, approximately 150,000 Americans will have a "silent" MI.
      6. 80% of deaths related to MI occur among individuals older than 65 years
      7. Classically, MI is precipitated by events that increase myocardial oxygen demand:
         a. Physical exertion (e.g., exercise and sex)
         b. Extreme weather conditions
         c. Consumption of a heavy meal (increases the risk by 4 times within a 2-hr period)
         d. Stressful events
   B. Predisposing factors
      1. Coronary artery disease/hyperlipidemia
      2. Hypertension
      3. Metabolic syndrome with increase in measured visceral fat
      4. Obesity (body mass index [BMI] greater than 30 kg/m^2)
      5. Cigarette smoking
      6. Diabetes (type 1 and type 2)
      7. Male gender (more prevalent until age 65 years, then incidence is equal in men and women)
      8. Family history

9. Sedentary lifestyle
C. General comments
1. For ST elevation myocardial infarction (STEMI), national recommendations stipulate that all emergency departments should treat patients with acute MI within 30 min (door to fibrinolytics) and 90 min (door to angioplasty) upon arrival at a hospital.
2. The occurrence of MI and sudden cardiac death peaks between 6:00 a.m. and noon. A significant number of deaths related to MI also occur between 4:00 a.m. and 6:00 a.m.

III. **Types of angina**
A. Stable (chronic or classic)
1. Intermittent chest pain or discomfort with a predictable pattern: the same onset, intensity, and duration
2. Usually induced by exercise, exertion, or emotional upset
3. Pain at rest is unusual. Pain usually lasts 1–5 min, with a maximum duration of 10–20 min
4. May radiate to upper chest, epigastrium, arm, jaw, neck, or back
5. ECG at the time of the angina may show ST segment depression (ischemia)
6. Results from atherosclerotic blockage (plaques) over time
7. Nitroglycerin usually relieves pain. Rest may also relieve symptoms.
8. Angina may be controlled through lifestyle changes (e.g., weight loss, cholesterol control, blood pressure control, and smoking cessation) and medications such as nitrates, β-blockers, or calcium channel blockers. Angina may be controlled without severe complications.
B. Prinzmetal's (variant angina)
1. Precipitating event is coronary artery spasms caused by an increase in intracellular calcium levels
2. Pain often occurs at rest and may last up to 30 min
3. Pain is not usually precipitated by an increase in oxygen demand.
4. Pain may, and commonly occurs in the absence of atherosclerosis.
5. ECG usually shows ST segment elevation at time of the event.
6. Calcium channel blockers are prescribed to manage coronary artery spasms
C. Unstable (preinfarction, rest or crescendo, and acute coronary syndrome [ACS])
1. Chest pain lasts longer than 20–30 min.
2. Pain may be new onset or more severe than with stable angina, and may occur at rest or with low activity levels
3. Pattern of attacks usually progresses with increased frequency, duration, and intensity
4. Pain may radiate to chest, epigastrium, arm, jaw, neck, or back.
5. ECG may show ST segment depression
6. Nitrates are usually insufficient to relieve pain
7. Management includes adherence to ACS protocols
8. Increased incidence of MI within 6 months after onset of angina
D. Microvascular angina (syndrome X/metabolic syndrome)
1. Chest pain mimics angina
2. Exercise stress test is positive
3. No evidence of abnormal angiogram or coronary spasm
4. Postulated defective mechanism resulting in dilatation of the coronary microcirculation

IV. **"P-Q-R-S-T" method of pain assessment**
1. P = Provocative: What activities elicit pain?
2. Q = Quality: What does the pain feel like? Do other symptoms occur simultaneously?
3. R = Region/radiation: Where is the pain? Does the pain radiate? If so, to where?
4. S = Severity: Rate the pain on a scale of 0–10. (Some institutions now use a 0–5 scale.)
5. T = Timing/treatment: When did the pain begin? How long does it last? What did you do to relieve the pain? Were such measures effective?

V. Pain of angina versus MI
A. Generally, anginal pain is more diffuse and vague than pain resulting from MI.
B. With MI, pain may be described as "vise-like"—"crushing" substernal pressure that may or may not radiate to the jaw and/or left arm.
C. Pain from MI may radiate to the jaw, back, shoulders, arms, or abdomen.
D. Other descriptors that patients may use include aching, cramping, grinding, burning, stinging, soreness, tearing, or gnawing.
E. Approximately 15% of patients who experience MI have no pain. Lack of pain is particularly common among diabetic patients and the elderly, secondary to neuropathies.
F. Generally, women who experience angina/MI complain of more gastrointestinal-like symptoms than are reported by men, or complain of pain radiating to the back.
   1. Because women present differently, unstable angina (UA) or MI should be considered appropriate differentials requiring a complete cardiac workup
   2. If the origin of the pain is related to acute GI causes such as esophagitis, gastritis, and gastric/duodenal ulcers, the administration of a "GI cocktail" consisting of Maalox or Mylanta, viscous lidocaine, and Donnatal should provide immediate relief.

VI. ACS: three subclassifications
A. UA: new onset of symptoms, or change in pattern or frequency of symptoms
B. Non-ST segment elevation MI (NSTEMI)
   1. May present with angina, or may be a "silent MI"
   2. Elevated enzymes
   3. No ST segment elevation on 12-lead ECG
C. ST segment elevation MI (STEMI)
   1. Chest pain or angina that is not relieved with nitroglycerin
   2. Elevated enzymes
   3. ST segment elevation on 12-lead ECG

VII. Subjective/physical examination findings of ACSs (UA, NSTEMI, and STEMI)
A. Note: Patient history and physical examination findings are very important for early detection and diagnosis.
B. Nausea
C. Vomiting
D. Diaphoresis
E. Cool, clammy skin
F. Chest pain, usually substernal; in MI, not relieved by nitroglycerin
G. Dyspnea
H. Feeling of impending doom

VIII. Diagnostics/laboratory findings of ACSs
A. Twelve-lead ECG changes
   1. UA and NSTEMI may present with ST segment depression (ischemia)
   2. STEMI will present with ST segment elevation (injury pattern)
   3. Signs of MI progression:
      a. Heightening or peaking of T waves
      b. ST segment elevation
      c. Inversion of T waves
      d. Formation of Q waves
      e. Diminished height of R waves
   4. Note: approximately 30% of patients who experience MI show no immediate 12-lead ECG changes
   5. Hallmarks of ischemia versus injury versus infarction include the following:
      a. Ischemia—T-wave inversion, peaked T waves, and ST segment depression. Note: With angina, cardiac changes usually do not persist once pain has been alleviated.
      b. Injury—ST segment elevation greater than 1 mm above baseline

c. Infarction—may produce Q waves (pathologic) greater than 25% of QRS complex height or more than 1 mm wide (0.04 s)
  6. Expected site of MI based on ECG changes
     a. Inferior: leads II, III, and aVF; diaphragmatic involving the right coronary artery (80%–90%) or the left circumflex artery (10%–20%)
     b. Inferolateral: leads II, III, aVF, V5, and V6; site = left circumflex artery
     c. Anterior: V3 and V4; site = left anterior descending artery
     d. Anterolateral and lateral: leads I, aVL, V5, and V6; site = left anterior descending artery or left circumflex artery
     e. Anteroseptal: V1, V2, and V3; site = left anterior descending artery
     f. Posterior: Reciprocal changes noted in V1 and V3, broad or tall R waves, and ST depression without T-wave inversion may be seen; site = right coronary artery or left circumflex artery
     g. Right ventricular: V4R to V6R (right-sided lead tracing), also associated with inferior infarction pattern and posterior infarction pattern
B. Serum cardiac enzymes (Table 14.1)
  1. Troponin is myocardial specific and is the preferred biomaker for ACS, with Troponin I rising slightly faster than Troponin T (3 hr vs. 6 hr)
  2. Other biomakers include creatine kinase isoenzyme MB (CK-MB) and myoglobin, with myoglobin rising within 1–2 hr and CK-MB rising 4–12 hr
  3. Because of the variability of the enzymes rising, serial enzyme testing is needed every 6–8 hr

Table 14.1	Serum cardiac enzymes			
Serum marker	Earliest increase, hours	Peak, hours	Duration	Other causes of elevation
Troponin T	4–6	10–24	14–21 days	Regenerative muscular disorders, unstable angina
Troponin I	4–6	10–24	5–7 days	100% specific for myocardial necrosis
Myoglobin	2–3	6–9	3–15 hr	Regenerative muscular disorders, unstable angina
CK-MB	4–8	15–24	48–72 hr	Post cardioversion, cardiac myocardial involvement and acute pericarditis with procedures, myocarditis, contusion, cardiac surgical
Total CK	3–6	24–36	18–30 hr	Smooth muscle injury, nonspecific
LD_1	8–12	72–144	7–12 days	Hemolytic and megaloblastic anemias, acute renal infarction, hemolysis, and testicular cancer
Total LD	10–12	48–72	10–14 days	Smooth muscle injury, nonspecific

Note: CK-MB = creatine kinase isoenzyme MB; CK = creatine kinase; LD1 = human heart LD1 isoenzyme; LD = human lactate dehydrogenase isoenzyme. Adapted with permission from "2010 American Heart Association Guidelines for Cardiopulmonary Resuscitation and Emergency Cardiovascular Care, Part 10: Acute Coronary Syndromes," by R.E. O'Connor, W. Brady, S.C. Brooks, D. Diercks, J. Egan, C. Ghaemmaghami, V. Menon, B.J. O'Neil, A.H. Travers, and D. Yannopoulos, 2010, Circulation, 122, Supple. 3 S787-S817. doi: 10.1161/CIRCULATIONAHA.110.971028. Accessed http://circ.ahajournals.org/content/122/18_suppl_3/S787/T.expansion.html , December 16, 2013. Copyright 2013 by the American Heart Association.

C. Laboratory analyses
   1. High levels of C-reactive protein (CRP) or high-sensitivity CRP (hs-CRP) in patients with UA and acute MI are indicators of future coronary events. Higher hs-CRP levels also are associated with lower survival rates; recent studies suggest that higher rates are associated with the reclosure of coronary arteries after angioplasty.
      a. Low risk: hs-CRP level less than 1 mg/L
      b. Average risk: hs-CRP level 1–3 mg/L
      c. High risk: hs-CRP level greater than 3 mg/L
   2. Elevated levels of B-type natriuretic peptide are strongly correlated with myocardial ischemia/damage and may serve to predict severity of future cardiac complications, including heart failure and mortality.
      a. Normal B-type natriuretic peptide levels vary with age and sex, with women having slightly higher normal values.
      b. Mean levels
         i. Ages 55–64 years: 26 pg/ml
         ii. Ages 65–74 years: 31 pg/ml
         iii. Ages 75 years and older: 63 pg/ml
      c. Expected levels associated with MI: 100–400 pg/ml
   3. Complete blood count
   4. Prothrombin time (PT) and partial thromboplastin time (PTT)
   5. Basic metabolic panel (BMP)
   6. Lipoprotein profile

IX. **Management of ACSs**
   A. See figure 14.1 for ACS treatment algorithm. See Table 14.2, 14.3, 14.4 for ACS treatment considerations
   B. Emergency management of ACS with or without PCI
      1. Aspirin, 162–325 mg PO; chew and swallow
         a. If the patient is allergic to aspirin, consider clopidogrel as a substitution.
      2. Nitroglycerin, sublingual 0.4 mg (1 every 5 min); intravenous nitroglycerin may subsequently be used after narcotic administration (e.g., morphine), yet it should be used with extreme caution in patients with inferior MI because hypotension related to dramatic preload changes may occur.
      3. Supplemental oxygen at 2–4 L/min per nasal cannula
      4. Bedside monitor: evaluate potentially life-threatening arrhythmias
      5. Intravenous access: blood for cardiac enzymes and other laboratory values may be drawn at this time
      6. Continuous pain assessment
      7. Pulse oximetry
      8. Twelve-lead ECG within 10 min of presentation
      9. If pain is not relieved, consider morphine (0.1 mg/kg) IV, 2–4 mg, to relieve chest pain or anxiety, and may repeat with 2–8 mg every 5–15 min until pain is relieved unless other adverse effects occur. This completes adherence to national recommendations for the use of morphine, oxygen, nitroglycerin, and aspirin (MONA) in the emergent pharmacological management of ACS.
      10. Admit the patient to the coronary care unit or 23-hr observation unit to rule out NSTEMI or STEMI, pending the results of cardiac enzymes
      11. If diagnosis of ACS is made or suspected, continue immediately as follows:
         a. For hemodynamically stable patients, institute β-blocker therapy. Current guidelines recommend starting oral β-blockers within the first 24 hr of admission. ACC/AHA no longer recommends routinely using intravenous β-blockers.

i. β-blockers such as metoprolol (Lopressor) can be started at 25–50 mg PO and then titrated slowly based on hemodynamics. Maintenance dosage is 50–100 mg BID.
ii. If β-blocker therapy must be stopped, taper dosage over 1–2 weeks before ending therapy.
iii. Consider heparin continuous intravenous drip (e.g., 60 units/kg IV bolus followed by 12 units/kg/hr continuous infusion) to maintain PTT between 1.5 and 2.
    (a) Note: The emergency antagonist for heparin is protamine sulfate. Low molecular weight heparin (e.g., enoxaparin [Lovenox], 1 mg/kg every 12 hr subcutaneously for 2–8 days) may be used as an alternative to unfractionated heparin, especially indicated in patients with NSTEMI and patients with UA. PTT should be monitored for unfractionated heparin and for both unfractionated heparin and Lovenox platelets should be monitored.
  b. Consider the administration of an antiplatelet agent glycoprotein IIb/IIIa inhibitor, such as tirofiban (Aggrastat), in combination with heparin for patients with NSTEMI. Initial dose should be 0.4 mcg/kg/min IV for 30 min and continued at 0.1 mcg/kg/min. Dosing should be continued through angiography and for 12–24 hr after angioplasty. Monitor for bleeding.
    i. Other preparations include abciximab (for PCI only, not ACS) (ReoPro), 0.25 mg/kg IV bolus, followed by 0.125 mcg/kg/min (maximum 10 mcg/min) for 12 hr; or eptifibatide (Integrilin), 180 mcg/kg IV (maximum, 22.6 mg) over 1–2 min, then 2 mcg/kg/min (maximum 15 mg/hr) by continuous infusion for up to 72 hr. If the patient is to undergo percutaneous coronary intervention (PCI), reduce infusion to 0.5 mcg/kg/min and continue for 20–24 hr after the procedure for up to 96 hr of therapy.
  c. Consider continuous nitroglycerin intravenous drip if pain is not relieved by sublingual nitroglycerin and morphine. Begin at 5–10 mcg/min nitroglycerin and titrate up by 5–10 mcg/min every 5 min until either pain is relieved, or if the patient becomes hypotensive (i.e., systolic blood pressure less than 90 mmHg).
12. Consider fibrinolytic/thrombolytic therapy for STEMI (see Fibrinolytic/Thrombolytic Therapy section below)
13. Consider the need for cardiac catheterization/percutaneous transluminal coronary angioplasty (PTCA)/PCI, or coronary artery bypass graft (CABG) surgery
14. Admit to critical care unit for continuous monitoring
15. Following emergent therapy, consider the steps presented in the following section.
C. After an acute ischemic event, consider additional testing.

Table 14.2	ST segment elevation or new or presumably new LBBB: evaluation for reperfusion
Step 1	**Assess time and risk**
Time since onset of symptoms	
Risk of STEMI	
Risk of fibrinolysis	
Time required to transport to skilled PCI catheterization suite	

Table 14.2 ST segment elevation or new or presumably new LBBB: evaluation for reperfusion

Step 2	Select reperfusion (fibrinolysis or invasive) strategy

If presentation less than 3 hr and no delay for PCI, then no preference for either strategy

Fibrinolysis generally preferred if:	An invasive strategy generally preferred if:
Early presentation (3 hr or less from symptom onset)	Late presentation (symptom onset longer than 3 hr ago)
Invasive strategy not an option (e.g., lack of access to skilled PCI facility or difficult vascular access) or would be delayed	Skilled PCI facility available with surgical backup
Medical contact-to-balloon or door-to-balloon is longer than 90 minutes	Medical contact-to-balloon or door-balloon is less than 90 minutes
(Door-to-balloon) minus (door-to-needle) is longer than 1 hr	(Door-to-balloon) minus (door-to-needle) is less than 1 hr
No contraindications to fibrinolysis	Contraindications to fibrinolysis, including increased risk of bleeding and ICH High risk from STEMI (CHF, Killip class is > 3) Diagnosis of STEMI is in doubt

Note. LBBB = left bundle branch block; STEMI = ST elevation myocardial infarction; PCI = percutaneous coronary intervention; ICH = intracerebral hemorrhage; CHF = congestive heart failure. Adapted with permission from "2010 American Heart Association Guidelines for Cardiopulmonary Resuscitation and Emergency Cardiovascular Care, Part 10: Acute Coronary Syndromes," by R.E. O'Connor, W. Brady, S.C. Brooks, D. Diercks, J. Egan, C. Ghaemmaghami, V. Menon, B.J., O'Neil, A.H. Travers, and D. Yannopoulos, 2010, *Circulation, 122*, Suppl. 3 S787-S817. Copyright 2010 by the American Heart Association.

1. Exercise/stress test: the use of a treadmill to monitor ECG changes for signs of ischemia as well as heart rate and BP
   a. Usually requires 10–15 min
   b. A maximal test requires that the patient exercise until at least 85% of the maximum heart for the patient's age is achieved.
   c. Exercise continues until chest pain, fatigue, or other adverse effects are experienced, including the following:
      i. Extreme weakness
      ii. Severe dyspnea
      iii. Syncope or dizziness
      iv. Ataxia
      v. Claudication
      vi. Appearance of S3 or S4 heart sounds
      vii. ST segment elevation or depression of 1 mm or greater
      viii. Systolic BP above 250 mmHg
      ix. Decrease in systolic BP greater than 10 mmHg
      x. Rise in diastolic BP to higher than 90 mmHg or by more than 20 mmHg over the patient's baseline measurement
      xi. "Glassy-eyed" appearance, cold sweats, or confusion
   d. Submaximal tests are usually conducted on patients 4–7 days after MI. Identify patients with reversible ischemia. The stress test is stopped once the patient reaches a specific calculated target heart rate. Usually, the targeted heart rate (THR) is calculated with use of this formula: $(220 - age) \times 0.85 = THR$.
   e. Abnormal results/positive stress test: downsloping or flat ST segment of 1 mm or greater than 1 mm from an originally depressed ST segment.
2. Thallium stress test: use of a radionuclide to detect perfusion of the myocardium

a. Test is conducted similarly to the treadmill test
b. During the final portion of the test, a radionuclide, such as thallium 201, or other tracing preparation, such as technetium-99m teboroxime (Cardiotec) or technetium-99m sestamibi (Cardiolite), is intravenously injected.
c. Patient is then placed on a nuclear imaging scanner, where the myocardium is scanned for distribution of the radionuclide/tracing agent
d. Scan is repeated in 3–4 hr
e. Abnormal results: Light distribution indicates decreased or absent perfusion on the first scan. Defects depicted on the first scan, but not on the second, indicate reversible ischemia. Defects on both scans indicate areas of scar tissue that have resulted from MI.

3. Pharmacological stress test: use of pharmacological agents to increase coronary blood flow in patients who are unable to exercise to the point of reaching their target heart rates.
   a. Drugs of choice to increase coronary artery perfusion include dipyridamole (Persantine) and adenosine (Adenocard). Dobutamine (Dobutrex) is given primarily to increase cardiac output rather than to increase coronary blood flow (i.e., perfusion); subsequently, coronary blood flow will increase.
   b. If dipyridamole (Persantine) is used, thallium 201 is administered approximately 5 min after the intravenous dose, followed by a nuclear scan. Aminophylline, 50–125 mg, is given to reverse the adverse effects of dipyridamole, which may include chest pain, nausea, dizziness, or headache. Two to three hours later, administer a second dose of thallium, then conduct a second scan.
   c. Abnormal results/positive test: downsloping or flat ST segment 1 mm or greater for longer than 0.08 seconds, or greater than 1 mm depression from an initial ST segment depression of the patient's baseline measurement.

4. Ultrasonographic testing—consider the use of the following:
   a. Echocardiogram
   b. Doppler echocardiogram
   c. Color flow Doppler imaging
   d. Transesophageal echocardiogram

D. Outpatient management of stable angina
   1. Nitrates—encourage the use of sublingual or buccal spray (0.4 mg) 5 min before exertion that may cause angina. Consider long-acting preparations such as the following:
      a. Isosorbide dinitrate (Isordil), 5–40 mg PO three times a day (most common)
      b. Isosorbide mononitrate (Imdur, Ismo)
         i. Imdur: 30–120 mg daily
         ii. Ismo: 20 mg PO BID (separated by 7 hr)
      c. Nitroglycerin sustained release, 2.5–6.5 mg every 8–12 hr
      d. Nitroglycerin transdermal patches (Nitro-Dur; Nitro-Derm), which deliver 5–40 mg every 24 hr
         i. Teach patient to take the patch off each morning for a nitrate-free interval—12–14 hr patch-on and 10–12 hr patch-off
   2. β-blockers: preparation/initial dose (dosage range)
      a. Metoprolol (Lopressor), initial dosage: 50 mg in two doses daily, then 100 mg in two or three doses for angina; Toprol XL, 50–100 mg PO each day in one dose
      b. Carvedilol (Coreg), 6.25 mg PO BID, titrating to 25 mg PO BID
      c. Nadolol (Corgard), 20 mg daily; titrate to 40–80 mg daily; maximum dosage is 240 mg daily
      d. Atenolol (Tenormin), 25 mg daily; titrate to 100 mg daily
      e. Propranolol starting dose: 40 mg, and titrate to 180–240 mg per day in divided dosages (TID or QID)

CHAPTER 14   Angina and Myocardial Infarction

   f. Major contraindications: bradyarrhythmias, severe bronchospastic disease, and heart failure
3. Calcium channel blockers are not first-line drugs for patients with ACS. They are recommended only for patients who have normal left ventricular function along with recurrent chest pain but cannot tolerate β blockers.
   a. Diltiazem (Cardizem SR), 90 mg BID (180–360 mg in two doses)
   b. Diltiazem (Cardizem CD), 180 mg daily (180–360 mg daily)
   c. Diltiazem (Dilacor XR), 180 or 240 mg daily (180–540 mg daily)
   d. Diltiazem (Tiazac SA), 240 mg daily (180–540 mg daily)
   e. Verapamil (Calan SR, Isoptin SR, and Verelan), 180 mg daily (180–480 mg in one or two doses)
   f. Dihydropyridine calcium channel blockers (e.g., amlodipine) may be used as adjunct therapy with β-blockers.
      i. Specifically, amlodipine and felodipine are used frequently for angina syndromes as these cause much less reflex tachycardia compared to other dihydropyridine CCBs and appear to preferentially vasodilate the coronary vasculature.
4. Ranolazine (Ranexa) 500–1000 mg PO BID; adjunct therapy for refractory angina with inadequate response to other antianginal drugs (amlodipine, β-blockers, and/or nitrates)
5. If the patient is unresponsive to a single agent, use an alternative classification of agent before progressing to combination therapy.
6. If the patient remains symptomatic, the use of either a β-blocker and a long-acting nitrate combination or a β-blocker and a calcium channel blocker (other than verapamil) combination is most effective.
7. Low-dose aspirin therapy (81–325 mg daily)
8. For patients who do not tolerate aspirin: clopidogrel (Plavix), 75 mg PO daily
9. For UA and NSTEMI, a combination of aspirin plus clopidogrel for 12 months

E. Post-MI outpatient management
   1. See patient for follow-up PRN immediately after discharge
   2. Future visits after initial follow-up should be scheduled every 2–6 months
   3. Consider stress testing 3–4 weeks after MI
   4. Repeat ECG at 3 months, then every 1–2 years thereafter
   5. Continue pharmacological therapy
      a. β-blocker, 50 mg once daily (e.g., metoprolol succinate [Toprol XL])
      b. Continue aspirin therapy, 81 mg daily, indefinitely
      c. ACE inhibitor in patients with left ventricular dysfunction and most patients with Q-wave MI for remodeling (e.g., captopril, 25–50 mg three times a day) is particularly recommended for patients with ejection fractions less than 40% beginning 3–16 days after infarction
   6. Cardiac rehabilitation as indicated
   7. Monitor lipoprotein profiles
   8. Statin therapy-atorvastatin (Lipitor), 80 mg once daily; rosuvastatin (Crestor), 20–40 mg once daily

FIBRINOLYTIC/THROMBOLYTIC THERAPY

I. Definition
   A. Pharmacological process in which agents are used to restore myocardial blood flow through the lysing of clots within the coronary arteries (90% of all STEMI involve a thrombus)
   B. Indications
      1. Preferred mode of treatment for STEMI if PCI is not available within 90 min
      2. Unrelieved chest pain of recent onset (longer than 30 min, but less than 6 hr); variations of this indication have been used, such as administration up to, but not beyond, 24 hr after initiation of pain

Table 14.3	Likelihood of ischemic etiology and short term risk		
Part I	Chest pain patients without ST segment elevation: likelihood of ischemic etiology		
	A. High likelihood	**B. Intermediate likelihood**	**C. Low likelihood**
	High likelihood that chest pain is of ischemic etiology if patient has any of the findings in the column below.	Intermediate likelihood that chest pain is of ischemic etiology if patient has NO findings in column A and any of the findings in the column below.	Low likelihood that chest pain is of ischemic etiology if patient has NO findings in column A or B. Patients may have any of the findings in the column below.
History	Chief symptom is chest or left arm pain or discomfort plus current pain reproduces pain of prior documented angina and known CAD, including MI	Chief symptom is chest or left arm pain or discomfort Older than age 70 Male sex Diabetes mellitus	Probable ischemic symptoms Recent cocaine use
Physical examination	Transient mitral regurgitation	Extracardiac vascular disease	Chest discomfort reproduced by palpation
	Hypotension - Diaphoresis - Pulmonary edema or rales	Palpitation	Diaphoresis
ECG	New (or presumed new) transient ST deviation (0.5 mm or more) or T-wave inversion (2 mm or more) with symptoms	Fixed Q waves Abnormal ST segments or T waves that are not new	Normal ECG or T-wave flattening or T-wave inversion in leads with dominant R waves
Cardiac markers	Elevated troponin I (or T)	Any finding in column B above PLUS:	Normal
	Elevated CK-MB	Normal	
Part II	Risk of death or nonfatal MI over the short term in patients with chest pain and high or intermediate likelihood of ischemia (column A or B in part I)		
	High risk	**Intermediate risk**	**Low risk**
	Risk is high if patient has any of the following findings.	Risk is intermediate if patient has any of the following findings.	Risk is low if patient has NO high-or intermediate-risk features; may have any of the following.
History	Accelerating tempo of ischemic symptoms over prior 48 hr	Prior MI or Peripheral artery disease or Cerebrovascular disease or CABG, prior aspirin use	
Character of pain	Prolonged, continuing (longer than 20 mintues) rest pain	Prolonged (longer than 20 minutes) rest angina is now resolved (moderate to high likelihood of CAD) Rest angina (less than 20 minutes) or relieved by rest or sublingual nitrates Older than age 70	New-onset functional angina (Class III or IV) in past 2 weeks without prolonged rest pain (but with moderate or high likelihood of CAD)

CHAPTER 14 Angina and Myocardial Infarction

Part II	Risk of death or nonfatal MI over the short term in patients with chest pain and high or intermediate likelihood of ischemia (column A or B in part I)		
	High risk	Intermediate risk	Low risk
Physical examination	Pulmonary edema related to ischemia New or worse mitral regurgitation murmur Hypotension, bradycardia, tachycardia S_3 gallop or new or worsening rales Older than age 75		
ECG	Transient ST segment deviation (0.5 mm or more) with rest angina New or presumably new bundle branch block Sustained VT	T-wave inversion 2 mm or greater Pathologic Q waves or T waves that are not new	Normal or unchanged ECG during an episode of chest discomfort
Cardiac markers	Elevated cardiac troponin I or T Elevated CK-MB	Any of the above findings PLUS: Normal	Normal

Note: If High (A) or Intermediate (B) Likelihood of Ischemia. CABG = coronary artery bypass graft; CAD = coronary artery disease; CK-MB = creatine kinase isoenzyme MB; MI = myocardial infarction; ECG = electrocardiography; VT = ventricular tachycardia; S3 = third heart sound. Adapted with permission from "2010 American Heart Association Guidelines for Cardiopulmonary Resuscitation and Emergency Cardiovascular Care, Part 10: Acute Coronary Syndromes," by R.E. O'Connor, W. Brady, S.C. Brooks, D. Diercks, J. Egan, C. Ghaemmaghami, V. Menon, B.J. O'Neil, A.H. Travers, and D. Yannopoulos, 2010, *Circulation, 122*, Suppl. 3 S787-S817. doi: 10.1161/CIRCULATIONAHA.110.971028. Accessed http://circ.ahajournals.org/content/122/18_suppl_3/S787/T.expansion.html , December 16, 2013. Copyright 2010 by the American Heart Association.

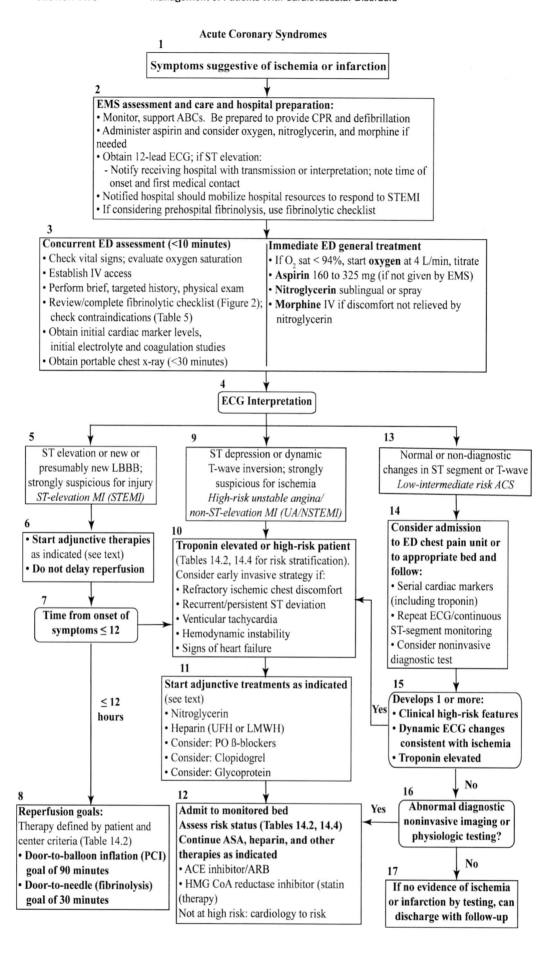

CHAPTER 14 Angina and Myocardial Infarction

Table 14.4	TMI risk score for patients with unstable angina and non-ST-segment elevation MI: predictor variables	
Predictor Variable	**Point value of variable**	**Definition**
Age 65 or older	1	
3 or more risk factors for CAD	1	Risk factors Family history of CAD Hypertension Hypercholesterolemia Diabetes Current smoker
Aspirin use in last 7 days	1	
Recent, severe symptoms of angina	1	2 or more anginal events in last 24 hr
Elevated cardiac markers	1	CK-MB or cardiac-specific troponin level
ST deviation 0.5 mm or greater	1	ST depression 0.5 mm or greater is significant; transient ST > 0.5 mm for < 20 minutes is treated as ST segment depression and is high risk; ST elevation 1 mm or greater for longer than 20 minutes places these patients in the STEMI treatment category
Prior coronary artery stenosis 50% or greater	1	Risk predictor remains valid even if this information is unknown
Calculated TIMI risk score	**Risk of 1 or more primary end points[a] in 14 days or less**	**Risk Status**
0 or 1	5%	Low
2	8%	
3	13%	Intermediate
4	20%	
5	26%	High
6 or 7	41%	

Note: MI, Myocardial infarction; CAD, Coronary artery disease; CK-MB, Creatine kinase isoenzyme MB; STEMI, ST elevation myocardial infarction; TIMI, Thrombolysis in myocardial infarction. Adapted with permission from "2010 American Heart Association Guidelines for Cardiopulmonary Resuscitation and Emergency Cardiovascular Care, Part 10: Acute Coronary Syndromes," by R.E. O'Connor, W. Brady, S.C. Brooks, D. Diercks, J. Egan, C. Ghaemmaghami, V. Menon, B.J. O'Neil, A.H. Travers, and D. Yannopoulos, 2010, Circulation, 122, Suppl. 3 S787-S817. Copyright 2010 by the American Heart Association. [a]Primary end points: death, new or recurrent MI, and need for urgent revascularization.

3. ECG changes—ST segment elevation (in two contiguous leads; 1-mm elevation in limb leads, or 2 mm elevation in precordial leads), Q waves, or bundle branch block
4. Greatest benefit occurs within 1–3 hr of onset of pain; mortality may be reduced by 50%

C. Contraindications (see Table 14.5)
D. Major complication: hemorrhage including intracranial hemorrhage
   a. Twofold increase in risk of intracranial hemorrhage in patients older than 75 years
   b. Increased risk of intracranial hemorrhage for patients weighting less than 70 kg, or patients with severe hypertension
E. Preparations
   1. Tissue plasminogen activator (t-PA) offers less risk of bleeding because it is fibrin specific and will not deplete clotting factors. This can be repeated later in life and is especially effective in the following types of patients:
      a. Patients with large/anterior wall MI
      b. Patients who have undergone previous CABG surgery
      c. Young patients
   2. Reteplase (rPA) is an agent very similar to t-PA, but it has a longer half-life.
   3. Tenecteplase (TNKase) binds to fibrin and converts plasminogen to plasmin
   4. Streptokinase is a synthetic protein derived from group C β-hemolytic streptococci that combines with plasminogen to activate the fibrinolytic process. It can be administered only once in a lifetime because of the development of antibodies, and it is especially effective in the following types of patients:
      a. Patients with small MI
      b. Patients at high risk for stroke
      c. Late treatment (more than 6 hr following onset of pain)
      d. Advanced patient age (older than 75 years)
      e. Young patients
F. Select fibrinolytic/thrombolytic choices (see Table 14.6)
G. Considerations during administration
   1. Observe for signs of tissue reperfusion.
      a. Abrupt pain relief
      b. ECG normalization and/or appearance of Q waves
      c. Reperfusion arrhythmias, especially accelerated idioventricular rhythm, sinus bradycardia, ventricular tachycardia, and ventricular fibrillation
      d. Improved capillary refill and oxygen saturation
   2. Monitor neurologic status for changes related to possible cerebrovascular accident.
   3. Monitor the patient for bleeding (e.g., gums, urine, and bruising), and check therapeutic coagulation values
H. Post-fibrinolytic/thrombolytic treatment
   1. Ensure adequate pain relief via the use of morphine, 4–8 mg IV
   2. For patients who are hypertensive, tachycardic or have ongoing ischemia, consider the short-term use of intravenous β-blockers immediately after infarction, followed by oral treatment when possible.
   3. Nitroglycerin is given for recurrent chest pain; routine administration as a single agent is not recommended
   4. Consider ACE inhibitors after thrombolysis and the use of β-blockers in patients with continuing ischemia despite the use of nitrates

PERCUTANEOUS TRANSLUMINAL CORONARY ANGIOPLASTY (PTCA)/ PERCUTANEOUS CORONARY INTERVENTION (PCI)

I. **Definition**
   A. PTCA/PCI is an invasive procedure whereby a narrow catheter with an inflatable balloon tip is inserted percutaneously into the aorta and up into the coronary arteries under fluoroscopy.

B. The balloon is temporarily inflated to compress atherosclerotic plaque against the arterial wall, resulting in dilatation of the lumen of the coronary artery.
C. PCIs, including intracoronary arterial stents (both bare metal and drug-eluting stents), are commonly used in conjunction with PTCA with the goal of restoring myocardial blood flow (Thrombolysis in myocardial infarction grade 3 [TIMI 3]).
   1. Bare metal stenosis stents are typically used for patients who are at high risk for bleeding, may require surgical procedures within the next 12 months, or are unlikely to be compliant with 12 months of dual antiplatelet therapy.
   2. Drug-eluting stents require 12 months of dual antiplatelet therapy (aspirin and clopidogrel)

II. Indications/criteria for use/incidence
A. PTCA is the preferred mode of treatment for MI only when immediately available to patients (i.e., less than 90 min of arrival in the emergency department), or when fibrinolytics are contraindicated
B. ECG changes, including ST segment depression or elevation, or onset of left bundle branch block (LBBB)
C. Evolving MI
D. Angina (recent onset, or condition is stable yet unresponsive to medical treatment)
E. Adequate ventricular function and collateral circulation
F. Relatively proximal, noncalcified lesions
G. Lesions less than 10 mm in length
H. Lesions not involving a major bifurcation
I. It is estimated that at least 400,000 PTCAs are performed annually in the United States.

III. Laboratory/diagnostics
A. Hemoglobin (Hgb), hematocrit (Hct), and platelets
B. Basic metabolic panel electrolytes
C. Coagulation profile
D. Type and cross match 2 units of packed red blood cells in case CABG surgery is necessary

IV. Special considerations
A. Patient teaching
   1. Chance of necessary CABG surgery if complications occur
   2. The patient will remain awake, receive local anesthesia to the groin, and must lie still.
   3. The procedure is not painful
   4. NPO after midnight (unless emergency)
   5. The patient must keep the leg straight, and a pressure bandage may be used after the procedure has been performed (follow hospital protocol).
   6. The patient will be walking within 4–6 hr after the procedure has been completed.
B. Observe for signs of reperfusion
   1. ECG changes
   2. Pain relief
   3. Other signs of improving clinical status
C. Monitor therapeutic coagulation values after the procedure has been performed (may vary depending on laboratory). Many institutions are monitoring only activated coagulation time (ACT) after PTCA for sheath removal (e.g., ACT less than 175); follow hospital protocol (see table 14.7)
D. Observe for complications
   1. Restenosis may occur in 30%–40% of patients. This is indicated by angina, ST segment elevation per 12-lead ECG, and/or arrhythmias. Emergency repeat PTCA or CABG surgery is warranted in this case.
   2. Contrast dye allergy (evidenced by signs of anaphylaxis; feeling warm or somewhat flushed during PTCA is normal)
   3. Hematoma formation at the groin site
   4. Coronary artery perforation/rupture, embolism, spasms of coronary arteries, and MI are possible

CORONARY ARTERY BYPASS GRAFT (CABG) SURGERY

I. Definition
   A. Procedure in which ischemic areas of the heart are revascularized through a grafting approach from the aortic root to a point distal to the ischemic lesion, using one of the following for the graft:
      1. Internal mammary artery (better for long-term patency)
      2. Saphenous vein
      3. Radial artery
      4. Gastroepiploic artery

II. Indications
   A. Refractory UA
   B. MI
   C. Failure of PTCA
   D. Greater than 50% left main coronary artery occlusion
   E. Triple-vessel coronary artery disease
   F. Left ventricular failure related to heart failure or cardiogenic shock

III. Expectations in the immediate postoperative period
   A. Continuous cardiac monitoring: Atrial fibrillation occurs in 20%–30% of patients, warranting consideration of anticoagulation if it persists longer than 24 hr
   B. Mechanical ventilation: extubation within 2–6 hr, or less in most patients
   C. Pulmonary artery catheter to measure hemodynamic profile
   D. Arterial line for continuous BP readings and laboratory analyses
   E. Pulmonary capillary wedge pressure, maintained slightly higher than normal (e.g., 18–20 mmHg)
   F. Hypotension: If warm cardioplegia was used, maintain BP and mean arterial pressure by volume loading with crystalloids, colloids, or packed red blood cells. Autotransfusion may also be used.
   G. Serum potassium level maintained in the high-to-normal range (e.g., 4.5–5.0 mEq/L; some protocols prefer higher ranges after CABG)
   H. Serum magnesium level maintained at approximately 2.0 mEq/L to assist in preventing arrhythmias
   I. Clotting factors: administering fresh frozen plasma and platelets as indicated for depletion
   J. Mediastinal chest tubes x 2: As a general rule, if output exceeds 400 ml within 2 consecutive hr or 300–500 ml within 1 hr, re-exploratory surgery is indicated. Chest tubes are commonly removed within 24 hr postoperatively as long as significant decreases in bleeding/output are noted.
   K. Epicardial pacing wires x 2 may be used if heart rate drops to below 80 bpm
   L. Nasogastric (NG) tube to lower wall suction for gastric decompression
   M. Foley catheter to ensure adequate (more than 30 ml/hr) urinary output, or per protocol
   N. Common vasopressors, inotropes, vasodilators and antiarrhythmic agents
      1. Vasopressors:
         a. Dopamine (Intropin): used for blood pressure support/hypotension
         b. Norepinephrine (Levophed) is a vasoconstrictor used for severe shock
      2. Inotropes:
         a. Dobutamine (Dobutrex): used to increase cardiac output, thereby increasing blood pressure
         b. Milrinone (Primacor): used to increase contractility and decrease preload and afterload via vasodilatation
      3. Vasodilators
         a. Nitroprusside (Nipride): used for transient hypertension resulting from vasoconstriction related to hypothermia during surgery

CHAPTER 14 Angina and Myocardial Infarction

   b. Nitroglycerin (Tridil): used for coronary and systemic vasodilatation to decrease preload and myocardial oxygen consumption
  4. Antiarrhythmics:
   a. Amiodarone: class II antiarrhythmic, prolongs the conduction through AV node; may be used for rate control in atrial fibrillation (AF) or converting AF to sinus rhythm
   b. Esmolol (Brevibloc): β-blocker used for tachycardia and afterload reduction
   c. Diltiazem (Cardizem): calcium channel blocker used for tachycardia
  O. Monitoring for neurologic changes: Cerebrovascular accidents may occur in 5%–10% of patients. Increased risk is seen in the following types of patients:
   1. Advanced age
   2. African American men
   3. Hypertension
   4. Obesity
   5. Diabetes mellitus
   6. Atrial rhythm disorders
   7. Cardiopulmonary bypass lasting longer than 2 hr
  P. Monitoring for infection: postoperative fever 101.3°F (38°C) or higher warrants suspicion for culture and sensitivity testing of blood, wound, urine, and sputum. Provide antibiotic therapy as indicated (see Infections chapter).
IV. **Potential complications of MI**
  A. Arrhythmias—see Ectopy and Arrhythmia Emergencies chapter
  B. Heart failure—see Heart Failure chapter
  C. Pulmonary edema—see Restrictive (Inflammatory) Lung Diseases and Congestive Heart Failure chapter
  D. Cardiogenic shock—most common fatal complication of MI (see Management of the Patient in Shock chapter)
  E. Pericarditis—see Inflammatory Cardiac Diseases chapter
  F. Infection—especially leg wound, sternotomy, or systemic (see Infections chapter)

CARDIAC TAMPONADE

I. **Definition**
  A. Accumulation of blood and/or fluid in the pericardial space, resulting in a life-threatening decrease in cardiac output
II. **Etiology/incidence/predisposing factors**
  A. Blunt/penetrating trauma to the upper chest
  B. Postoperative cardiac surgical patients or following cardiac catheterization
  C. Patients with pericarditis
  D. Acute MI
  E. May be caused by viral, bacterial, or fungal infections
III. **Subjective findings—unremarkable**
IV. **Physical examination findings**
  A. Beck's triad
   1. Jugular venous distention—rarely present with traumatic injury related to hypovolemia
   2. Narrowing pulse pressure
   3. Distant heart tones
  B. Tachycardia
  C. Pulsus paradoxus
  D. Changes in level of consciousness (e.g., anxiety and confusion)
  E. Oliguria
  F. Other signs of shock
V. **Diagnostics/laboratory findings**
  A. Echocardiogram is used to confirm diagnosis
  B. Chest x-ray may show widening mediastinum
VI. **Management**
  A. Pericardiocentesis

B. Symptomatic treatment of shock (e.g., oxygen, fluid resuscitation, and inotropic agents) (see Management of the Patient in Shock chapter)

IMPLICATIONS FOR THE ELDERLY

I. **General Implications**
   A. The majority of elderly patients presenting with an acute MI either have nondiagnostic ECG changes, or they present with an NSTEMI
   B. Individuals older than 75 years are more likely to have a silent MI
   C. Individuals older than 85 years are more likely to present with LBBB or signs of heart failure
   D. Clopidogrel dose is 75 mg for individuals older than 75 years and who are to receive fibrinolytic therapy rather than the normal clopidogrel loading dose of 300 mg

II. **Management**
   A. Individuals older than 75 years have better outcomes with PCI than with thrombolytic therapy
   B. The risk of a hemorrhagic stroke following thrombolytic therapy is greater for individuals older than 85 years

Table 14.5 Contraindications and Cautions for Fibrinolytic Therapy in STEMI

Absolute contraindications
Any prior ICH
Known structural cerebral vascular lesion (e.g., arteriovenous malformation)
Known malignant intracranial neoplasm (primary or metastatic)
Ischemic stroke within 3 months (except acute ischemic stroke within 4.5 hr)
Suspected aortic dissection
Active bleeding or bleeding diathesis (excluding menses)
Significant closed-head or facial trauma within 3 months
Intracranial or intraspinal surgery within 2 months
Severe uncontrolled hypertension (unresponsive to emergency therapy)
For streptokinase, prior treatment within the previous 6 months
Relative contraindications
History of chronic, severe, poorly controlled hypertension
Significant hypertension on presentation (SBP > 180 mmHg or DBP > 100 mmHg)
History of prior ischemic stroke > 3 months
Dementia
Known intracranial pathology not covered in absolute contraindications
Traumatic or prolonged (> 10 minutes) CPR
Major surgery (< 3 weeks)
Recent (within 2 to 4 weeks) internal bleeding
Noncompressible vascular punctures
Pregnancy
Active peptic ulcer
Oral anticoagulant therapy

Note. Viewed as advisory for clinical decision making and may not be all-inclusive or definitive. CPR=cardiopulmonary resuscitation; DBP=diastolic blood pressure; ICH=intracranial hemorrhage; SBP=systolic blood pressure; STEMI=ST-elevation myocardial infarction. Adapted from "2010 American Heart Association Guidelines for Cardiopulmonary Resuscitation and Emergency Cardiovascular Care, Part 10: Acute Coronary Syndromes," by R.E. O'Connor, W. Brady, S.C. Brooks, D. Diercks, J. Egan, C. Ghaemmaghami, V. Menon, B.J., O'Neil, A.H. Travers, and D. Yannopoulos, 2010, *Circulation, 122*, Suppl. 3 S787-S817. Copyright 2010 by the American Heart Association.

Table 14.6	Fibrinolytic therapy			
	Alteplase; tissue plasminogen activator (t-PA)	**Streptokinase**	**Reteplase (r-PA)**	**Tenecteplase (TNKase)**
Peak effect	45 min	20 min–2 hr	NA	NA
Duration	6 hr–2 days	6–24 hr	NA	Half-life 20 min
Fibrin specific	Yes	No	Yes	Yes
Dosage/Infusion	15-mg bolus followed by 50 mg over 30 min, then 35 mg over 1 hr (not to exceed 100 mg)	750,000 units over 20 min, followed by 750,000 units over 40 min	10-unit bolus over 20 min, repeated in 30 min	Give IV bolus over 5 seconds, using body weight; not to exceed 50 mg Less than 60 kg: 30 mg (6 ml) 60–70 kg: 35 mg (7 ml) 70–80 kg: 40 mg (8 ml) 80–90 kg: 45 mg (9 ml) More than 90 kg: 50 mg (10 ml)
Anticoagulation following administration	Aspirin, 325 mg every day; heparin, 5000-unit bolus followed by 1000-unit/hr infusion (maintain PTT 1.5–2 × control)	Aspirin, 325 mg every day; no evidence shown to improve outcome with use of heparin	Aspirin, 325 mg every day; heparin 5000-unit bolus followed by 1000-unit/hr infusion (maintain PTT 1.5–2 × control)	Baby aspirin, 160 mg + heparin, 5000 units IV, followed by 750–1000 mg continuous IV infusion
Allergic reactions	No	Yes	No	
Reocclusion	10%–30%	5%–20%	Unknown	5%–20%

Note. APSAC = asinoylated plasminogen streptokinase activator complex; PTT = partial thromboplastin time.

Table 14.7	Therapeutic coagulation values	
Coagulation test	**Normal values, seconds**	**Therapeutic values**
International normalized ratio (INR)	0.8–1.2	MI or mechanical heart valve: 2.5–3.5 × normal Chronic atrial fibrillation: 2.0–3.0 × normal, or less than 2.5 × normal if patient is older than age 70 Deep vein thrombosis or pulmonary embolus treatment: 2.0–3.0 × normal
Activated coagulation time (ACT)	70–120	150–190 seconds, or longer than 300 seconds after PTCA/stent application
Activated partial thromboplastin time (APTT)	28–38	1.5–2.5 = normal
Prothrombin time (PT)	11–16	1.5–2.5 = normal
Partial thromboplastin time (PTT)	60–90	1.5–2.5 = normal

Note. MI = myocardial infarction; PTCA = percutaneous transluminal coronary angioplasty.

BIBLIOGRAPHY

American College of Cardiology Foundation/American Heart Association. (2012, December 17). 2013 ACCF/AHA guideline for the management of ST-elevation myocardial infarction: Executive summary. *Circulation, 127*, 529–555. Retrieved December 15, 2013, from http://circ.ahajournals.org/content/127/4/529.full

American Heart Association. (2010, November 2). 2010 American Heart Association guidelines for cardiopulmonary resuscitation and emergency cardiovascular care science. Part 10: Acute coronary syndromes. *Circulation, 122*(Suppl 3), S787-S817. Retrieved December 16, 2013, from http://circ.ahajournals.org/content/122/18_suppl_3/S787.full

Bonow, R., Mann, D. L., Zipes, D.P., & Libby, P. (2011). *Braunwald's heart disease: A textbook of cardiovascular medicine* (9th ed.). Philadelphia, PA: Elsevier Saunders.

Brady, W., Brooks, S.C., Diercks, D., Egan, J., Ghaemmaghami, C., Menon, V., O'Neill, B.J., Travers, A.H., & Yannopoulos, D. (2010). 2010 American Heart Association guidelines for cardiopulmonary resuscitation and emergency cardiovascular care, part 10: acute coronary syndromes. In Robert E O'Connor (Chair), *Circulation 122, Suppl. 3,* S787-S817. doi: 10.1161/CIRCULATIONAHA.110.971028.

Chisholm-Burns, M., Wells, B., Schwinghammer, T., Malone, P., Kolesar, J., & DiPiro, J. (2013). *Pharmacotherapy: Principles and practice* (3rd ed.). New York, NY: McGraw Hill Medical.

Foreman, M., Milisen, K., & Fulmer, T (Eds.). (2009). *Critical care nursing of older adults, best practices* (3rd ed.). New York, NY: Springer Publishing Company.

Foster, J., & Prevost, S. (Eds.). (2012). *Advanced practice nursing of adults in acute care*. Philadelphia, PA: F.A. Davis Company.

Godara, H., Hirbe, A., Nassif, M., Otepka, H., & Rosenstock, A. (Eds.). (2014). *The Washington manual of medical therapeutics* (34th ed.). Philadelphia, PA: Wolters Kluwer Health/Lippincott, Williams & Wilkins.

Goldman, L., & Schafer, A.I. (2012). *Goldman's Cecil medicine* (24th ed.). Philadelphia, PA: Elsevier Saunders.

Griffin, B., Callahan, T., & Menon, V. (Eds.). (2012). *Manual of cardiovascular medicine* (4th ed.). Philadelphia, PA: Wolters Kluwer Health/Lippincott, Williams & Wilkins.

Guy, Jeffrey. (2012). *Pharmacology for the prehospital professional* (Rev. Ed.). Sudbury, MA: Jones and Bartlett Publishers.

Judge, E. P., Phelan, D., & O'Shea, D. (2010). Beyond statin therapy: a review of the management of residual risk in diabetes mellitus. *Journal of the Royal Society of Medicine, 103*(9), 357–362.

Marini, J.J., & Wheeler, A.P. (2009). *Critical care medicine: The essentials* (4th ed.). Philadelphia, PA: Wolters Kluwer Health/Lippincott, Williams & Wilkins.

Marino, P. (2013). *The ICU book* (4th ed.). Philadelphia, PA: Wolters Kluwer Health/Lippincott, Williams & Wilkins.

McPhee, S. J., Papadakis, M. A., & Rabow, M. W. (Eds.). (2012). *Current medical diagnosis and treatment* (51st ed.). New York, NY: McGraw Hill.

Mittleman, M. A., & Mostofsky, E. (2011). Physical, psychological, and chemical triggers of acute cardiovascular events: Preventive strategies. *Circulation, 124,* 346–354.

Parrillo, J. E., & Delllinger, R. P. (2013). *Critical care medicine: Principles of diagnosis and management in the adult* (4th ed.). Philadelphia, PA: Mosby Elsevier Saunders.

Seiden, S. W. (2009). Evaluating patients with persistent chest pain and no obstructive coronary artery disease. *Journal of the American Medical Association, 302*(6).

Urden, L. D., Stacy, K. M., & Lough, M. E. (2009). *Critical care nursing: Diagnosis and management* (6th ed.). St. Louis, MO: Mosby Elsevier Saunders.

CHAPTER 15

Adjunct Equipment/Devices

SHEILA D. MELANDER • THOMAS W. BARKLEY JR.

INTRA-AORTIC BALLOON PUMP (IABP)

I. **Overview**
   A. Introduced in late 1960s, primarily for patients with cardiogenic shock
   B. Classified as an assist device and designed to do the following:
      1. Increase coronary artery perfusion
      2. Decrease oxygen consumption

II. **Indications**
   A. Preinfarction angina refractory to pharmacological therapy
   B. Acute myocardial infarction
   C. Refractory ventricular arrhythmias related to ischemia
   D. Severe mitral valve regurgitation
   E. Severe ventriculoseptal defect
   F. Before or after heart surgery
   G. Low cardiac output states, such as septic shock

III. **Contraindications**
   A. Absolute
      1. Aortic aneurysm
      2. Bypass grafting from the aorta to peripheral vessels
      3. Aortic insufficiency
   B. Relative
      1. Peripheral or central atherosclerosis
      2. Bleeding disorders
      3. History of embolic event
      4. Ethical considerations (e.g., advanced age, severe left ventricular failure, and multisystem failure), weighing the benefits of intra-aortic balloon pump therapy against quality-of-life issues

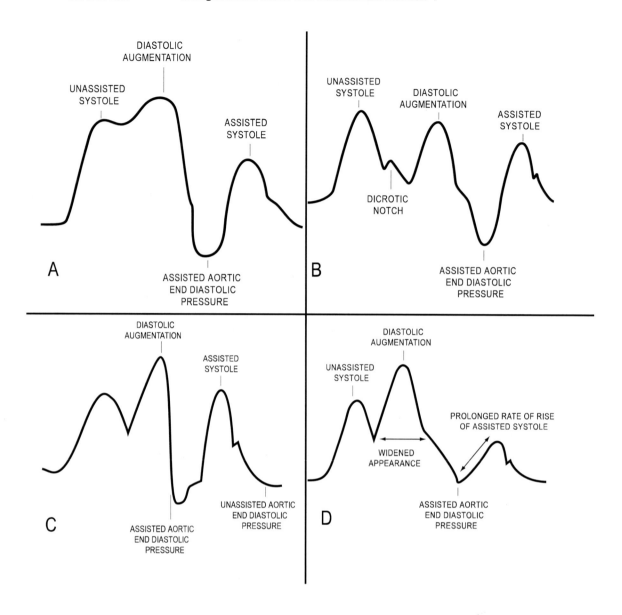

Figure 15.1. Wave form characteristics. (A) Waveform characteristics: inflation of IAB before dicrotic notch; diastolic augmentation encroaches onto systole, may be unable to distinguish. Physiological effects: potential premature closure of the aortic valve, potential increase in LVEDV and LVEDP or PCWP, increased LV wall stress or afterload, aortic regurgitation, and increased MVO2 demand. (B) Waveform characteristics: inflation of IAB after the dicrotic notch, absence of a sharp V. Physiological effects: suboptimal coronary artery perfusion. (C) Waveform characteristics: deflation of IAB is seen as a sharp decrease after diastolic augmentation, suboptimal diastolic augmentation, assisted aortic end-diastolic pressure may be equal to or less than the unassisted aortic end-diastolic pressure, and assisted systolic pressure may increase. Physiological effects: suboptimal coronary perfusion, potential for retrograde coronary and carotid blood flow, suboptimal afterload reduction, and increased MVO2 demand. (D) Waveform characteristics: Assisted aortic end-diastolic pressure may be equal to the unassisted aortic end-diastolic pressure, rate of increase of assisted systole is prolonged, and diastolic augmentation may appear widened. Physiological effects: afterload reduction is essentially absent, increased MVO2 consumption because of the left ventricle ejecting against a greater resistance and a prolonged isovolumetric contraction phase, and IAB may impede LV ejection and increase the afterload. Reproduced with permission from Datascope®. Adapted with permission from "Principles of Intra-aortic Balloon Pump Counterpulsation," by Krishna, M., & Zacharowski, K. (2009). Continuing Education in Anaesthesia, *Critical Care and Pain, 9*(1), pp. 24–28.

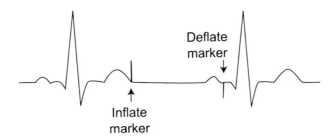

Figure 15.2. Use of timing markers as a reference on th electrocardiogram (ECG) tracing. Adapted with permission from *Introduction to Critical Care Nursing* (4th ed.), by M. L. Sole, D. Klein, and M. Moseley, 2004. Copyright 2004 by Saunders Elsevier.

IV. **Components**
   A. Consists of a thin, polyurethane balloon mounted on a catheter
   B. The catheter is surgically or percutaneously inserted into the patient's aorta by threading it up through the femoral artery into the descending aorta. Note that the coronary arteries originate from the aorta immediately above the aortic valve.
   C. The catheter is connected to a bedside console that shuttles helium into and out of the balloon "in concert" with the cardiac cycle.

V. **Therapeutic effects**
   A. The IABP improves coronary artery perfusion, reduces afterload, and improves perfusion to vital organs.
   B. Inflation and deflation of the balloon are automatically timed with the cardiac cycle.
   C. The IABP inflates during diastole (when the aortic valve is closed). This displaces blood backward, which increases perfusion to the coronary arteries, and also displaces blood forward, which increases perfusion to vital organs.
   D. The balloon deflates just before contraction (systole—when the aortic valve opens). This sudden deflation reduces the pressure in the aorta, decreases afterload, and reduces myocardial oxygen demand. These, in turn, assist the heart during systole.

VI. **Management considerations**
   A. Vital signs and hemodynamics should be frequently monitored.
   B. Ensure accurate timing/pump operation based on any of the following:
      1. R-wave of the ECG (Figure 15.2)
      2. Upstroke (dicrotic notch) of the arterial line tracing
      3. Spike from a pacemaker
      4. Waveform on the balloon pump (Figure 15.3); the following checklist may be used to ensure optimal balloon inflation/deflation:
         a. Inflated at the dicrotic notch
         b. Should see a clear V at the inflation point
         c. Peak diastolic pressure should be greater than or equal to the peak systolic pressure
         d. Should see a clear U reflecting the balloon aortic end-diastolic pressure (BAEDP)
         e. Ensure that the BAEDP is 5–15 mmHg less than the patient's aortic end-diastolic pressure (PAEDP)
         f. Note that the assisted peak pressure is less than the peak systolic pressure
         g. Calculate the end-diastolic dip to reflect the decreased workload of the heart: BAEDP – PAEDP = 5–15 mmHg
         h. Involved leg must be kept straight
   C. Head of the bed should be elevated only slightly
   D. Monitor for complications
      1. Lower extremity ischemia related to occlusion of the femoral artery by the catheter or by emboli from catheter thrombus formation
      2. Displacement of the catheter related to patient movement

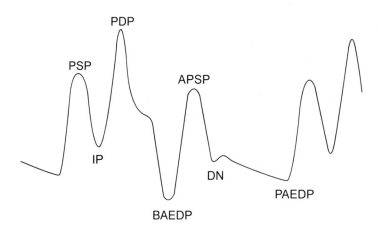

Figure 15.3. Timing the waveform to check for proper timing of counter pulsation. PSP = peak systolic pressure; PDP = peak diastolic pressure; APSP = assisted peak systolic pressure; IP = inflation point; BAEDP = balloon aortic end-diastolic pressure; DN = diacrotic notch; PAEDP = patient end-diastolic pressure. Reproduced with permission from Datascope Corp. Copyright 2013 by Datascope Corp.

       3. Balloon perforation
       4. Infection
   E. Weaning parameters: hemodynamically stable vital signs, including the following:
       1. Normal cardiac index (2.5 L/minute or greater)
       2. Normal mean arterial pressure (MAP), greater than 70 mmHg
       3. Normal pulmonary capillary wedge pressure (6–12 mmHg)
       4. Absence of chest pain
       5. Absence of other signs of inadequate perfusion
   F. Weaning method: either
       1. Decrease the volume in the balloon with each inflation (e.g., in periods of 25% reduction), or
       2. Decrease the frequency of inflation (e.g., from every cardiac sequence to every other, to every third)

VII. Complications
   A. Balloon rupture
   B. Embolus
   C. Arterial occlusion
   D. Destruction of red blood cells caused by the pump
   E. Inability to wean the patient from the pump

PACEMAKERS

I. Definition
   A. Electronic devices that deliver stimuli (i.e., impulses) to the cardiac muscle in an effort to maintain adequate heart rate and cardiac output when the patient's intrinsic pacemaker becomes insufficient
   B. May be used for single (atrial or ventricular) or dual (atrial, ventricular, or atrioventricular [AV]-sequential) biventricular (right and left ventricle) chamber pacing

II. Primary indications—with symptomatic patients or those refractory to pharmacological therapy
   A. Bradyarrhythmias
   B. Heart block
   C. Sick sinus syndrome
   D. Asystole
   E. Atrial tachyarrhythmias

F. Ventricular tachyarrhythmias
III. **Components**
   A. The pacing system consists of a power source, called the pulse generator, which senses the patient's intrinsic cardiac activity and delivers stimuli to the cardiac muscle on the basis of the patient's intrinsic cardiac activity.
   B. The pacemaker contains a unipolar or bipolar lead/electrode catheter that is placed in the right atrium or right or left ventricle, in contact with the endocardium.
   C. The tip of the lead/electrode makes contact with the cardiac muscle and is responsible for transferring electrical stimuli from the pulse generator to the heart.
   D. Temporary pacemakers usually have a pulse generator that is external to the body, but the pulse generator of permanent pacemakers is usually internal.
IV. **Operational definitions**
   A. Capture—a process that occurs when the pulse generator's delivered impulse/stimulus is adequate to depolarize cardiac muscle
      1. A single-chamber pacemaker will depolarize the atrium or the ventricle, resulting in a large P-wave (atrial) or a large QRS complex (ventricular), following the respective pacing artifact (Figure 15.4).
      2. A dual-chamber pacemaker will depolarize the right atrium and the right ventricle as needed (Figure 15.5).
   B. Spike/artifact—vertical line that is seen before the P-wave or the QRS complex, indicating pacemaker firing (i.e., before the P-wave [atrial pacemaker] and before the QRS complex [ventricular pacemaker])
   C. Sensing—activity that occurs when the pacemaker recognizes intrinsic electrical activity of the heart; the pacemaker then "resets" the timing mechanism, resulting in inhibition of the pacing stimulus
      1. Sensing is designed to prevent potentially life-threatening competition between the artificial pacemaker and the patient's intrinsic pacemaker.
   D. Rate responsiveness—refers to a special modulation that enables the pacemaker to increase or decrease the rate of firing as needed
   E. Programmability—ability to painlessly and noninvasively change pacemaker settings or parameters on the basis of the patient's needs
   F. Programmable settings/parameters—it is possible to program three settings/parameters in all pacemakers
      1. Rate—number of times each minute that the pacemaker will fire if the patient's intrinsic rate drops to less than the set rate
      2. Energy output (mA)—strength of electrical current needed to depolarize the myocardium, usually set at 2–3 times the pacemaker threshold
      3. Sensitivity (mV)—adjustment of the amplitude of myocardial electrical impulses that the pacemaker can detect; reflects the ability of the pacemaker to detect the patient's intrinsic cardiac activity; usually set at a low number (e.g., 2–3 mV); the lower the number, the more sensitive the pacemaker
   G. Additional settings/parameters for dual-chamber pacemakers
      1. AV interval—milliseconds of time between the beginning of atrial depolarization and the beginning of ventricular depolarization caused by the pacemaker; the usual setting is 120–200 ms
      2. Maximum rate—upper limit of how fast the ventricle can be paced to accompany atrial activity
      3. Atrial refractory period—millisecond interval denoting when the pacemaker will not respond to the patient's atrial activity
V. **Types of pacemakers**
   A. Four basic types of pacemakers are available:

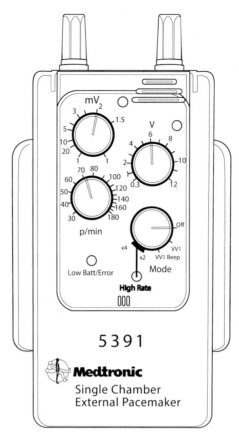

Figure 15.4. Medtronic single-chamber pacemaker, model 5391. Adapted with permission. Copyright 2014 by Medtronic.

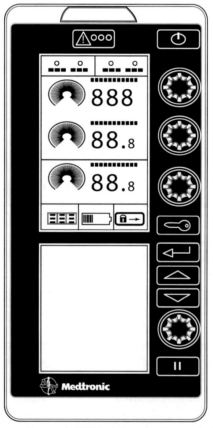

Figure 15.5. Medtronic dual-chamber pacemaker, model 5392. Adapted with permission. Copyright 2014 by Medtronic.

1. Transcutaneous—external pacemaker used to produce ventricular pacing; indicated in cardiac emergencies such as severe bradycardia and asystole; temporary
   a. An anterior and a posterior electrode (pad) are placed on the thorax.
   b. Sedation is warranted because of painful chest wall stimulation
   c. Rate, energy output, and sensitivity are programmable
2. Transthoracic—temporary ventricular pacemaker used only as a "last resort" during cardiac emergencies such as asystole; requires a subxiphoid insertion via a long needle into the right ventricle, through which a pacing wire is threaded to the endocardium
3. Transvenous—most common type of pacemaker used permanently, yet may be used temporarily; produces atrial, ventricular, or AV-sequential pacing.
   a. The pulse generator is implanted under the skin, usually in the upper chest; the lead is inserted via the subclavian vein into the right atrium and the right ventricle.
4. Epicardial—commonly used after cardiac surgery; leads are sewn lightly to the epicardium and appear externally on the chest through puncture sites; leads are "grounded" with the use of some form of rubber, such as a glove or a glass test tube with a rubber cap
   a. Use is discontinued several days after cardiac surgery is performed
B. Description codes—each type of pacemaker is programmed by means of a five-position generic code, although the first three letters are most commonly used. Each letter in the code has a special meaning (Table 15.1).
   1. I: chamber paced
   2. II: chamber sensed
   3. III: mode of response
   4. IV: programmable functions
   5. V: special tachyarrhythmia functions
      a. AAI: atrial pacing, atrial sensing, and inhibited by atrial activity (i.e., P-waves)
      b. VVI: ventricular pacing, ventricular sensing, and inhibited by ventricular activity (i.e., QRS complexes)
      c. DDD: atrial and ventricular pacing, atrial and ventricular sensing, and inhibited by responses from the atria or the ventricles

VI. Operation and threshold measurement
A. Pacemaker settings—Table 15.2 shows settings that should be checked for each type of pulse generator or pacing mode
B. Measuring the pacing threshold—to ascertain the smallest number of milliamperes needed for depolarization
   1. The rate should be set on demand mode and at approximately 10 beats per minute faster than the patient's intrinsic rate
   2. Check the ECG for 1:1 capturing (i.e., QRS complex and T-wave after every pacemaker spike)
   3. Check the pace indicator on the pulse generator—it should be flashing at the set rate
   4. Decrease the milliampere output slowly until a loss of capture occurs (i.e., spike occurs without a QRS complex or T-wave following it)
   5. Then slowly increase the milliampere output until capturing returns, and note the setting at that time
   6. The resulting setting is indicative of the pacing threshold
   7. Increase the milliampere output to two to three times the pacing threshold
   8. Return the rate to the original setting
   9. Repeat this process to determine the atrial pacing threshold by changing the atrial mA output setting; capture will be seen by a P-wave following the atrial pacemaker spike
C. Measuring the sensing threshold—to ascertain a measurement of the smallest electrical impulse (millivolt) that the pacemaker can detect

Table 15.1	Five-Position Generic (NASPE/BPEG) Pacemaker Code			
I. Chamber Paced	II. Chamber Sensed	III. Mode of Response	IV. Programmable Functions	V. Special Tachyarrhythmia Functions
O—none	O—none	O—none	O—none	O—none
A—atrium	A—atrium	T—triggered	P—simple programmable	P—pacing
V—ventricle	V—ventricle	I—inhibited	M—multiprogrammable	S—shock
D—dual	D—dual	D—dual	C—communicating R—rate modulation	D—dual

Note. NASPE = North American Society of Pacing and Electrophysiology; BPEG = British Pacing and Electrophysiology Group. Adapted with permission from *Introduction to Critical Care Nursing* (4th ed.), by M. L. Sole, D. Klein, and M. Moseley, 2004. Copyright 2004 by Saunders Elsevier.

1. The sensing threshold is measured to ensure that the pacemaker will sense intrinsic beats and will not fire at the same time.
    a. Adjust the sensitivity to the lowest millivolt number (i.e., most sensitive setting)
    b. Adjust the rate to 10 pulses less than the patient's intrinsic rate
        i. Note: do not perform this procedure if the patient's intrinsic rate is unsatisfactory
    c. The pacemaker should not be firing at this time, and the patient's intrinsic activity should be visible on the monitor.
    d. Ensure that the patient can tolerate the new rate
    e. Check the sense indicator on the pulse generator—it should be flashing in concert with each intrinsic beat
    f. Increase the millivolts slowly (i.e., decreasing the sensitivity) until a loss of sensing is indicated, evidenced by a sense indicator that is no longer flashing
    g. Ensure that the pace indicator flashes as the pacemaker fires asynchronously
    h. Then increase the sensitivity slowly (i.e., decrease the millivolts) until flashing of the sense indicator is noted with each intrinsic beat
    i. The resultant setting is indicative of the sensing threshold
    j. Adjust the sensitivity to a setting that is less than half of the sensing threshold, or to the lowest number (most sensitive)
    k. Ensure that the rate is set back at the original position
    l. Repeat this process to determine the atrial sensing threshold by changing the atrial sensitivity; sensing of the P-wave should be noted on the monitor.
VII. Major complications and treatment
    A. Failure to capture—evidenced by appearance of pacemaker artifact without the appropriate complex following the spike (Figure 15.6)
        1. Position the patient on the left side
        2. Assess the chest x-ray for displacement
        3. Reprogram to increase the pacemaker amplitude
        4. Increase the milliampere output to maximum
        5. Change the battery (temporary) or the generator (permanent)
    B. Failure to pace—evidenced by absence of pacemaker artifact when firing of the pacemaker should have occurred (Figure 15.7)
        1. Position the patient on the left side
        2. Assess the chest x-ray for displacement
        3. Distance the patient from possible sources of electromagnetic interference such as MRI scanners and radio towers
        4. Warm the patient if the failure to pace is related to patient shivering
        5. Decrease the sensitivity by increasing the millivolts

6. Change the battery (temporary) or the generator (permanent)
C. Failure to sense—evidenced by random pacemaker spikes/artifacts throughout the patient's cardiac cycle that occur in competition with the patient's intrinsic cardiac rhythm (Figure 15.8)
   1. Position the patient on the left side
   2. Assess the chest x-ray for displacement
   3. Enhance sensitivity by decreasing the millivolts
   4. Use a magnet for a minimum length of time to check pacemaker function
   5. To prevent further competition and potentially life-threatening arrhythmias such as ventricular tachycardia, ventricular fibrillation, and asystole, turn off the pacemaker if the patient's cardiac output is stable
   6. Change the battery (temporary) or the generator (permanent)

Table 15.2 Pacemaker Settings to be Checked for Each Type of Pulse Generator or Pacing Mode

Type of Pulse Generator	Common Pacing Mode(s)	Controls/Relevant Settings
Single chamber	Ventricular demand (VVI)	Rate Output/mA Sensitivity—should be on a low number, not on asynchronous
Dual chamber	Atrial asynchronous (AOO)	AV interval Ventricular rate (will reflect atrial rate in this mode) Atrial output Ventricular output—should be set at minimum level (0.1 mA), as the ventricle is not paced in this mode Ventricular sensitivity—not relevant for this mode
	Ventricular demand (VVI)	Ventricular rate Ventricular sensitivity—should be set on a low number Ventricular output Atrial output—should be set at minimum level (0.1 mA), as the atrium is not placed in this mode AV interval—Note: should be set at minimum level (0 ms), as the atrium is not paced in this mode.
DDD	Atrial demand pacing (AAI)	Base pacing rate Atrial output Atrial sensitivity Atrial refractory (automatic set at 200 ms)
	Ventricular demand pacing (VVI)	Base pacing rate Ventricular output Ventricular sensitivity
	AV-sequential demand (DVI)	Base pacing rate Ventricular output Ventricular sensitivity
	Physiologic pacing (DDD)	Base pacing rate Maximum pacing rate Atrial output Ventricular output Atrial sensitivity Ventricular sensitivity Atrial refractory AV interval

Note. AV = atrioventricular. Adapted with permission from *Critical Care Skills: A Clinical Handbook* (2nd ed.), by B. C. Mims, M. K. Roberts, K. H. Toto, J. D. Brock, L. E. Leuke, and T. E. Tyner. Copyright 2004 by Saunders Elsevier.

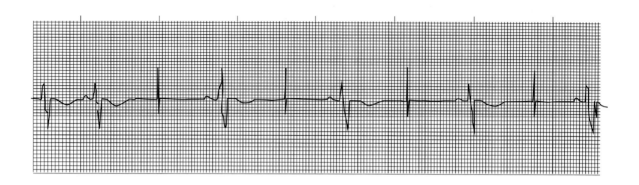

Figure 15.6. VVI mode. Rate = 71; V-V interval = 840 ms. Spikes occur at the appropriate time (the end of the V-V interval), but are not follwed by a QRS complex. The pacemaker is firing appropriately but is failing to capture. Adapted with permission from *Critical Care Skills: A Clinical Handbook* (2nd ed.), by B. C. Mims, M. K. Roberts, K. H. Toto, J. D. Brock, L. E. Leuke, and T. E. Tyner. Copyright 2004 by Saunders Elsevier.

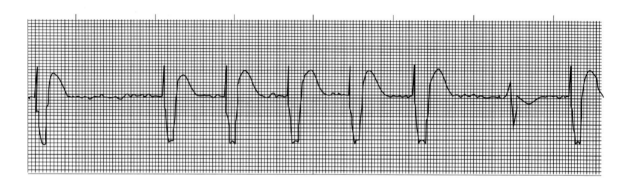

Figure 15.7. Ventricular pacemaker shows two long pauses where the pacemaker failed to pace as soon as it should have.

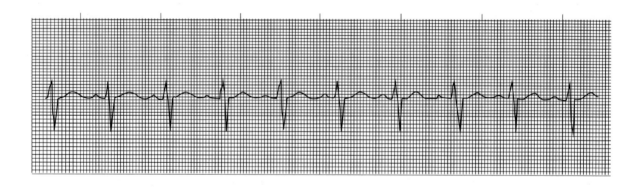

Figure 15.8. Pacing spikes falling at random: failure to sense. From Critical Care Skills: A Clinical Handbook (2nd ed.), by B. C. Mims, K. H. Toto, L. E. Leuke, et al., 2004, St. Louis: WB Saunders. Adapted with permission.

AUTOMATIC INTERNAL CARDIOVERTER/DEFIBRILLATOR (AICD)

I. **Definition**
   A. Electronic device implanted subcutaneously to automatically treat life-threatening arrhythmias

II. **Indications/general comments**
   A. Survival of sudden cardiac arrest unrelated to myocardial infarction
   B. Primary prevention for sudden cardiac death was approved by the Centers for Medicare and Medicaid Services in 2005 to include patients with coronary artery disease and an EF less than 35%, known dilated and other cardiomyopathies with EF less than 35%
   C. Patients with life-threatening ventricular arrhythmias that are refractory to pharmacological therapy
   D. It is estimated over 120,000 people worldwide have AICDs.

III. **Equipment**
   A. The AICD consists of a pulse generator and a lead system, similar to those of a pacemaker.
   B. The pulse generator, designed to last longer than 5 years, is usually implanted subcutaneously in the patient's subclavian area. Older AICDs were placed in the abdomen.
   C. The transvenous lead system is inserted through the left subclavian vein into the right ventricle and then is tunneled and connected to the pulse generator. One ventricular patch is also connected to the pulse generator. Some models have two transvenous leads (that use the right and the left subclavian veins) and two ventricular patches.

IV. **Programmability**
   A. Defibrillation
   B. Cardioversion
   C. Antitachycardia pacing
   D. Antibradycardia pacing

V. **Codes—two types depict the functions of the AICD (Tables 15.3 and 15.4)**

Table 15.3	NASPE/BPEG defibrillator (NBO) code		
Antitachycardia	**Tachycardia**	**Antibradycardia Shock Chamber**	**Pacing Chamber**
O = None	O = None	E = Electrogram	O = None
A = Atrium	A = Atrium	H = Hemodynamic	A = Atrium
V = Ventricle	V = Ventricle		V = Ventricle
D = Dual (A + V)	D = Dual (A + V)		D = Dual (A + V)

Note. NASPE = North American Society of Pacing and Electrophysiology; BPEG = British Pacing and Electrophysiology Group. From Andreoli's Comprehensive Cardiac Care (8th ed.), by M. Kinney, D. Packa, K. Andreoli, et al., 1995, St. Louis: Mosby; and "The NASPE/BPEG Defibrillator Code," by A. Bernstein, A. J. Camm, J. D. Fisher, et al., 1993, *PACE, 16*, p. 1776. Adapted with permission.

Table 15.4	NASPE/BPEG defribillator (NBD) code, short form
ICD-S	ICD with schock capability only
ICD-B	ICD with bradycardia pacing, as well as shock
ICD-T	ICD with tachycardia (and bradycardia) pacing, as well as shock

Note. NASPE = North American Society of Pacing and Electrophysiology; BPEG = British Pacing and Electrophysiology Group; ICD = internal cardioverter-defibrillator. From Andreoli's Comprehensive Cardiac Care (8th ed.), by M. Kinney, D. Packa, K. Andreoli, et al., 1995, St. Louis: Mosby; and "The NASPE/BPEG Defibrillator Code," by A. Bernstein, A. J. Camm, J. D. Fisher, et al., 1993, PACE, 16, p. 1776. Adapted with permission.

VI. Patient teaching
   A. Document device-related events
   B. Maintain MedicAlert identification
   C. Families and significant others should be trained in cardiopulmonary resuscitation
   D. Magnets may activate or deactivate the device. Monitor for tones emitted from the device that signal deactivation after exposure to external magnets

BIBLIOGRAPHY

Birnie, D. H., Healey, J. S., Wells, G. A., Verma, A., Tang, A. S., Krahn, A. D., . . . Essebag, V. (2013). Pacemaker or defibrillator surgery without interruption of anticoagulation. *New England Journal of Medicine, 368*(22), 2084–2093. doi:10.1056/NEJMoa1302946

Braunschweig, F., Boriani, G., Bauer, A., Hatala, R., Herrmann-Lingen, C., Kautzner, J., . . . Schalij, M. J. (2010). Management of patients receiving implantable cardiac defibrillator shocks: Recommendations for acute and long-term patient management. *Europace, 12*(12), 1673–1690. doi:10.1093/europace/euq316

Centers for Medicare and Medicaid Services. (2005). *NCD for Implantable Automatic Defibrillator. CMS Manual System*. Retrieved from http://www.cms.gov/medicare-coverage-database/details/ncd-details.aspx?NCDId=110&ncdver=3&IsPopup=y&NCAId=102&NcaName=Implantable+Defibrillators+-+Clinical+Trials&bc=AAAAAAAAIAAA&

Epstein, A. E., DiMarco, J. P., Ellenbogen, K. A., Estes, N. A. M., III, Freedman, R. A., Gettes, L. S., . . . Varosy, M.D. (2013). 2012 ACCF/AHA/HRS focused update incorporated into the ACCF/AHA/HRS 2008 guidelines for device-based therapy of cardiac rhythm abnormalities. *Journal of the American College of Cardiology, 61*(3), e6–75.

Goldberger, J. J., Buxton, A. E., Cain, M., Costantini, O., Exner, D. V., Knight, B. P., . . . Zipes, D. P. (2011). Risk stratification for arrhythmic sudden cardiac death: Identifying the roadblocks. *Circulation, 123*(21), 2423–2430.

Healey, J. S., Connolly, S. J., Gold, M. R., Israel, C. W., Van Gelder, I. C., Capucci, A., . . . ASSERT Investigators. (2012). Subclinical atrial fibrillation and risk of stroke. *New England Journal of Medicine, 366*(2), 120–129. doi:10.1056/nejmoa1105575

Hillis, L. D., Smth, P. K., Anderson, J. L., Bittl, J. A., Bridges, C. R., Byrne, J. G., . . . Winniford, M. D. (2011). 2011 ACCF/AHA guideline for coronary artery bypass graft surgery. A report of the American College of Cardiology Foundation/American Heart Association Task Force on Practice Guidelines. Developed in collaboration with the American Association for Thoracic Surgery, Society of Cardiovascular Anesthesiologists, and Society of Thoracic Surgeons. *Journal of the American College of Cardiology, 58*(24), 123–210.

Kushner, F. G., Hand, M., Smith, S. C., Jr., King, S. B., III, Anderson, J. L., Antman, E. M., . . . American College of Cardiology Foundation/American Heart Association Task Force on Practice Guidelines. (2009). 2009 focused updates: ACC/AHA guidelines for the management of patients with ST-elevation myocardial infarction (updating the 2004 guideline and 2007 focused update) and ACC/AHA/SCAI guidelines on percutaneous coronary intervention (updating the 2005 guideline and 2007 focused update) a report of the American College of Cardiology Foundation/American Heart Association Task Force on Practice Guidelines. *Circulation, 120*(22), 2271–2306. doi:10.1161/circulationaha.109.192663

Krishna, M., & Zacharowski, K. (2009). Principles of intra-aortic balloon pump counterpulsation. *Continuing Education in Anaesthesia, Critical Care and Pain, 9*(1), 24–28. doi:10.1093/bjaceaccp/mkn051

Perera, D., Stables, R., Thomas, M., Booth, J., Pitt, M., Blackman, D., . . . BCIS-1 Investigators. (2010). Elective intra-aortic balloon counterpulsation during high-risk percutaneous coronary intervention: A randomized controlled trial. *JAMA, 304*(8), 867. doi:10.1001/jama.2010.1190

Perera, D., Stables, R., Clayton, T., De Silva, K., Lumley, M., Clack, L., . . . BCIS-1 Investigators. (2013). Long-term mortality data from the balloon pump-assisted coronary intervention study (BCIS-1): A randomized, controlled trial of elective balloon counterpulsation during high-risk percutaneous coronary intervention. *Circulation, 127*(2), 207. doi:10.1161/circulationaha.112.132209

Rassin, M., Zilcha, L., & Gross, D. (2009). 'A pacemaker in my heart' - classification of questions asked by pacemaker patients as a basis for intervention. *Journal of Clinical nursing, 18*(1), 56–62.

Theologou, T., Bashir, M., Rengarajan, A., Khan, O., Spyt, T., Richens, D., & Field, M. (2011). Preoperative intra aortic balloon pumps in patients undergoing coronary artery bypass grafting. *Cochrane Database of Systematic Reviews, 19*(1). doi:10.1002/14651858.cd004472.pub3

Zipes, D. P., Camm, A. J., Borggrefe, M., Buxton, A. E., Chaitman, B., Fromer, M., . . . Tracy, C. (2006). ACC/AHA/ESC 2006 guidelines for management of patients with ventricular arrhythmias and the prevention of sudden cardiac death: A report of the American College of Cardiology/American Heart Association Task Force and the European Society of Cardiology Committee for Practice Guidelines (writing committee to develop guidelines for management of patients with ventricular arrhythmias and the prevention of sudden cardiac death). *Circulation*, 114, e385–e484. doi:10.1161/circulationaha.106.178233

CHAPTER 16

Peripheral Vascular Disease

THERESA M. WADAS • THOMAS W. BARKLEY, JR.

PERIPHERAL VASCULAR DISEASE: OVERVIEW

I. **Definition/incidence/prevalence**
   A. Definition: disorders of the peripheral arteries and veins
   B. Affects approximately 1:5 adults
      1. Prevalence increases with age; increases 15% to 20% among individuals older than 70 years
      2. Often coexists with other atherosclerotic disorders
   C. Includes two categories of disease:
      1. Peripheral arterial disease (PAD) or peripheral arterial occlusive disease (PAOD)
      2. Chronic venous insufficiency (CVI)

II. **Etiology/predisposing factors**
   A. Same as for coronary artery disease (see Coronary Artery Disease and Hyperlipidemia chapter)
   B. Strongest associations demonstrated with diabetes mellitus and smoking
   C. More common in the lower extremities than in the upper extremities because of the higher incidence of obstructive lesions in this region

III. **Peripheral arterial disease**
   A. Subjective/physical exam findings
      1. Only half of men and a quarter of women have symptoms or recognize their symptoms
      2. The six P's:
         a. Pain-intermittent claudication (i.e., pain to calf, thigh, or buttock)
         b. Pallor
         c. Pulse absent or diminished distal to the obstruction
         d. Paresthesias
         e. Paralysis
         f. Poikilothermia
      3. Presence of bruits over the narrowed artery
      4. Loss of hair on toes or lower legs
      5. "Glossy," thin, cool, dry skin
      6. Reduced skin temperature

CHAPTER 16   Peripheral Vascular Disease

7. Peripheral edema if extremity is kept in dependent position
8. Atypical leg pain is often seen in the elderly.
   a. Limb heaviness, numbness, or soreness

B. Classification
   1. The two most widely used clinical classifications are the following:
      a. Fontaine's (stages of PAD), used in Europe
      b. Rutherford's (categories of PAD), used in the United States
         i. Stage 0—Asymptomatic
         ii. Stage 1—Mild claudication
         iii. Stage 2—Moderate claudication: The distance that delineates mild, moderate and severe claudication is not specified in the Rutherford classification, but is mentioned in the Fontaine classification as 200 meters.
         iv. Stage 3—Severe claudication
         v. Stage 4—Rest pain
         vi. Stage 5—Ischemic ulceration not exceeding ulcer of the digits of the foot
         vii. Stage 6—Severe ischemic ulcers or frank gangrene

C. Diagnostic testing
   1. Ankle-brachial index (ABI): 1.0 or higher in normal individuals and less than 1.0 in patients with PAD; individuals with long-standing diabetes, chronic renal failure, and/or the very elderly often have dense calcified vessels that are poorly compressible, which may result in high ankle pressures and ABI values
   2. Doppler ultrasonography: does not provide visualization of arterial anatomy
   3. Duplex ultrasonography: accuracy diminished in certain individuals such as obesity
   4. Treadmill testing: assesses functional limitations; decline in ABI after exercise supports the diagnosis of PAD
   5. Magnetic resonance angiography (MRA): contraindicated in patients with certain devices, such as implantable cardiac devices, intracranial metallic stents, clips, coils, and other devices
   6. Computed tomographic angiography (CTA): useful for individuals where magnetic resonance angiography (MRA) is contraindicated, such as elderly with implantable cardiac devices; disadvantages include image interference from calcified arteries, radiation exposure, and use of contrast dye.
   7. Contrast angiography: useful in defining anatomy and determining hemodynamic significance of arterial lesions to assist in planning revascularization procedures; associated with risk of bleeding, infection, vascular access complications, contrast allergy, and contrast nephropathy

D. Management
   1. Supportive measures
      a. Meticulous care of feet, which must be kept clean and protected against excessive drying with moisturizing creams
      b. Protective shoes that fit well to reduce trauma
      c. Patient should avoid the use of elastic support hose because it reduces blood flow
      d. Supervised exercise program
   2. Medications
      a. Cilostazol (Pletal), 100 mg PO BID to treat claudication by inhibiting platelet aggregation and inducing vasodilation; contraindicated in elderly with heart failure
      b. Pentoxifylline (Trental), 400 mg PO TID; considered second-line therapy as an alternative therapy to cilostazol (Pletal) to improve walking distance; decreases viscosity and increases red blood cell flexibility

c. Aspirin (acetylsalicylic acid, 81–325 mg daily) or clopidogrel (Plavix, 75 mg daily) to reduce risk of myocardial infarction, stroke, or thrombotic complications; dual therapy can be considered for individuals with increased cardiovascular risk, but not for individuals with increased bleeding risk.
3. Revascularization interventions: indicated for patients with disabling, progressive, or severe symptoms despite medical therapy, for those with critical limb ischemia, and a very favorable risk-benefit ratio
    a. Percutaneous transluminal angiography, stent placement, atherectomy, cutting balloons, thermal devices, and lasers are particularly useful for elderly and frail patients.
    b. Bypass surgery depends on the location and extent of obstruction as well as overall medical condition of the patient; not suitable for those with diffuse arterial occlusions, veins that are not suitable for grafting, and multiple comorbidities
4. Risk factor modification
    a. Diabetes
    b. Smoking cessation
    c. Hypertension
    d. Hyperlipidemia
5. Refer to vascular specialist for patients with progressive reduction of walking distance despite risk factor modification and consistent walking programs for those with limitations that interfere with their activities of daily living

IV. **Chronic venous insufficiency**
   A. Results from venous outflow disturbance of the limbs; may or may not be associated with venous valvular insufficiency and involves the superficial and/or deep venous system of the lower extremities
   B. Subjective/physical exam findings
      1. Dull ache in the leg that worsens with prolonged standing and resolves with leg elevation
      2. Tingling, burning, muscle cramps, sensation of throbbing, or heaviness in affected leg
      3. Restless legs
      4. Fatigue
      5. Dependent edema to the feet
      6. Leg swelling or "tightness"
      7. Increased leg circumference
      8. Shiny, taut, hyperpigmented skin
      9. Brown blotches
      10. Ulcerations or varicosities on legs or feet
   C. Classification and scoring
      1. Clinical, etiologic, anatomic, and pathophysiologic (CEAP) classification schema: characterizes severity based on range of symptoms and signs; includes seven categories that indicate presence or absence of symptoms
      2. Venous severity score: provides a numeric score based on three components:
         a. Venous clinical severity score
         b. Anatomic segment disease score
         c. Disability score
   D. Diagnostic testing
      1. Venous duplex imaging: confirms the diagnosis of CVI and assesses its etiology and severity
      2. Photoplethysmography: assesses the overall physiological function of the venous system; venous refill time less than 18–20 seconds depending on patient's position, indicative of CVI

3. Air plethysmography: measures the components of the pathophysiological mechanisms of CVI; includes the components of reflux, obstruction, and muscle pump dysfunction
4. Phlebography or venography: performed if venous reconstruction is planned or if duplex scan results are inconclusive
   a. Ascending: injection of contrast in the dorsum of the foot with the visualization of contrast traveling up the lower extremity in the deep venous system; determines patency of veins
   b. Descending: proximal injection of contrast in a semivertical posture on a tilt table with the use of the Valsalva maneuver; useful to identify reflux in the common femoral vein and at the saphenofemoral junction
5. Computed tomography and magnetic resonance venography: used to identify pelvic venous obstruction or iliac venous stenosis in patients with lower limb varicosity when a proximal obstruction or iliac vein compression is suspected
6. Intravascular ultrasound: used to evaluate iliac vein compression or obstruction and to monitor patient after venous stenting

E. Management
   1. The specific treatment is based on disease severity.
      a. CEAP Classes 4–6 often require reconstructive treatment.
      b. CEAP Classes 4–6 and Class 3 with edema indicate referral to vascular specialist.
   2. Supportive measures
      a. Elevate legs to minimize edema and decrease intra-abdominal pressure
      b. Compressive stockings
         i. Prescription for elastic compression stockings; tension is based on clinical severity
            (a) CEAP Classes 2–3: 20–30 mmHg
            (b) CEAP Classes 4–6: 30–40 mmHg
            (c) Recurrent ulcers: 40–50 mmHg
         ii. Length: most common is knee length
      c. Meticulous wound and skin care
      d. Weight reduction as appropriate
      e. Review medications for agents that may potentially cause edema (e.g., calcium channel blockers).
      f. Graded exercise program
   3. Reconstructive interventions
      a. Sclerotherapy: used for obliterating telangiectases, varicose veins, and venous segments with reflux; may be used as primary intervention or in conjunction with other interventions
      b. Ablative therapy with radiofrequency and/or laser
         i. Radiofrequency
            (a) Frequently used for great saphenous vein reflux as an alternative to stripping
      c. Complications
         i. Saphenous vein nerve injury
         ii. Deep vein thrombosis (DVT): requires the use of duplex ultrasound surveillance
      d. Endovascular or stent therapy
         i. Indicated to restore outflow of venous system and obstruction relief
         ii. Commonly used with iliac vein stenosis and obstruction
         iii. Close follow-up is required to ensure stent patency
         iv. Surgical treatment indicated for individuals who are refractory to medical therapy; also considered for individuals who are unable to comply with medical therapy
      e. Ligation and stripping, and venous phlebectomy

                i. Used with CEAP Classes 2–6 with superficial venous reflux
                ii. Commonly used with great saphenous vein
            f. Subfascial endoscopic perforation surgery
                i. Ligate incompetent perforator veins from a remote site on the leg that is away from ulcer area
            g. Valve reconstruction
                i. Performed for individuals with advanced CVI who have recurrent ulcerations with severe and disabling symptoms
            h. Valvoplasty: open and closed technique
            i. Refer to:
                i. Vascular specialist: patients with significant saphenous reflux for ablation
                ii. Wound care specialist: patients with ulcers

SPECIFIC DISORDERS

I. **Occlusive arterial disease**
    A. Arteriosclerosis obliterans
        1. Definition/incidence/prevalence
            a. Definition: stenosis or occlusion of arterial lumen that results from atherosclerosis, may be acute or chronic
            b. Increased incidence in men (3:1 male-to-female ratio), commonly between 50 and 70 years of age
            c. Higher incidence among diabetic patients
            d. Prevalence increases with age
        2. Etiology/predisposing factors
            a. Same as for coronary artery disease (see Coronary Artery Disease and Hyperlipidemia)
            b. Strongest associations demonstrated with diabetes mellitus and smoking
            c. CAD is more common in the lower extremities than in the upper extremities (femoropopliteal, popliteal-tibial, and aortoiliac vessels); thus, the lower extremities are most commonly affected
        3. Subjective/physical examination findings
            a. Same as for PAD
            b. Acute limb ischemia
                i. Acute and sudden severe pain, paresthesia, numbness, and coldness of involved extremity
                ii. Paralysis with severe and persistent ischemia; sensory and motor function preserved if sufficient collateral circulation present
                iii. Loss of distal pulse to the occlusion
                iv. Cyanosis, pallor, or mottling of affected extremity
                v. Decreased skin temperature
                vi. Weakened or absent deep tendon reflexes
        4. Diagnostic testing
            a. Same as for PAD
        5. Management
            a. Chronic: same as for PAD
            b. Acute limb ischemia
                i. Initiate anticoagulation with heparin IV immediately
                ii. Revascularization interventions

(a) Intra-arterial thrombolysis with recombinant tissue plasminogen activator (rt-PA) is often effective in management of occlusive arterial disease. This treatment is also indicated when a patient's overall condition contraindicates surgical intervention or when the patient's smaller distal vessels are occluded.
(b) Endovascular clot removal techniques (e.g., percutaneous mechanical thrombectomy)
(c) Surgery: thromboembolectomy

B. Thromboangiitis obliterans (Buerger's disease)
1. Definition/incidence/prevalence
   a. Definition: non-atherosclerotic-inflammatory vasculopathy involving small- and medium-sized arteries and veins in the distal upper and lower extremities caused by an inflammatory, highly cellular intraluminal thrombus
   b. More common in men (ages 20–40 years); rarely occurs in women
   c. Prevalence is higher in Asians and Eastern Europeans
   d. Strongly associated with smoking
2. Etiology/predisposing factors
   a. The etiology is unknown, but it is postulated that the immune system plays a central role in the etiology.
   b. Smoking plays a major role in initiation and progression of disease.
   c. Potential genetic disposition
3. Phases
   a. Acute phase: characterized by acute inflammation involving all layers of the vessel wall, especially the veins in association with occlusive thrombosis; microabscesses in the periphery of the thrombus
   b. Intermediate phase: progressive development of occlusive thrombus in the arteries and veins; prominent inflammatory cell infiltrates within the thrombus, less inflammation in the vessel wall
   c. Chronic phase: end-stage lesion characterized by occlusive thrombus with extensive recanalization, prominent vascularization of the media, and adventitial, perivascular fibrosis
4. Subjective/physical exam findings
   a. Intermittent claudication, particularly calf pain, which often begins in the arch of the foot
   b. Pain at rest
   c. Pain relieved by dependent positioning
   d. Coldness, numbness, or pallor of the extremity or extremities
   e. Absent or diminished pulse, especially distal pulses
   f. Ulcerations
5. Diagnostic testing
   a. Physical examination is the most accurate method for diagnosis
   b. Same as for PAD
   c. Laboratory tests to exclude autoimmune or connective tissue diseases and diabetes mellitus
   d. Transthoracic echocardiography and arteriography to exclude proximal source of emboli
6. Management
   a. Same as for PAD; smoking cessation is the only definitive treatment to prevent the disease's progression
   b. Vasodilators promote vasodilation and may improve blood flow.
      i. Vasodilators, such as α-blockers, calcium channel blockers, and sildenafil may be helpful but have not been studied in prospective clinical trials.

ii. Prostaglandins, administered intravenously or intra-arterially; may be beneficial
  c. Surgical interventions
    i. Surgical revascularization: rarely possible because of the diffuse vascular damage and the distal nature of disease
    ii. Sympathectomy decreases arterial spasm, provides short-term pain relief, and promotes ulcer healing; it is usually performed laparoscopically
    iii. Ilizavor's technique induces neoangiogenesis.
    iv. Spinal cord stimulators are used to provide pain relief and promote peripheral microcirculation.
    v. Stem cell therapy induces angiogenesis.
    vi. Amputation occurs at a rate of 50% for individuals who continue to smoke.

VENOUS DISEASE

I. **Definition**
   A. Condition in which alteration in the character of veins results in thrombosis or decreased venous return
   B. Manifests as superficial thrombophlebitis or DVT
II. **Etiology/incidence**
   A. Stasis of blood (e.g., immobility)
   B. Hypercoagulability
   C. Other
   D. DVT is more common in women than in men.
III. **Superficial thrombophlebitis**
   A. Etiology/incidence
      1. Intravenous cannulation of veins—most common cause
      2. Trauma to preexisting varices
      3. Infection: Staphylococcus, most common cause
      4. Accounts for 10% of all nosocomial infections
      5. One in five cases associated with DVT
   B. Physical exam findings
      1. Palpable, cordlike, and reddened vein (i.e., linear appearance of redness)
      2. Involved area is tender and warm
      3. Absence of significant swelling of the extremities
      4. Fever in 70% of patients
   C. Management
      1. Elevation of affected limb
      2. Warm compresses
      3. Nonsteroidal anti-inflammatory drugs (e.g., indomethacin [Indocin SR]) once or BID
IV. **Deep vein thrombosis**
   A. Risk factors: internal and acquired
      1. Internal: Virchow's triad
         a. Stasis of blood flow
         b. Endothelial injury
         c. Hypercoagulability
      2. Acquired factors
         a. Increased age (greater than 40 years)
         b. Major surgery
         c. Trauma (especially to pelvis or lower extremities)
         d. Malignancy
         e. Lupus anticoagulant

CHAPTER 16   Peripheral Vascular Disease

   f. Female hormones
   g. Obesity
   h. Chronic heart failure
   i. The elderly are particularly susceptible because of limited or restricted mobility and comorbidities; furthermore, 60% of first time DVT occurs in nursing home residents.
B. Physical exam findings
   1. Aching/"throbbing" pain
   2. Tenderness to palpation
   3. Positive Homans' sign (pain upon dorsiflexion of the foot) occurs in approximately 40% of patients
   4. Increased body temperature
   5. Localized edema/swelling distal to the occlusion
   6. Other signs of inflammation (e.g., redness, swelling, fever, and extremity warm to touch) may be present.
C. Pretest probability/laboratory/diagnostic findings
   1. Assessment of pretest clinical probability
      a. Includes nine clinical parameters with scores of 0 points or higher
      b. If the d-dimer is elevated and the score is 3 or higher, duplex ultrasonography is indicated.
   2. Laboratory findings
      a. The d-dimer level may be normal or elevated; 90% of hospitalized elderly have elevated d-dimer levels secondary to infections and tissue damage.
      b. Clotting factor studies
   3. Duplex ultrasonography is used for suspected symptomatic proximal lower extremity DVT; accuracy may be lower for distal DVT, asymptomatic DVT, and upper extremity thrombosis.
   4. Venography is indicated if ultrasonography results are inconclusive, laboratory findings are unclear, and no other explanation for symptoms can be found.
D. Management
   1. Supportive measures
      a. Bed rest with elevation of involved extremity; mobilize as soon as clinically feasible
      b. Local heat to affect area
      c. Compression stocking for acute DVT in lower extremity, use below the knee compression stocking (30–40 mmHg at the ankle)
   2. Anticoagulation therapy may vary from institution to institution.
      a. Unfractionated heparin
         i. Weight-based nomogram: bolus of 80 units/kg ideal body weight, followed by continuous intravenous drip of 18 units/kg/hr
         ii. Fixed dose: 5000 units bolus followed by 1000 units/hr
         iii. The literature supports an activated partial thromboplastin time (aPTT) goal range of 1.5–2.5 x baseline aPTT.
         iv. Disadvantages: higher incidence of heparin-induced thrombocytopenia (HIT), variable bioavailability, bone demineralization, and the need for inpatient treatment
      b. Low molecular weight heparin
         i. Enoxaparin (Lovenox), 1 mg/kg subcutaneous BID or 1.5 mg/kg subcutaneous once daily
            (a) Advantages: lower incidence of HIT; more predictable pharmacokinetics and bioavailability, does not require laboratory monitoring
            (b) Contraindicated in patients with severe renal dysfunction
         ii. Dalteparin (Fragmin), 200 units/kg SQ every 24 hr

iii. Tinzaparin (Innohep), 175 units/kg SQ daily
- (a) May be contraindicated in morbidly obese patients or those with severe renal impairment
- c. Factor Xa inhibitors
    - i. Fondaparinux (Arixtra)
        - (a) Weight based: general dose to 5 mg SQ once daily (if body weight less than 50 kg), 7.5 mg SQ once daily (if body weight 50–100 kg), 10 mg SQ daily (if body weight greater than 100 kg)
        - (b) Advantages: 100% bioavailability, daily dosing, and does not cause HIT
    - ii. Rivaroxaban (Xarelto), 15 mg PO BID for 21 days, followed by 20 mg PO once daily
- d. Warfarin (Coumadin), initiate at time of diagnosis of VTE, typically first dose is 5–10 mg PO daily
    - i. Continue heparin/LMWH/fondaparinux until therapeutic anticoagulant levels are achieved with warfarin. Or administer dabigatran (Pradaxa), 150 mg PO BID once warfarin has been administered for 5–10 days.
    - ii. Monitor international normalized ratio (INR) after initial daily doses of warfarin
    - iii. Adequate oral anticoagulant effect is achieved when INR is at least 2–2.5 (goal INR is 2–3)
- e. Duration of therapy is usually 3–6 months for first time episode and indefinitely for recurrent DVT and/or individuals with the following: cancer, anticardiolipin antibodies, lupus anticoagulant, homozygous factor V, prothrombin (factor II) gene mutation, antithrombin deficiency, protein C or S deficiency, or combination of two or more thrombophilias
- f. Catheter-directed thrombolytic therapy
    - i. Regimens may vary depending on institution, size of thrombus, vessel occluded, etc.
    - ii. Used for thrombosis less than 1 week, extends above the inguinal ligament or proximally in an upper limb, associated with severe symptoms and significant edema
    - iii. Contraindicated if patient has an increased risk of bleeding
- g. Inferior vena cava (IVC) filter: used in patients for whom anticoagulation is contraindicated for prevention of pulmonary embolus, especially elderly, who may be susceptible to frequent falls, or in patients with recurrent DVT despite adequate anticoagulation

BIBLIOGRAPHY

Anderson, J. L., Halperin, J. L., Albert, N., Bozkurt, B., Brindis, R. G., Curtis, L. H., . . . Shen, W. K. (2013). Management of patients with peripheral artery disease (compilation of 2005 and 2011 ACCF/AHA guideline recommendations). A report of the American College of Cardiology Foundation/American Heart Association Task Force on Practice Guidelines. *Journal of the American College of Cardiology, 61*(14), 1555–1570.

Chang, R. N., Wang, S., Kirsner, R. S., & Federman, D. G. (2011). The elderly and peripheral arterial disease. *Clinical Geriatrics, 19*(7). Retrieved from http://www.clinicalgeriatrics.com/articles/Elderly-and-Peripheral-Arterial-Disease

Creager, M. A., & Loscalzo, L. (2012). Vascular disease of the extremities. In D. L. Longo, A. S. Fauci, D. L. Kasper, J. Hauser, L. Jameson, and J. Loscalzo (Eds.), *Harrison's principles of internal medicine* (18th ed.). Retrieved from http://accessmedicine.mhmedical.com/content.aspx?bookid=331&sectionid=40727028

Gloviczki, P., Comerota, A. J., Dalsing, M. C., Eklof, B. G., Gillespie, D. L., Gloviczki, M. L., . . . American Venous Forum. (2011). The care of patients with varicose veins and associated chronic venous diseases: Clinical practice guidelines of the Society for Vascular Surgery and the American Venous Forum. *Journal of Vascular Surgery, 53*(5 Suppl), 2S–48S. doi:10.1016/j.jvs.2011.01.079

Jones, W. S., Schmit, K. M., Vemulapalli, S., Subherwal, S., Patel, M. R., Hasselblad, V., . . . Dolor, R. J. (2013). *Treatment strategies for patients with peripheral artery disease.* Comparative Effectiveness Reviews, No. 118. (Prepared by the Duke Evidence-based Practice Center under Contract No. 290-2007-10066-I.) . Rockville, MD: Agency for Healthcare Research and Quality (US). Retrieved from https://www.ncbi.nlm.nih.gov/books/NBK148574/

Kane, R. L., Ouslander, J. G., Abrass, I. B., & Resnick, B. (2013). Peripheral vascular disease. In R. L. Kane, J. G. Ouslander, I. B. Abrass, & B. Resnick (Eds.), *Essentials of clinical geriatrics* (7th ed.). New York, NY: McGraw-Hill Medical. Retrieved from http://accessmedicine.mhmedical.com.libdata.lib.ua.edu.aspx?bookid=678

Lambert, M. A., & Belch, J J. F. (2013). Medical management of critical limb ischemia: Where do we stand? *Journal of Internal Medicine, 274*, 295–307. doi:10.1111/joim.12102

Piazza, G., & Creager, M. A. (2010). Thromboangiitis obliterans. *Circulation, 121,* 1858–1861.

Rapp, J. H., Owens, C. D., & Johnson M. D. (2014). Blood vessel & lymphatic disorders. In M. A. Papadakis, S. J. McPhee, & M. W. Rabow (Eds.), *CURRENT medical diagnosis and treatment.* New York, NY: McGraw-Hill Medical.

Shanmugasundaram, M., Ram, V. K., Luft, U. C., Szerlip, J., & Alpert, J. S. (2011). Peripheral arterial disease—What do we need to know? *Clinical Cardiology, 34*(8), 478–482. doi:10.1002/clc.20925

Veli-Pekka, H. (2011). *Deep vein thrombosis.* Helsinki, Finland: Wiley Interscience.

Vijayakumar, A. K., Tiwari, R., & Prabhuswamy, V. K. (2013). Thromboangiitis obliterans (Buerger's disease): Current practices. *International Journal of Inflammation, 2013.* doi:10.1155/2-13/156905

Wennber, P. W., & Rooke, T. W. (2011). Diagnosis and management of diseases of the peripheral arteries and veins. In V. Fuster, R. A. Walsh, & R. A. Harrington (Eds.), *Hurst's the heart* (13th ed.). New York, NY: McGraw-Hill Medical.

CHAPTER 17

Inflammatory Cardiac Diseases

SHEILA MELANDER • THOMAS W. BARKLEY, JR.

PERICARDITIS

I. **Definition/general comments**
   A. Acute, painful inflammation of the pericardium
   B. May be mild or life-threatening
   C. May also be subacute, chronic, recurrent, or constrictive
   D. Accurate patient history is of paramount importance in making the diagnosis

II. **Etiology/predisposing factors/incidence**
   A. Viruses: most common cause, especially infections with coxsackieviruses and echoviruses, Epstein-Barr virus, influenza, hepatitis, HIV, varicella, and mumps
   B. MI: affects 10%–15% of patients within the first week after MI
   C. Higher incidence among males
   D. Cardiac surgery
   E. Rheumatic fever
   F. Neoplasia
   G. Radiation therapy
   H. Uremia
   I. Tuberculosis
   J. Idiopathic
   K. Trauma
   L. Other causes, such as drug allergy or autoimmune disease
   M. Acutely affects 2%–6% of the general population

III. **Subjective findings**
   A. Reports of precordial/retrosternal, localized, "pleuritic" chest pain; pain that usually lasts for only a few seconds; patient may report pain under the breast
   B. Pain reports as being intensified with coughing, swallowing, inspiration (patient may complain of shortness of breath), or recumbent positioning; relieved by sitting in a forward position
   C. Fever may or may not be present (underlying cause)

IV. Physical examination findings
   A. Pericardial friction rub—classically heard best with the patient sitting up and leaning forward
   B. Pleural friction rub may or may not be present
   C. Dyspnea

V. Laboratory/diagnostic findings
   A. ST segment elevation: concave ST segment elevation in multiple, if not all, leads mimicking "smiling face"—ST segment elevation is not specific enough for differentiation between AMI and pericarditis
      1. Needs to be noted in multiple leads with smiling face appearance
      2. Elevation will return to normal in a few days; this is followed by possible T-wave inversion
   B. Depressed PR interval: highly diagnostic of pericarditis
   C. Elevated erythrocyte sedimentation rate
   D. Leukocytosis
   E. Consider ordering the following:
      1. CBC (to rule out infection/leukemia)
      2. Electrolytes or basic metabolic profile
      3. BNP (can help differentiate if cardiac or pulmonary in etiology)
      4. Blood cultures (if bacteria/infection is suspected)
      5. Echocardiogram (to confirm pericardial fluid)

VI. Management
   A. Depends on underlying cause (i.e., tuberculous pericarditis or other)
   B. Colchicine (Colcrys), 0.6 mg PO twice a day
   C. NSAIDs
      1. Ibuprofen (Motrin), 600 mg PO three times a day with meals
         a. Preferred regimen, better tolerated than aspirin or indomethacin, less expensive than naproxen and available OTCs
      2. Aspirin (acetylsalicylic acid [ASA]), 650 mg PO every 6–8 hr for 2 weeks
      3. Naproxen, 500 mg BID with meals
      4. Ketorolac (Toradol), 60 mg IV/IM for 1 dose, followed by 15–30 mg IV/IM every 6 hr PRN for pain (max 120 mg/day, not to exceed 5 days)
         a. In adults 65 or older, or those who weigh less than 50 kg, recommended dose is 15 mg IV single dose or 15 mg IV every 6 hr (max 60 mg/day)
      5. Indomethacin (Indocin), 25–50 mg every 8 hr with meals
      6. PPI therapy may be required due to the risk of gastrointestinal toxicity (i.e., pantoprazole 40 mg PO daily)
   D. Corticosteroids—indicated only after contraindication to NSAID therapy or failure of high-dose NSAIDs of several weeks' duration because corticosteroids may enhance viral replication
      1. Prednisone (Deltasone), 60 mg daily
      2. Then, taper and discontinue; lack of taper may cause recurrent pericarditis
   E. Antibiotics—as indicated for bacterial infections
   F. Hydrocodone 5 mg/acetaminophen 325 mg (Norco) PO every 4 hr PRN for pain
   G. Monitor patient closely for cardiac tamponade

ENDOCARDITIS

I. Definition
   A. Inflammation/infection of the endothelial layer of the heart, usually involving the cardiac valves
   B. Endocarditis should be ruled out in any patient who presents with fever of unknown origin and development of a new heart murmur.

II. Etiology/incidence/predisposing factors
  A. Most commonly caused by bacteria
   1. *Staphylococcus aureus*
   2. *Streptococcus pyogenes*
   3. *Pneumococcus*
   4. *Neisseria* organisms
  B. May also be caused by fungi and viruses, especially in immunocompromised patients
  C. Increased incidence associated with congenital heart disease and with valvular disease
  D. Predisposing factors include recent invasive procedures such as dental surgery, genitourinary surgery, the use of invasive catheters, hemodialysis, or burn treatment.

III. Subjective findings
  A. Fever lasting for several weeks
  B. Headache
  C. Weight loss
  D. Fatigue
  E. Night sweats
  F. Exertional dyspnea
  G. Cough
  H. General malaise

IV. Physical examination findings
  A. Fever—medium to high grade
  B. Murmur—may not be detectable in some patients, especially those with right-sided endocarditis
  C. Skin changes
   1. Pallor, purpura, petechiae
   2. Osler's nodes—painful, red nodules in distal phalanges
   3. Splinter hemorrhages—linear, subungual; resembling splinters
   4. Janeway's lesions—macules on palms and soles; rarely observed; smaller than Osler's nodes and not painful
   5. Roth's spots—small, white retinal infarcts, encircled by areas of hemorrhage
   6. Pallor
   7. Splenomegaly

V. Diagnostics/laboratory findings
  A. Patient may have normochromic, normocytic anemia
  B. WBC count may be elevated; always a "left shift" in the differential with band formation
  C. Erythrocyte sedimentation rate is usually elevated.
  D. Microscopic hematuria and proteinuria may be present.
  E. Consider ordering the following:
   1. Blood cultures—most important diagnostic test; perform three cultures from three different sites
   2. Echocardiogram to assess valvular involvement
   3. Basic metabolic panel (BMP)
  F. Duke Criteria bases diagnosis on the following:
   1. Direct evidence based on histological findings, or
   2. Positive Gram stain or culture from surgery/autopsy, or
   3. Two major clinical criteria: positive blood culture of common causative organisms, vegetations/abscesses found on echocardiogram, endocardial damage, *Coxiella burnetii* infection, or
   4. Five minor clinical criteria: fever, predisposing valvular condition/IV drug abuse, vascular phenomenon, immunologic phenomenon, other positive blood cultures, or
   5. Combination of one major and three minor criteria

VI. Management
A. Infectious disease consultation
B. Generally, while results are pending, empiric therapy may be necessary if the patient is critically ill.
C. Empiric therapy
1. Vancomycin dose adjusted to achieve vancomycin trough level of 15–20 mcg/ml (provides coverage for staphylococci [MSSA & MRSA] and enterococci) PLUS or MINUS
   a. Cefotaxime, 1–2 grams IV every 6 hr or ceftriaxone 1–2 grams IV every 12 hr (provides coverage for streptococci [PCN susceptible and PCN resistant], as well as the HACEK and non-HACEK Gram-negative bacilli)
2. When pathogens have been identified and susceptibility data is available, the antimicrobial regimen is adjusted accordingly.
   a. Penicillin-susceptible viridans group Streptococci and *Streptococcus bovis*
      i. Penicillin G, 3 million units IV every 4 hr (12–18 million units per 24 hr), plus or minus gentamicin; dose adjusted to achieve peak of 3–4 mcg/ml and trough of 1–1.5 mcg/ml
   b. Staphylococci (methicillin-susceptible strains: MSSA)
      i. Nafcillin or oxacillin, 12 grams every 24 hr IV in 4–6 equally divided doses, PLUS or MINUS
      ii. Gentamicin dose adjusted to achieve peak of 3–4 mcg/ml and trough of 1–1.5 mcg/ml
      iii. For penicillin-allergic patients:
         (a) Cefazolin (Ancef), 2 grams IV every 8 hr, or vancomycin (Vancocin), dose adjusted to achieve vancomycin trough level of 15–20 mcg/ml
   c. Enterococci:
      i. Ampicillin, 2 grams IV every 4 hr, PLUS or MINUS
      ii. Gentamicin dose adjusted to achieve peak of 3–4 mcg/ml and trough of 1–1.5 mcg/ml
      iii. For penicillin-allergic patients:
         (a) Vancomycin, dose adjusted to achieve vancomycin trough level of 15–20 mcg/ml PLUS or MINUS
         (b) Gentamicin dose adjusted to achieve peak of 3–4 mcg/ml and trough of 1–1.5 mcg/ml

VII. Endocarditis prophylaxis
A. Endocarditis prophylaxis recommendations have been revised and are a major departure from previous AHA recommendations.
1. Infective endocarditis (IE) is much more likely to result from frequent exposure to random bacteremia associated with daily activities than from bacteremia caused by a dental, GI tract, or GU tract procedure.
2. The risk of antibiotic-associated adverse events exceeds the benefit, if any, from prophylactic antibiotic therapy. Maintenance of optimal oral health and hygiene may reduce the incidence of bacteremia from daily activities and is more important than prophylactic antibiotics for a dental procedure to reduce the risk of IE.
B. According the latest recommendations, there are no prospective, randomized, placebo-controlled studies that exist on the efficacy of antibiotic prophylaxis to prevent IE in patients who undergo a dental procedure.
1. Although the absolute risk for IE from a dental procedure is impossible to measure precisely, the best available estimates are that less than 1% of all cases result in streptococcal IE annually in the United States.

2. The overall risk in the general population is estimated to be as low as one case of IE per 14 million dental procedures.

C. Cardiac conditions associated with the highest risk of adverse outcomes from endocarditis for which prophylaxis with dental procedures is reasonable include:
   1. Prosthetic cardiac valve or prosthetic material used for cardiac valve repair
   2. Previous IE
   3. Congenital heart disease (CHD)
      a. Unrepaired cyanotic CHD, including palliative shunts and conduits
      b. Completely repaired congenital heart defect with prosthetic material or device, whether placed by surgery or by catheter intervention, during the first 6 months after the procedure
      c. Repaired CHD with residual defects at the site or adjacent to the site of a prosthetic patch or prosthetic device (which inhibits endothelialization)
   4. Cardiac transplantation recipients who develop cardiac valvulopathy
   5. Mitral valve prolapse (MVP) is the most common underlying condition for which antibiotics have previously been prescribed for in the Western world; however, the absolute incidence of endocarditis is extremely low for the entire population with MVP, and it is not usually associated with the grave outcome associated with the conditions identified above.

D. Procedures in which prophylaxis is recommended:
   1. Dental procedures for patients with underlying cardiac condition
      a. All dental procedures that require or involve manipulation of the gingival tissue
      b. All dental procedures that involve the periapical region of the teeth
      c. Any procedure that involves perforation of the oral mucosa
   2. Gastrointestinal tract procedures
      a. The administration of prophylactic antibiotics solely to prevent endocarditis is not recommended for those undergoing GU or GI procedures, including diagnostic esophagogastroduodenoscopies or colonoscopies.
      b. Latest recommendations suggest that due to increasing antibiotic-resistant strains, unless the above discussed cardiac situations exist in conjunction with a procedure, or if there is an established GI or GU tract infection, antibiotic prophylaxis does not decrease risk
   3. Respiratory tract procedures
      a. Tonsillectomy and/or adenoidectomy
      b. Surgical procedures that include respiratory mucosa
      c. Bronchoscopy, only if incision of the respiratory mucosa is involved
   4. See Table 17.1 for indications for antibiotic use

Table 17.1	Indications for antibiotic use	
Situation	**Agent**	**Regimen—Single Dose 30–60 minutes before procedure**
Oral	Amoxicillin	2 grams
Unable to take oral medication	Ampicillin OR Cefazolin or ceftriaxone	2 grams IV/IM 1 gram IV/IM
Allergic to penicillins or ampicillin—Oral regimen	Cephalexin[a] OR Clindamycin OR Azithromycin or clarithromycin	2 grams 600 mg 500 mg
Allergic to penicillins or ampicillin and unable to take oral medication	Cefazolin or Ceftriaxone* OR Clindamycin	1 gram IV/IM 600 mg IV/IM

[a]Cephalosporins should not be used in an individual with a history of anaphylaxis, angioedema, or urticaria with penicillins or ampicillin.

BIBLIOGRAPHY

Ballweg, R., Sullivan, E. M., Brown, D., & Vetrosky, D. (2012). *Physician assistant: A guide to clinical practice* (5th ed.). Philadelphia, PA: Elsevier Saunders.

Burton, M. A., & Ludwig, L. J. M. (2010). *Fundamentals of nursing care: Concepts, connections, & skills.* Philadelphia, PA: F.A. Davis.

Domino, F. J., Baldor, R. A., Grimes, J. A., & Golding, J. (2013). *The 5 minute clinical consult* (22nd ed.). Philadelphia, PA: Lippincott Williams & Wilkins.

Ferri, F. F. (2011). *Ferri's clinical advisor: Instant diagnosis and treatment* (1st ed.). Philadelphia, PA: Elsevier Mosby.

Fowler, V. G., Jr., Scheld, W. M., & Bayer, A. S. (2009). Endocarditis and intravascular infections. In G. L. Mandell, J. E. Bennett, & R. Dolin (Eds.), *Principles and practice of infectious diseases* (7th ed.). Philadelphia, PA: Elsevier Churchill Livingstone.

Imazio, M., Spodick, D. H., Brucato, A., Trinchero, R., & Adler, Y. (2010). Controversial issies in the management of pericardial diseases. *Circulation, 121*(7), 916–928. doi:10.1161/CIRCULATIONAHA.108.844.753

Karchmer, A. W. (2011). Infective endocarditis. In R. O. Bonow, D. L. Mann, D. P. Zipes, & P. Libby (Eds.), *Braunwald's heart disease: A textbook of cardiovascular medicine* (9th ed.). Philadelphia, PA: Saunders Elsevier.

Khandaker, M., Espinosa, R., Nishimura, R., Sinak, L., Hayes, S., Melduni, R., & Oh, J. (2010). Pericardial disease: Diagnosis and management. *Mayo Clinic Proceedings, 85*(6), 572–593. Retrieved from http://www.ncbi.nlm.nih.gov/pmc/articles/PMC2878263/

Nel, S. H., & Naidoo, D. P. (2014). An echocardiographic study of infective endocarditis, with special reference to patients with HIV. *Cardiovascular Journal of Africa, 25*(2), 50–57. doi: 10.5830/CVJA-2013-084

Palraj, R., Knoll, B. M., Baddour, L. M., & Wilson, W. R. (2014). Prosthetic valve endocarditis. In J. E. Bennett, R. Dolin, and M.J. Blaser (Eds.), *Mandell, Douglas, and Bennett's principles and practice of infectious diseases* (pp. 1029–1040). Philadelphia, PA: Elsevier Saunders.

Rajendram, R., Ehtisham, J., & Forfar, C. (2011). *Oxford case histories in cardiology.* Oxford: Oxford University Press.

Sexton, D. J. (2013). Infective endocarditis: Historical and Duke criteria. In S. B. Calderwood & E. L. Baron (Eds.), *UpToDate*. Waltham, MA: UpToDate. Retrieved from http://www.uptodate.com/contents/infective-endocarditis-historical-and-duke-criteria?source=search_&search=Infective+endocarditis%3A+Historical+and+Duke+criteria&selectedTitle=1~150

Sharif, N. & Dehghani, P. (2013). Acute pericarditis, myocarditis, and worse! *Canadian Family Physician, 59*(1), 39–41. Retrieved from http://www.cfp.ca/content/59/1/39.full?sid=59957acb-83a1-4a59-975b-731815481c6b

CHAPTER 18

Heart Failure

JOAN KING • ROBERT FELLIN • THOMAS W. BARKLEY, JR.

I. **Definition/general comments**
   A. Heart failure (HF) is a clinical syndrome, rather than a disease, caused by a variety of pathophysiologic processes in which the heart is unable to pump an adequate amount of blood to meet the metabolic demands of tissues.
   B. HF may be defined as left-sided HF, right-sided HF, or combined failure, in which there is dysfunction of both ventricles. Characteristics include the following:
      1. Dilatation or hypertrophy of either the left or right ventricle or both
      2. Elevated cardiac filling pressure
      3. Inadequate oxygen delivery caused by cardiac dysfunction
      4. Most commonly, left-sided HF occurs first. After one side of the heart fails, the other may eventually fail because of increased strain and workload.
      5. Two classification systems exist:
         a. The New York Heart Association (NYHA) classification classifies HF into four groups that differ by symptoms (Table 18.1).
         b. The American Heart Association (AHA) has developed four stages with the focus of the first two stages on identifying patients who are at high risk for asymptomatic HF (Table 18.2).
   C. Current practice divides HF in terms of the type of ventricular dysfunction
      1. Systolic HF: defined as signs of failure (Table 18.1)
         a. With an ejection fraction (EF) less than 40%
         b. Impaired contractility that leads to reduced stroke volume and cardiac output
         c. Associated with eccentric hypertrophy
      2. Diastolic HF: defined as signs of failure
         a. With an EF of greater than 50%
         b. A nondilated left ventricle (LV) but elevated LV filling pressures
         c. Normal contractility but impaired ventricular filling related to impairment of ventricular relaxation
         d. Associated with concentric hypertrophy but with a cardiothoracic ratio less than 55% on anteroposterior chest radiograph

CHAPTER 18 Heart Failure

Table 18.1 New York Heart Association Heart Failure Functional Classification

Functional Class	Patient Description	Manifestations
Class I	No limitation of activity	Suffer no symptoms from ordinary activities
Class II	Slight, mild limitation of activity	Comfortable at rest or with mild exertion
Class III	Marked limitation of activity	Comfortable only at rest
Class IV	Should be at complete rest, confined to bed or chair	Any activity brings discomfort, and symptoms occur at rest

Table 18.2 American Heart Association Stages of Heart Failure

Stage of HF	Definition	Manifestations
Stage A	High risk for HF without structural heart disease	HTN, CAD, DM, obesity, metabolic syndrome
Stage B	Structural heart disease present and strongly associated with HF, but asymptomatic	Previous MI Left ventricular remodeling, including LVH and low EF; asymptomatic valvular disease
Stage C	Structural heart disease with current or prior symptoms	Structural heart disease and symptoms of HF
Stage D	Refractory heart failure	Marked symptoms of HF at rest Recurrent hospitalizations despite guided directed medical therapy

Note. HF = heart failure; HTN = hypertension; CAD = coronary artery disease; DM = diabetes mellitus; MI = myocardial infarction; LVH = left ventricular hypertrophy; EF = ejection fraction.

      e. Also referred to as heart failure with preserved ejection fraction (HFpEF)
      f. HFpEF (borderline refers to individuals who have an EF between 41% and 49%, and they are treated with protocols similar to HFpEF)
      g. May be caused by valvular disease or other conditions
   D. Other terms that may be used to describe HF include the following:
      1. Myocardial remodeling—pathologic myocardial hypertrophy or dilatation
      2. HF with a dilated LV
      3. Asymptomatic left ventricle dysfunction—EF less than 40% but no clinical signs or symptoms of HF

II. **Incidence/etiology/predisposing factors**
   A. Affects more than 6 million persons in the United States
   B. Estimated 550,000 new cases diagnosed each year
   C. Most common inpatient diagnosis in patients older than 65 years
   D. Single largest Medicare hospitalization expenditure; cost estimated at $32 billion per year
   E. HF is more common in men than in women until age 75; at that time, incidence becomes approximately equal in both genders
   F. Estimated death rate among African Americans is 50% higher than among Caucasians.
   G. Predisposing factors
      1. Left ventricular dysfunction from coronary artery disease (CAD) is the most common cause; patients experiencing myocardial infarction (MI) with atherosclerotic cardiovascular disease have an 8–10 times increased risk for subsequent HF.
      2. Hypertension—risk is 3 times higher in patients with hypertension; leading risk factor for acute HF; CAD is the most common cause of chronic HF
      3. Diabetes
      4. Physical inactivity
      5. Obesity
      6. Excessive alcohol intake

7. Smoking

H. Other precipitating factors/disease states
1. Infections such as pericarditis and viral or bacterial systemic infections
2. Endocrine abnormalities such as hyperthyroidism, thyrotoxicosis, and pheochromocytoma
3. Nutritional disorders such as beriberi (thiamine deficiency) and kwashiorkor (protein deficiency)
4. Preeclampsia
5. Cardiomyopathy including dilated cardiomyopathy, restrictive cardiomyopathy, and takotsubo cardiomyopathy (broken heart syndrome)
6. Musculoskeletal disorders such as muscular dystrophy and myasthenia gravis
7. Autoimmune disorders such as lupus erythematosus, sarcoidosis, and amyloidosis
8. Genetic factors leading to hypertrophic cardiomyopathy
9. Valvular heart disease
10. Rheumatic or congenital heart disease

III. **Compensatory mechanisms common with heart failure**
A. Hypertrophy
1. Cardiac wall thickens with increased muscle mass over time because of increased strain and workload
2. Wall thickening leads to higher myocardial oxygen demands.
B. Dilatation
1. Chambers enlarge to compensate for increased blood volume.
2. Because of increased volume, muscle fibers become stretched and, up to a point, increase contractile force (Frank Starling law)
3. However, overstretching of cardiac muscle fibers impairs appropriate actin-myosin interaction, and there is a decrease in contractile force.
C. Sympathetic nervous system: Inadequate cardiac output activates the sympathetic nervous system to release epinephrine and norepinephrine. As a result, there is:
1. An increase in heart rate
2. An increase in systemic vascular resistance, which increases afterload, and
3. An increase in myocardial oxygen demand
D. Renal response (renin-angiotensin-aldosterone cascade)
1. Blood filtration in the kidneys decreases when cardiac output decreases.
2. The kidneys respond to a falsely decreased blood volume with an increased release of renin.
3. Renin activates release of angiotensin I and angiotensin II.
4. Angiotensin causes peripheral vasoconstriction (increase in systemic vascular resistance) and release of aldosterone.
5. Aldosterone causes sodium retention.
6. Sodium retention is detected by the posterior pituitary, and antidiuretic hormone is secreted.
7. Antidiuretic hormone increases water absorption in the renal tubules, resulting in water retention.

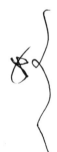

IV. **Right- versus left-sided HF: Physical examination findings**
A. Right-sided HF: The right ventricle is impaired and blood backs up into the right ventricle, the right atrium, and the systemic venous circulation. Signs include the following:
1. Increased central venous pressure
2. Jugular venous distention
3. Peripheral edema
4. Hepatomegaly (liver enlargement) and presence of hepatojugular reflux
5. Ascites
6. S3 and/or S4 heart sounds

CHAPTER 18   Heart Failure

   B. Left-sided heart failure: The LV is impaired, and blood backs up into the left ventricle, left atrium, pulmonary veins, and lungs. Signs include the following:
      1. Increased pulmonary capillary wedge pressure
      2. Crackles (rhonchi and/or rales)
      3. Adventitious breath sounds (crackles)
      4. Dyspnea
      5. Atrial fibrillation related to atrial distention
      6. Pulsus alternans (every other pulse beat is diminished)
      7. S3 common and, rarely, S4 heart sounds
      8. Bilateral infiltrates on chest radiograph
      9. Evidence of pulmonary edema

V. **Subjective/physical examination findings of HF**
   A. Fatigue—may be an early sign
   B. Dyspnea—related to poor gas exchange associated with fluid retention
   C. Orthopnea
   D. Paroxysmal nocturnal dyspnea (PND) or nocturnal cough
   E. Tachycardia—related to the sympathetic nervous system response to decreased cardiac output
   F. Edema
      1. Legs (peripheral)
      2. Liver (hepatomegaly) along with hepatojugular reflux
      3. Spleen (splenomegaly)
      4. Abdominal cavity (ascites)
      5. Lungs (pulmonary edema)
   G. Nocturia—at night, when the body is in the supine position, fluid shifts from the interstitial spaces back into the intravascular space, resulting in increased renal blood flow and diuresis
   H. Skin changes—related to increased tissue capillary oxygen extraction; skin may look dusky and may also be diaphoretic
   I. Behavioral changes—related to impaired cerebral circulation, especially in the presence of atherosclerosis (e.g., unexplained fatigue, restlessness, confusion, delirium, decreased attention span, and decreased memory)
   J. Chest pain—in the presence of atherosclerosis, chest pain is related to decrease of coronary perfusion
   K. Weight gain with an increase in weight of 1 kg, representing 1 liter of fluid retention

VI. **Laboratory/diagnostics**
   A. History and physical examination are very important for diagnosis and follow-up treatment
   B. Arterial blood gases (respiratory alkalosis due to compensatory hyperventilation is common; as the failure progresses, the patient may develop metabolic and respiratory acidosis)
   C. B-type natriuretic peptide (BNP) indicates LV dysfunction, and elevated levels are correlated with myocardial ischemia/damage; may serve to predict severity of current/future cardiac complications, including HF and mortality
      1. Normal BNP levels vary with age and sex, with women having slightly higher normal values.
      2. Mean levels are as follows:
         a. Ages 55–64 years = 26 pg/ml
         b. Ages 65–74 years = 31 pg/ml
         c. 75 years and older = 63 pg/ml
      3. Expected levels associated with concurrent MI = 100–400 pg/ml
      4. With HF, monitoring of trends in elevation is appropriate.

5. When the diagnosis of HF is uncertain with patients in whom the condition is suspected, the N-terminal portion of the pro-BNP peptide nasotracheal (NT-proBNP) levels should be assessed. (The assessment is necessary because BNP is rapidly eliminated from the body.)
   a. Normal range for NT-proBNP for individuals younger than 75 years is less than 125 pg/ml
   b. Normal range for NT-proBNP for individuals 75 years or older is less than 450 pg/ml
   c. NT-proBNP levels will increase with both age and renal dysfunction.
6. BNP is not recommended for routine evaluation of structural heart disease in patients at risk for, but without signs of HF.

D. Erythrocyte sedimentation rate (decreased)
E. Electrolyte analyses via basic metabolic panel
F. BUN, creatinine levels, and glomerular filtration rate (GFR) to assess for renal insufficiency
G. Chest radiograph (may reveal cardiomegaly and/or congestion)
H. ECG to assess for the following:
   1. Evidence of current or previous myocardial infarction
   2. Dysrhythmias such as atrial fibrillation or atrial flutter
   3. Ectopy such as premature ventricular contractions
   4. Evidence of left or right bundle branch block or prolonged conduction time
   5. Reduced ECG complex size
I. Echocardiogram to assess valvular function, wall motion abnormalities, and EF
J. Nuclear stress test to assess baseline tolerance and evidence of areas of reversible ischemia

VII. **Management considerations (Figure 18.1)**
   A. The management of asymptomatic patients with reduced LVEF focuses on controlling cardiovascular risk factors and preventing/reducing ventricular modeling.
      1. Regular exercise (American College of Cardiology Foundation/American Heart Association 2013 Guidelines)
      2. Smoking cessation
      3. Discouraging alcohol consumption
      4. Aggressive blood pressure control
      5. Angiotensin-converting enzyme (ACE) inhibitor therapy is recommended for all patients with reduced LVEF less than 40% who do not have renal insufficiency.
      6. Angiotensin receptor blockers (ARBs) are recommended for asymptomatic patients with reduced LVEF who cannot take ACE inhibitors because of cough or angioedema.
      7. β-blocker therapy is recommended for all patients with reduced LVEF regardless of DM status.
      8. Diuretic therapy if patient begins to show evidence of fluid retention
   B. Nonpharmacologic management for patients with chronic heart disease
      1. Patients should receive carbohydrate and caloric restraint teaching.
      2. Sodium restriction
         a. Two to 3 grams of sodium daily is recommended for patients with the clinical syndrome of HF and preserved or depressed LVEF
         b. Less than 2 grams of sodium daily should be considered in moderate to severe HF
      3. Fluid restriction: less than 2 L is recommended for patients with severe hyponatremia (Na less than 130 mEq/L) and for all patients with fluid retention, regardless of diuretic therapy
      4. Specifically monitor caloric intake, prealbumin, BUN for patients with unintentional weight loss/wasting
      5. Daily multivitamin recommended, especially for those on restricted diets or diuretic therapy

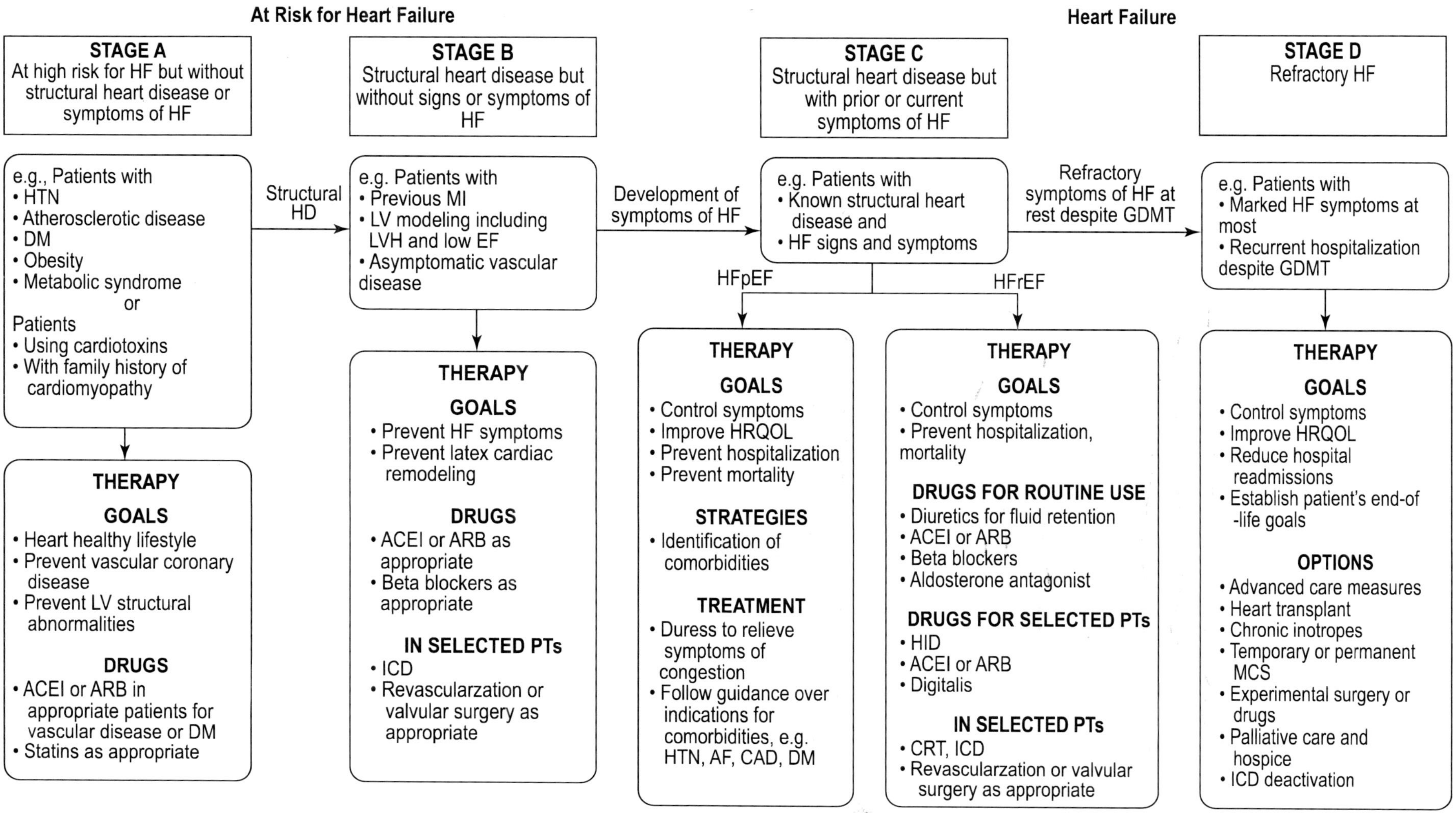

Heart Failure

At Risk for Heart Failure

STAGE A
At high risk for HF but without structural heart disease or symptoms of HF

e.g., Patients with
- HTN
- Atherosclerotic disease
- DM
- Obesity
- Metabolic syndrome

or

Patients
- Using cardiotoxins
- With family history of cardiomyopathy

↓

THERAPY

GOALS
- Heart healthy lifestyle
- Prevent vascular coronary disease
- Prevent LV structural abnormalities

DRUGS
- ACEI or ARB in appropriate patients for vascular disease or DM
- Statins as appropriate

STAGE B
Structural heart disease but without signs or symptoms of HF

Structural HD →

e.g., Patients with
- Previous MI
- LV modeling including LVH and low EF
- Asymptomatic vascular disease

↓

THERAPY

GOALS
- Prevent HF symptoms
- Prevent latex cardiac remodeling

DRUGS
- ACEI or ARB as appropriate
- Beta blockers as appropriate

IN SELECTED PTs
- ICD
- Revascularzation or valvular surgery as appropriate

Development of symptoms of HF →

Heart Failure

STAGE C
Structural heart disease but with prior or current symptoms of HF

e.g. Patients with
- Known structural heart disease and
- HF signs and symptoms

HFpEF ↙   ↘ HFrEF

THERAPY

GOALS
- Control symptoms
- Improve HRQOL
- Prevent hospitalization
- Prevent mortality

STRATEGIES
- Identification of comorbidities

TREATMENT
- Duress to relieve symptoms of congestion
- Follow guidance over indications for comorbidities, e.g. HTN, AF, CAD, DM

THERAPY

GOALS
- Control symptoms
- Prevent hospitalization, mortality

DRUGS FOR ROUTINE USE
- Diuretics for fluid retention
- ACEI or ARB
- Beta blockers
- Aldosterone antagonist

DRUGS FOR SELECTED PTs
- HID
- ACEI or ARB
- Digitalis

IN SELECTED PTs
- CRT, ICD
- Revascularzation or valvular surgery as appropriate

Refractory symptoms of HF at rest despite GDMT →

STAGE D
Refractory HF

e.g. Patients with
- Marked HF symptoms at most
- Recurrent hospitalization despite GDMT

↓

THERAPY

GOALS
- Control symptoms
- Improve HRQOL
- Reduce hospital readmissions
- Establish patient's end-of-life goals

OPTIONS
- Advanced care measures
- Heart transplant
- Chronic inotropes
- Temporary or permanent MCS
- Experimental surgery or drugs
- Palliative care and hospice
- ICD deactivation

Figure 18.1. Stages in the development of HF and recommended therapy by stage. ACEI = angiotensin-converting enzyme inhibitor; ARB = angiotensin-receptor blocker; CAD = coronary artery disease; CRT = cardiac resynchronization therapy; DM = diabetes mellitus; EF = ejection fraction; GDMT = guideline-directed medical therapy; HD = heart disease; HF = heart failure; HFpEF = heart failure with preserved ejection fraction; HFrEF = heart failure with reduced ejection fraction; HID = Hydralazine isosorbide dinitrate ; HRQOL = health-related quality of life; HTN = hypertension; ICD = implantable cardioverter-defibrillator; LV = left ventricular; LVH = left ventricular hypertrophy; MCS = mechanical circulatory support; and MI = myocardial infarction; PTs = patients. Adapted from "2013 ACCF/AHA Guideline for the Management of Heart Failure. A Report of the American College of Cardiology Foundation/American Heart Association Task Force on Practice Guidelines," by C. W. Yancy, M. Jessup, B. Bozkurt, J. Butler, D. E. Casey Jr, M. H. Drazner, G. C. Fonarow, . . . B. L. Wilkoff, 2013, *Circulation, 128.*

6. Assess quality-of-life issues (e.g., depression, sexual dysfunction, and impact on daily activities of living) at regular intervals.
7. Pneumococcal vaccine and annual flu vaccine, as appropriate

C. Basic management considerations for patients with LV systolic dysfunction (Table 18.3)
   1. ACE inhibitors are recommended for symptomatic and asymptomatic patients with LVEF 40% or less, with doses titrated as tolerated during concomitant; up titration of β-blockers
   2. Substitute other therapies for ACE inhibitors in the following circumstances:
      a. If the patient cannot tolerate ACE inhibitors because of cough, ARBs are recommended. If the patient cannot tolerate ARBs, the combination of hydralazine plus oral nitrate may be considered.
      b. If the patient cannot tolerate ACE inhibitors because of hyperkalemia or renal insufficiency, a similar response is expected in terms of adverse effects as with ARBs. A combination of hydralazine plus an oral nitrate should be considered.
   3. β-blockers, along with ACE inhibitors, are established routine therapy in patients with LV systolic dysfunction. Further, this combination is recommended as routine therapy for asymptomatic patients with an LVEF 40% or less.
      a. β-blockers are recommended for all patients with an LVEF 40% or less.
      b. β-blockers are recommended in most patients and in those with LV systolic dysfunction, even if diabetes, chronic obstructive pulmonary disease, or peripheral vascular disease is present.
      c. β-blockers should be used with caution in patients with diabetes who have recurrent hypoglycemia, asthma, or resting limb ischemia; considerable caution is warranted in those with bradycardia or hypotension.
      d. β-blockers are not recommended in patients who have asthma with active bronchospasms.
   4. ARBs are recommended for routine therapy in asymptomatic and symptomatic patients with an LVEF 40% or less who are intolerant to ACE inhibitors for reasons other than hyperkalemia or renal insufficiency.
      a. Individual ARBs, rather than ACE inhibitors, are considered initial therapy for the following patients:
         i. HF after MI
         ii. Chronic HF and systolic dysfunction
      b. ARBs should be considered in patients with angioedema while on ACE inhibitors; the combination of hydralazine plus oral nitrates may be considered when patients do not tolerate ARB therapy.
      c. In patients with recent MI and LV dysfunction, routine administration of ARBs is not recommended when in addition to ACE inhibitors and β-blockers.
   5. Aldosterone antagonists (or mineralocorticoid receptor antagonists) are recommended for patients with the NYHA Class II-IV (previously Class IV or Class III) HF with a LVEF of 35% or less, unless contraindicated, to reduce morbidity and mortality.
      a. Patients with NYHA class II HF should have a history of prior cardiovascular hospitalization or elevated plasma natriuretic peptide levels to be considered for aldosterone receptor antagonists.
      b. Creatinine should be 2.5 mg/dl or less in men or 2.0 mg/dl or less in women (or estimated glomerular filtration rate greater than 30 ml/min/1.73 m^2)
      c. Potassium should be less than 5.0 mEq/L
      d. Careful monitoring of potassium, renal function, and diuretic dosing should be performed at initiation and closely followed thereafter to minimize risk of hyperkalemia and renal insufficiency.
   6. For African Americans with LV systolic dysfunction, the combination of hydralazine plus oral nitrates is recommended as part of standard therapy (in addition to β-blockers and ACE inhibitors).

a. NYHA Class II, III, or IV HF
b. Hydralazine plus oral nitrates may be considered in others (i.e., non-African Americans) with LV systolic dysfunction, which remains symptomatic despite optimal standard therapy.
7. Polypharmacy in patients with LV systolic dysfunction—required for optimal management
   a. ACE inhibitor plus β-blocker = standard therapy
   b. An ARB can be substituted for an ACE inhibitor as indicated.
   c. An ARB can be added to an ACE inhibitor in patients for whom β-blockers are contraindicated or are not tolerated.
      i. Additional agents should be considered in patients with systolic dysfunction HF who have persistent symptoms or worsening of the disease despite optimal therapy with an ACE inhibitor and a β-blocker, as well as in those who are unable to tolerate a β-blocker.
      ii. The specific agent chosen should be selected on the basis of numerous entities, including clinical considerations, renal status, chronic K+ levels, blood pressure, and volume status, among others.
      iii. Triple combination therapy of an ACE inhibitor, an ARB, and an aldosterone agonist is not recommended because of the potential risks associated with hyperkalemia (Box 18.1).
      iv. Example regimens include the following:
         (a) Addition of an ARB
         (b) Addition of an aldosterone antagonist for moderate or severe HF
         (c) Addition of the combination of hydralazine plus isosorbide dinitrate for African Americans and perhaps others

Box 18.1	Guidelines for minimizing the risk of hyperkalemia in patients treated with aldosterone antagonists
1.	Impaired renal function is a risk factor for hyperkalemia during treatment with aldosterone antagonists. The risk of hyperkalemia increases progressively when serum creatinine exceeds 1.6 mg/dL. *In elderly patients and others with low muscle mass in whom serum creatinine does not accurately reflect glomerular filtration rate, the determination that glomerular filtration rate or creatinine clearance exceeds 30 ml/min is recommended.
2.	Aldosterone antagonists should not be administered to patients with baseline serum potassium in excess of 5.0 mEq/L.
3.	An initial dose of spironolactone 12.5 mg or eplerenone 25 mg is recommended, after which the dose may be increased to spironolactone 25 mg or eplerenone 50 mg, if appropriate.
4.	The risk of hyperkalemia is increased with the concomitant use of higher doses of ACEIs (e.g., captopril, 75 mg or more daily; enalapril or lisinopril, 10 mg or more daily).
5.	Nonsteroidal anti-inflammatory drugs and cyclooxygenase-2 inhibitors should be avoided.
6.	Potassium supplements should be discontinued or reduced.
7.	Close monitoring of serum potassium is required; potassium levels and renal function should be checked in 3 days and at 1 week after initiation of therapy and at least monthly for the first 3 months.
8.	Diarrhea or other causes of dehydration should be addressed immediately.

Note. Although the entry criteria for the trials of aldosterone antagonists included creatinine greater than 2.5 mg/dl, the majority of patients had creatinine much lower; in one trial (335a), 95% of patients had creatinine less than or equal to 1.7 mg/dl. ACEI = angiotensin converting enzyme inhibitor. Adapted from "2009 Focused Update Incorporated Into the ACC/AHA 2005 Guidelines for the Diagnosis and Management of Heart Failure in Adults: A Report of the American College of Cardiology Foundation/American Heart Association Task Force on Practice Guidelines Developed in Collaboration With the International Society for Heart and Lung Transplantation," by F. G. Kushner, M. Hand, S. C. Smith, et al., 2009, *Journal of the American College of Cardiology, 53,* p. e30. Copyright 2009 by the American College of Cardiology Foundation and the American Heart Association, Inc. Adapted with permission.

Table 18.3 Cardiovascular Medications Useful for Treatment of Patients at Various Stages of Heart Failure

Drug	Stage A	Stage B	Stage C
ACE inhibitors			
Benazepril	H	–	–
Captopril	H, DN	Post-MI	HF
Enalapril	H, DN	Asymptomatic LVSD	HF
Fosinopril	H	–	HF
Lisinopril	H, DN	Post-MI	HF
Moexipril	H	–	–
Perindopril	H, CV risk	–	–
Quinapril	H	–	HF
Ramipril	H, CV risk	Post-MI	Post-MI
Trandolapril	H	Post-MI	Post-MI
Angiotensin receptor blockers			
Candesartan	H	–	HF
Eprosartan	H	–	–
Irbesartan	H, DN	–	–
Losartan	H, DN	CV risk	–
Olmesartan	H	–	–
Telmisartan	H	–	–
Valsartan	H, DN	Post-MI	Post-MI, HF
Aldosterone blockers			
Eplerenone	H	Post-MI	Post-MI
Spironolactone	H	–	HF
β-blockers			
Acebutolol	H	–	–
Atenolol	H	Post-MI	–
Betaxolol	H	–	–
Bisoprolol	H	–	HF
Carteolol	H	–	–
Carvedilol	H	Post-MI	HF, Post-MI
Labetalol	H	–	–
Metoprolol succinate	H	–	HF
Metoprolol tartrate	H	Post-MI	–
Nadolol	H	–	–
Penbutolol	H	–	–
Pindolol	H	–	–
Propranolol	H	Post-MI	–
Timolol	H	Post-MI	–
Digoxin	–	–	HF

Note. Stage A = patients at high risk for developing heart failure; Stage B = patients with cardiac structural abnormalities who have not developed HF symptoms; Stage C = patients with current of prior symptoms of HF; CV risk = cardiovascular risk; DN = diabetic neuropathy; H = hypertension; HF = heart failure; LVSD = left ventricular systolic dysfunction; Post-MI = reduction in heart failure or other cardiac events following myocardial infarction. Adapted from "2009 Focused Update Incorporated Into the ACC/AHA 2005 Guidelines for the Diagnosis and Management of Heart Failure in Adults: A Report of the American College of Cardiology Foundation/ American Heart Association Task Force on Practice Guidelines Developed in Collaboration With the International Society for Heart and Lung Transplantation," by F. G. Kushner, M. Hand, S. C. Smith, et al., 2009, Journal of the American College of Cardiology, 53, p. e30. Copyright 2009 by the American College of Cardiology Foundation and the American Heart Association, Inc. Adapted with permission.

blockers, along with ACE inhibitors, are established routine therapy in patients with LV systolic dysfunction. Further, this combination is recommended as routine therapy for asymptomatic patients with an LVEF 40% or less

8. Diuretic therapy: Loop and distal tubular agents are necessary adjuncts for HF when symptoms are due to sodium and water retention (Tables 18.4 and 18.5).
   a. Loop diuretics are considered the class of choice for HF treatment.
   b. Diuretic therapy is recommended to restore and maintain normal volume status in patients with symptomatic HF; again, loop diuretics, rather than thiazide types, are typically necessary.
   c. Initial doses are usually increased as necessary to relieve signs/symptoms; after initial therapy with short-acting loop diuretics; increasing administration frequency (e.g., twice or thrice daily) provides greater diuresis with fewer physiologic adverse effects than are produced by larger, single doses.
   d. For patients with poor absorption of oral medication or with erratic diuretic effects, oral toresmide may be considered, particularly in a patient who has right-sided HF and refractory fluid retention despite high doses of other loop diuretics.
   e. Once or BID addition of chlorothiazide or metolazone to loop diuretic regimens should be considered in patients with persistent fluid retention, despite high-dose loop therapy;
   long-term daily use, especially of metolazone, should be avoided because of potential electrolyte shifts and volume disturbances; rather, consider using these agents periodically (e.g., every other day or weekly).
   f. Because chlorothiazide diuretics delete potassium, electrolytes should be monitored frequently, especially when starting chlorothiazide diuretics or adjusting dosages
   g. Patients requiring diuretic therapy to treat fluid retention will generally require long-term treatment, yet at lower doses than those initially required to promote diuresis; monitor for electrolyte abnormalities, hypotension, and renal dysfunction.
9. Digoxin: Debate and lack of consensus are noted in the literature regarding the use of digoxin in patients with normal sinus rhythm; most agree to the benefits of use in patients with symptomatic LV systolic dysfunction who have atrial fibrillation or in patients who remain symptomatic and are in AHA Stage C or D of HF.
   a. Digoxin should be considered in patients with symptomatic LV systolic dysfunction (LVEF occurs in 40% or less) who are receiving standard therapy, including ACE inhibitors and β-blockers (i.e., NYHA Classes II-IV).
   b. On the basis of lean body mass, renal function, and other current medications, the dose of digoxin should be 0.125 mg daily in most patients, with maintenance of a digoxin level below 1 nanogram/ml.
   c. Maintained rate control of the ventricular response to atrial fibrillation is recommended, although high doses of digoxin (greater than 0.25 mg daily) are not recommended to achieve this result.
   d. Digoxin has a narrow therapeutic range. Digoxin levels and potassium levels should be monitored closely in patients assessed for signs of digoxin toxicity, especially in patients in with a history of hypokalemia.
10. Anticoagulants and antiplatelet agents: warfarin, aspirin, and clopidogrel all have potential benefits in treating patients with HF
    a. Warfarin treatment to maintain a goal international normalized ratio (INR) of 2:3 is recommended for all patients with HF; the same treatment is also recommend for patients with chronic or documented atrial fibrillation with a CHADS2 score of 1 or greater, a history of pulmonary embolus, and stroke or transient ischemic attack, unless otherwise contraindicated. Also considered when patient's EF falls below 20%–25%
    b. In some instances, dabigatran (Pradaxa) may be prescribed for anticoagulation in atrial fibrillation. However, extreme caution must be taken when used in a patient with renal or liver impairment.

c. Patients with asymptomatic or symptomatic cardiomyopathy and documented recent large anterior MI or recent MI with documented LV thrombus should also be treated with warfarin to maintain a goal INR of 2:3, or another oral anticoagulation agent, for the initial 3 months after MI, unless otherwise contraindicated.
 d. In the absence of the indicators above, warfarin may be considered in those with cardiomyopathy and an LVEF 35% or less.
   i. Long-term treatment with an antithrombotic agent is recommended for patients with HF with ischemic cardiomyopathy, regardless of whether they are receiving ACE inhibitors.
   ii. Aspirin is recommended in most patients for whom anticoagulation therapy is not specifically indicated.
   iii. Warfarin (INR; goal, 2:3) and clopidogrel, 75 mg, may be considered as alternatives to aspirin.
   iv. Routine use of aspirin and an ACE inhibitor in combination may be considered for patients with HF when simultaneous indications for both drugs exist.
D. Electrophysiologic testing and use of devices in HF
 1. Electrophysiologic testing
  a. Immediate evaluation is recommended in patients with HF who present with syncope.
  b. Routine electrophysiologic testing is not recommended in patients with LV systolic dysfunction who have asymptomatic nonsustained ventricular tachycardia in the absence of prior infarction.
 2. Implantable cardioverter defibrillator (ICD) placement
  a. In patients with or without CAD (including MI longer than 40 days postinfarction), prophylactic ICD placement should be considered (LVEF 30% or less) and may be considered (LVEF 31%–35%) for patients with mild to moderate HF (NYHA Classes II-III).
  b. Concomitant ICD placement should be considered in patients undergoing implantation of a biventricular pacing device.
  c. ICD placement is recommended for survivors of cardiac arrest from ventricular fibrillation or hemodynamically unstable ventricular tachycardia without evidence of MI. ICD placement is also recommended if cardiac arrest occurs longer than 48 hr after onset of infarction in the absence of a recurrent ischemic event.
  d. ICD placement is not recommended in chronic, severe refractory HF when no reasonable expectation for improvement exists.
 3. Biventricular resynchronization pacing improves hemodynamics in patients in which an echocardiogram reveals asynchronous contractions of the right and left ventricles.
  a. For patients who have persistent, moderate to severe HF (NYHA Class II and Class III) despite optimal therapy, biventricular pacing therapy should be considered if the following signs are also present: sinus rhythm, left bundle branch block with a quantitative reference standard complex (120–150 or more milliseconds), and severe LV systolic dysfunction (LVEF 35% or less, with LV dilatation greater 5.5 cm).
  b. Some ambulatory NYHA Class IV patients may be considered for biventricular pacing if ambulatory.
  c. Biventricular pacing is not recommended in patients who are asymptomatic, have mild symptoms of HF, or have quantitative reference standard that is fewer than 120 ms.
 4. Dual-chamber (atrioventricular) pacemakers
  a. Routine use is not recommended for patients with HF in the absence of symptomatic bradycardia or high-grade atrioventricular block.
E. Basic management considerations for patients with HF and preserved left ventricular function, defined as having an LVEF greater than 41%–50%

1. Ischemic heart disease evaluation is recommended
2. Aggressive blood pressure control
3. Low-sodium diet/sodium restriction
4. Diuretic therapy: Treatment may begin with a low-thiazide or loop preparation; for patients with more severe fluid retention, loop therapy should be implemented. Avoid excessive diuresis.
5. ARBs or ACE inhibitors should be considered in patients with HF and preserved LVEF.
    a. ACE inhibitors should be considered in all patients with HF and preserved LVEF who have symptomatic atherosclerotic cardiovascular disease, diabetes, and one additional risk factor; for those intolerant to ACE inhibitors, ARBs should be considered.
6. β-blocker therapy is recommended in patients with HF and preserved LVEF who have had prior MI, hypertension, or atrial fibrillation requiring ventricular rate control.
7. Calcium channel blockers are contraindicated in patients with systolic HF; diltiazem or verapamil should be considered in patients with the following conditions:
    a. Symptom-limiting angina
    b. If hypertension is present, then consider amlodipine
8. Continuous positive airway pressure is recommended to address obstructive sleep apnea

F. Basic management considerations for patients with acute decompensated HF (ADHF)
   1. Diagnosis should be made primarily on the basis of signs and symptoms; when unsure, obtain BNP or NT-proBNP in patients who have dyspnea and comparable HF signs; BNP should not be interpreted in isolation but rather within the context clinical data.
   2. Hospitalization is recommended or should be considered for symptomatic patients with ADHF.
       a. Recommended hospitalization: hypotension, worsening renal function, altered mental status, dyspnea at rest (primarily reflected as tachypnea first, then falling oxygen saturation), hemodynamically significant arrhythmia (including new-onset atrial fibrillation), acute coronary syndromes, and so on
       b. Hospitalization considered: worsened congestion (even without dyspnea; typically reflected by 5 kg or more weight gain), signs or symptoms of pulmonary/systemic congestion (even in the absence of weight gain), PND, major electrolyte disturbances, associated comorbidities (e.g., pneumonia, pulmonary embolus, diabetic ketoacidosis, symptoms suggestive of transient ischemic attack, cerebrovascular accident, repeated ICD firings, previously undiagnosed HF with signs systemic or pulmonary congestion, and so on.
   3. Inpatient monitoring considerations
       a. Daily weight: determine after morning void, noting that a 1-kg increase in weight reflects a liter of fluid retained. Increase in weight needs to be correlated with other signs of fluid retention.
       b. Daily intake and output
       c. Vital signs, including orthostatic blood pressure measurements
       d. Daily electrolyte assessment, especially serum potassium, magnesium, and sodium
       e. Daily renal function assessment (BUN and serum creatinine)
       f. Monitor potential signs (e.g., edema, ascites, rales, hepatomegaly, jugular venous distention, hepatojugular reflux, liver tenderness, etc.)
       g. Monitor potential symptoms (e.g., orthopnea, PND, nocturnal cough, dyspnea, fatigue, etc.)
   4. Recommended initial treatment of fluid overload with loop diuretics intravenously, then orally. Upon an inadequate response to diuretic therapy, consider sodium and fluid restriction, increased doses of loop diuretics, continuous loop diuretic infusion, or addition of a second type of oral (e.g., metolazone) or intravenous (e.g., chlorothiazide) diuretic; finally, ultrafiltration may be considered.

Table 18.4	Oral diuretics Recommended for Use in the Treatment of Patients in Chronic Heart failure		
Drug	Initial Daily Dose	Maximum Total Daily Dose	Duration of Action
Loop diuretics			
Bumetanide	0.5–1.0 mg once or twice	10 mg	4–6 hr
Furosemide	20–40 mg once or twice	600 mg	6–8 hr
Torsemide	10–20 mg once	200 mg	12–16 hr
Thiazide diuretics			
Chlorothiazide	250–500 mg once or twice	1000 mg	6–12 hr
Chlorthalidone	12.5–25 mg once	100 mg	24–72 hr
Hydrochlorothiazide	25 mg once or twice	200 mg	6–12 hr
Indapamide	2.5 mg once	5 mg	36 hr
Metolazone	2.5 mg once	20 mg	12–24 hr
Potassium-sparing diuretics			
Amiloride	5 mg once	20 mg	24 hr
Spironolactone	12.5–25 mg once	50 mg	2–3 days
Triamterene	50–75 mg twice	200 mg	7–9 hr
Sequential nephron blockade			
Metolazone	2.5–10 mg once plus loop diuretic		
Hydrochlorothiazide	25–100 mg once or twice plus loop diuretic		
Chlorothiazide (IV)	500–1000 mg once plus loop diuretic		

Note. Higher doses may occasionally be used with close monitoring. IV = intravenous. Adapted from "2009 Focused Update Incorporated Into the ACC/AHA 2005 Guidelines for the Diagnosis and Management of Heart Failure in Adults: A Report of the American College of Cardiology Foundation/American Heart Association Task Force on Practice Guidelines Developed in Collaboration With the International Society for Heart and Lung Transplantation," by F. G. Kushner, M. Hand, S. C. Smith, et al., 2009, Journal of the American College of Cardiology, 53, p. e21. Copyright 2009 by the American College of Cardiology Foundation and the American Heart Association, Inc. Adapted with permission.

Table 18.5 Intravenous Diuretic Medications Useful for the Treatment of Patients With Severe Heart Failure

Drug	Initial Dose	Maximum Single Dose
Loop diuretics		
Bumetanide	1 mg	4–8 mg
Furosemide	40 mg	160–200 mg
Torsemide	10 mg	100–200 mg
Thiazide diuretics		
Chlorothiazide	500 mg	1000 mg
Sequential nephron blockade	Chlorothiazide, 500–1000 mg IV once or twice, plus loop diuretics once—multiple doses per day	
	Metolazone (as Zaroxolyn or Diulo), 2.5–5 mg PO, once or BID with loop diuretic	
IV infusions		
Bumetanide	1-mg IV load, then 0.5–2 mg/hr infusion	
Furosemide	40-mg IV load, then 10–100 mg/hr infusion	
Torsemide	20-mg IV load, then 5–20 mg/hr infusion	

Note. IV = intravenous; PO = per os (by mouth). Adapted from "2009 Focused Update Incorporated Into the ACC/AHA 2005 Guidelines for the Diagnosis and Management of Heart Failure in Adults: A Report of the American College of Cardiology Foundation/American Heart Association Task Force on Practice Guidelines Developed in Collaboration With the International Society for Heart and Lung Transplantation," by F. G. Kushner, M. Hand, S. C. Smith, et al., 2009, Journal of the American College of Cardiology, 53, p. e25. Copyright 2009 by the American College of Cardiology Foundation and the American Heart Association, Inc. Adapted with permission.

5. Fluid restriction (less than 2 L/day) is recommended for patients with moderate hyponatremia (Na less than 130 mEq/L) and should be considered in other patients to assist in treatment of fluid overload; more strict fluid restriction may be warranted for patients with Na less than 125 mEq/L.
6. In the absence of hypoxia, routine oxygen administration is not recommended.
7. For patients without hypotension, intravenous nitroglycerin, nitroprusside, or nesiritide may be considered because of their vasodilation properties, in addition to diuretic therapy, to rapidly improve congestive symptoms; intravenous vasodilator agents such as nitroglycerin or nitroprusside and diuretics are recommended for rapid improvement in patients with acute pulmonary edema or severe hypertension.
8. Continuous positive airway pressure, in an emergent or urgent situation, may decrease venous return to the heart and decrease preload while waiting for diuretics to relieve fluid overload.
9. Intravenous inotropes such as milrinone or dobutamine may be considered in patients with advanced HF characterized by LV dilatation, reduced LVEF, diminished peripheral perfusion, or end-organ dysfunction, particularly if these patients are hypotensive or have an inadequate response/intolerance to intravenous vasodilators.
    a. Administration of vasodilators instead of intravenous inotropes (e.g., milrinone, dobutamine) should be considered when adjunct therapy is needed in other patients with ADHF
    b. Agents such as milrinone and dobutamine are not recommended unless HF filling pressures are known to be elevated on the basis of direct measurement or clear clinical signs.

10. Routine invasive hemodynamic monitoring in patients with ADHF is not recommended. However, it should be considered for ADHF patients who are refractory to initial therapy, whose volume status and cardiac filling pressures are unclear, who present with significant hypotension or worsening renal function, and who need adequate documentation of hemodynamic response to inotropic agents.
11. Patients who are refractory to therapy placement of a left ventricular assist device (LVAD) may be considered as candidates for either destination therapy or bridge to transplantation.

G. Basic management considerations for patients with HF in the setting of ischemic heart disease:
   1. CAD risk factor assessment is recommended in all patients with chronic HF, regardless of EF because CAD is the most common cause of chronic HF.
   2. Cardiac catheterization is recommended for patients with HF and angina.
   3. Patients with HF and no angina but with known CAD (and those at high risk for CAD) should undergo noninvasive stress imaging and/or coronary angiography.
   4. Examples of imaging tests to be used include exercise or pharmacologic stress myocardial perfusion imaging, exercise or pharmacologic stress echocardiography, cardiac magnetic resonance imaging, and positron emission tomography scanning.
   5. Management of risk factors (e.g., lipids, smoking, physical inactivity, weight, and hypertension) is of primary importance.
   6. Specific therapies for patients with HF and CAD:
      a. Antiplatelet therapy is recommended in patients with HF and CAD, unless contraindicated.
      b. ACE inhibitors are recommended in all patients with systolic dysfunction or preserved systolic dysfunction after MI.
      c. β-blockers are recommended for management of all patients with reduced LVEF or post-MI.
      d. ACE inhibitors and β-blockers are recommended to be started within 48 hr during hospitalization in hemodynamically stable post-MI patients with LV dysfunction or HF.
      e. Nitrates should be considered in patients with HF when additional anti-anginal pain relief is needed.
      f. Amlopidine (calcium channel blocker) should be considered in HF patients with angina, despite the optimal use of β-blockers and nitrates, especially in patients with both angina and decreased systolic function.
      g. Drugs that should be avoided in HF patients, or withdrawn if possible, include most antiarrhythmic drugs, calcium channel blockers except for amlodipine, NSAIDs, and thiazolidinediones (ACCF/AHA guidelines).
      h. Coronary revascularization is recommended in patients with HF for relief of refractory angina or acute coronary syndromes, when possible.

H. The basic management considerations for patients with hypertension and HF are as follows:
   1. Aggressive blood pressure control (less than 130/80 mmHg is preferred in clinical practice; however, current heart failure guidelines do not identify a goal blood pressure)
   2. The use of several agents should be considered; usually, an ACE inhibitor or an ARB, a diuretic, and often, a β-blocker or amlodipine should be included.
   3. For asymptomatic LV dysfunction with LV dilatation and low EF, the following treatments are suggested:
      a. An ACE inhibitor (20 mg enalapril daily) is recommended
      b. Addition of a β-blocker is recommended even if blood pressure is controlled.
      c. If BP remains elevated, the addition of a diuretic is recommended followed by another antihypertensive agent.

4. For symptomatic LV dysfunction with LV dilatation and low EF (Table 18.6), the following recommendations apply:
   a. Target doses of the following are recommended: ACE inhibitors, ARBs, β-blockers, aldosterone inhibitors, and isosorbide dinitrate/hydralazine in various combinations (with a diuretic if needed).
   b. If BP remains above 130/80 mmHg, a non-cardiac depressing calcium antagonist, such as amlodipine, may be considered, or consider increasing the doses of other antihypertensive medications.

I. Specific considerations for special populations experiencing HF include the following:
   1. Elderly
      a. Cardiovascular changes with aging, including a decrease in peak contractility, responsiveness of heart rate to sympathetic nervous system stimulation, peripheral vasodilation, and decrease in renal function, all contribute to increase incidence of ADHF in the elderly.
      b. β-blocker and ACE inhibitor therapy is also standard in all patients with HF from LV systolic dysfunction; however, these medications need to be titrated slowly, and therapeutic goals should be adjusted appropriately.
      c. Monitor carefully for fluid overload, noting jugular venous distension, S3 gallop, and peripheral edema as the hallmark signs of ADHF in elderly
   2. Women: β-blocker therapy and ACE inhibitor therapy are recommended for HF that results from symptomatic or asymptomatic LV systolic dysfunction.
   3. African Americans with HF: β-blocker therapy and, to some extent, ACE inhibitor therapy are recommended as part of standard care for patients with HF due to symptomatic or asymptomatic LV systolic dysfunction.
      a. ARBs may be substituted for African Americans with HF who are intolerant to ACE inhibitors.
      b. A combination of hydralazine and isosorbide dinitrate is recommended as a standard therapy, in addition to β-blockers and ACE inhibitors, for African Americans with LV systolic dysfunction and NYHA Class III or IV HF (and may be considered for some with NYHA Class II HF).

Table 18.6	Inhibitors of the Renin-Angiotensin-Aldosterone System and β-Blockers Commonly Used for the Treatment of Patients With HF With Low Ejection Fraction	
Drug	Initial Daily Dose(s)	Maximum Dose(s)
ACE inhibitors		
Captopril	6.25 mg 3 times	50 mg 3 times
Enalapril	2.5 mg twice	10–20 mg twice
Fosinopril	5–10 mg once	40 mg once
Lisinopril	2.5–5 mg once	20–40 mg once
Perindopril	2 mg once	8–16 mg once
Quinapril	5 mg twice	20 mg twice
Ramipril	1.25–2.5 mg once	10 mg once
Trandolapril	1 mg once	4 mg once
Angiotensin receptor blockers		
Candesartan	4–8 mg once	32 mg once
Losartan	25–50 mg once	50–100 mg once
Valsartan	20–40 mg twice	160 mg twice
Aldosterone antagonists		
Spironolactone	12.5–25 mg once	25 mg once or twice
Eplerenone	25 mg once	50 mg once
β-blockers		
Bisoprolol	1.25 mg once	10 mg once
Carvedilol	3.125 mg twice	25 mg twice (50 mg twice for patients weighing more than 85 kg)
Carvedilol CR	10 mg once daily	80 mg once daily
Metoprolol succinate extended release (metoprolol CR/XL)	12.5–25 mg once	200 mg once

Note. ACE = angiotensin-converting enzyme; HF = heart failure. Adapted from "2009 Focused Update Incorporated Into the ACC/AHA 2005 Guidelines for the Diagnosis and Management of Heart Failure in Adults: A Report of the American College of Cardiology Foundation/American Heart Association Task Force on Practice Guidelines Developed in Collaboration With the International Society for Heart and Lung Transplantation," by F. G. Kushner, M. Hand, S. C. Smith, et al., 2009, *Journal of the American College of Cardiology, 53,* p. e29. Copyright 2009 by the American College of Cardiology Foundation and the American Heart Association, Inc. Adapted with permission.

BIBLIOGRAPHY

Chisholm-Burns, M. A., Wells, B. G., Schwinghammer, T. L., Malone, P. M., Kolesar, J. M., & Dipiro, J. T. (2013). *Pharmacotherapy: Principles and practice* (3rd ed.). New York, NY: McGraw Hill Medical.

Foreman, M. D., Milisen, K., & Fulmer, T. T. (2009). *Critical care nursing of older adults: Best practices* (3rd ed.). New York, NY: Springer Publishing Company.

Foster, J. G. W. & Prevost, S. S. (Eds.). (2012). *Advanced practice nursing of adults in acute care.* Philadelphia, PA: F.A. Davis Company.

Go, A. S., Mozaffarian, D., Roger, V. L., Benjamin, E. J., Berry, J. D., Borden, W. B., . . . Turner, M. B. (2013). Heart Disease and Stroke Statistics—2013 Update: A Report from the American Heart Association. *Circulation, 127*(1), e6-e245. doi: 10.1161/CIR.0b013e31828124ad

Godara, H., Hirbe, A., Nassif, M., Otepka, H., & Rosenstock, A. (Eds.). (2014). *The Washington manual of medical therapeutics* (34th ed.). Philadelphia, PA: Wolters Kluwer/Lippincott, Williams, & Wilkins.

Griffin, B. P., Callahan, T. D., & Menon, V. (Eds.). (2012). *Manual of cardiovascular medicine* (4th ed.). Philadelphia, PA: Wolters Kluwer/Lippincott, Williams, & Wilkins.

Heidenreich, P. A., Trogdon, J. G., Khavjou, O. A., Butler, J., Dracup, K., Ezekowitz, M. D., . . . Woo, Y. J. (2011). Forecasting the future of cardiovascular disease in the United States: A policy statement from the American Heart Association. *Circulation, 123*(8), 933-944. doi: 10.1161/CIR.0b013e31820a55f5

Management of patients with cardiovascular disorders. (2014.) In T. W. Barkley Jr. (Ed.), *Adult nurse practitioner certification review manual.* West Hollywood, CA: Barkley & Associates.

Marini, J. J., & Wheeler, A. P. (2009). *Critical care medicine: The essentials* (4th ed.). Philadelphia, PA: Wolters Kluwer/Lippincott, Williams, & Wilkins.

Marino, P. L. (2013). *The ICU book* (4th ed.). Philadelphia, PA: Wolters Kluwer Health/Lippincott, Williams, & Wilkins.

Parrillo, J. E., & Dellinger, R. P. (2013). *Critical care medicine: Principles of diagnosis and management in the adult* (4th ed.). Philadelphia, PA: Elsevier Saunders.

Yancy, C. W., Jessup, M., Bozkurt, B., Butler, J., Casey, D. E., Drazner, M. H., . . . Wilkoff, B. L. (2013). 2013 ACCF/AHA guideline for the management of heart failure: Executive summary: A report of the American College of Cardiology Foundation/American Heart Association Task Force on Practice Guidelines. *Circulation, 128*(16), 1810–1852. doi: 10.1161/CIR.0b013e31829e8807

Yancy, C. W., Jessup, M., Bozkurt, B., Butler, J., Casey, D. E., Drazner, M. H., . . . Wilkoff, B. L. (2013). 2013 ACCF/AHA guideline for the management of heart failure: A report of the American College of Cardiology Foundation/American Heart Association Task Force on Practice Guidelines. *Journal of the American College of Cardiology, 62*(16), e147–e239. doi:10.1016/j.jacc.2013.05.019.

CHAPTER 19

Valvular Disease

THERESA M. WADAS • ROBERT FELLIN • THOMAS W. BARKLEY, JR.

I. **Definition**
   A. Impairment of unidirectional flow that results from damaged cardiac valves
   B. Two types
      1. Stenosis ("narrowing: obstructed forward blood flow")
      2. Regurgitation ("insufficiency: backward blood across the valve")
   C. May occur with all cardiac valves
   D. Aortic stenosis and mitral regurgitation: most common valvular disease in the elderly

II. **Mitral stenosis**
   A. Definition: narrowing of the mitral valve that results in obstructed forward blood flow
   B. Etiology/incidence
      1. Rheumatic heart disease, including endocarditis from rheumatic fever, is most common
      2. Fibrosis and calcification of the valve with scarring
      3. Valve leaflets become immobilized and narrow the orifice
      4. Approximately two thirds of patients are female
   C. Subjective and physical examination findings
      1. Fatigue
      2. Dyspnea
      3. Orthopnea
      4. Hemoptysis—associated with pulmonary venous hypertension and elevated left atrial pressures
      5. Other findings consistent with left-sided heart failure
      6. Palpitations—associated with atrial fibrillation
      7. Loud S1 heart sound with low-pitched, mid-diastolic murmur; does not radiate, heard best at the apex and in the left lateral position
      8. Apical crescendo rumble
      9. Mitral facies with malar flush
   D. Diagnostic tests
      1. Echocardiogram (two-dimensional)—confirms diagnosis; demonstrates restricted motion of the valve and quantifies severity

CHAPTER 19 Valvular Disease

2. Doppler echocardiogram—prolonged pressure half-time across the valve; quantifies severity
3. Transesophageal echocardiogram (TEE)—check for valvular measurements, estimates of transvalvular peak and mean gradients, assessment of LV and RV function, chamber sizes estimate of pulmonary artery pressure, and presence of thrombus
4. ECG—check for atrial fibrillation; if in sinus rhythm, tall and peaked P waves in lead II and upright in V1 seen with severe pulmonary hypertension
5. Chest X-ray—check for the appearance of a straight left-sided heart border or large left atrium, prominence of main pulmonary arteries, dilation of the upper lobe pulmonary vein, and posterior displacement of the esophagus, and Kerley B lines
6. Cardiac catheterization to assess associated lesions and presence of coronary artery disease

E. Medical therapy
   1. Anticoagulation: warfarin or heparin is indicated in patients with:
      a. Mitral stenosis (MS) and atrial fibrillation (AF) (paroxysmal, persistent, or permanent)
      b. MS and a prior embolic event
      c. MS and a left atrial thrombus
      d. Efficacy of oral anticoagulant agents in preventing embolic events has not been studied in patients with MS. It is controversial as to whether long-term anticoagulation should be given to patients with MS in normal sinus rhythm on the basis of left atrial enlargement or spontaneous contrast on TEE.
   2. Heart rate control: can be beneficial in patients with MS and atrial fibrillation and fast ventricular response
   3. Heart rhythm control: cardioversion may be necessary to improve hemodynamic instability in select patients
      a. In stable patients, the decision for rate versus rhythm, control depends on multiple factors (duration, left atrial size, etc.). It is much more difficult to achieve rhythm control in patients with MS because of the rheumatic process.
   4. Antibiotic prophylaxis for surgical or dental procedures (refer to Inflammatory Cardiac Disease chapter section on endocarditis prophylaxis for appropriate indications/criteria and definitive therapy)

F. Intervention
   1. Percutaneous mitral balloon commissurotomy (PMBC) is recommended for symptomatic patients with severe MS. There is no role for percutaneous mitral balloon or surgical commissurotomy for patients with MS due to calcification.
   2. Mitral valve surgery (replacement or repair) is indicated in severely symptomatic patients who are not high risk for surgery and who are not candidates for or failed previous PMBC.
      a. Patients with calcification are often elderly and debilitated, have multiple comorbidities, and are at high risk for surgery; therefore, intervention should be delayed until symptoms are severely limiting and cannot be managed with medical therapy.

III. **Mitral regurgitation**
   A. Definition: backflow of blood into the left atrium as a result of deficient mitral valve closure
   B. Etiology
      1. Rheumatic disease
      2. "Floppy" mitral valve
      3. Papillary muscle dysfunction related to ischemic heart disease
      4. Infective endocarditis
      5. Ruptured chordae tendineae
      6. Hypertrophic obstructive and dilated cardiomyopathy

7. Systemic lupus erythematosus
8. Commonly associated with heart failure in the elderly

C. Subjective and physical examination findings
1. Fatigue
2. Weakness
3. Exertional dyspnea
4. Palpitations—associated with atrial fibrillation
5. S3 heart sound with holosystolic murmur at the fifth intercostal space/midclavicular line (apex)—may radiate to base or left axilla; blowing, musical, or high-pitched at times
6. Apical thrill may be palpable (grade IV/VI).

D. Diagnostic tests
1. Echocardiogram (two-dimensional)—thickened valve with or without flailing leaflets or vegetation; indicated to assess the mechanism of the MR and its hemodynamic severity, also provides rapid assessment of clinical change
2. Doppler echocardiogram—regurgitant flow into the left atrium
3. Transesophageal echocardiogram
4. ECG—check for atrial fibrillation and left ventricular hypertrophy, if in sinus rhythm, tall and peaked P waves in lead II and upright in VI/VI seen with severe pulmonary hypertension
5. Chest X-ray—check for enlarged left atrium and/or ventricle.
6. Cardiac catheterization—same as for mitral stenosis

E. Management
1. Acute MR
   a. Vasodilating agents (sodium nitroprusside or nicardipine): decreases MR while simultaneously increasing forward output
   b. Intra-aortic balloon counterpulsation: temporizing measure for achieving hemodynamic stability until definitive mitral surgery can be performed
   c. Mitral valve surgery (repair or replacement) is recommended for symptomatic patients with acute severe primary MR
2. Chronic MR
   a. Primary MR
      i. Standard regimen for HF: β-blockers, ACE inhibitors, or ARBs
      ii. Vasodilator therapy not indicate for normotensive asymptomatic patients with chronic primary MR and normal systolic LV function
      iii. MV surgery (repair or replacement) recommended for symptomatic patients with chronic severe primary MR
      iv. Transcatheter MV repair may be considered for severely symptomatic patients with chronic severe primary MR who have a reasonable life expectancy, but a prohibitive surgical risk because of severe comorbidities
   b. Secondary MR
      i. Standard regimen for HF: β-blockers, ACE inhibitors, or ARBs
      ii. Cardiac resynchronization therapy with biventricular pacing is recommended for symptomatic patients with chronic severe secondary MR who meet the indications for device therapy.
      iii. MV surgery may be considered for severely symptomatic patients with chronic severe secondary MR. MV repair may be considered for patients with chronic moderate secondary MR who are undergoing other cardiac surgery.
3. Antibiotic prophylaxis for surgical or dental procedures (refer to Inflammatory Cardiac Disease chapter section on endocarditis prophylaxis for appropriate indications/criteria and definitive therapy)

CHAPTER 19 Valvular Disease

IV. **Mitral valve prolapse**
   A. Definition/etiology/incidence
      1. Protrusion of the mitral valve into the left atrium during systole as the result of damaged leaflets of the valve
      2. Cause often unknown; appears to have genetic disposition to collagen disorders such as Marfan syndrome, osteogenesis imperfecta, and Ehlers-Danlos syndrome
      3. Usually benign
      4. Affects up to 2%–6% of the population
      5. More prevalent in women between the ages of 15 and 30 than in men; if observed in men, often older (older than 50 years of age)
      6. Familial incidence for some—suggesting autosomal dominant form of inheritance
   B. Physical examination findings
      1. Often asymptomatic
      2. Fatigue
      3. Dizziness or lightheadedness
      4. Dyspnea
      5. Chest pain or palpitations may occur
      6. Syncope
      7. Dysrhythmias—most commonly ventricular premature contractions, paroxysmal supraventricular and ventricular tachycardia, and atrial fibrillation
      8. Midsystolic click frequently followed by a late systolic crescendo-decrescendo murmur, medium to high pitched sound, heard best at the apex
         a. Increases during the straining phase of the Valsalva maneuver or any intervention that increases LV volume
         b. Decreases during squatting and isometric exercises
   C. Diagnostic tests
      1. Same as for other mitral disorders
   D. Management
      1. Antibiotic prophylaxis for procedures only for those with a prior history of endocarditis (refer to Inflammatory Cardiac Disease chapter section on Endocarditis prophylaxis for appropriate indications/criteria and definitive therapy)
      2. Avoid stimulants in patients with palpitations
      3. β blockers for patients with mild tachyarrhythmias
      4. Aspirin, 81–325 mg daily for patients with documented neurological focal events who are in sinus rhythm with no atrial thrombi
      5. Same additional treatment as for mitral stenosis and regurgitation
      6. Monitor patient for complications
         a. Mitral regurgitation—most common complication
         b. Bacterial endocarditis—risk is 2–3 times that of the general population
         c. Supraventricular arrhythmias

V. **Aortic stenosis (AS)**
   A. Definition: narrowing of the aortic valve resulting in obstructed forward blood flow
   B. Etiology/incidence
      1. ~~Rheumatic disease is the most common cause~~.
      2. Degenerative or senile calcific disease most common cause in elderly
      3. Idiopathic calcification of the aortic valve
      4. Congenital
      5. Most common valvular disorder in the U.S. and among the elderly
   C. Subjective and physical examination findings
      1. Dyspnea—may be marked
      2. Angina—occurs in approximately 70% of patients
      3. Syncope—occurs in approximately 20% of patients

4. Murmur—systolic, "blowing," rough, harsh at the second right intercostal space, usually radiating to the neck and apex; classic crescendo-decrescendo quality; may especially radiate to the apex in elderly patients
5. A thrill or anacrotic "shudder" may be palpable over carotid arteries—commonly found on left; may be normal due to concurrent atherosclerosis and increased vascular stiffness in elderly patients
6. Pulsus parvus et tardus—peripheral arterial pulse rises slowly to a delayed peak
7. Presence of S4—reflects LV hypertrophy and elevated LV end-diastolic pressure
8. LV impulse displaced laterally
9. Absence of A2 component of second heart sound (absence of aortic component); intensity of S2 is a reliable marker of AS severity (softer the S2 sound, the more severe the AS)
10. Because onset of symptoms may be subtle, elderly may not have any limitations or may unconsciously alter habits to avoid symptoms

D. Diagnostic tests
1. Echocardiogram—same as for mitral disorders
2. ECG—check for LV hypertrophy seen with severe AS
3. Chest X-ray—check for concentric hypertrophy of the left ventricle with a calcified valve, dilated proximal ascending aorta along the upper right heart border, enlargement of heart chambers, and pulmonary artery
4. Cardiac catheterization: same as for mitral disorders

E. Management
1. Surgery—mortality rate is dependent upon preoperative clinical and hemodynamic state; for elderly, pay particular attention to pulmonary, renal, and hepatic function
   a. 10-year survival rate is 60%
   b. 30% of bioprosthetic valves demonstrate valve failure in 10 years, requiring re-replacement
   c. Equal percentage of patients develop hemorrhagic complications secondary to anticoagulants, particularly among the elderly and frail elderly
2. Percutaneous balloon aortic valvuloplasty—preferred approach in young adults with congenital, noncalcific AS
3. Transcatheter Aortic Valve Implantation (TAVI)
   a. Implantation procedure involves accessing a femoral artery, performing balloon valvuloplasty, and then advancing the device across the native valve. During rapid right ventricular pacing, a balloon is inflated to deploy the valve and the frame.
4. Nitrates should be used with caution in patients with symptomatic coronary artery disease with AS due to their effect on coronary artery perfusion.
5. Medical therapy for hypertension should follow standard guidelines, starting at a low dose and gradually titrating upward PRN to achieve BP control. There are no studies addressing specific antihypertensive medications in patients with AS, but diuretics should be avoided if the LV chamber is small, because even smaller LV volumes may result in a fall in cardiac output.
6. Avoid strenuous physical activity and competitive sports; avoid dehydration and hypovolemia to safe guard against significant reduction in cardiac output
7. Antibiotic prophylaxis for procedures for patients with prior history of endocarditis (refer to Inflammatory Cardiac Disease chapter section on endocarditis prophylaxis for appropriate indications/criteria and definitive therapy)

VI. **Aortic regurgitation**
A. Definition: backflow of blood into the left ventricle as a result of deficiencies of the aortic valve leaflets or the aorta
B. Etiology
1. Rheumatic fever

2. Rheumatoid arthritis
3. Infectious endocarditis is the most common cause of acute presentation.
4. Idiopathic valve calcification

C. Subjective and physical examination findings
1. Fatigue
2. Dyspnea
3. Syncope
4. Sinus tachycardia during exertion or with emotion
5. Feeling of head pounding or palpitations
6. Chest pain even in the absence of coronary artery disease
7. Jarring of the entire body and the bobbing motion of the head with each systole and abrupt distention and collapse of the larger arteries
8. Corrigan's pulse—rapidly rising "water-hammer" pulse, which collapses suddenly as arterial pressure falls rapidly during late systole and diastole
9. Quincke's pulse—alternate flushing and paling of the skin at the root of the nail while pressure is applied to the nail tip
10. Widened pulse pressure—result of both systolic hypertension and a lowering of the diastolic pressure
11. S3 heart sound
12. LV impulse—heaving and laterally displaced
13. Murmur—high pitched, blowing, decrescendo diastolic, murmur at the third left intercostal space along the left sternal border; heard best with patient sitting up, leaning forward, and with the breath held in forced expiration
14. Signs of congestive heart failure

D. Diagnostic tests
1. Same as for mitral disorders
2. Chest X-ray—check for moderate to severe left ventricular enlargement

E. Management
1. Surgical—guided by the stage of AR as well as clinical setting (i.e., aortic dissection or hemodynamic instability)
   a. Acute AR: in presence of hemodynamic instability, surgery is usually not delayed
      i. Intra-aortic balloon counterpulsation is contraindicated in patients with acute severe AR
      ii. AVR (repair or replacement) is indicated for symptomatic patients with severe AR regardless of LV systolic function
   b. Chronic AR: requires staging/surgical risk assessment
      i. AVR is indicated for asymptomatic patients with chronic severe AR and LV systolic dysfunction
2. Pharmaceutical
   a. Acute AR:
      i. Vasodilating agents: sodium nitroprusside
      ii. β blockers, diltiazem and verapamil; unless treating aortic dissection, these agents should be used cautiously, if at all, because they will block the compensatory tachycardia and could precipitate a marked reduction in BP
      iii. Antibiotic prophylaxis against bacterial endocarditis for dental or other surgical procedures (refer to Inflammatory Cardiac Disease chapter section on endocarditis prophylaxis for appropriate indications/criteria and definitive therapy)
   b. Chronic AR:
      i. Treatment of hypertension (systolic BP greater than 140 mmHg) is recommended in patients with chronic AR, preferably with dihydropyridine calcium channel blockers or ACE inhibitors/ARBs

ii. β blockers less effective because reduction in heart rate is associated with an even higher stroke volume, which contributes to elevated systolic pressure in patients with chronic severe AR

iii. ACE inhibitors/ARBs and β blockers are reasonable in patients with severe AR who have symptoms and/or LV dysfunction when surgery is not performed because of comorbidities.

iv. Vasodilating drugs are effective in reducing systolic BP in patients with chronic AR, however they are not routinely recommended in patients with chronic asymptomatic AR and normal LV systolic function.

BIBLIOGRAPHY

Adams, D. H., Carabello, B. A., & Castillo, J. G. (2011). Mitral valve regurgitation. In V. Fuster, R. A. Walsh, & R. A. Harrington (Eds.), *Hurst's the heart* (13th ed.). [E-reader version]. Retrieved from http://accessmedicine.mhmedical.com.libdata.lib.ua.edu/content.aspx?bookid=376&sectionid=40279811

Carbello, B. A. (2011). Mitral stenosis. In V. Fuster, R. A. Walsh, & R. A. Harrington (Eds.), *Hurst's the heart* (13th ed.). [E-reader version]. Retrieved from http://accessmedicine.mhmedical.com.libdata.lib.ua.edu/content.aspx?bookid=376&sectionid=40279812

Cawley, P. J., & Otto, C. M. (2011). Valvular heart disease in the elderly. *Current Cardiovascular Risk Reports, 5*(5), 413–421. doi:10.1007/s12170–011–0187–z

Chikwe, J., Filsoufi, F., & Carpentier, A. (2011). Prosthetic heart valves. In V. Fuster, R. A. Walsh, & R. A. Harrington (Eds.), *Hurst's the heart* (13th ed.). [E-reader version]. Retrieved from http://accessmedicine.mhmedical.com.libdata.lib.ua.edu/content.aspx?bookid=376&sectionid=40279814

Cupido, B. J., & Commerford, P. J. (2013). Rheumatic fever and valvular heart disease. In C. Rosendorff (Ed.), *Essential cardiology: Principles and practice*. New York, NY: Springer.

Freeman, R. V. & Otto, C. M. (2011). Aortic valve disease. In V. Fuster, R. A. Walsh, & R. A. Harrington (Eds.), *Hurst's the heart* (13th ed.). [E-reader version]. Retrieved from http://accessmedicine.mhmedical.com.libdata.lib.ua.edu/content.aspx?bookid=376&sectionid=40279810

Gongidi, V. R. & Hamaty, J. N. (2011). Aortic stenosis: A focused review in the elderly. *Clinical Geriatrics, 19*(3), 19–22.

Lazar, H. L. (2012). The year in review: The surgical treatment of valvular disease-2011. *Journal of Cardiac Surgery, 27*(4), 493–510. doi:10.1111/j.1540–8191.2012.01494.x

Nishimura, R. A., Otto, C. M., Bonow, R. O., Carabello, B. A., Erwin, J. P., Guyton, R. A. . . . Thomas, J. D. (2014). 2014 AHA/ACC guideline for the management of patients with valvular heart disease: A report of the American College of Cardiology/American Heart Association Task Force on Practice Guidelines. *Circulation.* doi:10.1161/CIR.0000000000000029

O'Gara, P. & Loscalzo, J. (2012). Valvular heart disease. In D. L. Longo, A. S. Fauci, D. L. Kasper, S. L. Hauser, J. L. Jameson, & J. Loscalzo (Eds.), *Harrison's principles of internal medicine* (18th ed.). [E-reader version]. Retrieved from ttp://accessmedicine.com/content/aspx?aID=9127003

Saikrishnan, N., Kumar, G., Sawaya, F. J., Lerakis, S. & Yoganathan, A. P. (2014). Accurate assessment of aortic stenosis: A review of diagnostic modalities and hemodynamics. *Circulation, 129*(2), 244–253. doi:10.1161/CIRCULATION AHA.113.002310

Vahanian, A., Alfierei, O., Andreotti, F., Antunes, M. J., Baron-Esquivias, G., Baumgartner, H., . . . Zembata, M. (2012). Guidelines on the management of valvular heart disease (version 2012). *European Heart Journal, 33*(19), 2451–2496. doi:10.1093/eurheartj/ehs109

Whitlock, R. P., Sun, J. C., Fremes, S. E., Rubens, F. D., & Teoh, K. H. (2012). Antithrombotic and thrombolytic therapy for valvular disease: Antithrombotic therapy and prevention of thrombosis, 9th ed: American College of Chest Physicians evidence-based clinical practice guidelines. *Chest, 141*(2 Suppl), 576S–600S. doi:10.1378/chest.11–2305

CHAPTER 20

Cardiomyopathy

SHEILA MELANDER • THOMAS W. BARKLEY, JR.

I. **Definition**
   A. Idiopathic disorder causing cardiac muscle dysfunction that may result in systolic or diastolic dysfunction not due to atherosclerosis, hypertension, or valvular disease
II. **Types**
   A. Dilated
      1. Abnormal systolic pump function
      2. Dilated ventricles without proportionate compensatory hypertrophy
      3. Systolic heart failure
   B. Hypertrophy
      1. Autosomal dominant disorder
      2. Stiff left ventricle during diastole that restricts ventricular filling
      3. Ventricular hypertrophy that occurs without dilatation or a thickening septum
      4. Diastolic heart failure
   C. Restrictive
      1. Inadequate diastolic filling
      2. Rigid ventricular walls
      3. Diastolic heart failure
III. **Etiology/incidence**
   A. Dilated
      1. Caused by ischemic heart disease, alcoholism, persistent tachycardia, that is, inappropriate sinus tachycardia or AFib with RVR, systemic lupus erythematosus, toxins, cocaine; also, idiopathic causes
      2. Most common type of cardiomyopathy
      3. Approximately 1% of the general population is affected; 10% of these patients are older than 80 years of age.
   B. Hypertrophic
      1. Cause is idiopathic
      2. Chronic hypertension has been associated with increased incidence.
   C. Restrictive

1. Related to a variety of conditions
   a. Sarcoidosis
   b. Endomyocardial fibrosis (after open heart surgery)
   c. Exposure
   d. Idiopathic causes
2. Relatively uncommon

IV. **Subjective/physical exam findings**
   A. Dilated cardiomyopathy is associated with left or biventricular congestive heart failure (CHF).
      1. Increased jugular venous distention
      2. Low pulse pressure
      3. S3 and/or S4 heart sounds
      4. Peripheral edema
      5. Rales
      6. Dyspnea
      7. Orthopnea
      8. Paroxysmal nocturnal dyspnea
      9. Mitral or tricuspid regurgitation
      10. Cardiomegaly
   B. Hypertrophic
      1. Dyspnea
      2. Chest pain
      3. Syncope
      4. Murmur—harsh, "diamond-shaped" (crescendo-decrescendo) systolic, at the left sternal border; decreases with squatting and increases with the Valsalva maneuver
      5. S4 heart sound
      6. Maximized apical pulse (double or triple)
   C. Restrictive—associated with right-sided heart failure
      1. Dyspnea
      2. Fatigue
      3. Weakness
      4. Edema
      5. Jugular venous distention
      6. Ascites
      7. Murmurs (regurgitant)
      8. Kussmaul breathing (possibly)

V. **Diagnostics**
   A. Dilated cardiomyopathy
      1. Chest x-ray
         a. Marked cardiac enlargement
         b. Pulmonary edema (interstitial)
      2. ECG
         a. ST segment/T-wave changes with left ventricular hypertrophy
         b. Right or left bundle branch block
         c. Arrhythmias common
            i. Atrial fibrillation
            ii. Premature atrial contractions
            iii. Premature ventricular contractions
            iv. Ventricular tachycardia
      3. Echocardiogram
         a. Left ventricular dilatation and dysfunction with low ejection fraction
      4. Routine blood and urine chemistries

B. Hypertrophic
   1. Chest x-ray
      a. Mild cardiomegaly or normal heart size
   2. ECG
      a. Abnormal Q waves in anterolateral and inferior leads
      b. Left ventricular hypertrophy
   3. Echocardiogram (diagnosis confirmed by two-dimensional approach)
      a. Left ventricular hypertrophy
      b. Increased or at times normal ejection fraction
   4. Exercise stress testing and 24-hr Holter monitor screening
   5. Routine blood and urine chemistries
C. Restrictive
   1. Chest x-ray
      a. Evidence of CHF, possibly including pleural effusion
      b. Cardiomegaly is usually mild to moderate.
   2. ECG
      a. ST segment/T-wave changes
      b. Atrial fibrillation, left axis deviation, and other arrhythmias are possible
   3. Echocardiogram
      a. Thickened cardiac valves
      b. Increased wall thickness
      c. Normal or small left ventricle size with mild to normal left ventricle function
   4. Routine blood and urine chemistries
   5. Cardiac catheterization/MRI to distinguish from constrictive pericarditis
      a. Impairment of the left ventricle is more evident than impairment of the right ventricle (e.g., pulmonary capillary wedge pressure is greater than central venous pressure) with restrictive cardiomyopathy.
      b. MRI reveals greater thickening of the pericardium with restrictive cardiomyopathy.
      c. With constrictive pericarditis, both ventricles are usually involved.
   6. Myocardial biopsy for definitive diagnosis

VI. **Management**
   A. Dilated cardiomyopathy
      1. Treatment of the underlying condition (e.g., discontinuing use of alcohol, treating endocrine causes, and rapid heart rate arrhythmias)
      2. For heart failure (see Heart Failure chapter)
         a. Rest
         b. Daily weights
         c. Restricted sodium
         d. Diuretics
         e. ACE inhibitors
         f. Digitalis if needed to reduce heart rate and thus workload in associated tachyarrhythmias
      3. Vasodilators, especially combined with ACE inhibitors and nitrates
      4. Oral anticoagulation for emboli prophylaxis
      5. β-blockers such as Carvedilol or Coreg, or Metoprolol (Lopressor; Toprol XL)—ow-dose β-blockade
      6. Diltiazem (Cardizem)—especially effective for idiopathic causes; however, not advocated for use in patients with left ventricular depression
      7. Antiarrhythmics PRN
   B. Hypertrophic

1. β-blocking drugs are recommended for the treatment of symptoms (angina or dyspnea) in adult patients with obstructive or nonobstructive HCM, but should be used with caution in patients with sinus bradycardia or severe conduction disease.
2. If low doses of β-blocking drugs are ineffective for controlling symptoms, titrate the dose to a resting heart rate of less than 60-65 bpm (up to generally accepted and recommended maximum doses of these drugs).
   a. Metoprolol, 25 mg PO every 12 hr (maximum 400 mg/day)
   b. Atenolol, 25 mg PO daily (maximum 200 mg/day)
   c. Verapamil (Calan), 120-480 mg daily to BID, for obstructive and nonobstructive disease in those for whom β-blockers are contraindicated/intolerable)
3. With acute heart failure, IV normal saline in addition to propranolol (Inderal) or verapamil (Calan)
4. Antibiotic prophylaxis for invasive procedures, may be indicated depending upon individual valvular diagnoses
5. Amiodarone (Cordarone) or other antiarrhythmics to prevent recurrence of atrial fibrillation
6. Avoidance of alcohol
7. Consider dual-chamber pacing to prevent progression of the disease, as indicated
   a. ACE inhibitors, nitrates, diuretics, and digoxin are contraindicated with hypertrophic obstructive disease
8. Consider implantation of internal cardioverter defibrillator for the prevention of sudden death

C. Restrictive
1. Control major cause(s) of death due to heart failure
   a. Restrict sodium intake
   b. Use diuretics PRN
   c. Administer antiarrhythmics as appropriate
2. Perform repeated phlebotomies to decrease iron deposition in the heart for patients with cardiomyopathy caused by hemochromatosis
3. Corticosteroids for sarcoidosis
4. Symptomatic treatment

BIBLIOGRAPHY

Bojar, R. M. (2011). *Manual of perioperative care in adult cardiac surgery* (5th ed.). Boston, MA: Wiley/Blackwell Publishing.

Carvalho, V. O., Bocchi, E. A., & Guimarães, G. V. (2009). Hydrotherapy in heart failure: A case report. *Clinics, 64*(8).

Dunphy, L. H. (2004). *Management guidelines for nurse practitioners working with adults* (2nd ed.). Philadelphia, PA: FA Davis.

England, B., Lee, A., Tran, T., Faw, H., Yang, P., Lin, A., . . . Ross, B. D. (2005). Magnetic resonance criteria for future trials of cardiac resynchronization. *Journal of Cardiovascular Magnetic Resonance, 7*(5), 827–834.

Ferri, F. F. (2011). *Ferri's clinical advisor 2011: Instant diagnosis and treatment.* Philadelphia, PA: Elsevier Health Sciences.

Gersh, B. J., Maron, B. J., Bonow, R. O., Dearani, J. A., Fifer, M. A., Link, M. S., . . . & Yancy, C. W. (2011). 2011 ACCF/AHA guideline of the diagnosis and treatment of hypertropic cardiomyopathy: Executive summary. *Circulation, 124,* 2761–2796.

Gheorghiade, M., Flaherty, J. D., Fonarow, G. C., Desai, R. V., Lee, R., McGiffin, D., . . . Ahmed, A. (2011). Coronary artery disease, coronary revascularization, and outcomes in chronic advanced systolic heart failure. *International Journal of Cardiology, 151*(1), 69–75.

Grimes, J. A. (2013). *The 5-minute clinical consult.* Philadelphia, PA: Lippincott Williams & Wilkins.

Hare, J. M. (2011). The dilated, restrictive, and infiltrative cardiomyopathies. In R. O. Bonow, D. L. Mann, D. P. Zipes, & P. Libby (Eds.). *Braunwald's heart disease: A textbook of cardiovascular medicine* (9th ed.). Philadelphia, PA: Saunders Elsevier.

Klabunde, R. E. (2004). *Cardiovascular physiology concepts*. Philadelphia, PA: Lippincott Williams & Wilkins.

Maron, B., & Maron, M. (2013). Hypertrophic cardiomyopathy. *Lancet, 381*(9862), 242-255. doi:10.1016/S0140-6736(12)60397-3

Schiros, C. G., Ahmed, M. I., Sanagala, T., Zha, W., McGiffin, D. C., Bamman, M. M., . . . Dell'Italia, L. J. (2013). Importance of 3-dimensional geometric analysis in the assessment of the athlete's heart. *American Journal of Cardiology, 111*(7), 1067–1072.

Wackett, A., & Fan, R. (2005). *Cardiomyopathy, restrictive*. Retrieved September 4, 2007, from www.emedicine.com/EMERG/topic81.htm

Wexler, R. K., Elton, T., Pleister, A., & Feldman, D. (2009). Cardiomyopathy: An overview. *American Family Physician, 79*(9), 778–784.

CHAPTER 21

Arrhythmias

FREDRICK CARLSTON • ROBERT FELLIN • THOMAS W. BARKLEY, JR

COMMON CARDIAC RHYTHMS/ARRHYTHMIAS AND TREATMENT

I. **Normal sinus rhythm (NSR) (Figure 21.1)**
   A. Characteristics
      1. Regular rate and rhythm
      2. PR interval and QRS complex normal
         a. PR interval 0.20 seconds or less
         b. QRS complex 0.12 seconds or less
   B. Rate is 60–100 beats/minute (bpm)

II. **Sinus bradycardia (SB) (Figure 21.2)**
   A. Characteristics
      1. Regular rate and rhythm
      2. PR interval and QRS complex normal
   B. Rate 60 bpm or less than expected relative to underlying condition or cause
   C. Etiology
      1. Increased vagal tone (e.g., in athletes)
      2. Medications: AV nodal blockers (e.g., digitalis, β blockers, calcium channel blockers)
      3. Recreational drug abuse
      4. Metabolic or electrolyte abnormalities
      5. Autonomic dysfunction or neurologic causes
      6. Ischemic or valvular heart disease
      7. Sinus node dysfunction; includes inappropriate sinus bradycardia and tachy-brady syndrome
   D. Clinical manifestations
      1. May be asymptomatic
      2. Presyncope or syncope, dizziness, orthostatic, fatigue, or weakness
      3. Signs of decreased perfusion, hypotension, or confusion
   E. Treatment
      1. Consult/refer to cardiologist or electrophysiologist
      2. If asymptomatic, treatment may not be indicated
      3. Diagnostic testing could include Holter monitor or rhythm patch, labs, and tilt-table test

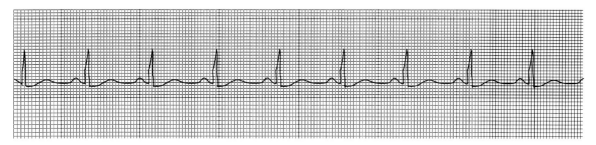

Figure 21.1. Normal sinus rhythm.

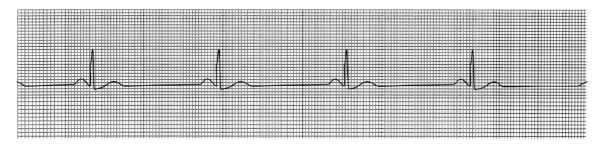

Figure 21.2. Sinus bradycardia.

        4. If indicated, may require permanent pacemaker
        5. For acute symptomatic bradycardia, initiate transcutaneous pacing Medication (e.g., atropine, dopamine, isoproterenol) can be used

III. Sinus arrhythmia (Figure 21.3)
    A. Characteristics
        1. Rate is variable (i.e., variable R-R interval)
        2. Normal PR interval and QRS complex
        3. Rate varies with respirations
    B. Etiology: common in children and the elderly
    C. Clinical manifestations: none known
    D. Treatment: none indicated

IV. Junctional rhythm (Figure 21.4)
    A. Characteristics
        1. Because the beat originates in the atrioventricular (AV) node, usually no P waves precede QRS complexes
        2. Occasionally, P waves are retrograde conducted, resulting in a downward deflection before or after the QRS complex.
        3. Rate is usually 40–60 bpm (i.e., the intrinsic AV node rate)
        4. Accelerated junctional rhythms have the same criteria, but rates range from 60–100 bpm.
        5. Rarely seen in adult patients
    B. Etiology (common causes)
        1. Digitalis toxicity
        2. Theophylline
        3. Dopamine
    C. Treatment
        1. Consult/refer to cardiologist or electrophysiologist
        2. Atropine, 0.5 mg intravenous push (IVP), to a maximum of 3 mg (for unstable patient)
        3. Consider pacing if patient is severely bradycardic (for unstable patient)

V. Sinus tachycardia (ST) (Figure 21.5)
    A. Characteristics
        1. Regular rate and rhythm

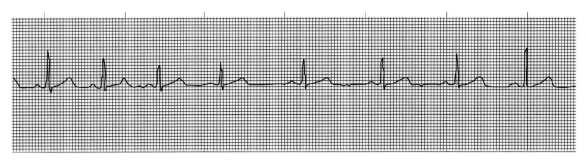

Figure 21.3. Sinus arrythmia

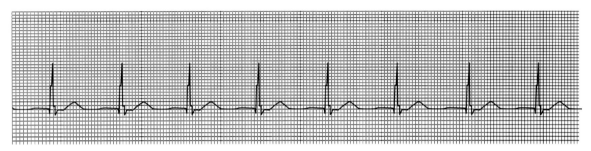

Figure 21.4. Accelerated junctional rhythm (strip is approximately 80 bpm)

        2. PR interval and QRS complex normal
- B. Rate 100 bpm or more and typically less than 150–160 bpm
- C. Etiology
    1. Usually reflects an underlying process, metabolic state, or medication use (e.g., fever, shock, CHF, pain, cocaine or other illicit drug use, hypovolemia)
    2. Inappropriate sinus tachycardia
- D. Clinical manifestations
    1. May be asymptomatic
    2. Chest tightness, SOB, palpitations, fatigue, facial flushing
    3. Hypertension
    4. If poor perfusion: hypotension, loss of consciousness (LOC)
- E. Treatment
    1. Treat the underlying problem or cause
    2. If all causes of sinus tachycardia have been excluded, consult/refer to cardiologist or electrophysiologist for evaluation of inappropriate sinus tachycardia
        - a. β-blockers or non-dihydropyridine calcium channel blockers (i.e., diltiazem or verapamil) may be indicated
        - b. Can lead to tachycardia-induced cardiomyopathy
        - c. Refractory cases may require SA node ablation

VI. Premature atrial contractions (PACs) (Figure 21.6)
- A. Characteristics
    1. Occur when an ectopic focus in the atria fires before the next sinus node impulse; P waves usually look different (i.e., either smaller or peaked)
    2. Rate usually "resets" itself, resulting in one premature beat followed by a normal series of beats in sinus rhythm
- B. Etiology: not considered an abnormal finding
- C. Clinical manifestations: usually asymptomatic; rarely can cause symptoms of palpitations and SOB
- D. Treatment: in general, none; in patients who are symptomatic, β-blockers or non-dihydropyridine calcium channel blockers (i.e., diltiazem or verapamil) are usually effective

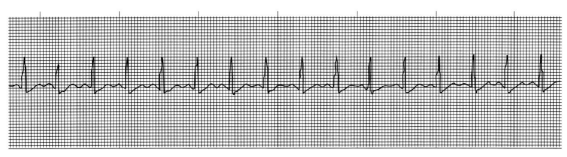

Figure 21.5. Sinus tachycardia.

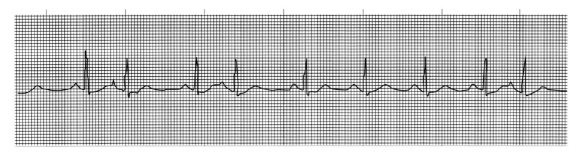

Figure 21.6. Premature atrial contractions

VII. Atrial tachycardia
    A. Characteristics
        1. Often sudden onset and sudden stop, sustained atrial tachycardia is relatively rare
        2. Rate of 140–220 bpm
        3. Ventricle is a "slave" to the atrium
        4. P wave morphology usually different; QRS remains unchanged
        5. Pacemaker is coming from a single ectopic focus that is outside the SA node
    B. Etiology
        1. Usually occurs in patients with abnormal automaticity or pulmonary problems
        2. Can be caused by medications including Digoxin excess
        3. Can be caused by increased catecholamine state or volume overload (atrial stretch)
    C. Clinical manifestations
        1. Patients can be asymptomatic
        2. Patients can report chest pressure, palpitations, syncope or presyncope, SOB, or fatigue
        3. Patients with poor perfusion may have hypotension, LOC, shock
    D. Treatment
        1. Consult/refer to cardiologist or electrophysiologist.
        2. Treat underlying cause
        3. Can try vagal maneuvers by asking the patient to cough, strain as though having a bowel movement, or elicit the patient's gag reflex
        4. AV nodal blockers (β-blockers, non-dihydropyridine calcium channel blockers [i.e., diltiazem or verapamil])
        5. Antiarrhythmics may be required if AV nodal blockers are not effective (see Table 21.1)
        6. Cardiac ablation of ectopic focus may be indicated and has a 95% success rate
        7. For unstable patient, follow ACLS guidelines

VIII. Multifocal atrial tachycardia
    A. Characteristics
        1. P waves of three or more different morphologies
        2. P-P, P-R, and R-R intervals vary
        3. Rates usually 100–180 bpm
        4. Irregular and is often mistaken for atrial fibrillation
        5. Can degenerate into atrial fibrillation

Table 21.1	Antiarrhythmic Agents	
Agent	**Indication**	**Adverse Effects**
Class IA: Sodium Channel Blockers All may cause new or worsen dysrhythmias Effective for atrial and ventricular arrhythmias, however infrequently used due to their significant toxicity		
Disopyramide phosphate (Norpace)	AF, PSVT, PVC, VT, WPW	constipation, nausea, muscle weakness, blurred vision, fatigue, heart failure
Procainamide HCl (Pronestyl)	AF, PVC, VT, WPW	agranulocytosis, SLE, hypotension, hepatotoxicity, ventricular arrhythmia,
Quinidine gluconate (Quinaglute)	AF, PVC, VT, WPW	nausea, abdominal pain, diarrhea, hemolytic anemia, thrombocytopenia, hepatitis, ventricular tachycardia (torsade de pointe)
Class IB: Sodium Channel Blockers Cannot be used to treat atrial arrhythmias		
Lidocaine	PVC, VT, VF	hypotension, nausea, blurred vision, methemoglobinemia, paresthesias, confusion, seizure, tremors
Mexiletine (Mexitil)	PVC, VT, VF	nausea, vomiting, dizziness, lightheadedness, tremor, blurred vision, visual disturbance, agranulocytosis, hepatotoxicity
Class IC: Sodium Channel Blockers Do not use in patients with structural heart disease		
Flecainide (Tambocor)	AF, PSVT, ventricular arrhythmias	palpitations, nausea, dizziness, headache, blurred vision, fatigue
Propafenone (Rythmol)	AF, ventricular arrhythmias, WPW	chest pain, edema, palpitations, constipation, altered sense of taste, vomiting, dizziness, anxiety, fatigue, agranulocytosis, heart failure
Class II: β-Adrenergic Blockers Primarily used for rate control		
Acebutolol (Sectral)	Atrial tachyarrhythmias AF (rate control; control ventricular rate)	hypotension, dizziness, bradycardia, 2nd or 3rd degree heart block, fatigue, insomnia, nausea
Atenolol (Tenormin)		
Esmolol (Brevibloc)		
Metoprolol (Lopressor)		
Propranolol (Inderal)		
Class III: Potassium Channel Blockers All may cause new or worsen dysrhythmias Effective for atrial and ventricular arrhythmias		
Amiodarone (Cordarone, Pacerone)	AF, PSVT, VF, ventricular arrhythmias	bradyarrhythmia, hypotension, photodermatitis, photosensitivity, thyroid dysfunction, nausea, vomiting, increased liver enzymes, dizziness, paresthesia, visual disturbance, optic neuritis, fatigue, toxic epidermal necrolysis, pulmonary fibrosis
Dofetilide (Tikosyn)	AF/atrial flutter	chest pain, dizziness, headache, heart block, ventricular arrhythmia
Ibutilide (Corvert)	AF/atrial flutter	bradyarrhythmia, heart block, ventricular arrhythmia, headache, hypotension

Table 21.1	Antiarrhythmic Agents	
Agent	**Indication**	**Adverse Effects**
Sotalol (βpace)	AF, PSVT, ventricular arrhythmias	dizziness, weakness, fatigue, nausea, vomiting, diarrhea, bradycardia, heart block, heart failure, bronchospasm
Dronedarone (Multaq)	AF	abdominal pain, diarrhea, indigestion, nausea, vomiting, heart failure, CVA, liver failure Doubles the risk of death in patients with symptomatic heart failure
Class IV: Calcium Channel Blockers **Primarily used for rate control**		
Diltiazem (Cardizem)	Atrial tachyarrhythmias, AF (rate control; control ventricular rate)	peripheral edema, hypotension, dizziness, bradycardia, 2nd or 3rd degree heart block, fatigue, insomnia, constipation
Verapamil (Calan)	Supraventricular tachycardia, PSVT	
Miscellaneous Agents **May produce new dysrhythmias or worsen existing ones**		
Adenosine (Adenocard)	PSVT	chest discomfort, flushing, abdominal discomfort, dizziness, headache, dyspnea
Digoxin (Lanoxin)	AF (rate control; control ventricular rate)	nausea, vomiting, headache, visual disturbances Monitor drug levels

Note. AF = atrial fibrillation; PAC = premature atrial complex; PSVT = paroxysmal supraventricular tachycardia; PVC = premature ventricular complex; VF = ventricular fibrillation; VT = ventricular tachycardia; WPW = Wolff-Parkinson-White syndrome

   B. Etiology
      1. Occurs in the elderly or acutely ill patients
      2. Common in patients with pulmonary disorders and associated with hypoxia
      3. Occasionally seen with sepsis, volume overload, and theophylline toxicity
   C. Treatment
      1. Rhythm itself is rarely associated with instability
      2. Treat the underlying disorder
      3. Magnesium, one dose of 2 grams followed by infusion of 1–2 grams per hr over 5 hr, may reduce atrial ectopy. Mg levels may rise to 2.5–3 mg/dl
      4. Verapamil or β-blockers for rate control; caution recommended when using β-blockers in patients with pulmonary disease
      5. No need for anticoagulation; no increased stroke risk
IX. **Atrial fibrillation (A-fib) (Figure 21.7; also see Figure 21.20 at the end of this chapter)**
   A. Characteristics
      1. No discernible P waves; fibrillatory waves are noted instead
      2. PR interval is not measurable (wavy baseline).
      3. QRS complex is regularly irregular.
      4. Atrial rate is commonly 400–700 bpm.
      5. Ventricular rate is usually 100–160 bpm or greater
      6. Most common sustained arrhythmia; estimated 2.2 million people in the U.S. have atrial fibrillation
   B. Classifications
      1. Lone atrial fibrillation
      2. Paroxysmal atrial fibrillation
      3. Post-operative atrial fibrillation

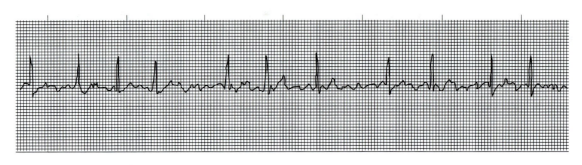

Figure 21.7. Atrial fibrillation.

  4. Persistent (longer than 7 days)
  5. Permanent or chronic atrial fibrillation
  6. Associated with increased morbidity, mortality, and preventable stroke
 C. Etiology
  1. Can be caused by various factors (e.g., catecholamine surges, volume overload causing atrial stretch, medications, hyperthyroidism, and autonomic tone)
  2. Etiology is unknown; irregular electrical signals from pulmonary veins entering the left atrium as a trigger source are becoming increasingly appreciated
  3. Prevalence increases with age with 0.4%–1% in the general population and as high as 8% in patients 80 years or older.
  4. Because the atrium is not contracting normally, blood clots could form in left atrium (left atrial appendage) and the patient is at higher risk of embolic stroke
  5. The HAS-BLED Bleeding Risk Score can be used to assess the risk of bleeding for atrial fibrillation management; comprised of evaluating the following clinical characteristics: hypertension, abnormal renal and liver function, stroke, bleeding tendency/predisposition, labile INRs for patients taking warfarin, elderly, and drugs/alcohol
  6. Use the CHADS2 score to assess the risk of atrial fibrillation by attributing and adding the specified number of points (see table 21.2)
  7. The CHADSVASC scoring is becoming the standard.
X. **Clinical manifestations**
  1. Patient may be asymptomatic
  2. Patient may report palpitations, SOB, presyncope, diaphoresis, fatigue, weakness, chest pressure or tightness
  3. Patient with decreased perfusion may have hypotension and LOC
 A. Treatment
  1. Referral to cardiologist or electrophysiologist
  2. Treatment is immediate direct-current cardioversion (DCC) for an unstable patient in rapid atrial fibrillation

Table 21.2	CHADS2 Score: Stroke risk assessment in atrial fibrillation
Score	**CHADS2 Risk Criteria**
1 point	Heart failure
1 point	Hypertension
1 point	Age greater than 75 years
1 point	Diabetes mellitus
2 points	Stroke/transient ischemic attack

3. Treatment strategy of the stable patient is individualized, decision is made to pursue rate control strategy vs rhythm control strategy; both strategies include stroke risk reduction (see Tables 21.4 & 21.5).
    a. AV nodal blockers for rate control (see Table 21.1)
    b. Antiarrhythmics (see Table 21.1) and/or planned TEE and cardioversion (see Tables 21.4 & 21.5) for rhythm control
    c. Anticoagulation for stroke risk reduction
        i. Aspirin vs Coumadin based on individual stroke risk
        ii. Newer direct thrombin inhibitors are becoming more prevalent in part because INR testing is not required (e.g., dabigatran).
4. Catheter ablation with pulmonary vein isolation is available to patients who are symptomatic and not responsive to AV nodal blockers or antiarrhythmics (has 75% success rate and often requires more than one ablation).
5. Treatment recommendations when using the CHADS2 Risk Assessment scoring guidelines (see table 21.3)

XI. **Atrial flutter (A-flutter) (Figure 21.8; also see Figure 21.20)**
   A. Characteristics
      1. Sawtooth appearance of flutter waves (F waves), especially if the rhythm strip is turned upside down
      2. PR interval is not measurable
      3. Atrial rate ranges from 240–340 bpm
      4. QRS complex is usually normal
      5. Incidence varies from 0.4%–1.2%
      6. Considered to have the same stroke risk as atrial fibrillation
   B. Etiology
      1. Same causative factors as atrial fibrillation; catecholamine surge, volume overload causing atrial stretch, medications, hyperthyroidism, or autonomic tone
      2. Manifested by reentrant electrical circuit that travels within the right atrium in a counter-clockwise rotation (typical atrial flutter); clockwise may also be seen (atypical atrial flutter)
   C. Clinical manifestations
      1. May be asymptomatic
      2. Symptoms include palpitations, SOB, diaphoresis, fatigue, weakness, presyncope, chest pressure or tightness
      3. Patients with decreased perfusion may have hypotension and LOC
   D. Treatment
      1. Similar to atrial fibrillation; atrial flutter does not often respond as well to rate control strategy
      2. Ablation of reentrant circuit has 95% success rate

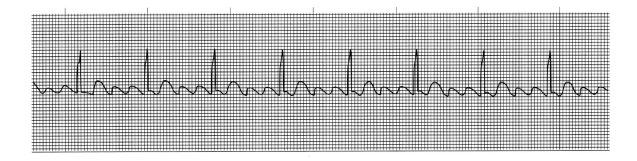

Figure 21.8. Atrial flutter.

XII. AV nodal re-entry tachycardia (AVNRT)
   A. Characteristics
      1. Most common SVT (excluding A-fib and A-flutter)
      2. An AV nodal dependent arrhythmia
      3. Rates 150–190 but can exceed 200
      4. Involves the slow and fast pathway within the AV node
      5. P waves are hidden within the QRS
      6. Usually found in patients without underlying heart disease; more common in women
   B. Etiology
      1. Caused by a PAC that travels down a slow pathway within the AV node, causing the conduction to create a re-entrant pathway within the AV node
   C. Clinical manifestations
      1. Patients may experience palpitations, SOB, presyncope, fatigue, or diaphoresis
      2. Patients with poor perfusion may experience hypotension, LOC, or shock
   D. Treatment
      1. Vagal maneuvers to attempt termination
      2. Adenosine, 6 mg rapid IV push; if not successful, increase to 12 mg
      3. Referral to cardiologist or electrophysiologist
      4. β-blockers and non-dihydropyridine calcium channel blockers (i.e., diltiazem, verapamil) help to prevent recurrence
      5. Ablation is the curative therapy with a 95% success rate (Heart block is the major complication risk with 0.8% of patients requiring permanent pacemaker due to the proximity of the AV node)
      6. Antiarrhythmics are used for patients not wanting ablation and not responding to AV nodal blockers (see Table 21.1)

XIII. AV reentrant tachycardia (AVRT)
   A. Characteristics
      1. Type of SVT that is AV node dependent
      2. Rates similar to AVNRT, however, more often greater than 200 bpm
      3. Relies on the presence of an accessory pathway; this abnormal conduction pathway between the atrium and the ventricle can be on the left or right sides of the heart, the free wall or septum
      4. P waves are usually within the ST segment or T wave
   B. Etiology
      1. Conduction through a reentry circuit that travels through the accessory pathway and back through the AV node
   C. Clinical manifestations
      1. Patients may experience palpitations, SOB, presyncope, fatigue, or diaphoresis.
      2. Patients with poor perfusion may experience hypotension, LOC, or shock.
   D. Treatment
      1. Vagal maneuvers to attempt termination
      2. Adenosine, 6 mg rapid IV push; if not successful, increase to 12 mg; can repeat once
      3. For unstable AVNRT, proceed to direct-current cardioversion.
      4. Referral to cardiologist or electrophysiologist
      5. β-blockers and non-dihydropyridine calcium channel blockers (i.e., diltiazem or verapamil) help to prevent recurrence
      6. Ablation of accessory pathway is the curative therapy with a 95% success rate. Heart block is a complication risk if the accessory pathway is close to septum.
      7. Antiarrhythmics used for patients not wanting ablation and not responding to AV nodal blockers (see Table 21.1)

Table 21.3 CHADS2 Risk Assessment scoring guidelines

CHADS2 Score	Risk	Recommendation
0	Low	Aspirin (81–325 mg) daily
1	Intermediate	Aspirin (81–324 mg) daily or warfarin (INR 2.0–3.0)
2 or more	High	Warfarin (INR 2.0–3.0) unless contraindicated

Table 21.4 Therapeutic interventions for cardioversion of atrial fibrillation

Intervention	Comments
Direct-Current Cardioversion	• Recommended for patients with AF or atrial flutter as a method to restore sinus rhythm. If cardioversion is unsuccessful, repeated direct-current cardioversion attempts may be made after adjusting the location of the electrodes or applying pressure over the electrodes, or following administration of an antiarrhythmic medication • Recommended when a rapid ventricular response to AF or atrial flutter does not respond promptly to pharmacological therapies and contributes to ongoing myocardial ischemia, hypotension or HF • Recommended for patients with AF or atrial flutter and pre-excitation when tachycardia is associated with hemodynamic instability
Amiodarone	• Maintains efficacy in patients with atrial fibrillation present for more than 7 days • Many drug-drug interactions and adverse effects
Dofetilide	• Dofetilide therapy should not be initiated out of hospital due to the risk of excessive QT prolongation that can cause Torsades de pointes. • MD must be registered by manufacturer to prescribe • Dofetilide is prescribed and dispensed only by healthcare providers, hospitals, and pharmacies that are certified to have received appropriate dofetilide dosing and treatment initiation education.
Flecainide	Avoid in patients with structural heart disease; increased risk of arrhythmia
Ibutilide (IV form only)	Avoid in patients with structural heart disease; increased risk of arrhythmia
Propafenone	Avoid in patients with structural heart disease; increased risk of arrhythmia

Table 21.5 Recommended antiarrhythmic drug therapy for maintenance of sinus rhythm in patients with recurrent paroxysmal or recurrent persistent atrial fibrillation

Condition	Recommendation
No structural heart disease	First line: flecainide, propafenone or sotalol Second line: amiodarone or dofetilide or catheter ablation
Heart Failure	First line: amiodarone or dofetilide Second line: catheter ablation
Coronary artery disease	First line: sotalol (should be used only if patients have normal left ventricular systolic function) Second line: amiodarone or dofetilide or catheter ablation
Hypertension without significant LVH	First line: flecainide, propafenone or sotalol Second line: amiodarone or dofetilide or catheter ablation
Hypertension with significant LVH	First line: amiodarone Second line: catheter ablation

Note. LVH = left ventricular hypertrophy

XIV. Wolff-Parkinson White syndrome (WPW)
  A. Characteristics
   1. Defined as the presence of short PR and Delta wave on EKG along with evidence of SVT
   2. Delta wave: short PR and "slurring" of initial portion of the QRS
   3. 0.2% of general population, about 70% asymptomatic
   4. 60%–70% men
   5. Predisposition to tachyarrhythmias
   6. In asymptomatic patients, a Delta wave does not confirm WPW syndrome but rather a "WPW pattern" (WPW pattern should not be treated, but can be monitored; these patients should be referred to a cardiologist)
  B. Etiology
   1. Conduction through an accessory pathway that can conduct both antegrade and retrograde; the antegrade conduction produces a Delta wave, due to "pre-excitation" of the ventricle.
   2. Can present as SVT and Delta waves after conversion back to NSR
  C. Clinical manifestations
   1. Patients may experience the same symptoms as SVT: palpitations, SOB, presyncope, fatigue, or diaphoresis.
   2. Patients who present with atrial fibrillation present with wide and bizarre QRS's d/t pre-excitation; ventricular rates can be as high as 200–300 and can degenerate to ventricular fibrillation; these patients can be very symptomatic.
  D. Treatment
   1. Referral to cardiologist or electrophysiologist
   2. WPW pattern on EKG: monitor, refer for expert consultation
   3. WPW that presents in SVT, treat the same as you would SVT; vagal maneuvers, adenosine
   4. WPW that presents in atrial fibrillation: avoid AV nodal blockers which can cause 1:1 conduction through the accessory pathway (e.g., HR's could be greater than 300 bpm).
   5. In stable patients with atrial fibrillation, use drugs that prolong the refractory period of the bypass tract (procainamide or amiodarone) or consider transesophageal echocardiogram (TEE) and direct-current cardioversion (DCCV); in the unstable patient, move directly toward DCCV.
   6. EP study and ablation of accessory pathway is the curative therapy and preferred choice.
   7. Can also use antiarrhythmics (see Table 21.1)

XV. Premature ventricular contractions (PVCs) (Figure 21.9)
  A. Etiology
   1. Irritability of the myocardium due to the following:
      a. Electrolyte imbalance
      b. Hypoxia
      c. Acidosis
      d. Myocardial infarction
      e. Other
   2. A stimulus from the ventricle replaces the sinoatrial (SA) node as the pacemaker for one or more beats, and contraction occurs without the usual transmission from the atrium.
  B. Clinical manifestations
   1. Patients may or may not be aware of PVCs
   2. Symptoms are usually related to the number and frequency of abnormal beats
   3. Patients may complain of "fluttering" or "palpitations" of the heart
   4. On the monitor, PVCs exhibit a wide QRS configuration that differs from that of the normal beat
  C. Implications

1. Unifocal PVCs that occur infrequently or have the same focus (i.e., have the same shape [Figure 21.10, A]), have limited significance, and may occur in the absence of heart disease
2. An increase in the frequency of these beats is more significant, especially if the PVCs occur more often than 6 times per minute, or if the patient has had a very recent myocardial infarction.
3. PVCs that are the result of more than one focus (i.e., multifocal [Figure 21.10, B]) are more serious and may precede ventricular tachycardia or ventricular fibrillation.
   a. The risk is minimal if the beats are isolated.
   b. The danger increases if beats do the following:
      i. Are frequent (i.e., more than six per minute)
      ii. Are multifocal (have different shapes) (Figure 21.11)
      iii. Occur with every other beat (bigeminal) (Figure 21.12)
      iv. Occur with every third beat (trigeminal) (Figure 21.13)
      v. Occur repetitively (pairs)
      vi. Appear on the downslope of the T wave (when the heart is relatively refractory and electrically unstable)
   c. If a PVC lands on the downslope of the T wave, the patient may experience ventricular tachycardia and/or ventricular fibrillation.
D. Treatment
   1. None if asymptomatic
   2. Check electrolytes and replace PRN
   3. First line treatment for symptomatic PVCs is β-blockers which help to decrease sympathetic tone
   4. For symptomatic treatment of PVCs, consult cardiologist or electrophysiologist for consideration of antiarrhythmics or VT ablation.

XVI. **Ventricular tachycardia (VT) (Figure 21.14)**
A. Etiology
   1. 3 or more wide complex QRS (greater than 120 ms) that are ventricular in origin with a rate greater than 100 bpm
   2. Can originate anywhere below the AV node
   3. Monomorphic is the most common; uniform QRS and regular
   4. Non-sustained is defined as less than 30 seconds
   5. Can be caused by ischemia, scar tissue, electrolyte disturbances, QT prolongation, cardiomyopathy, or be idiopathic
B. Clinical manifestations
   1. Patient can be asymptomatic
   2. Patients may feel palpitations, SOB, chest pain, or presyncope
   3. Patients could have VT arrest or sudden cardiac death
C. Implications
   1. If untreated, VT produces rapid hemodynamic decompensation caused by inadequate filling and emptying of the ventricles
   2. If untreated, VT leads to VF, asystole, and death
D. Treatment of VT
   1. Consult cardiologist or electrophysiologist—causes should be ruled out and treatment guided by experts; for stable VT and nonsustained VT, β-blockers are the mainstay
      a. Blocks the sympathetic response
      b. Slows sinus rate
   2. Treatment with amiodarone, sotalol, and mexiletine is used frequently to reduce the number and frequency of shocks.
      a. May be controversial due to a high side effect profile
      b. Blocks potassium repolarization which increases wavelength for reentry

3. Consider magnesium, 1–2 grams IV if torsades de pointes with prolonged QT interval is present
4. Be prepared for cardioversion
5. Treat underlying cause
   a. If ischemia is the cause, may need to go to cath lab or OR for revascularization
   b. Monitor and replace electrolytes
   c. Monitor QT for prolongation; if prolonged (general rule greater than 500), look for QT medication offenders
   d. Patients with cardiomyopathy may require ICD placement (e.g., primary prevention of sudden cardiac death in patients with an ejection fraction less than 35%)
6. Consult electrophysiologist for consideration of EP study, ablation, and/or AICD placement
   a. AICD placement has supplanted the use of antiarrhythmics for the chronic management of ventricular arrhythmias. Concomitant antiarrhythmic therapy can be used in patients who often receive shocks to reduce the incidence of appropriate shocks from VT or VF, reduce the VT rate so that it can be terminated with antitachycardia pacing, reduce the incidence of inappropriate shocks triggered by the AF or atrial flutter and prolong the device's battery life.
E. Treatment of unstable VT. Follow ACLS guidelines:
   1. Begin high quality CPR with interruptions kept to a minimum; early defibrillation; CPR resumed for 5 cycles between shocks
   2. Epinephrine 1 mg every 3–5 minutes; vasopressin 40 units can replace 1st or 2nd dose of epinephrine; consider amiodarone 300 mg IVP after 3rd shock, 2nd dose of amiodarone 150 mg IVP.
   3. Lidocaine, 1–1.5 mg/kg with a 2nd dose of 0.5–0.75 mg/kg for refractory VT that does not respond to amiodarone
   4. Consider magnesium, 1–2 grams IV if torsades de pointes with prolonged QT interval is present
   5. For airway management, consider capnography

XVII. **Ventricular fibrillation (V-fib) (Figure 21.15)**
   A. Etiology
      1. Often precipitated by VT
      2. No organized electrical activity
      3. Chaotic "wavy" baseline
      4. Characterized as course vs fine
      5. Same causes as VT
   B. Clinical manifestations
      1. Sudden loss of consciousness and/or seizure-like activity
      2. Absence of pulse or respirations
      3. Cyanosis
      4. Dilated pupils
   C. Implications
      1. V-fib results in sudden death unless the arrhythmia is immediately terminated.
      2. Although V-fib may be reversed, irreversible brain damage may result from lack of perfusion.
   D. Treatment of unstable V-fib. Follow ACLS guidelines:
      1. Begin high quality CPR with interruptions kept to a minimum; early defibrillation; CPR resumed for 5 cycles between shocks
      2. Epinephrine 1 mg every 3–5 minutes; vasopressin 40 units can replace 1st or 2nd dose of epinephrine; consider amiodarone 300 mg IVP after 3rd shock, 2nd dose of amiodarone 150 mg IVP

3. Lidocaine, 1–1.5 mg/kg with a 2nd dose of 0.5–0.75 mg/kg for refractory VT that does not respond to amiodarone
4. Consider magnesium, 1–2 grams IV if torsades de pointes with prolonged QT interval is present
5. Airway management, consider capnography

XVIII. **First-degree AV block (Figure 21.16)**
   A. Characteristics
      1. Delay in the impulse from the atria to the ventricles characterized by a PR interval of longer than 0.20 seconds
      2. Rhythm is regular, and the QRS complex is not affected
   B. Etiology
      1. Occurs in all ages in both normal and diseased hearts
      2. Drugs
         a. Digoxin
         b. β-blockers
         c. Calcium channel blockers
         d. Damage to the junction
   C. Clinical manifestations: usually asymptomatic
   D. Treatment
      1. Rarely, if ever, needs treatment; untreated if asymptomatic
      2. If PR interval prolonged greater than 0.4 seconds and/or the patient is symptomatic, consult a cardiologist or electrophysiologist for consideration of permanent pacemaker.

XIX. **Second-degree block (Mobitz type I) (Wenckebach) (Figure 21.17)**
   A. Characteristics
      1. Usually transient and occurs at the AV node
      2. Progressive prolongation of the PR interval until an impulse is completely blocked (dropped)
      3. Then, the pattern usually repeats
      4. R-R interval decreases prior to the blocked beat
      5. Atrial rhythm is usually regular, and the ventricular rhythm is usually irregular, with progressive shortening of the R-R interval before the blocked impulse.
      6. QRS complex is not affected
   B. Etiology
      1. Usually from drug effects (e.g., digitalis, verapamil, propranolol)
      2. Myocardial infarction
      3. Sometimes seen in young athletes
   C. Clinical manifestations
      1. Often asymptomatic
      2. If symptomatic, may see the following:
         a. Decreased cardiac output
         b. Hypotension
         c. LOC
   D. Treatment
      1. Rarely an unstable arrhythmia, often no treatment needed
      2. If symptomatic consult expert
      3. Can progress to complete heart block; patients should be monitored for worsening conduction disease. This can be done as outpatient at regular intervals
      4. Evaluation of all medications, electrolytes, and thyroid function may be indicated. Echocardiogram to rule out structural heart disease

XX. **Second-degree block (Mobitz type II) (Figure 21.18)**
   A. Characteristics
      1. Usually occurs below the level of the AV node

2. Commonly associated with an organic lesion in the conduction pathway
3. Associated with poorer prognosis than Mobitz type I
4. PR interval does not lengthen prior to a dropped beat
5. More than one dropped beat may occur in succession
6. Sometimes associated with widened QRS complex
7. Overall, the atrial rate is unaffected, but the ventricular rate is less than the atrial rate.

B. Etiology
1. Failure of conduction below the AV node; generally secondary to structural damage to the conduction system (e.g., infarction, fibrosis, necrosis).

C. Clinical manifestations: same as second-degree type 1

D. Treatment
1. Urgent cardiologist or electrophysiologist consultation for permanent pacemaker
2. While waiting for cardiologist or electrophysiologist, patient should be hospitalized, on telemetry with transcutaneous pacemaker and closely monitored
3. Work up of alternative causes (e.g., Lyme's disease, medications, metabolic abnormalities); echocardiogram to rule out structural heart disease
4. IV atropine, 0.5 mg given every 3–5 minutes with a maximum of 3 mg, should be administered to patients with signs or symptoms of poor perfusion (altered mental status, chest pain, hypotension, shock).
5. For treatment of symptomatic bradycardia, dopamine, epinephrine, and isoproterenol are alternatives when patient unresponsive to atropine, or as a temporizing measure while waiting for an available pacemaker.

XXI. **Third-degree AV block (complete heart block) (Figure 21.19)**
A. Characteristics
1. Complete absence of conduction between the atria and the ventricles
2. Atrial rate is unaffected, and the ventricular rate is slower than the atrial rate
3. Ventricular rate is usually 40–60 bpm
4. PR interval will vary because the atria and the ventricles are depolarized from different pacemakers.

B. Etiology
1. Myocardial ischemia or scar is the most common cause
2. May also be caused by medications (e.g., digitalis), metabolic abnormalities, or any other degeneration of the conduction system

C. Clinical manifestations
1. Asymptomatic if the ventricular rate is adequate
2. Otherwise, progressive decrease in cardiac output leads to LOC

D. Treatment
1. Urgent cardiologist or electrophysiologist consultation for permanent pacemaker
2. While waiting for expert, patient should be hospitalized, on telemetry, with transcutaneous pacemaker and close monitoring.
3. Work up for alternative causes (e.g., Lyme's disease, medications, metabolic abnormalities); echocardiogram to rule out structural heart
4. IV atropine, 0.5 mg given every 3–5 minutes with a maximum of 3 mg, should be administered to patients with signs or symptoms of poor perfusion (altered mental status, chest pain, hypotension, shock)
5. For treatment of symptomatic bradycardia, dopamine, epinephrine, and isoproterenol are alternatives when patient is unresponsive to atropine, or as a temporizing measure while waiting for an available pacemaker

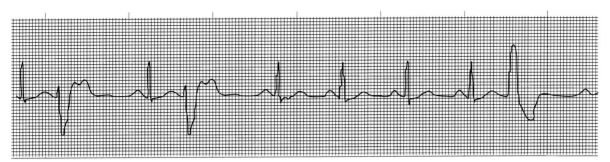

Figure 21.9. Premature ventricular contractions.

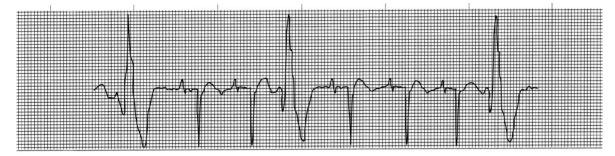

Figure 21.10A. Onifocal premature ventricular contractions

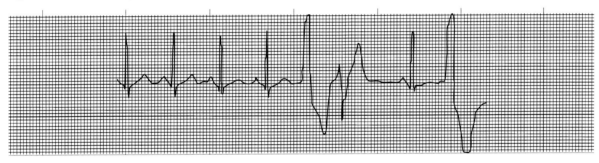

Figure 21.10B. Multifocal premature ventricular contractions

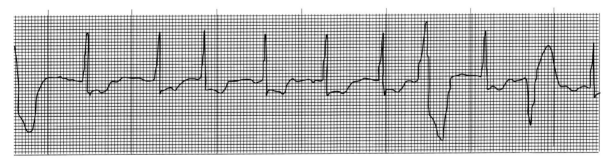

Figure 21.11. Multifocal premature ventricular contractions.

SECTION TWO Management of Patients With Cardiovascular Disorders

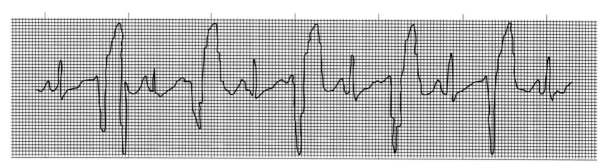

Figure 21.12. Regular sinus rhythm with bigeminal premature ventricular contractions.

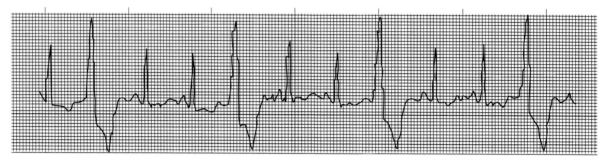

Figure 21.13. Regular sinus rhythm with trigeminal premature ventricular contractions.

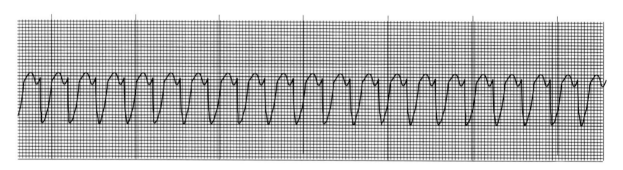

Figure 21.14. Ventricular tachycardia.

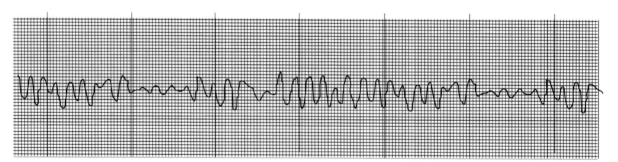

Figure 21.15. Ventricular fibrillation.

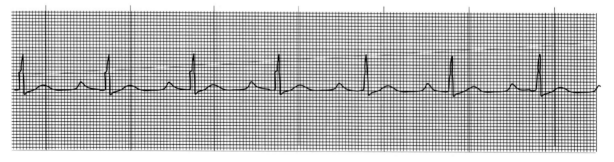

Figure 21.16. First-degree AV block

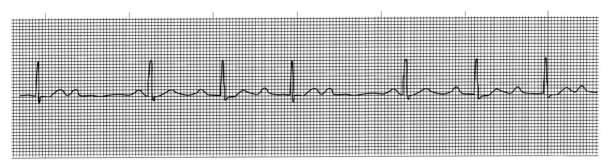

Figure 21.17. Second-degree block, Mobitz type I.

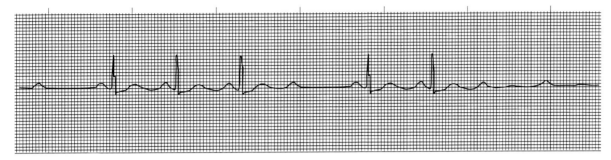

Figure 21.18. Second-degree block, Mobitz type II.

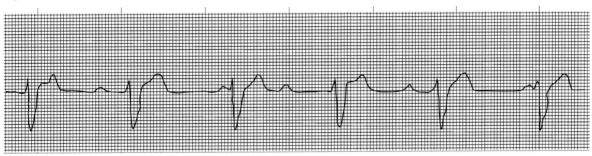

Figure 21.19. Third-degree AV block (complete heart block)

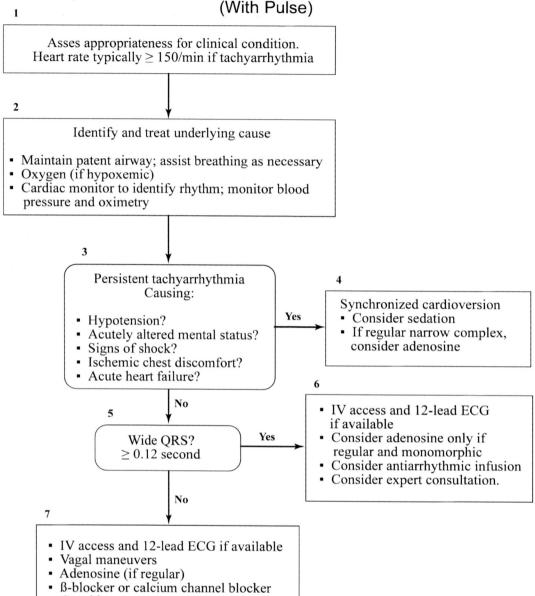

Figure 21.20. Tachycardia Algorithm. QRS = ventricular complex; IV = intravenous; ECG = electrocardiogram. Adapted from "2010 American Heart Association Guidelines for Cardiopulmonary Resuscitation and Emergency Cardiovascular Care Science," by R. W. Neumar, C. W. Otto, M. S. Link, S. L. Kronick, C. W. Callaway, P.J. Krudenchuck . . . L. J. Morrison, 2010, *Circulation, 122*.

BIBLIOGRAPHY

Anderson, J. L., Halperin, J. L., Albert, N. M., Bozkurt, B., Brindis, R. G., Curtis, L. H., . . . Shen, W. (2013). Management of patients with atrial fibrillation (compilation of 2006 ACCF/AHA/ESC and 2011 ACCF/AHA/HRS recommendations). *Journal of the American College of Cardiology, 61*(18), 1935–1944.

Cohn, E. G. (2012). *Flip and see ECG* (4th ed.). Philadelphia, PA: Elsevier Health Sciences.

Hazinski, M. F., Samson, R., & Schexnayder, S. (2010). *2010 Handbook of Emergency Cardiovascular Care for Healthcare Providers*. Dallas, TX: American Heart Association.

Sinz, E. (2013). *ACLS for experienced providers: Manual and resource text*. Dallas, TX: American Heart Association.

January, C. T., Wann, S., Alpert, J. S., Calkins, H., Cleveland, J. C., Cigarroa, J. E., . . . Yancy, C. W. (2014). 2014 AHA/ACC/HRS guideline for the management of patients with atrial fibrillation: Executive summary. *Journal of the American College of Cardiology*. doi:10.1016/j.jacc.2014.03.021

Karch, A. M. (2013). *2014 Lippincott's nursing drug guide*. Riverwoods, IL: Lippincott Williams & Wilkins.

Kee, J. L., Hayes, E. R., & McCuistion, L. E. (2012). *Pharmacology: A nursing process approach* (7th ed.). St. Louis, MO: Elsevier Saunders.

Levine, E. (2014). *CHADS2 score for stroke risk assessment in atrial fibrillation*. Retrieved from http://emedicine.medscape.com/article/2172597-overview

Lip, G. Y. (2014). Anticoagulation in older adults. In L. Leung, K. E. Schmader, & J. S. Tirnauer (Eds), *Uptodate*. Waltham, MA: UpToDate.

Peberdy, M. A., Callaway, C. W., Neumar, R. W., Geocadin, R. G., Zimmerman, J. L., Donnino, M., . . . Kronick, S. L. (2010). American Heart Association guidelines for cardiopulmonary resuscitation and emergency cardiovascular care. *Circulation, 122*, 5640–5933.

Poldermans, D., Bax, J. J., Boersma, E., Hert, S. D., Eeckhout, E., Fowkes, G., . . . Vermassen, F. (2009). Guidelines for pre-operative cardiac risk assessment and perioperative cardiac management in non-cardiac surgery. The task force for preoperative cardiac risk assessment and perioperative cardiac management in non-cardiac sugery of the European Society of Cardiology (ESC) and endorsed by the European Society of Anaesthesiology (ESA). *European Heart Journal, 30*(22), 2769–2812.

Tracy, C. M., Epstein, A. E., Darbar, D., DiMarco, J. P., Dunbar, S. B., Estes, M., . . . Varosy, P. D. (2012). 2012 ACCF/AHA/HRS focused update of the 2008 guidelines for device-based therapy for cardiac rhythm abnormalities: A report of the American College of Cardiology Foundation/American Heart Association Task Force on Practice Guidelines and the Heart Rhythm Society. *Circulation, 126*, 1784–1800.

Urden, L. D., Stacy, K. M., & Lough, M. E. (2010). *Critical care nursing: Diagnosis and management* (6th ed.). St. Louis, Mo.: Mosby/Elsevier.

SECTION THREE

Management of Pulmonary Disorders

CHAPTER 22

Diagnostic Concepts of Oxygenation and Ventilation

AMITA AVADHANI • CHARLENE M. MYERS

PULMONARY PERFUSION

I. **Definition**
   A. Movement of mixed venous blood through the pulmonary capillary bed for the purpose of gas exchange between the blood and the alveolar air
II. **The pulmonary vascular system is a high-volume system with low capillary resistance.**
   A. Pulmonary blood flow is about 6 L/minute.
   B. Mean pulmonary arterial pressure is 15 mmHg.
III. **Regional differences in blood flow in the lungs**
   A. Lung bases receive a greater percentage of blood flow than do the apices.
   B. Factors that affect the distribution of pulmonary blood flow:
      1. Gravity and hydrostatic pressure differences within the blood vessels: a patient's blood must flow against gravity to the apices when the person is in the upright position.
      2. Effect of alveolar pressure: alveolar pressure may be greater than pulmonary capillary pressure in the apical and middle regions of lungs because of the following:
         a. Positive pressure ventilation
         b. Decreased right ventricular preload (decreased hydrostatic pressure), dehydration, and hemorrhage
         c. Air trapping in chronic obstructive pulmonary disease
      3. Effect of decreased PaO_2 (partial pressure of oxygen in arterial blood) (alveolar gas): local reflex that causes vasoconstriction of pulmonary arterioles supplying hypoxic alveoli

VENTILATION

I. **Definition**
   A. Mechanical movement of air into and out of the alveoli for the purpose of gas exchange between the atmosphere and capillary blood
   B. Gas flows from higher atmospheric to lower intrapulmonary pressure during inhalation.
II. **Regulation of ventilation**
   A. Central nervous system control

1. Brain stem centers (medulla and pons): cells fire automatically to trigger inhalation, others fire to halt inhalation, and exhalation occurs passively.
   2. Cerebral cortex: allows voluntary control to override brain stem centers in response to chemical stimuli and lung inflation changes
B. Chemical regulation
   1. Central chemoreceptors in medulla respond to increased partial pressure of carbon dioxide in arterial blood ($PaCO_2$) (hypercapnia) and decreased pH (acidosis) through medullary stimuli by increasing ventilatory depth and rate; hypercapnia is the major stimulus to alter ventilation.
   2. Peripheral chemoreceptors in aortic and carotid bodies respond to decreased PaO_2 (hypoxemia) by stimulating medullary centers to enhance ventilation.
   3. Patients with chronically high $PaCO_2$: hypercapnic ventilatory drive is lost; these patients respond only to changes in PaO_2 by stimulation of peripheral receptors to adjust ventilation (hypoxemic respiratory drive)
      a. Supplemental O_2: Administer low liter flows very carefully to prevent apnea (e.g., begin with 1–2 L/minute and assess).
      b. Do not withhold O_2 if needed; be prepared to assist with mechanical ventilation if respiratory drive is depressed.

III. Work of breathing (WOB)
A. Definition: amount of effort required to overcome the elastic and resistive properties of the lungs and chest wall
B. Elasticity (elastic recoil): tendency of the lungs to return to their original shape
   1. Lungs try to collapse because of tension between the interstitial elastic fibers and the surface of the alveoli
   2. Chest wall attempts to resist inward-moving recoil
C. Compliance: measure of distensibility, or how easily the lungs and thorax can be stretched; describes resistance as a result of elastic properties. Increased compliance means less pressure is needed to stretch the lungs and/or thorax
   1. High compliance: easier to expand lung tissue (e.g., chronic obstructive pulmonary disease)
   2. Low compliance: stiff lungs; chest wall less distensible (e.g., pneumonia and acute respiratory distress syndrome)
D. Resistance is determined by the radius of the airway through which air is flowing. Increased resistance means increased effort for ventilation and increased WOB.

IV. Alveolar ventilation: amount of air that reaches alveoli and participates in gas exchange
A. $PaCO_2$: best indicator of alveolar ventilation
B. Normal: $PaCO_2$ is 35–45 mmHg

ALVEOLAR DIFFUSION

I. Definition
A. Exchange of O_2 and CO_2 across the alveolocapillary membrane
B. Oxygen diffuses down the concentration gradient from higher alveolar pressure (PAO_2) to lower pulmonary capillary pressure (PaO_2).
C. CO_2 diffuses at a rate 20 times greater than that of O_2 from capillary to alveolus

II. A-a gradient: alveolar-to-arterial oxygen gradient; $AaDO_2$: alveolar-to-arterial oxygen difference
A. A calculation to aid in diagnosing the degree of a patient's hypoxemia
B. Formula: difference between partial pressure of O_2 in the alveoli (PAO_2) and partial pressure of O_2 in arterial blood (PaO_2)
   1. PAO_2: calculated
   2. PaO_2: from arterial blood gases

CHAPTER 22 Diagnostic Concepts of Oxygenation and Ventilation

3. Note: A-a gradient OR $AaDO_2 = PAO_2 - PaO_2$
4. Formula to calculate PAO_2

$$PAO_2 = \frac{PIO_2 - PaCO_2}{0.8 \text{ (respiratory quotient)}}$$

PIO_2 = Partial pressure of inspired oxygen: 21%–100%
Pb = Barometric pressure: 760 mmHg (at sea level)
PH_2O = Water vapor pressure: 47 mmHg

$$PAO_2 = \frac{[0.21 \times (760 - 47)] - 40}{0.8}$$

$PAO_2 = 0.21 \times 713 - 50$
$PAO_2 = 100$ mmHg
Normal $PAO_2 = 60 - 100$ mmHg

C. Normal values: difference between alveolar and arterial oxygen
 1. Young adult breathing room air ($FIO_2 = 21\%$): less than 10 mmHg difference
 2. Adult older than age 60 on room air: less than 20 mmHg difference
 3. Breathing FIO_2 100% = less than 50 mmHg difference

OXYGEN TRANSPORT IN THE CIRCULATION

I. **O_2 Carried in the blood**
   A. O_2 dissolved in plasma (3% of total) = PaO_2 (normal is 80–100 mmHg)
   B. O_2 bound to hemoglobin (Hgb) (97% of total) = SaO_2 (oxygen saturation) (normal is 95%–100%)
   C. Note: reserve for times of increased demand
   D. Note: assess Hgb level for oxygen-carrying capacity. If Hgb level is decreased yet adequately saturated, the patient is not adequately oxygenated

II. **PaO_2 and SaO_2: indirect measurement of O_2 available to tissues**

III. **O_2 that stays bound to Hgb is useless to body cells.**
   A. Affinity: ability of Hgb to release O_2
     1. Weak affinity: easily releases O_2 to tissues
     2. Strong affinity: easily accepts and retains O_2

IV. **Oxyhemoglobin dissociation curve: demonstrates affinity of Hgb for O_2**
   A. Flat part of curve: binding portion in lungs
     1. Increased affinity; binds easily: PAO_2 is 60–100 mmHg, with SaO_2 greater than 90%
   B. Steep part of curve: dissociation portion at the tissue level
     1. Weaker affinity: Hgb readily dissociates O_2 when PAO_2 falls to below 60 mmHg.

V. **Shifts in oxyhemoglobin dissociation curve: other patient variables affect affinity of Hgb for O_2**
   A. Shift to the left: greater affinity
     1. Binds easily in the lung; less unloading to tissues
     2. Increased affinity leads to possible tissue hypoxia due to strong bond between Hgb and O_2; need for O_2 may have decreased
     3. Causes:
        a. Alkalosis
        b. Hypothermia
        c. Decreased 2,3-diphosphoglycerate
   B. Shift to the right: decreased affinity
     1. Hgb unloads more O_2 to tissues
     2. Delivery of O_2 to tissues improves as long as loading of O_2 in lungs is adequate
     3. Causes:
        a. Acidosis

b. Increased tissue metabolism, anaerobic metabolism, and hyperthermia
c. Increased 2,3-diphosphoglycerate

VI. Continuous SvO_2 (mixed venous oxygen saturation) monitoring: monitoring O_2 transport and extraction

A. Measure of mixed venous O_2 saturation by the pulmonary artery catheter
 1. Continuous measure and display of mixed venous oxygen saturation
 2. Hgb reflects light, which can be measured according to its saturation.
B. Normal SvO_2: 75%; Hgb unloads 25% of its O_2 before returning to the heart.
 1. Normal ratio of supply of O_2 to demand: 4:1
 2. Acceptable SvO_2 range: 60%–80%

Venous blood gases	Arterial blood gases
pH = 7.36	pH = 7.4
$PvCO_2$ = 47 mmHg	$PaCO_2$ = 40 mmHg
HCO_2 = 24 mEq/L	HCO_3 = 24 mEq/L
PvO_2 = 40 mmHg	PaO_2 = 100 mmHg
SvO_2 = 75%	SaO_2 = 99%
Hgb = 15 grams	Hgb = 15 grams

C. Trends in changes in SvO_2: assesses the effectiveness of peripheral oxygen delivery; may signal need to assess cardiac profile
 1. SvO_2 less than 60% or trend downward: patient has tapped the venous reserve of O_2
  a. Implies increased tissue extraction of O_2
   i. Note: greater risk for anaerobic metabolism
  b. Causes
   i. Decreased O_2 supply (e.g., decreased FIO_2, anemia, and decreased CO)
   ii. Increased O_2 demand (e.g., fever, increased WOB, shivering, pain, and agitation)
  c. SvO_2 less than 40% = anaerobic metabolism leading to organ dysfunction
 2. SvO_2 greater than 80%: implies decreased tissue extraction of oxygen
  a. High return of O_2 is often an earlier indicator of change in patient status than change in hemodynamic parameters
  b. Causes:
   i. Increased O_2 supply (e.g., FIO_2 greater than need and polycythemia)
   ii. Decreased O_2 demand (e.g., sleep and hypothermia)
   iii. Decreased effective O_2 delivery and uptake by cells (e.g., sepsis, cyanide toxicity, and shift of O_2/Hgb curve to left)

VII. Oxygen supply/demand balance: calculations

ROI_2 = venous O_2 return to heart
 = CI × (venous O_2 content) × 10
 = CI × (1.34 × Hgb × Svo_2) × 10
 = 3 × (1.34 × 15 × .75) × 10
 = 3 × (15) × 10
 = 450 mL/min/m²

DOI_2 = arterial O_2 delivery to tissues
 = CI × (arterial O_2 content) × 10
 = CI × (1.34 × Hgb × SaO_2) × 10
 = 3 × (1.34 × 15 × 0.98) × 10
 = 3 × (20) × 10
 = 600 mL/min/m²

VO_2 = tissue O_2 demand
$DOI_2 - ROI_2 = VO_2$
600 mL − 450 mL = 150 mL/min/m²

Note. CI = cardiac index; Prolonged Svo_2 and/or prolonged Vo_2 are poor prognosis.

VENTILATOR ADJUSTMENTS

I. **Respiratory acidosis**
   A. The goal is to decrease PCO_2
   B. Make the following ventilator adjustments:
      1. Increase the respiratory rate; watch for auto-PEEP with high respiratory rate (beware of hypotension from reduced preload)
      2. Increase the tidal volume:
         a. In assist control mode, directly increase the tidal volume.
         b. In pressure control or pressure support modes, increase the inspiratory pressure to increase tidal volume.
      3. In acute lung injury, some extent of hypercapnia/respiratory acidosis should be generally tolerated, rather than raising the tidal volume greater than 8 ml/kg.

II. **Respiratory alkalosis**
   A. The goal is to increase PCO_2
   B. Make the following ventilator adjustments:
      1. Decrease the respiratory rate
      2. Decrease the tidal volume
      3. If the patient is breathing faster than the set rate, these strategies will not work.
   C. Determine the cause of respiratory alkalosis and correct the cause, for example, sepsis, pulmonary embolism, pain, and so forth.

III. **Hypoxemia**
   A. The goal is to improve tissue oxygenation by improving SaO_2, PO_2, and PaO_2.
   B. Increase FiO_2; increase PEEP. (Watch out for the drop in cardiac output from decreased preload associated with increase in PEEP. Preload can be augmented with IV fluids.)

IV. **Difficult ventilation may first manifest itself as increase in peak inspiratory pressure, resulting from the following:**
   A. Bronchospasm
   B. Secretions in the airways, endotracheal tube, and ventilator tubing
   C. Pulmonary edema
   D. Pneumothorax
   E. Intubation in the right mainstem
   F. Mucus plug
   G. Worsening airspace disease (adult respiratory distress syndrome, pneumonia, and pulmonary edema)
   H. Agitated patient with ventilator dyssynchrony
   I. Therefore, it would be important to address the cause to correct the ventilatory issue.

BIBLIOGRAPHY

Andreoli, T. E., & Cecil, R. L. (2010). Andreoli and Carpenter's Cecil essentials of medicine (8th ed.). Philadelphia, PA: Saunders/Elsevier.

Criner, G. J., Barnette, R. E., & Alonzo, G. E. (2010). Critical care study guide text and review (2nd ed.). New York, NY: Springer.

Cyna, A. M. (2011). Handbook of communication in anaesthesia and critical care: A practical guide to exploring the art. Oxford: Oxford University Press.

Galvagno, S. M. (2014). Emergency pathophysiology clinical applications for prehospital care. Hoboken: Teton NewMedia, Inc.

George, R. B. (2005). Chest medicine: Essentials of pulmonary and critical care medicine. Philadelphia, PA: Lippincott Williams & Wilkins.

Goroll, A. H., & Mulley, A. G. (2009). Primary care medicine: Office evaluation and management of the adult patient (6th ed.). Philadelphia: Wolters Kluwer Health/Lippincott Williams & Wilkins.

CHAPTER 23

Measures of Oxygenation and Ventilation

BIMBOLA AKINTADE • CHARLENE M. MYERS

OXYGENATION AND VENTILATION

I. **Definition**
   A. Closely interrelated terms that collectively refer to the processes by which oxygen (O_2) and carbon dioxide (CO_2) are transported between atmosphere and tissue via concentration gradients, perfusion, and affinity of hemoglobin for oxygen
   B. Oxygenation refers to movement of oxygen into the blood and its transport and delivery to tissue.
      1. Diffusion pressures, determined by gradients between the respective partial pressures of alveolar, plasma, and tissue oxygen, allow for movement of oxygen from alveoli to blood to tissue.
      2. Hemoglobin and its affinity for oxygen allows for blood transport of far more oxygen than could be dissolved in plasma alone.
      3. Perfusion, determined by cardiac output and vascular tone, affects oxygen delivery to tissue capillaries.
   C. Ventilation refers to the exchange of extrapulmonary and intra-alveolar gas mixtures.
      1. Resupply of oxygen diffused into blood and removal of CO_2 diffused from blood allow for maintenance of their respective alveolar-capillary pressure gradients
      2. Patent airway(s), neuromuscular function, and structural integrity of chest wall allow for inspiratory and expiratory air flow.
II. **Clinical measurements**
   A. Exercise tolerance: Ability to perform a normal exercise load (e.g., climb a flight of stairs without stopping) suggests adequate oxygenation and ventilation.
   B. Dyspnea, air hunger, work of breathing
      1. Does the patient report distress?
      2. Does the patient appear distressed?
   C. Cyanosis
      1. Dusky bluish tint from excessive amounts of unsaturated hemoglobin
      2. The more central the cyanosis, the greater its severity. For example, cyanosis evident on the face and chest is more severe than cyanosis limited to the fingertips.
   D. Arterial blood gases (ABGs)

1. Partial pressures of oxygen and carbon dioxide
2. Oxygen saturation of arterial hemoglobin
3. pH
4. Presence or absence of metabolic imbalance
5. Normal values for arterial blood gas
   a. pH = 7.35–7.45
   b. Partial pressure of oxygen in arterial blood (PaO_2) = 80–97 mmHg
   c. Partial pressure of carbon dioxide in arterial blood ($PaCO_2$) = 35–45 mmHg
   d. Bicarbonate (HCO3) = 22–26 mEq/L
   e. Base excess, -3 to +3 mEq/L
   f. Saturation of arterial oxygen (SaO_2) greater than 98%
6. Partial pressures of arterial oxygen and carbon dioxide and arterial oxygen saturation decline as altitude above sea level increases.
7. Oxygenation
   a. Interpret PaO_2 in light of fraction of inspired oxygen (FIO_2). As a general rule, PaO_2 should be 4–5 times the percentage of O_2 (e.g., the FIO_2 of room air is 21%, and a normal PaO_2 is 80–97 mmHg).
   b. PaO_2/FiO_2 ratio describes the degree of impairment in pulmonary gas exchange. Normal ratios are 300–500 mmHg. Low ratios indicate impaired oxygen exchange, while ratios less than 200 mmHg indicated severe hypoxemia.
8. Ventilation
   a. Ventilation is reciprocally reflected by $PaCO_2$. For example, a rising $PaCO_2$ means that a decrease in ventilation has occurred (and vice versa).
   b. Every 10 mmHg shift in $PaCO_2$ should produce a reciprocal 0.08 shift in pH. A $PaCO_2$ of 50 mm would thus predict a pH of 7.32. Any difference from that predicted shift must be attributed to a concurrent metabolic imbalance or compensation.

III. Limitations
A. Invasiveness
   1. Drawing blood for an ABG measurement is often painful for the patient and involves significant risk of injury and compromise of perfusion distal to the site.
   2. If frequent measurements are required, as in a critically ill or mechanically ventilated patient, an indwelling arterial catheter should be placed.
B. An ABG is not a continuous measurement, and its accuracy is specific only to the time it was drawn.
   1. A more continuous measurement would be peripheral oxygen saturation, measured by a pulse oximeter or an end-tidal CO_2 measurement device.
C. The ABG sample must be handled with care.
   1. The sample must not be allowed to clot and must be heparinized.
   2. Excessive amounts of heparin in a small blood sample will alter the pH.
   3. Any air bubbles must be expelled from the syringe because oxygen and carbon dioxide in the sample will equilibrate with the air bubble.
   4. If more than a few minutes may pass before the sample is measured, it must be chilled to limit the ongoing metabolism of cellular components.
D. Sample may inadvertently be taken from a vein in close proximity to the intended arterial site.
   1. The clinician must make an astute analysis for results inconsistent with an arterial sample.

PULSE OXIMETRY

I. **Definition**
   A. Pulse oximetry is a noninvasive, continuous, and relatively inexpensive method for transcutaneous measurement of the degree to which hemoglobin in arterial blood is saturated with oxygen (SaO_2).

II. **Mechanism**
   A. Pulse oximetry (SpO_2) uses a light-emitting diode to transmit light in the trans-red and near-infrared wavelengths through perfused tissue to a receiving sensor.
   B. The device compares light emitted versus light received by the sensor to calculate light absorbed by oxyhemoglobin and thus, the saturation of hemoglobin with oxygen.
   C. The device can detect a pulsatile fluctuation in saturation and can selectively display the highest measurement as the SpO_2 (presumed to reflect the SaO_2).
   D. The pulse oximetry probe may be applied for intermittent or continuous measurements. It is typically placed on a digit but can be placed on an earlobe, cheek, nose, or toe.
   E. The accuracy of the displayed reading may be affected by several factors.
      1. Abnormal hemoglobins
      2. Movement of the probe may create artifact, causing the measurement to be rejected. Alternative placement or stabilization with tape may be required.
      3. It is recommended but not always necessary that nail polish be removed so an accurate reading is obtained.

III. **Normal values are variable and must be interpreted in light of altitude, the patient's age, and cardiopulmonary function.**
   A. Remember that the relationship between oxygen saturation and partial pressure of oxygen is nonlinear. It is prudent to commit to memory the following:
      1. SpO_2 of 90% represents a PaO_2 of 60 mmHg
      2. SpO_2 of 75% is a PaO_2 of 40 mmHg
      3. SpO_2 of 50% is a PaO_2 of 27 mmHg
   B. Factors that can distort the normal relationship between oxygen saturation and partial pressure of oxygen must be considered.
      1. With alkalosis or hypothermia, the PaO_2 may be lower than predicted by the SpO_2.
      2. With acidosis or hyperthermia, the PaO_2 may be higher than predicted by the SpO_2.

IV. **Limitations of pulse oximetry**
   A. Pulse oximetry is only a presumptive reflection of SaO_2 and does not provide information regarding pH, $PaCO_2$, or respiratory rate.
   B. Pulse oximetry is confounded by the presence of carbon monoxide.
      1. The device will misinterpret carboxyhemoglobin as oxyhemoglobin and thereby provide a false elevation.
      2. When carbon monoxide poisoning is suspected, an ABG analysis is a more reliable measurement of oxygenation.
   C. Methylene blue dye and, similarly, methemoglobinemia will be misinterpreted by the oximeter as deoxygenated hemoglobin, thus falsely indicating a lowered oxygen saturation.
   D. Pulse oximetry is most valuable as a reading of central oxygenation.
      1. In some circumstances (e.g., shock, hypothermia, severe peripheral vascular disease, use of high-dose vasopressors), a peripherally placed oximeter will not accurately reflect central oxygenation.
      2. Remember that pulse oximetry measures oxygen saturation, not oxygen content. For example, an anemic patient may have high oxygen saturation, but low oxygen content. (100% of half is still half!)

MEASUREMENT OF CLINICAL PERFUSION

I. Definition
A. Technique of using blood flow to direct a balloon-tipped catheter from the central venous circulation through the right side of the heart into the pulmonary artery (PA) for the purpose of hemodynamic monitoring

II. General description
A. The most basic PA catheter consists of three lumina, each accessed by its separate respective port.
  1. A distal lumen opens at the tip of the catheter.
  2. A proximal lumen opens approximately 30 cm from the distal tip.
  3. A lumen opens into a balloon immediately proximal to the distal tip.
B. The catheter is approximately 100–110 cm long and has markings every 10 cm to allow measurement of how far the catheter has been inserted.
C. Most PA catheters have a temperature sensor at the tip that provides an accurate core temperature and permits calculation of cardiac output via a thermodilution technique.
  1. A known temperature change is induced in the blood flow upstream from the probe.
     a. Rapid manual injection of 10 ml of room temperature saline via the proximal port for intermittent measurements
     b. Frequent sequential heating via a heating coil located 10–20 cm from the distal tip for "continuous" measurements
  2. As ongoing blood flow dilutes the temperature change (thermodilution), cardiac output is calculated on the basis of rate of return to baseline blood temperature.
     a. A faster return to baseline will result in a higher cardiac output calculation (and vice versa).
D. Common versions of the catheter may incorporate additional ports and functions.
  1. A venous infusion port is usually located within a centimeter of the proximal port and may be used interchangeably.
  2. An oximetry sensor on the distal tip can allow measurement of mixed venous oxygen saturation (SvO_2).
  3. SvO_2 is an important value in guiding resuscitation, and supplies information about both respiratory and circulatory systems.
  4. It is a valuable measure of systemic oxygenation. It reflects the relationship between supply and demand, and tissue oxygenation.
  5. Measure of less than 70% indicates systemic delivery is impaired.
  6. Pacing capabilities may be provided via integrated pacing electrodes or a dedicated port through which a pacing wire may be inserted.

III. Catheter placement
A. Central venous access, most commonly at an internal jugular, subclavian, or femoral site, is first attained with a large-bore (6–8.5 French) introducer catheter.
B. The PA catheter is advanced through the introducer and is positioned by flow-directed balloon flotation.
C. The catheter is positioned with the distal tip in a branch of the pulmonary artery.
  1. The most common placement leaves the distal tip in the right branch.
  2. With normal anatomy, the proximal port will be positioned in the right atrium.
  3. Ongoing assessment of catheter placement is essential.
     a. Proper placement will most commonly occur with the catheter inserted approximately 50–60 cm
     b. Astute analysis of chest X-ray and pressure waveforms measured at distal and proximal ports can confirm placement.

IV. Indications for placement
A. PA catheterization is indicated only in the following circumstances:

1. Specific hemodynamic parameters cannot be adequately inferred by less invasive clinical assessment
   a. Differentiation between cardiogenic (high pulmonary capillary wedge pressure [PCWP], normal pulmonary artery pressure [PAP]) and pulmogenic (normal PCWP, high PAP) pulmonary edema
   b. Cardiac output/cardiac index (CO/CI), systemic vascular resistance (SVR), pulmonary vascular resistance (PVR), SvO_2
2. Accurate, direct measurements are required to guide titration of therapy.

V. **Contraindications to placement of a PA catheter**
   A. No absolute contraindications
   B. Relative contraindications include the following:
      1. Coagulopathies (for fear of uncontrolled bleeding at deep central vascular puncture site)
      2. Left bundle branch blocks (for fear of complete heart block resulting from interruption of right bundle branch function during catheter placement)
      3. Presence of temporary pacing catheter (for fear of disruption of pacing)

VI. **Information provided by the pulmonary catheter is extensive; however, the quality of this information is highly dependent on the integrity of the monitoring system (monitor, transducers, tubing) and the ability of the clinician to assess the reliability of the information and the system that generates it.**
   A. Pressure in the central venous space (CVP) is measured though the proximal port.
      1. Reflects right ventricular (RV) end-diastolic filling pressure (RV preload)
      2. Most often used to infer general systemic volume status
      3. Used in calculation of SVR
   B. Pressure measured at the distal port is dependent on whether the balloon is inflated
      1. When the balloon is not inflated, the pressure measured is the PAP.
      2. When the balloon is inflated (and properly positioned), it occludes ("wedges") the branch of the PA in which it is positioned.
      3. Pressure measured is the PCWP
      4. Reflects left ventricular (LV) end-diastolic filling pressure (LV preload)
      5. Most often used to infer left ventricular function
      6. Used in calculation of PVR
   C. The temperature probe accurately measures core temperature.
   D. Directly measured pressures and temperature are used as variables included in calculation of hemodynamic parameters, most prominently CO/CI, SVR, and PVR

VII. **Complications**
   A. Sepsis
      1. Limit risk by scrupulous site care/protection
      2. Limit duration at site to 7–10 days
   B. Pulmonary hemorrhage
      1. Use minimal inflation of balloon that achieves wedge
      2. Inflate only as long as required to get the measurement
      3. Do not inflate against resistance.
      4. Avoid unnecessary inflations.
      5. Pulmonary hemorrhage is usually heralded by hematemesis.
   C. Cardiac rhythm disturbances—associated with ventricular stimulation by catheter tip
      1. Usually occurs during placement as catheter passes through RV
      2. May herald displacement of catheter from PA into RV
   D. Thrombocytopenia—may be associated with prolonged catheter placement

FLUID RESUSCITATION

I. **Definition**
   A. Process by which optimal cardiac output, and thus adequate perfusion to vital organs, is restored by increasing intravascular volume from exogenous or endogenous sources

II. **Indicators of inadequate intravascular volume**
   A. No reason to suspect cardiogenic or neurogenic shock
   B. Evidence of inadequate ventricular filling pressures (preload)
      1. Hypotension, tachycardia, low CVP, low PCWP
      2. Flat neck veins in the Trendelenburg position
   C. Decreased urine output—less than 0.5 ml/kg/hour
   D. Obvious history of significant volume wasting disease
      1. Hemorrhage
      2. Prolonged emesis or diarrhea
      3. Prolonged diaphoresis
      4. Excess diuresis
      5. Sepsis
   E. Poor response to early goal-directed therapy

III. **Fluid resuscitation in a seriously ill patient should be managed in a critical care setting.**
   A. Consideration should be given to the placement of adequate monitoring devices, including the following:
      1. Arterial catheter for monitoring and sampling purposes
      2. CVP which is a hemodynamic parameter to measure and monitor fluid status
      3. Urinary bladder catheter to provide an accurate measurement of urine production
   B. Body temperature should be monitored during large-volume resuscitations
      1. Substantial amounts of room temperature fluids or chilled blood products can rapidly chill a patient.
      2. Fluids should be warmed before administration, if hypothermia is evident.
      3. In actively bleeding patients or patients with hemorrhagic shock, administration of cool/cold blood products may lead to coagulopathy.
   C. At least two large-bore (at least 16-gauge) intravenous catheters may be lifesaving.
      1. Catheter should be placed in as large a vessel as can be accessed readily
      2. Peripheral access should be no more distal than the antecubital veins

IV. **Choices for Fluid Resuscitation**
   A. Crystalloid solutions
      1. Normal saline (0.9% NS) is a good choice for routine fluid resuscitation.
         a. When administering 1 L, only approximately 250 ml remain intravascular; the rest remains in the interstitial space.
      2. Lactated Ringer's solution has a wider variety of elemental constituents than normal saline and is commonly employed in the operating suite.
         a. When infused in large volumes, can lead to hyperchloremic acidosis due to high concentration of chloride
      3. Dextrose-containing solutions come in a wide variety of concentrations.
         a. These should be used only after the patient's need for dextrose is considered.
         b. Dextrose-containing solutions are not first-line agents for volume expansion.
   B. Packed RBCs
      1. Fluid of choice for major hemorrhage after PRBCs
      2. Each unit of red cells typically increases the hematocrit of a 70-kg person by 3%.
   C. Colloid solutions, such as albumin, may be thought of as intravascular sponges that, through oncotic attraction, absorb volume from the extravascular space and hold it within the intravascular space.

1. Use with caution because this effect is transient and does little to correct the primary problem of decreased intravascular volume.
2. Colloid solutions should be reserved for specific indications, such as refractory hypovolemia, among others.
D. Fresh frozen plasma, platelets, and cryoprecipitate are not useful in fluid resuscitation, except as these relate to correction of underlying hemorrhagic conditions.
V. **Adequacy of fluid resuscitation may be judged by clinical indicators such as the following:**
   A. Normalization of blood pressure and heart rate
   B. Increasing urinary output
   C. Normalization of hemodynamic parameters such as CVP, PCWP, CO/CI, and SVR

BIBLIOGRAPHY

Dries, D. J. (2013). Traumatic shock and tissue hypoperfusion: Nonsurgical management. In J. E. Parrillo & R. P. Dellinger (Eds.), *Critical care medicine: Principles of diagnosis and management in the adult* (4th ed., pp. 409–431). Philadelphia, PA: Elsevier Saunders.

Eskaros, S. M., Papadakos, P. J., & Lachmann, B. (2009). Respiratory monitoring. In R. D. Miller, L. I. Eriksson, L. A. Fleisher, J. P. Weiner-Kronish, & W. L. Young (Eds.), *Miller's anesthesia* (7th ed., pp. 1411–1442). Philadelphia, PA: Churchill Livingstone Elsevier.

Fontes, M. L., Skubas, N., & Osorio, J. (2011). Cardiac tamponade. In F. F. Yao, M. L. Fontes, & V. Malhotra (Eds.), *Yao and Artusio's anesthesiology: Problem-oriented patient management* (7th ed.). Philadelphia, PA: Wolters Kluwer/Lippincott, Williams & Wilkins.

Gadepalli, S. K., & Hirschl, R. B. (2014). Mechanical ventilation in pediatric surgical disease. In G. W. Holcomb, P. J. Murphy, & D. J. Ostlie (Eds.), *Ashcraft's pediatric surgery* (6th ed.). Philadelphia, PA: Elsevier Saunders.

Galvagno, S. M. (2013). *Emergency pathophysiology: Clinical applications for prehospital care.* Jackson, WY: Teton NewMedia.

Green, D., & Paklet, L. (2010). Latest developments in peri-operative monitoring of the high-risk major surgery patient. *International Journal of Surgery, 8*(2), 90–99. doi:10.1016/j.ijsu.2009.12.004

Kieninger, A. N., & Lipsett, P. A. (2009). Hospital-acquired pneumonia: Pathophysiology, diagnosis, and treatment. *Surgical Clinics of North America, 89*(2), 439–461.

Kraft, M. (2011). Approach to the patient with respiratory disease. In L. Goldman & A. I. Schafer (Eds.), *Goldman's Cecil medicine* (24th ed.). Philadelphia, PA: Elsevier Saunders.

Leppikangas, H., Järvelä, K., Sisto, T., Maaranen, P., Virtanen, M., Lehto, P., . . . Lindgren, L. (2011). Preoperative levosimendan infusion in combined aortic valve and coronary bypass surgery. *British Journal of Anaesthesia.* doi:10.1093/bja/aeq402

Mishra, N., & Pothal, S. (2013). Pulmonary manifestations of liver diseases. *World Clinics: Pulmonary and Critical Care Medicine, 2*(2), 424–443.

Murphey, E. D., Sherwood, E. R., & Toliver-Kinsky, T. (2012). The immunological response and strategies for intervention. In D. N. Herndon (Ed.), *Total Burn Care* (4th ed., pp. 265–276). Philadelphia, PA: Elsevier Saunders.

Ohye, R. G., & Hirsch, J. C. (2012). Congenital heart disease and anomalies of the great vessels. In A. G. Coran, N. S. Adzick, T. M. Krummel, J. M. Laberge, R. C. Shamberger, & A. A. Caldamone (Eds.), *Pediatric Surgery* (7th ed., pp. 1647–1672). Philadelphia, PA: Elsevier Saunders Mosby.

Schroeder, R. A., Barbeito, A., Bar-Yosef, S., & Mark, J. B. (2009). Cardiovascular monitoring. In R. D. Miller, L. I. Eriksson, L. A. Fleisher, J. P. Weiner-Kronish, & W. L. Young (Eds.), *Miller's Anesthesia* (7th ed., pp. 1267–1328). Philadelphia, PA: Churchill Livingstone Elsevier.

Tamura, T. (2014). Sensing technologies for biomedical telemetry. In K. S. Nikita (Ed.), *Handbook of Biomedical Telemetry* (pp. 76–107). Hoboken, NJ: John Wiley and Sons.

Villar, J., Blanco, J., Añón, J. M., Santos-Bouza, A., Blanch, L., Ambrós, A., . . . Kacmarek, R. M. (2011). The ALIEN study: Incidence and outcome of acute respiratory distress syndrome in the era of lung protective ventilation. *Intensive Care Medicine, 37*(12), 1932–1941. Retrieved from http://icmjournal.esicm.org/Journals/abstract.html?doi=10.1007/s00134-011-2380-4

Weinberger, S. E., Cockrill, B. A., & Mandel, J. (2013). *Principles of pulmonary medicine* (6th ed.). Philadelphia, PA: Elsevier Saunders.

West, J. B. (2012). *Pulmonary pathophysiology: The essentials* (8th ed.). Philadelphia, PA: Wolters Kluwer Health/Lippincott, Williams, & Wilkins.

CHAPTER 24

The Chest X-ray

VICTORIA F. KU • THOMAS W. BARKLEY, JR.

GENERAL PRINCIPLES

I. **Most common views as an inpatient**
   A. Anteroposterior (AP) films with back against the film plate
      1. Usually obtained with a portable x-ray machine
         a. Indicated when patient's condition precludes prudent travel
         b. Most often done supine unless specified as upright
      2. May limit attainment of optimal image
         a. Increase magnification and decrease sharpness of the image
         b. Supine position
            i. May limit inspiration and lead to misinterpretation
            ii. Unable to accurately assess free pleural fluid level due to distribution of fluid throughout the whole lung
            iii. Flattening of posterior surface of heart, causing heart to be falsely widened up to 15%
   B. Posteroanterior (PA) films with chest against film plate
      1. Usually obtained in the x-ray suite
      2. Allows for optimal image
         a. Less magnification, with sharper image
         b. Done in the upright position
            i. Deeper inspiration shows more of the lung
            ii. Dependent free pleural fluid level more evident
            iii. Less distortion (widening) of cardiac silhouette
   C. Lateral films
      1. Most often done with film against left side
      2. Particularly useful in evaluating structures in the posterior mediastinal and retrocardiac spaces
      3. Also useful in evaluating the thoracic vertebrae
      4. May reveal free pleural fluid level not evident in supine AP

CHAPTER **24** The Chest X-ray

II. **Adequacy of the film**
   A. Some portion of the x-ray beam is absorbed by the material(s) it passes through before reaching the film plate
      1. Air, fat, soft tissue (water), and bone (metal) absorb progressively more radiation
   B. Only the portion of the beam that penetrates the material and is not absorbed will create a darker image on the film
      1. A high degree of penetration (low absorption) will create a black or radiolucent area on the film.
      2. A low degree of penetration (high absorption) will create a white or radiopaque area on the film.
   C. Sufficient detail in the image is largely determined by the intensity of the x-ray beam
      1. Optimal penetration is generally judged by the clarity of the vertebral bodies on the image
         a. Overpenetration: beam too intense, resulting in an overly dark image with subtle details rendered invisible
         b. Underpenetration: beam insufficiently intense, producing an overly white image; all details are lost in the glare
   D. The x-ray beam should be perpendicular to the film and/or anatomic plane, so as to avoid distortion of structural relationships and sizes. The x-ray should also be taken a minimal of six feet away to decrease magnification and increase sharpness.
      1. In the PA/AP view, clavicular symmetry is a general indicator of chest rotation from the perpendicular plane
         a. Clavicles should be approximately equal in length
         b. Clavicular heads should be equal distances from the spinal process
   E. The film should be exposed during a deep inspiration to produce good alveolar inflation and avoid diaphragmatic displacement of the heart.
      1. A general indicator of adequate inspiration is the seventh rib visible at or above the diaphragm
      2. Inadequate inspiration flattens the inferior border of the heart, causing the lateral borders to falsely widen

READING A CHEST X-RAY

I. **Keys to consistent accuracy**
   A. Understanding of normal anatomic relationships in three dimensions
   B. Understanding the impact of pathologic changes on image
   C. Organized search pattern and persistent repetition of this ordered approach film after film
   D. Always compare with previous films, when available
II. **Basic impact of disease on image**
   A. Silhouette sign
      1. A loss of the normal border between different densities, such as when lungs with normal air density become filled with fluid and, therefore, become water dense
      2. Useful in localizing infiltrate or fluid; for example, any anterior pulmonic process might blur the adjacent heart border. If an area of increased density in the right lung field obscures the border of the hemidiaphragm, the infiltrate is in the basal segment of the right lower lobe; if only the border of the right heart is lost, the infiltrate is in the right middle lobe
   B. Interstitial pattern
      1. As the pulmonary interstitium or tissues in the lungs outside of the alveoli, the bronchial tree, and vasculature acquire more water (more density), such become more distinct.
      2. Appears as aerated lung with distinct linear or nodular markings
      3. Diseases with interstitial pattern include idiopathic pulmonary fibrosis, radiation pneumonitis, and scleroderma.

C. Alveolar pattern
   1. As alveoli fill, consolidate, or collapse, interstitial markings become less distinct (similar to silhouette sign).
   2. Remaining air-filled bronchi may show up in contrast against otherwise non-aerated lung (air bronchogram)
   3. Alveolar patterns are likely acute whether focal, multifocal, or diffuse.
   4. Diseases with alveolar pattern may include pulmonary edema, bronchopneumonia, hemorrhage, and atelectasis, among others.

III. **Reviewing the x-ray with an organized approach**
   A. Ensure that you are looking at the proper film
      1. Identify the patient
      2. Verify the date and time of the film
   B. Examine the film for orientation, rotation, and image quality
      1. PA/AP views should be hung as if facing the patient's front
      2. Clavicles should be of equal length with heads astride chest midline
      3. Outline of separate vertebral bodies should be evident
      4. Compare side by side with prior x-rays
      5. Check the film for adequate inspiration
   C. Use systematic ways to examine the x-ray, by using the ABCDEHI pneumonic
      1. Airway
         a. The trachea should be midline
            i. A displaced trachea can indicate thyroid enlargement
         b. The carina should be between T4 and T6 and should be examined when the patient is intubated to ensure inflation of both lungs.
         c. The right main bronchus is straighter than the left main bronchus.
            i. Aspiration pneumonia is suspected when the consolidation occurs in the right lower lobe.
      2. Bones
         a. Include spine, clavicle, ribs, and scapula
         b. Anterior ribs appear more flat versus the posterior ribs, which have a sharper downward angle
         c. Each rib should be examined for fracture
         d. Intercostal spaces should be noted for widening or asymmetry, which can indicate diseases that cause hyperinflation of the lungs or chest wall tumors
      3. Circulation or cardiac
         a. Examine the mediastinum
            i. A widened mediastinum can indicate heart failure or aortic aneurysm
         b. Calcification is indicative of atherosclerosis
         c. The normal cardiac to thoracic ratio should be less than 50%
         d. The left mediastinal border consists of the brachiocephalic vein, the aortic arch, the pulmonary artery, the atrial appendage, and the left ventricle
         e. The right mediastinal border consists of the brachiocephalic vein, the superior vena cava, the ascending aorta, the right pulmonary artery, the right atrium, and the inferior vena cava
      4. Diaphragm
         a. The right diaphragm is normally 1–3 cm higher than the left diaphragm due to the liver elevating the left diaphragm.
         b. The costophrenic angles should be sharp
         c. Air under the diaphragm can be indicative of a perforated portion of the bowels, and such is a medical emergency
      5. Edges

a. Examine the edges of the lung and chest wall. Disease processes to keep in mind include the following:
    i. Subcutaneous emphysema
    ii. Pneumothorax
    iii. Hemothorax
    iv. Pleural effusions, and others
        (a) Pleural effusions require 175–250 ml of fluid to blunt at least one of the costophrenic angles
6. Fields
    a. Lung parenchyma is examined for density changes or consolidations that are incongruent with the rest of the lung fields.
7. Gastric bubble
    a. Loss of the gastric air bubble can indicate a hiatal hernia
    b. A large gastric bubble can be correlated with bloating
    c. Air density outside of the gastric bubble and gastrointestinal tract can indicate pneumoperitoneum
8. Hilum
    a. The hilar is the overlapping of pulmonary arteries and veins, and the left hilum is usually 1–2 cm above the right.
    b. Widening of the hilum can be indicative of pulmonary hypertension
9. Invasive lines
    a. Assess tubes, lines, drains, catheters, and wires
    b. Please refer to table 24.1 for correct positioning of invasive devices

SPECIFIC DISEASE ENTITIES

I. **Congestive heart failure**
   A. It often manifests as an enlarged cardiac shadow, along with increased pulmonary vascular markings
   B. Cardiogenic pulmonary edema can be seen on the chest x-ray as Kerley B lines, which are horizontal lines that are less than 2 cm long, found near the costophrenic angle of the lungs.
   C. Pleural effusions often occur along with the diagnosis of congestive heart failure.

II. **Pericardial effusion**
   A. The chest x-ray is not sensitive enough to detect pericardial effusion.
      1. Changes in the size and/or hazy borders of the cardiac silhouette seen in serial films may, however, be suggestive of an effusion
      2. Previous films should be reviewed for recognition and documentation of subtle changes
   B. Cardiac echocardiography is more reliable than chest x-ray for detection of pericardial effusions

III. **Emphysema**
   A. Pulmonary parenchyma tends to be more lucent than normal, reflecting the loss of tissue and hyperinflation.
   B. The cardiac silhouette is often narrow
   C. Diaphragmatic domes are often flattened
   D. Lung volumes appear larger

IV. **Pneumonia**
   A. A chest x-ray is an essential part of the initial workup of a suspected diagnosis of pneumonia.
   B. Pneumonia is suspected when an infiltrate is seen in a specific segment of the lung. The diagnosis of pneumonia requires clinical and laboratory findings as well.
   C. Improvement in the appearance of a chest film often lags behind clinical improvement by a factor of weeks

Table 24.1	Invasive devices and positioning on chest X-ray
Devices	**Proper Location on the CXR**
Endotracheal tube	2–4 cm above the carina, not deviating to one bronchus
Chest tubes	All opening of the chest tube are inside the chest wall, tube travels up to drain air, down to drain fluids
Nasogastric tube	Below the diaphragm with tip and side holes 10 cm into the antrum of the stomach, without looping back to the fundus
Small-bore feeding tube	Tip should be into the duodenum, pass the pylorus, confirmed with abdominal film
Central venous catheter	Tip should be in the superior vena cava, above the right atrium
Dialysis catheters	Tip ends in the superior vena cava
Pulmonary artery catheter	Travels around the heart into the left or more commonly, the right pulmonary artery, 2–4 cm from midline, not in the periphery of the lung
Peripherally inserted center catheter	Tip should be within the superior vena cava above the right atrium
Intra-aortic balloon pump	Tip should be in the aorta, 2 cm below the aortic arch
Pacemakers	Lead touching the right atrium and right ventricle. Pacemaker catheters should lie along lower right cardiac (right ventricular) border
Automatic internal cardiac defibrillator	Lead in the superior vena cava or brachial cephalic vein, and apex of the right ventricle.

V. **Pulmonary nodules (also called coin lesions)**
   A. A nodule is defined as "a lesion smaller than 3 cm in size." Larger lesions are referred to as "masses."
   B. Solitary nodules should always be evaluated
   C. The most valuable method for evaluation of a pulmonary nodule involves comparison with earlier films.
      1. Nodules should be followed by serial chest x-rays and yearly computed tomography scans
      2. Benign nodules are often found in nonsmokers younger than 35 years
      3. Benign nodules tend to be calcified
      4. Calcifications in benign nodules are typically described as central, laminar, diffuse, or popcorn
      5. Nodules described as eccentric or stippled may be benign or malignant
      6. Benign nodules tend to remain unchanged over time
   D. Computerized tomography and positron emission tomography are useful in evaluating questionable nodules.
   E. Persons ages 55–74 years old, are current smokers or have quit smoking within the past 15 years, and/or have a smoking history of 30 pack-years should receive lung cancer screening
      1. A pack-year is calculated by the number of packs smoked per day multiplied by the years smoked.
      2. Screening should be performed with low dose computed tomography scan and has been shown to decrease mortality by 20%.

BIBLIOGRAPHY

Antin-Ozerkis, D., Rubinowitz, A., Evans, J., Homer, R. J., & Matthay, R. A. (2012). Interstitial lung disease in the connective tissue diseases. *Clinics in Chest Medicine, 33*(1), 123–149.

Bejan, C. A., Xia, F., Vanderwende, L., Wurfel, M.W., Yetisgen-Yildiz, M. (2012). Pneumonia identification using statistical feature selection. *Journal of the American Medical Informatics Association*. Advance online publication. doi:10.1136/amianjnl-2011–000752

Castañer, E., Gallardo, X., Ballesteros, E., Andreu, M., Pallardó, Y., Mata, M. M., & Riera, L. (2009). CT diagnosis of chronic pulmonary thromboembolism 1. *Radiographics, 29*(1), 31–50. doi:10.1148/rg.291085061.

Daffner, R. H., & Hartman, M. S. (2014). *Clinical radiology: The essentials* (4th ed.). Philadelphia, PA: Lippincott, Williams & Wilkins.

Erkonen, W. E., & Smith, W. L. (2010). *Radiology 101: The basics and fundamentals of imaging* (3rd ed.). Philadelphia, PA: Lippincott Williams & Wilkins.

Gorgan, M., Bockorny, B., Lawlor, M., Volpe, J., & Fiel-Gan, M. (2013). Pulmonary hemorrhage with capillaritis secondary to mycophenolate mofetil in a heart-transplant patient. *Archives of Pathology and Laboratory Medicine, 137*(11), 1684–1687.

Hasegawa, N., Nishimura, T., Ohtani, S., Takeshita, K., Fukunaga, K., Tasaka, S., . . . & Ishizaka, A. (2009). Therapeutic effects of various initial combinations of chemotherapy including clarithromycin against mycobacterium avium complex pulmonary disease. *Chest Journal, 136*(6), 1569–1575.

Herrmann, C. (2009). *As easy as black and white: CXR interpretation*. Retrieved from http://www.aacn.org/wd/nti2009/nti_cd/data/papers/main/30978.pdf

Jiang, M., Chen, Y., Liu, M., Rosenbloom, S. T., Mani, S., Denny, J. C., Xu, H. (2011). *Journal of the American Medical Informatics Association, 18*, 601–606. doi:10.1136/amiajnl-2011-000163

Joarder, R., & Crundwell, N. (Eds.). (2009). *Chest x-ray in clinical practice*. New York, NY: Springer.

Li, F., Hara, T., Shiraishi, J., Engelmann, R., MacMahon, H., & Doi, K. (2011). Improved detection of subtle lung nodules by use of chest radiographs with bone suppression imaging: Receiver operating characteristic analysis with and without localization. *American Journal of Roentgenology, 196*(5), W535-W541.

Light, R. W. (2007). *Pleural diseases*. Philadelphia, PA: Lippincott Williams & Wilkins.

Napolitano, L. M., (2010). Use of severity scoring and stratification factors in clinical trials of hospital-acquired and ventilator-associated pnemonia [Supplemental material]. *Clinical Infectious Diseases, 51*(S1), S67-S80. doi:10.1086/653052

National Cancer Institute. (2010). *National lung screening trials*. Retrieved from: http://www.cancer.gov/clinicaltrials/noteworthy-trials/nlst/updates

Ozawa, Y., Hara, M., Kato, M., Shimizu, S., & Shibamoto, Y. (2014). Contrast enhancement of posterior mediastinal ganglioneuromas—Correlation between the level of enhancement and histopathological features. *Open Journal of Radiology, 4*(1), 123–129. doi:10.4236/ojrad.2014.41016

Pezzotti, W. (2014). Chest x-ray interpretation: Not just Black & White. *Nursing2014, 44*(1), 40–47.

del Portillo, I. P., Vázquez, S. T., Mendoza, J. B., & Moreno, R. V. (2014). Oxygen therapy in critical care: A double-edged sword. *Health, 6*(15), 2035–2046. doi:10.4236/health.2014.615238

Sussmann, A. R., & Ko, J. P. (2009). Understanding chest radiographic anatomy with MDCT reformations. *Clinical Radiology, 65*(2), 155–166.

Test, M., Shah, S. S., Monuteaux, M., Ambroggio, L., Lee, E. Y., Markowitz, R. I., . . . & Neuman, M. I. (2013). Impact of clinical history on chest radiograph interpretation. *Journal of Hospital Medicine, 8*(7), 359–364. doi:10.1002/jhm.1991

Tozzetti, C., Adembri, C., & Modesti, P. A. (2009). Pulse oximeter, the fifth vital sign: A safety belt, or a prison of the mind? *Internal and emergency medicine, 4*(4), 331–332.

West, J. B. (2012). *Pulmonary pathophysiology. The essentials* (7th ed.). Philadelphia, PA: Lippincott Williams & Wilkins.

CHAPTER 25

Pulmonary Function Testing

HALEY M. HOY • THOMAS W. BARKLEY, JR. • CHARLENE M. MYERS

I. **Purpose of a pulmonary function test (PFT)**
   A. To determine the existence of pulmonary function that may then be used to do the following:
      1. Assign a potential diagnosis to explain a patient's symptoms
      2. Differentiate between obstructions of airways and decreased pulmonary parenchymal compliance as the source of a patient's symptoms
      3. Evaluate the response to treatment of a pulmonary disease process
   B. Indications for a PFT
      1. Evaluate unexplained dyspnea and cough
      2. Assess severity of pulmonary dysfunction
      3. Determine potential reversibility of airway obstruction
   C. Limitations of the PFT
      1. The patient must be able to cooperate with the testing (inadequate cooperation negates the value of the testing), the person administering the test must be skilled, and the person interpreting the test must be knowledgeable in PFT interpretation.
      2. The patient should be relatively stable with respect to symptoms. Temporary worsening of symptoms may invalidate the severity of the dysfunction assessed.

II. **Types of PFTs**
   A. Spirometry continues to be recommended as the objective measurement of pulmonary function and for the diagnosis and management of respiratory dysfunction.
      1. Determines forced vital capacity (FVC) and forced expiratory flow rates
         a. Forced expiratory volume in one second (FEV_1) is considered the gold standard by which obstructive airway disease is measured. More specifically, the ratio of FEV_1/FVC is diagnostic for obstructive lung disease.
         b. Values are compared with predicted values derived from population-based reference groups
         c. Decreased FEV_1/FVC (less than 70% of normal) indicates the presence of airflow obstruction or an obstructive disorder
      2. If expiratory airflow obstruction is defined, the response to an aerosolized bronchodilator should be measured

CHAPTER 25   Pulmonary Function Testing

      a. An increase of 12% or 200 ml or greater is often accepted as a reason to use a bronchodilator
      b. However, although controversial, a smaller improvement in flow rate in the presence of more severe obstruction is often a reason to consider using a bronchodilator.
   3. Graphic display of inspiration and exhalation (flow volume loops) provides a comprehensive view of respiratory mechanics, allows the identification of subtle changes, can identify the location of airflow obstruction, and aids in differentiating between obstructive and restrictive disease.
   4. Results correlate with morbidity and life expectancy
   5. Safe, inexpensive, and fast
   6. Spirometry, however, is effort dependent, and some patients have difficulty performing the process because of advanced age or acute illness.
B. Spirometry with bronchodilator therapy (evaluation for bronchospasm)
   1. Determines the vital capacity and expiratory flow rates before and after aerosolized bronchodilator therapy
   2. Degree of responsiveness may be useful in determining the need for bronchodilator therapy
C. Body plethysmography (volume displacement techniques)
   1. Useful in determining all lung volumes, including the following:
      a. Vital capacity (measured during spirometry)
      b. Residual volume in the chest after expiration
      c. Total lung capacity (TLC)
   2. More completely differentiates between a restrictive ventilatory defect (lowered lung volumes) and an obstructive ventilatory defect (increased total lung volume and residual volume)
      a. TLC is decreased with restrictive disorders
      b. TLC is normal or increased with obstructive disorders
      c. Interpret cautiously in patients with neuromuscular weakness because this can sometimes decrease TLC and may prevent differentiation between restrictive and obstructive disorders
D. Measurement of exhaled nitrous oxide
   1. Noninvasive marker of airway inflammation
      a. Appears to reflect lower airway inflammation—a hallmark of the asthma disease process
      b. Useful in recognizing inflammation in symptom-free asthmatic patients who have normal lung function
      c. Helps with the titration of inhaled steroid therapy, in that inhaled steroids quickly reduce exhaled nitrous oxide levels, indicating a reduction in airway inflammation
E. Diffusing capacity of the lung for carbon monoxide (CO) (single-breath technique)
   1. Uses CO as a substitute for O_2 to assess the gas transfer function of the lungs
      a. Decreased diffusion capacity of carbon monoxide in the lung (DLCO) may indicate disorders of pulmonary parenchyma, vascular problems, or decreases in alveolar function (such as occur with lung resection or emphysema)
      b. Increased DLCO may indicate asthma, obesity, polycythemia, or cardiac left-to-right shunting
   2. Modified techniques to measure DLCO must be used for patients with end-stage heart disease and after heart transplant
F. Maximal (inspiratory) respiratory pressures
   1. Helps in the diagnosis of neuromuscular causes of respiratory dysfunction
      a. Decreased inspiratory and expiratory pressures indicate generalized neuromuscular diseases such as amyotrophic lateral sclerosis
      b. Decreased inspiratory pressures suggest dysfunction of the diaphragm

c. Decreased expiratory pressures are often seen with spinal cord injuries
  2. Important in the prognosis of neuromuscular dysfunction
     a. Helps in the evaluation of airway protective capacity (adequate cough)
     b. Helps predict successful weaning from mechanical ventilators
     c. Helps assess severity and progression of neuromuscular weakness
  G. Bronchial provocation testing (challenge)
     1. Aids in the identification of suspected asthma
        a. Useful test when spirometry is normal and cough is unexplained
     2. Involves the inhalation of methacholine, histamine, or other chemical stimulants to induce bronchial smooth muscle constriction
        a. Bronchial smooth muscle constriction occurs in asthmatic patients at much lower doses than that in nonasthmatic patients.
        b. Positive results for asthma are indicated by an FEV_1 that has decreased by 20% or more at a dose of 16 mg/ml or less.
        c. The test is 95% sensitive for the diagnosis of asthma; negative results make a diagnosis of asthma unlikely.
  H. High-resolution computed tomography
     1. Useful in examining specific individual airways and structural alterations associated with pathologic change
        a. Provides a way to view airways during expansion and contraction and to assess changes in airway size with changes in lung volume
     2. May show lesions missed on plain radiography
III. Understanding "normal" values or "predicted" values
   A. Pulmonary function testing laboratories compare the patient being studied versus a larger population of persons of similar age, race, gender, height, and weight.
   B. The nomograms used vary among laboratories and may prevent absolute comparison when testing is done in different locations.
IV. Lung volume measurements and the meaning of lung "capacities" (See table 25.1 and 25.2)
   A. Lung volume is reported as a single value
   B. Lung capacity refers to the combination of lung volumes
V. Determination of the presence of obstructive and restrictive ventilatory defects
   A. Obstructive ventilatory defects
      1. Flow rates are reduced when compared with normal values for similar persons
      2. Lung volumes generally are within the normal range or are larger than the normal range because of air trapping and hyperinflation (with increased reserve volume and TLC).
   B. Restrictive ventilatory defects
      1. Flow rates are normal or increased
      2. Lung volumes are proportionately reduced
VI. Determining severity of defects (lung volumes and flow rates)
   A. Values greater than 70% of predicted volumes/flow rates are considered within normal limits
   B. Values 60%–70% of predicted volumes/flow rates are mildly reduced
   C. Values 50%–60% of predicted volumes/flow rates are moderately reduced
   D. Values lower than 50% of predicted volumes/flow rates are severely reduced
   E. When values for residual volume and TLC exceed 120% of predicted, air trapping and hyperinflation are present
   F. When airflow obstruction is present, bronchodilator responsiveness is considered significant if expiratory airflow measurements improve by at least 15% over baseline values
      1. The absence of such a response is, by itself, not justification for withholding these medications
      2. Bronchodilators may improve other parameters of lung function, including secretion clearance.

VII. Peak expiratory flowmeter and asthma
   A. Simple and inexpensive device (indeed, usually provided by pharmaceutical companies that manufacture bronchodilators) intended for home use by asthmatic patients and those with other forms of potentially reversible airway obstruction
      1. Still recommended for daily monitoring
   B. Ideally, the patient will measure his or her peak expiratory flow rate (PEFR) at least once daily initially, at the same time each day, to provide a measure of functional airflow limitation over time.
      1. Values are recorded in a diary provided with the device
         a. Patients may demonstrate low compliance in terms of accurately and consistently recording results
      2. The patient's "best" flow rate, typical flow rates, and altered flow rates may then be used to determine the need for additional medication.
         a. PEFR 80%–100% of baseline
            i. The "green" zone
            ii. No change in therapy is needed
         b. PEFR 50%–80% of baseline
            i. The "yellow" zone
            ii. Temporary increase in intensity of therapy, or additional therapy, should be considered
         c. PEFR below 50% of baseline
            i. The "red" zone
            ii. Urgent/emergency care is advised

VIII. Implications for geriatric patients
   A. Many older adults experience changes in elastic recoil and musculoskeletal changes of the chest wall
      1. TLC usually remains constant but vital capacity decreases because residual volume increases
      2. Tidal volume may be decreased
      3. Alveoli collapse more easily
      4. Number of cilia diminish
      5. Decreased cough reflex
   B. It is important to allow extra time when performing lung function testing on older adults.

Table 25.1	Lung Volumes and Lung Capacities	
Lung volume	**Lung capacity**	
Inspiratory reserve volume (IRV) The amount of air that can be inhaled after a full inspiration	Vital capacity (forced) (FVC)	Total lung capacity (TLC)
Tidal volume (VT) The amount of air that is inhaled or exhaled during a normal breath		
Expiratory reserve volume (ERV) The amount of air that can be forced out of the lungs after a full expiration		
Residual volume (from plethysmography) RV The amount of air remaining in the lungs after a forced expiration		

Table 25.2	Expiratory Flow Rates
Flow rate measurement	
FEV_1 Forced expiratory volume in one second	Parameter assessed, comment on effort dependency Central and smaller airways
$FEV_1\%$ (FEV_1/FVC) FEV_1 as a percentage of forced vital capacity	How much of the vital capacity can be exhaled forcibly in one second? Effort dependent
FEF_{25-75} Forced expiratory flow rate over the midportion of exhalation	Small airways Relatively effort independent

BIBLIOGRAPHY

Chang, J. E., White. A. A., & Simon, R. A. (2014). Non-steroidal anti-inflammatory drug hypersensitivity and sinus disease. In C. C. Chang, G. A. Incaudo, & M. E. Gershwin (Eds.), *Diseases of the sinuses: A comprehensive textbook of diagnosis and treatment* (2nd ed., pp. 195–208). New York, NY: Springer.

Goldman, L., & Schafer, A. (2011). *Goldman's Cecil Medicine* (24th ed.). Philadelphia, PA: Elsevier Saunders.

King, G. G. (2011). Cutting edge technologies in respiratory research: Lung function testing. *Respirology, 16*(6), 883–890. doi:10.1111/j.1440–1843.2011.02013.x

Liang, B. M., Lam, D. C., & Feng, Y. L. (2012). Clinical applictions of lung function tests: A revisit. *Respirology, 17*(4), 611–619. doi:10.1111/j.1440–1843.2012.02149.x

MacIntyre, N. R. (2012). The future of pulmonary function testing. *Respiratory Care, 57*(1), 154–161. doi:10.4187/respcare.01422

Meiner, S. E. (2010). *Gerontologic nursing* (4th ed.). St. Louis, MO: Elsevier Mosby.

Pretto, J. J., Brazzale, D. J., Guy, P. A., Goudge, R. J., & Hensley, M. J. (2013). Reasons for referral for pulmonary function testing: An audit of 4 adult lung function laboratories. *Respiratory Care, 58*(3), 507–510. Retrieved from http://rc.rcjournal.com/content/58/3/507.full.pdf

Ruppel, G. L., & Enright, P. L. (2012). Pulmonary function testing. *Respiratory Care, 57*(1), 165–175. doi:10.4187/respcare.01640

West, J. B. (2012). *Pulmonary pathophysiology* (8th ed.). Philadelphia, PA: Wolters Kluwer Health/Lippincott, Williams, & Wilkins.

Wheaton, A. G., Ford, E. S., Thompson, W. W., Greenlund, K. J., Presley-Cantrell, L. R., & Croft, J. B. (2013). Pulmonary function, chronic respiratory symptoms, and health-related quality of life among adults in the United States—National Health and Nutrition Examination Survey 2007–2010. *BMC Public Health, 13*(854). Retrieved from http://www.biomedcentral.com/1471–2458/13/854

CHAPTER 26

Obstructive (Ventilatory) Lung Diseases

DAVID A. MILLER • THOMAS W. BARKLEY, JR. • ROBERT FELLIN • TOBIAS P. REBMANN

CHRONIC OBSTRUCTIVE PULMONARY DISEASE (COPD)

I. **Definition**
   A. COPD is a mixture of diseases, including emphysema, chronic bronchitis, and bronchospastic airway disease, all of which are characterized by limitation of expiratory airflow
   B. Acute exacerbations are superimposed upon chronic symptoms
II. **Etiologies/incidence**
   A. Tobacco smoking (cigarettes, cigars, and pipes) is the most common cause
      1. Most persons who smoke a pack of cigarettes per day for longer than 40 years will have manifestations of COPD.
      2. Note: One pack of cigarettes per day multiplied by the number of years smoked equals the number of pack-years of cigarettes smoked
   B. Inhalation of environmental pollutants (e.g., oxides of sulfur and nitrogen)
      1. Incidence depends on duration and concentration of exposure in heavily polluted areas
   C. Occupational exposure to inorganic chemicals (chlorine and fluorine) and organic chemicals (e.g., toluene) may result in obstructive airway disease.
III. **Subjective findings**
   A. Cough, dry and occasionally productive, especially in the early morning
   B. Sputum production
      1. Usually clear in color but may be discolored (e.g., yellow, purulent, and green)
      2. A change in the amount produced or the color of the sputum is important in management decisions
         a. Exertional dyspnea
   C. Weight loss with progressive disease due to early satiety and difficulty breathing after food is consumed, especially in the elderly
   D. Fatigue
   E. Complaints of chest tightness, owing to one of the following:
      1. Alterations that are slowly occurring in the chest wall (e.g., increase in anteroposterior chest diameter)
      2. Acute air retention within the thorax

IV. Physical exam findings
   A. General
   1. Respiratory rate is normal or increased
   2. Mental status should be alert and oriented
   3. Note sitting position for the presence of classic "emphysema stance"
      a. The patient sits with the chest forward and the arms straightened
      b. The upper body is lifted to allow for greater expansion of the chest, as gravity pulls the abdominal contents downward and away from the diaphragm
   4. Inspect for clubbing of the nail beds and for pursed-lip breathing
   B. Chest inspection
   1. Increase in the anteroposterior diameter of the chest
      a. Gives rise to a "barrel" configuration
      b. Normally, the diameter of the chest from axilla to axilla is about twice the anteroposterior diameter
      c. Loss of muscle strength in elderly may accelerate this
   2. Use of accessory muscles of respiration
      a. Sternocleidomastoids
      b. Intercostals
   C. Chest percussion
   1. Hyperresonance
   2. Low diaphragm
   D. Chest auscultation
   1. Diminished breath sounds throughout the chest
   2. Prolonged forced expiratory time (auscultation while the patient forcibly exhales shows that the effort needed to exhale the air requires longer than 3 seconds)
   3. Rhonchi on inspiration and/or expiration, especially when secretions are increased
   4. Occasional wheezing on expiration
      a. Asthma
      b. Chronic bronchitis

V. Laboratory/diagnostics
   A. Pulmonary function testing
   1. Expiratory flow rates are reduced
      a. Early disease: reduction in small airway flow rates
      b. Late disease: reduction in FEV_1 (forced expiratory volume in 1 second, a measure of the potential for severe complications of COPD)
   2. Lung volume changes
      a. Air trapping indicated by increased residual volume
      b. Hyperinflation indicated by increased total lung capacity
      c. Forced vital capacity (FVC) may be reduced by air trapping.
      d. The reduction in FVC is, on a percentage of a normal basis, less than the percentage reduction in predicted expiratory airflow.
   B. Arterial blood gases (ABGs) and pulse oximetry
   1. Earlier in the course of disease, and often during the later stages, both studies show normal oxygenation, and ABGs show no evidence of chronic respiratory acidosis
   2. Seen more frequently later in the course of disease, or during exacerbations of moderately severe disease
      a. Hypoxemia (partial pressure of oxygen in arterial blood [PaO_2] less than 55 mmHg)
      b. Hypercarbia (chronic respiratory acidosis)
   3. During acute exacerbations of COPD, hypoxemia and acute hypercarbia may be seen.
      a. Assessment requires at least one ABG analysis
      b. Increasing respiratory distress and changes in mental status (confusion, stupor) require more frequent checks of ABGs

4. Pulse oximetry
   a. Used frequently to assess for adequacy of oxygen transport within the blood at rest and during exertion
   b. Adequate oxygenation is implied when SaO_2 (oxygen saturation) is greater than 88% when the hemoglobin level is above 10 grams/dl
C. Other laboratory values
   1. Hemoglobin and hematocrit
      a. Hemoglobin less than 10 grams/dl may be suboptimal for oxygen transport
      b. Hematocrit greater than 55 ml/dl indicates secondary polycythemia is due to chronic hypoxemia
   2. Serum bicarbonate is often elevated with chronic hypercarbia
D. Chest x-ray
   1. Air trapping
   2. Blebs and bullae (dilated air spaces within the pulmonary parenchyma) may be seen, although usually require CT imaging to be recognized
   3. Flattened diaphragm
   4. Hyperinflation is noted by the following:
      a. Hyperlucency in upper lung zones
      b. Widening of intercostal spaces
      c. Ten or more ribs identified above diaphragm
   5. Retrosternal air noted on lateral view

VI. Nonpharmacological management

A. Smoking cessation (perhaps most difficult to achieve)
   1. Behavioral modification
   2. Nicotine replacement therapy (gum, lozenges, and transdermal) are all available over the counter. Decisions regarding the initial dosing should rely on the product chosen and the daily nicotine exposure. The provider should discuss this with the patient.
   3. Pharmacological
      a. Bupropion (Zyban), 150 mg daily for 3 days, then BID for 7–12 weeks
      b. Varenicline (Chantix) available in a starter month pack, then 1 mg BID for 8–16 additional weeks
B. Nonpharmacological therapy provided with heated or cooled aerosols of water in combination with chest physiotherapy may help thin airway secretions.
C. The value of chest physiotherapy (percussion and postural drainage) in COPD is controversial, but it may be worthwhile when patients perceive a benefit from it.

VII. Pharmacological management

A. All pharmacotherapy must take into consideration comorbid conditions, concomitant use of other medications, and dose adjustments for age, renal and hepatic function, and body mass where indicated
B. Symptom assessment in patients with COPD can be made using a standard assessment tool such as the COPD Assessment Tool (CAT, 2012) with its User Guide for Healthcare Professionals (CAT User Guide, 2012). The test evaluates cough, phlegm production, perceived chest tightness, dyspnea, impact on ADLs and IADLs, sleep, and energy; it is at least semiquantitative over time.
   1. Classifying the degree of severity of COPD by severity of airflow obstruction (GOLD, 2014)
      a. Four categories
         i. GOLD 1: Mild—FEV_1 80% or greater of predicted
         ii. GOLD 2: Moderate—50% or less FEV_1 less than 80% predicted
         iii. GOLD 3: Severe—30% or less FEV_1 less than 50% predicted
         iv. GOLD 4: Very severe—FEV_1 less than 30% predicted
      b. Exacerbation of COPD (GOLD, 2014)

i. Worsening of symptoms that leads to a change in therapy
ii. Two or more exacerbations per year is suggestive of deteriorating lung function (a higher GOLD category)
   c. Evaluate for possible worsening or co-existing conditions (comorbidities)
      i. Cardiovascular, depression/anxiety, muscle weakness, metabolic syndrome, coexisting lung disease
      ii. Treat these as indicated.
C. Drug management, stable COPD (GOLD, 2014)
   1. Anticholinergic agents
      a. Decrease airway secretions and airway smooth muscle tone
      b. Anticholinergic agents of choice in COPD
         i. Ipratropium bromide (Atrovent), two puffs 4 times a day; also premixed in saline for use in handheld nebulizer, or
         ii. Tiotropium bromide (Spiriva) 18 mcg, once daily by HandiHaler
         iii. Aclidinium (Tudorza) 400 mcg inhaled BID
         iv. Umeclidinium (Incruse Ellipta) 62.5 mcg inhaled daily
      c. Mainstay of therapy for COPD
      d. Adverse effects: dry mouth and dry, hacking cough, oral candidiasis (teach patient to rinse mouth after use), and urinary retention (especially elderly males with concomitant prostate hypertrophy)
   2. Bronchodilators
      a. Beta$_2$-adrenergic receptor agonists
         i. Relax smooth muscle tone and improve airflow
         ii. Stimulate ciliary motion to promote secretion mobilization
      b. Short-acting inhaled β_2 agonists: used for episodic symptom exacerbations
         i. Albuterol (Proventil, Ventolin), also premixed in saline for handheld nebulizer use
         ii. Levalbuterol (Xopenex); metered dose inhalers and nebulizer solutions, possibly less tachycardia and tremor effect than albuterol
      c. Other agents available (caution urged if severe coronary artery disease, history of rapid supraventricular or ventricular arrhythmias, or cardiomyopathy). These are maintenance drugs in the therapy of COPD.
         i. Long-acting inhaled β_2 agonists (LABA): used for maintenance therapy only; bronchodilation for up to 12 hr, currently not recommended without concomitant use of inhaled corticosteroid (GOLD, 2014)
            (a) Salmeterol (Serevent Diskus): prolonged receptor binding requires patient education about proper use to avoid induction of cardiac arrhythmias. (Advair: contains salmeterol 50 mcg, and fluticasone, 100, 250, or 500 mcg; dosage, 1 puff BID)
            (b) Formoterol (Foradil inhaler): similar prolonged receptor binding (Symbicort: contains formoterol 4.5 mcg and budesonide, 80 or 160 mcg; dosage, 2 puffs BID maximum. Dulera contains formoterol 5 mcg and mometasone 100 mcg; dosage, 2 puffs BID)
            (c) Vilanterol/fluticasone (Breo Ellipta): similar prolonged receptor binding; contains vilanterol (25 mcg) and fluticasone (100 mcg); dosage, 1 puff daily; NOT for patients with asthma
            (d) Vilanterol/umeclidinium (Anoro Ellipta): combination of long-acting β agonist and an anticholinergic agent; vilanterol (25 mcg) and umeclidinium (62.5 mcg), 1 inhalation daily; NOT for patients with asthma

3. Combination corticosteroid and LABA inhalation is recommended and should be administered at a standard dose of LABA with various doses of corticosteroid. This regimen is primarily indicated for asthma, although it does cross over to COPD with bronchospastic component (bronchitis).
    a. The 2014 GOLD report reiterates that when the FEV_1 less than 60% of predicted, inhaled corticosteroids improve symptoms, lung function, and quality of life, and reduce frequency of exacerbations.
4. Anti-inflammatory corticosteroids (can be used alone when stable after using with long-acting β agonist bronchodilators)
    a. Reduce acute and chronic effects of inflammation
    b. Can improve lung function
    c. Provide symptomatic relief of emphysema but do not improve lung function (FEV_1)
    d. Patients taking systemic doses of corticosteroids need to be warned of adverse effects that may result from the abrupt withdrawal of these agents, such as Addisonian crises (e.g., weakness, headache, fever, tachycardia, hypotension, tachypnea, and others).
    e. Oral (enteral) and parenteral doses should generally be rapidly tapered over several days until it is clear such agents have contributed to improving the patient's general condition.
        i. Oral tablets
            (a) Prednisone (Deltasone), 60 mg/day, tapered quickly to less than 20 mg/day
            (b) Methylprednisolone (Medrol), 64 mg/day, tapered to less than 16 mg/day
        ii. Intravenous preparations
            (a) Methylprednisolone sodium succinate (Solu-Medrol), 20–40 mg IV every 6–8 hr for severe exacerbations of COPD; tapered as patient condition allows
        iii. Intramuscular preparations (evidence of effectiveness above oral dosing is questionable)
            (a) Methylprednisolone (Depo-Medrol), 80–240 mg IM in divided doses to decrease discomfort
    f. Caution use of systemic corticosteroids in elderly due to immunosuppressive, hyperglycemic, and bone demineralization effects, even in short-term use if repeated frequently due to exacerbations.
5. Phosphodiesterase 4 inhibitors
    a. Used in later stages of disease
    b. Increases intracellular cAMP in lung tissue
    c. Reduces neutrophil and eosinophil counts in the lung
    d. Roflumilast (Daliresp), 500 mcg daily

D. COPD Stepwise treatment plans
  1. GOLD 0: at risk
     a. Normal lung function
     b. Cough and sputum production
     c. Remove toxins
  2. GOLD I: mild
     a. FEV_1 greater than 80% (see Pulmonary Function Testing chapter)
     b. Asymptomatic or may have chronic cough and sputum
     c. Short-acting beta agonist
  3. GOLD II: moderate
     a. FEV_1 50%–80%
     b. Asymptomatic or may have chronic cough and sputum
     c. Add long-acting $β_2$ agonist
  4. GOLD III: severe

a. FEV_1 30%–50%
b. Some symptoms daily
c. Add inhaled corticosteroid
5. GOLD IV: very severe
a. FEV_1 less than 30% or less than 50% with severe respiratory failure
b. Multiple symptoms
c. Long-term oxygen for severe hypoxia
d. Consider surgical treatment
E. Exacerbations: most common cause is bronchial infection
1. Systemic corticosteroids and antibiotics
2. Positive pressure noninvasive ventilation (BiPAP) helps decrease CO_2 retention and prevent intubation
3. Mechanical ventilation
F. Palliative care and end-of-life issues should be discussed and offered to patients with patients who have COPD, especially those who have severe disease, significant symptoms and are of advanced age.
G. Periodic review of proper use of metered dose inhalers is strongly recommended
H. Drugs for respiratory muscles (i.e., diaphragm and intercostals) and bronchodilator activity
1. Theophylline
a. Theo-Dur, 300 mg BID
b. Uni-Dur, 400–600 mg in the evening
c. Theophylline timed-release (Uniphyl), 400–600 mg in the evening
2. Therapeutic drug levels are recommended to be lower than 20 mg/L
a. Note: Evening doses acknowledge the circadian increase in airway smooth muscle tone.
b. Monitor for side effects, especially in elderly. Systemic adverse effects can occur even with serum levels within therapeutic range
I. Comments
1. Maintenance therapy for COPD may incorporate as many different classes of pharmacological agents PRN to maintain the patient's usual performance status. From a step-wise point of view, short-acting bronchodilators are used for mild disease, and then adding regular doses of anticholinergics, long-acting bronchodilators with inhaled corticosteroids, and then considering theophylline, 4-phosphodiesterase inhibitors, and other medications for more severe disease.
2. During exacerbations, inhaled bronchodilators may be needed more frequently than every 4 hr
3. Parenteral steroids should be added and rapidly tapered over several days until it is clear whether or not these preparations have contributed to improving the patient's general condition.
J. Antimicrobial agents
1. Indications
a. Changes in sputum quantity and color are considered important
i. Gram's stain may be helpful
ii. Sputum culture is not indicated for initiation of treatment
iii. In most instances, sputum and blood cultures should be obtained prior to initiation of antimicrobial therapy if pneumonia is suspected.
b. Recent upper respiratory infection (Note: upper respiratory infection is the most common cause of COPD exacerbation)
c. Radiographic evidence compatible with pneumonia is present
d. Bacteremia is suspected

2. Agents chosen should cover usually expected respiratory pathogens (see Lower Respiratory Tract Pathogens chapter), without being unnecessarily broader in spectrum than is required.
K. Agents to thin the sputum:
   1. Guaifenesin (Mucinex, Robitussin) may be of help to thin respiratory secretions, although total body hydration is clearly more important. Thus, these agents should be combined with adequate hydration.
   2. Acetylcysteine (Mucomyst 10% or 20%)
      a. Reduces sputum viscosity
      b. 1–10 ml of solution is inhaled every 6–8 hr, generally after a β_2 agonist is inhaled (see Bronchodilator section under pharmacological management of COPD)
      c. Can provoke bronchospasm
      d. "Tastes like rotten eggs" because of sulfur content
L. Supplemental oxygen (see Oxygen Supplementation chapter)
M. Antitussives are generally contraindicated for long term or chronic use in stable COPD
N. Risk prevention
   1. Flu vaccine
   2. Pneumonia vaccine
O. Surgical treatment: referral to a pulmonologist experienced with lung transplantation in COPD is recommended
   1. Lung transplantation
   2. Lung volume reduction surgery may help to relieve dyspnea and improve exercise tolerance
   3. Surgical intervention may be associated with significant adverse effects in elderly
P. Therapy: realities
   1. No treatment will restore lung function
   2. Removing toxins, including tobacco, occupational chemicals, and pollutants, is the only method of preventing continued deterioration of lung function
   3. Exercise training may help to improve respiratory function but does show improvement in exercise tolerance and symptoms
   4. Treatment will not change decline in lung function; treatment is based on preventing symptoms
Q. Special considerations in pharmacological management of COPD in the elderly
   1. Increased risk of adverse drug events (reduced hepatic metabolism and renal excretion)
      a. Short-acting β_2 agonist bronchodilators can induce tremor and tachycardia. Consider using an anticholinergic (ipratropium) with the β_2 adrenergic agent
      b. Inhaled corticosteroids: increased risk of cataracts
      c. Theophylline toxicity risk increases after age 75, especially due to drug interactions (e.g., with cimetidine)
      d. Systemic corticosteroids increase the risk of confusion, agitation, poor glycemic control, and osteoporosis (especially with less mobility due to breathing problems
   2. Increased risk for non-adherence due to difficulty with using hand-activated metered dose inhalers (arthritis) or forgetfulness (dementia)
   3. Polypharmacy increases the risk for non-adherence and for overuse of inhaled medications, requiring medication reconciliation at every encounter
   4. Those with comorbid conditions
      a. Gastroesophageal reflux
      b. Overweight or obese status
      c. Diabetes mellitus
      d. Obstructive sleep apnea
      e. Allergic rhinitis or sinusitis
      f. Cardiovascular disease

ASTHMA

I. **Definition**
   A. Clinical disorder characterized by periodic cough often with episodic wheezing, although wheezing less commonly heard among the elderly
   B. Sputum is usually described as "plugs" of sputum
   C. When the disorder is exacerbated, the patient may report "tightness" in the chest and dyspnea
      1. Symptoms may worsen with certain "triggers" (exercise; viral infection; strong emotions; weather changes)
      2. Symptoms may persist with exposure to animal dander, house dust, mold (home or external environment), smoke, pollen, airborne chemicals
   D. Patient often has a family history of asthma
   E. Inflammatory reaction
      1. Hypertrophy of bronchial smooth muscle and mucous glands
      2. Hyperactive airway and inflammation
      3. Causes bronchospasm and mucous production with airway edema
   F. Usually begins in childhood, with or without genetic predisposition
   G. Increased incidence in areas with environmental pollutants

II. **Physical exam findings**
   A. Reduced air entry sounds
   B. Prolonged expiration with expiratory wheezing
   C. Associated symptoms of hay fever or allergic rhinitis

III. **Differential diagnosis in older adults**
   A. COPD
   B. Heart failure
   C. Pulmonary embolism
   D. Endobronchial obstruction (tumor)
   E. Cough related to co-administration of certain medications (e.g., angiotensin converting enzyme inhibitors and β adrenergic blockers)
   F. Vocal cord dysfunction

IV. **Diagnostics**
   A. Diagnosis is based upon symptoms (due to episodic airflow obstruction), at least partially reversible airflow obstruction (based on spirometry), and exclusion of other diagnoses (especially important among elderly patients)
   B. Chest x-ray can be entirely normal or may show hyperinflation; among the elderly it may show evidence of comorbid cardiopulmonary conditions
   C. Spirometry to demonstrate the severity airflow obstruction and reversibility after inhalation of a short-acting bronchodilator
      1. Peak expiratory flow meters are used in monitoring asthma, not in diagnosing asthma
      2. Spirometry should be measured using American Thoracic Society standards.

V. **Management (see tables 26.1 & 26.2)**
   A. Engage the elderly patient as a partner in self-management
      1. Understanding which medications are for quick relief (See SABAs, step 1; systemic corticosteroids, steps 5 and 6) and which are for long-term control (see ICS, leukotriene modifiers, LABAs)
      2. Report changes in symptom patterns/exacerbations (nighttime awakenings; more frequent short-acting β adrenergic inhaler use; work absence; alteration in daily activities; worsening quality of life)
      3. Report significant changes, following the patient's asthma action plan, if used
      4. Report visits to the emergency room or hospitalizations for asthma

CHAPTER 26   Obstructive (Ventilatory) Lung Diseases

B. Stepwise Management of Asthma (assessment for hypoxemia should be done if health assessment and/or co-morbidities warrant this during any step in asthma management of elderly patients.) See figure 26.1.
C. Step 1—Intermittent: symptoms less than or equal to 2 days/week, less than or equal to 2 nighttime awakenings/month, less than or equal to 2 days/week use of SABA for symptom relief, no interference with normal activity, normal FEV_1 between exacerbations, FEV_1 greater than 80% predicted, and normal FEV_1/FVC
  1. Management
      a. SABA PRN. Examples include
          i. Albuterol HFA inhaler; 2 inhalations every 4 hr PRN
          ii. Albuterol 2.5 mg via nebulizer every 4 hr PRN
          iii. Levalbuterol inhaler; 2 inhalations every 4–6 hr PRN
          iv. Levalbuterol 0.63–1.25 mg every 4–6 hr PRN
          v. Pirbuterol inhaler; 2 inhalations every 4–6 hr PRN
      b. Patient education (including about proper use of inhaler or nebulizer), environment control, and management of comorbidities
      c. Reevaluate level of asthma control and adjust therapy in 2–6 weeks
D. Step 2—Mild persistent: symptoms greater than 2 days/week but not daily, 3–4 nighttime awakenings/month, greater than 2 days/week but not daily and not more than one time per day use of an SABA for symptom relief, minor limitation with normal activity, FEV_1 greater than 80% predicted, and normal FEV_1/FVC
  1. Management
      i. Preferred: low-dose inhaled corticosteroid (ICS). Examples include:
          (a) Budnesonide (Pulmicort Flexhaler), 180–360 mcg BID
          (b) Ciclesonide (Avlesco), 80 mcg BID
          (c) Fluticasone (Flovent HFA), 88 mcg BID
          (d) Mometasone (Asmanex), 220 mcg daily or BID
      ii. Alternative: leukotriene modifier (less effective than inhaled corticosteroids)
          (a) Leukotriene modifiers. Examples include:
              1. Montelukast (Singulair), 10 mg orally daily
              2. Zafirlukast (Accolate), 20 mg orally BID
      a. Consider subcutaneous allergen immunotherapy for patients with possible allergic asthma (based upon history)
      b. Assess for medication and treatment adherence
      c. Patient education (including about proper use of inhalers), environment control, and management of comorbidities
      d. Reevaluate level of asthma control and adjust therapy in 2–6 weeks
E. Step 3—Moderate persistent: daily symptoms, more than 1 time/week that the patient experiences nighttime awakening but not nightly awakening; daily use of an SABA for symptom relief, some limitation with normal activity, FEV_1 greater than 60% but less than 80% predicted, FEV_1/FVC reduced 5%
  1. Management
      i. Preferred: low-dose ICS plus LABA or medium-dose ICS (prolonged receptor binding requires patient education about proper use and frequency to avoid induction of cardiac arrhythmias)
          (a) Advair (100 mcg), one inhalation BID
          (b) Symbicort (80 mcg), two inhalations BID
          (c) Dulera, 2 inhalations BID
      ii. Consider a short course of oral systemic corticosteroids
      iii. Consider consulting asthma specialist
      a. Consider subcutaneous allergen immunotherapy for patients with allergic asthma
      b. Assess for medication and treatment adherence

c. Patient education (including for all inhalers used), environment control, and management of comorbidities
            d. Reevaluate level of asthma control and adjust therapy in 2–6 weeks
      F. Steps 4, 5, and 6—severe persistent: symptoms throughout the day, often to seven nighttime awakenings per week, several times per day use of an SABA for symptom relief, extremely limited normal activity, FEV_1 less than 60% predicted, FEV_1/FVC reduced by more than 5%. Assessment for hypoxemia should be done for steps 4, 5, and 6
         1. Management
            a. Step 4
               i. Preferred: medium-dose ICS plus LABA
                  (a) Advair 250 mcg, 1 inhalation BID
                  (b) Symbicort 160 mcg, 2 inhalations BID
               ii. Consider a short course of oral systemic corticosteroids
               iii. Assess for medication and treatment adherence
               iv. Consider asthma specialist (allergist; pulmonologist) consultation
               v. Consider subcutaneous allergen immunotherapy for patients with allergic asthma
               vi. Patient education, environment control, and management of comorbidities
               vii. Reevaluate level of asthma control and adjust therapy in 2–6 weeks or sooner
            b. Step 5:
               i. Preferred: high-dose ICS plus LABA (Advair 500)
               ii. Consider omalizumab (Xolair)
               iii. Strongly consider a short course of oral, systemic corticosteroids
               iv. Assess for medication and treatment adherence
               v. Consult an asthma specialist
               vi. Patient education (including for all inhalers), environment control, and management of comorbidities
               vii. Reevaluate the patient's level of asthma control and adjust therapy in 2–6 weeks or sooner
            c. Step 6:
               i. Preferred: high-dose ICS plus LABA (Advair 500) plus higher dose oral corticosteroid
               ii. Consideration for omalizumab (Xolair) for patients who have allergies and frequent exacerbations
               iii. Consideration for hospitalization should be made
               iv. Assess for medication and treatment adherence
               v. Consult an asthma specialist
      G. Step down therapy if possible and if asthma has been well controlled for at least 3 months
      H. Special considerations in the pharmacological management of asthma in the elderly (See special considerations in pharmacological management in the elderly in Pharmacological Management section of COPD, above)
         1. If the older patient has not been evaluated for reversible airway obstruction, consideration of three weeks of oral corticosteroids (20 mg. prednisone daily) and repeat spirometry to assess for reversible component.
         2. Periodic review of proper use of metered dose inhalers is strongly recommended

COPD AND ASTHMA DUAL DIAGNOSIS

I. Special consideration for the elderly patient
   A. Over 40% of COPD patients self-report a history of asthma, and the prevalence of the dual diagnosis increases with age.
      1. The dual diagnosis patients tend to progress more rapidly than either diagnosis alone.

CHAPTER 26   Obstructive (Ventilatory) Lung Diseases

   2. Dual diagnosis patients have increased comorbid diagnoses and rates of healthcare utilization.
  B. Current understanding of those at most risk for dual diagnosis of COPD and asthma
   1. Occurrence earlier in life
   2. African-Americans
   3. Female gender
   4. Less inhaled tobacco use that those with just COPD
   5. Higher rates of exacerbation
II. **Need greater attention to preventing exacerbations (see COPD and Asthma sections on management)**

BRONCHIECTASIS

I. **Definition**
  A. Clinical disorder characterized by periodic cough with production of copious sputum
  B. Copious sputum means one or more cups per day and occasionally bloody
  C. Often postinflammatory
   1. After severe pneumonia or obstruction of a bronchus by a foreign body
   2. After healing of tuberculosis
II. **Physical exam findings**
  A. Inspiratory rhonchi during acute exacerbations
  B. Noisy expiration
III. **Diagnostics**
  A. Chest x-ray may show fibrotic changes
  B. Chest CT scan will usually document dilatation of airways and thickening of bronchial walls.
IV. **Management**
  A. See Pharmacological Management section of COPD (above)
  B. Strong role for percussive therapy and postural drainage (airway clearance and pulmonary toilet)
   1. Flutter valve
   2. Percussive nebulizers
   3. Percussive garment (VEST)
   4. Positive expiratory pressure devices
  C. Generous use of mucolytics
  D. Emphasis is placed on use of antibiotics (even prophylactically)

OBSTRUCTIVE AIRWAY LESIONS

I. **Endobronchial lesions (e.g., tumors and foreign bodies)—seen on chest x-ray or suspected because of atelectasis**
  A. Subjective findings
   1. Cough
   2. Dyspnea
   3. Hemoptysis
   4. Weight loss
   5. May include findings outside the chest in other regions of the body when metastatic from another organ
  B. Diagnostics
   1. Computed tomographic scan showing a solid mass or irregularly shaped cavity within one lung
   2. Chest x-ray demonstrating a mass
   3. Fiberoptic bronchoscopy with biopsy
   4. Positron emission tomography scan to assist in identifying areas of metastasis

C. Treatment: based on discovered pathology; may include the following:
1. Surgical removal
2. Chemotherapy
3. Radiation therapy
4. Combination of the preceding

BIBLIOGRAPHY

GlaxoSmithKline. (2012). *COPD Assessment Test (CAT) Health Professional User Guide.* Retrieved June 1, 2014, from http://www.catestonline.org/images/UserGuides/ CATHCPUser%20guideEn.pdf

GlaxoSmithKline. (2012). *COPD Assessment Test (CAT)*. Retrieved June 1, 2014, from http://www.catestonline.org/images/pdfs/CATest.pdf

Global Institute for Chronic Obstructive Lung Disease (GOLD). (2014). *Global strategies for the diagnosis, management, and prevention of COPD, updated May, 2014*. Retrieved June 1, 2014, from http://www.goldcopd.org/Guidelines/guidelines-resources.html

Hanania, N. A., Sharma, G., & Sharafkhaneh, A. (2010). COPD in the elderly patient. *Seminars in Respiratory and Critical Care Medicine, 31*(5), 596–606.

Hardin, M., Silverman, E. K., Barr, R. G., Hansel, N. N., Schroeder, J. D., Make, B. J., . . . D., & Hersh, C. P. (2011). The clinical features of the overlap between COPD and asthma. *Respiratory Research, 12*, 127. doi:10.1186/1465-9921-12-127

U.S. Department of Health and Human Services. National Institutes of Health: National Heart, Lung, and Blood Institute. (2007). *Expert panel report 3: Guidelines for the diagnosis and management of asthma*. Retrieved from http://www.nhlbi.nih.gov/files/docs/guidelines/asthgdln.pdf

Wechsler, M. E. (2009). Managing asthma in primary care: Putting new guideline recommendations into context. *Mayo Clinic Proceedings, 84*(8), 707–717.

CHAPTER 26 Obstructive (Ventilatory) Lung Diseases

Step UP if needed (first check inhaler technique, adherence, environmental control, and comorbid conditions)

ASSESS CONTROL

Step DOWN if possible (and asthma is well controlled for at least 3 months)

	Step 1	Step 2	Step 3	Step 4	Step 5	Step 6
	Intermittent Asthma	Persistent Asthma: Daily Medication				
			Consult with asthma specialist if step 4 care or higher is required. Consider consultation at step 3.			
Preferred	SABA as needed	Low-dose ICS	Low-dose ICS + LABA *or* Medium-dose ICS	Medium-dose ICS + LABA	High-dose ICS + LABA	High-dose ICS + LABA + Oral Corticosteroid
Alternative		Cromolyn, LTRA, nedrocromil, or theophylline	Low-dose ICS + LTRA, theophylline, or zileuton	Medium-dose ICS + LTRA, theophylline, or zileuton	Consider omalizumab for patients who have allergic asthma	Consider omalizumab for patients who have allergic asthma
	Patient education and environmental control, and management of comorbidities at each step.					
	Step 2–4: Consider subcutaneous allergen immunotherapy for patients who have allergic asthma					
Rescue Medication	• SABA as needed for symptoms—up to 3 treatments at 20-minute intervals initially. Treatment intensity depends on symptom severity. • Short course of corticosteroids may be needed. • Use of SABA > 2 days a week for symptom relief (not prevention of EIB) generally indicates inadequate control and the need to step treatment.					

Figure 26.1. Stepwise approach for managing asthma in those ≥ 12 years of age. SABA = short-acting beta$_2$-agonist; ICS = inhaled corticosteroids; LTRA = leukotreine recepter antagonist; LABA = long-acting inhaled beta$_2$-agonist. Adapted from "Expert Panel Report 3: Guidelines for the Diagnosis and Management of Asthma" by the National Institutes of Health, National Heart, Lung, and Blood Institute, 2007.

Table 26.1 Classifying asthma severity and initiating treatment in youths ≥ 12 and adults

Components of Severity		Classification of Asthma Severity ≥ 12 years of age			
		Intermittent	Persistent		
			Mild	Moderate	Severe
Impairment Normal FEV$_1$/FVC: 8-19 yr 85% 20-39 yr 80% 40-59 yr 75% 60-80 yr 70%	Symptoms	≤ 2 days/week	> 2 days/week but not daily	Daily	Throughout the day
	Nighttime awakenings	≤ 2x/month	3-4x/month	1x/week but not nightly	Often 7x/week
	Short-acting beta$_2$ agonist use for symptom control (not prevention of EIB)	≤ 2 days/week	> 2 days/week but not daily, and not more than 1x on any day	Daily	Several times per day
	Interference with normal activity	None	Minor limitation	Some limitation	Extremely limited
	Lung function	-Normal FEV$_1$ between exacerbations -FEV$_1$ > 80% predicted -FEV$_1$/FVC normal	-FEV$_1$ > 80% predicted -FEV$_1$/FVC normal	-FEV$_1$ > 60% but < 80% predicted -FEV$_1$/FVC reduced 5%	-FEV$_1$ < 60% predicted -FEV$_1$/FVC reduced > 5%
Risk	Exacerbations requiring oral systemic corticosteroids	0-1/year (see notes)	≥ 2/year (see notes)		
		Consider severity and interval since last exacerbation. Frequency and severity may fluctuate over time for patients in any severity category. Relative annual risk of exacerbations may be related to FEV1.			
Recommended Step for Initiating Treatment See figure 26.1 for treatment steps		Step 1	Step 2	Step 3	Step 4
				And consider short course of oral systemic corticosteroids	
		In 2-6 weeks, evaluate level of asthma control that is achieved and adjust therapy accordingly.			

Notes: FEV$_1$ forced expiratory volume in 1 second; FVC: forced vital capacity

From the National Heart, Lung, and Blood Institute, Department of Health and Human Services, National Institutes of Health: Guidelines for the diagnosis and management of asthma (EPR-3), Section 4, Managing asthma long term: youth ≥ 12 years and adults, 2007: http://www.nhlbi.nih.gov/guidelines/asthma/09_sec4_lt_12.pdf, Tables 4.5, 4.6, 4.7. Accessed December 3, 2014.

Table 26.2	Assessing asthma control in those ≥ 12 years of age			
Components of Control		Well Controlled	Not Well Controlled	Very Poorly Controlled
Impairment	Symptoms	≤ 2 days/week	> 2 days/week	Throughout the day
	Nighttime awakenings	≤ 2x/month	1–3x/week	≥ 4x/week
	Interference with normal activity	None	Some limitation	Extremely limited
	SABA use for symptom control (not prevention of EIB)	≤ 2 days/week	> 2 days/week	Several times per day
	FEV_1 or peak flow	> 80% predicted/personal best	60%–80% predicted/personal best	< 60% predicted/personal best
	Validated questionnaires			
	ATAQ	0	1–2	3–4
	ACQ	≤ 0.75[a]	≥ 1.5	n/a
	ACT	≥ 20	16–19	≤ 15

Note. SABA = short-acting beta$_2$ agonist; EIB = exercised-induced bronchospasm; FEV_1 = forced expiratory volume in 1 second; ATAQ = asthma therapy assessment questionnaire; ACQ = asthma control questionnaire; ACT = asthma control test. Adapted from "Expert Panel Report 3: Guidelines for the Diagnosis and Management of Asthma" by the National Institutes of Health, National Heart, Lung, and Blood Institute, 2007.

[a]ACQ values of 0.76–1.4 are indeterminate regarding well-controlled asthma.

[b]The level of control is based on the most severe impairment or risk category. Assess impairment domain by patient's recall of previous 2–4 weeks and by spirometry/or peak flow measures. Symptom assessment for longer periods should reflect a global assessment, such as inquiring whether the patient's asthma is better or worse since the last visit. At present, there are inadequate data to correspond frequencies of exacerbations with different levels of asthma control. In general, more frequent and intense exacerbations (e.g., requiring urgent, unscheduled care, hospitalization, or ICU admission) indicate poorer disease control. For treatment purposes, patients who had ≥ 2 exacerbations requiring oral systemic corticosteroids in the past year may be considered the same as patients who have not-well-controlled asthma, even in the absence of impairment levels consistent with not-well-controlled asthma

Table 26.2 Assessing asthma control in those ≥ 12 years of age

Components of Control		Well Controlled	Not Well Controlled	Very Poorly Controlled
Risk	Exacerbations requiring oral corticosteroids	0–1/year	≥ 2/year[b]	
	Progressive loss of lung function	Consider severity and interval since last exacerbation. Evaluation requires long-term followup care		
	Treatment-related adverse effects	Medication side effects can vary in intensity from none to very troublesome and worrisome. The level of intensity does not correlate to specific levels of control but should be considered in the overall assessment of risk.		
Recommended Action for Treatment (see figure 26.1 for treatment steps)		Maintain current steps Regular followups every 1–6 months to maintain control. Consider step down if well controlled for at least 3 months	Step up 1 step and Reevaluate in 2–6 weeks. For side effects consider alternative treatment options	Consider short course of oral systemic corticosteroids Step up 1–2 steps, and Reevaluate in 2 weeks. For side effects, consider alternative treatment options

CHAPTER 27

Restrictive (Inflammatory) Lung Diseases

THOMAS W. BARKLEY, JR. • TOBIAS P. REBMANN • DAVID A. MILLER

PNEUMONIA

I. **Definition of pneumonia**
   A. Acute febrile inflammatory disorder of the lung(s), associated with cough and exertional dyspnea
   B. Infiltrate is present on chest x-ray; the appearance of the infiltrate may lag behind the appearance of symptoms by 24–48 hr, justifying a repeat chest x-ray at that time
   C. Leukocytosis may be present

II. **Incidence/etiology**
   A. Pneumonia is one of the most common of all serious lung conditions and a frequent cause of acute care hospitalization and mortality.
   B. Elderly are especially at risk due to poor immune systems, debilitation, and weakness preventing adequate airway clearance
   C. Organisms that are potential causes of community-acquired pneumonia:
      1. Bacteria
         a. *Streptococcus pneumoniae* (most common bacterial cause in adults)
         b. *Haemophilus influenza*
         c. *Klebsiella pneumoniae*
         d. Gram-negative organisms
      2. "Atypical" pathogens
         a. *Chlamydia pneumoniae*
         b. *Mycoplasma pneumoniae*
         c. *Mycobacterium tuberculosis*
      3. Viruses
         a. Respiratory syncytial virus
         b. Adenovirus
         c. Rhinovirus
   D. Overzealous treatment of mild respiratory infection in the past has contributed to the development of antimicrobial drug resistance, especially to *S. pneumoniae*
   E. Comorbidity from the following conditions contributes to high mortality from pneumonia:
      1. Chronic obstructive pulmonary disease (COPD)

2. Heart failure
3. Diabetes mellitus
4. Chronic liver and renal disease
F. The very young and the very old are at increased risk of death from pneumonia, despite the remarkable array of antimicrobial agents available to treat this disorder.

III. **Classification of pneumonia**
  A. "Typical" pneumonias manifest with "classic" findings
     1. Fever
     2. Chills
     3. Leukocytosis
     4. Cough
     5. Sputum production
     6. Increased fremitus
  B. "Atypical" pneumonias vary in their presentation
     1. Fever may be high
     2. Leukocytosis
        a. May be absent
        b. May be associated with a "left shift" in the differential white blood cell count (WBC) to include a high number of "band" forms
     3. Cough is often dry
     4. Headache
     5. Sore throat
     6. Excessive sweating
     7. Soreness in the chest
  C. Both forms demonstrate an infiltrate on chest x-ray
     1. Atypical pneumonias are more often diffuse
     2. Atypical pneumonias may particularly involve more than one lung segment or both lungs
  D. Occurrence information may assist in defining the type of pneumonia present
     1. Time of year
     2. Known epidemic disease
     3. Presence of comorbid conditions
  E. Community-acquired pneumonias (CAPs) are those acquired within the community setting
  F. Nosocomial pneumonias result from exposure to infection during a stay in a health care facility
     1. Hospital-acquired pneumonia (HAP)
        a. Pneumonia that occurs 48 hr or more after admission, which was not incubating at the time of admission (includes VAP and HCAP). *Staphylococcus aureus*, *Streptococcus pneumoniae*, and *Haemophilus influenzae* are the most common causative organisms.
     2. Ventilator-acquired pneumonia (VAP)
        a. Pneumonia that arises more than 48–72 hr after endotracheal intubation
        b. *Pseudomonas* is the most common causative organism
     3. Healthcare-associated pneumonia (HCAP)
        a. Includes any patient who was hospitalized in an acute care hospital for two or more days within 90 days of the infection; resided in a nursing home or long-term care facility; received recent intravenous antibiotic therapy, chemotherapy, or wound care within the past 30 days of the current infection; or attended a hospital or hemodialysis clinic
        b. Organisms in HCAP are more similar to those of HAP than CAP (e.g., higher rates of *Staphylococcus aureus* and *Pseudomonas aeruginosa*, and less *Streptococcus pneumoniae*, *Haemophilus influenzae*, and MRSA)

G. Pneumonias are often categorized by risk factors present that predispose the patient to pneumonia
   1. Aspiration pneumonias (related to altered mental status or dysphagia from stroke or neuromuscular disease, i.e., Parkinson's disease)
   2. Obstructive lesions of the airway
      a. Tumor
      b. Retained bronchopulmonary secretions
   3. Inhalation injury-related pneumonia
      a. Hypersensitivity pneumonia
      b. Near drowning
H. Pneumonia Index Severity Index may be helpful; grades severity based on age, sex, comorbid diseases, physical exam, and labs

IV. **Evaluation for possible pneumonia**
   A. Historical information
   B. Physical examination
      1. Tachypnea
      2. Tachycardia
      3. Fever
      4. Discomfort
      5. Rales (or "crackles") on auscultation over the affected area(s)
      6. Mental status changes and confusion
   C. Chest x-ray, in a search for new pulmonary infiltrates
   D. Laboratory/diagnostics
      1. Complete blood count (CBC), including differential WBC count
      2. Blood cultures
      3. Gram stain and culture of sputum
      4. Arterial blood gases (ABGs) and/or pulse oximetry
      5. Procalcitonin levels, when available, may aid in diagnosis of bacterial pneumonia and guide duration of antimicrobial therapy

V. **Treatment**
   A. Antimicrobial therapy with cultures pending (for specific treatment guidelines, see Lower Respiratory Tract Pathogens chapter)
   B. Antimicrobial therapy should be revised as culture information becomes available and as improvement occurs. In general, the narrowest spectrum antimicrobial to which known organisms are expected to respond should be used.
   C. Need to cover anaerobic organisms in cases of known or suspected aspiration
   D. Simultaneous treatment of coexisting illnesses is needed
      1. COPD
      2. Heart failure
      3. Diabetes
      4. Dehydration
   E. Not all patients, especially young adults, need hospitalization for pneumonia
      1. The decision to hospitalize a patient with pneumonia should be guided by the following:
         a. The possibility of rapidly progressive disease
         b. The overall status of the patient (coexisting problems)
         c. The patient's ability to reliably self-administer medication for this illness
      2. If in doubt, it is reasonable to observe the patient in hospital during initial therapy and to reassess early response to treatment

VI. **Prevention of pneumonia**
   A. Vaccination against influenza: Influenza virus vaccine
      1. Repeated annually
      2. Some revaccinate within a season if the patient:

    i. Is immunocompromised
    ii. Has severe underlying COPD or heart disease
  B. Vaccination against *S. pneumoniae*: pneumococcal vaccine polyvalent (Pneumovax)
    1. PCV13: pneumococcal conjugate vaccine for infants, children, and adults older than 19 years at high risk for disease
    2. PPSV23: pneumococcal polysaccharide vaccine for adults older than 65 years and those older than 2 years at high risk for disease
    3. If giving both vaccines, start with PCV 13 and give PPSV23 at least 8 weeks later
    4. Guidelines change frequently; refer to the Centers for Disease Control and Prevention for the latest recommendations

TUBERCULOSIS (TB)

I. **Etiology:** *Mycobacterium tuberculosis*
II. **Incidence**
  A. The rates of new infection by *M. tuberculosis* are increasing, especially among the homeless and among those living in crowded conditions, such as nursing homes and prisons in larger metropolitan areas.
  B. Alarmingly, the incidence of multidrug-resistant TB (defined as resistant to isoniazid and rifampin) also appears to be rising, especially along the East and West Coasts of the United States.
  C. This rise has coincided with increased numbers of patients with HIV and AIDS
III. **Clinical findings**
  A. Symptoms
    1. Most patients are asymptomatic
    2. Fever
    3. Cough, generally productive of purulent sputum that may contain blood
    4. Weight loss
    5. Night sweats that may require changing of bed linen
  B. Physical exam findings
    1. Body temperature elevation
    2. Cachexia may be noted.
    3. Rales over the affected areas: apical posttussive rales for apical disease
  C. Laboratory/diagnostics
    1. Normal CBC
    2. Low serum cortisol level if disseminated disease to the adrenal glands has destroyed the adrenal cortices
    3. Sputum
      a. Acid-fast smears are often positive, but therapy may have to be started empirically if other findings are suggestive of TB in the absence of positive smears
      b. Cultures for *M. tuberculosis* are usually positive within 6 weeks
    4. TB skin testing (intradermal purified protein derivative [PPD])
      a. Indicates only exposure, not necessarily active infection
      b. PPD (0.1 ml) injected intradermally; read 48 hr later
      c. Interpretation based on measurement of the largest diameter of the indurated area (not including flat but erythematous area):
        i. Less than 5 mm: negative test
        ii. 5 mm or more: positive test in an HIV-infected patient, recent TB exposure, immunocompromised, or patient with chest film typical for TB
        iii. 10 mm or more: positive test in health care workers, HIV-negative injection drug users, residents of nursing homes/homeless shelters, recent immigrants, etc.
        iv. 15 mm or more: positive test in any person

CHAPTER 27   Restrictive (Inflammatory) Lung Diseases

5. QuantiFERON TB Gold test
   a. Serum test used for diagnosis of TB, either latent or active, instead of PPD
   b. Not affected by prior exposure to bacille Calmette-Guérin (BCG) vaccination
D. Chest x-ray
   1. Infiltrate
      a. Especially present in the upper lobes of the lungs or in the superior segments of the lower lobes
      b. Can be present in any portion of the lungs
   2. Cavity within the lungs

IV. **Treatment**
   A. Patient isolation during initial evaluation and treatment, according to the Occupational Safety and Health Administration standards, is mandatory
   B. Suspected disease, or smear-positive disease, pending the return of sputum cultures
      1. Four-drug therapy
         a. Isoniazid, 300 mg PO daily (or 5 mg/kg; maximum, 300 mg daily), with pyridoxine, 50 mg PO, to prevent INH-induced peripheral neuropathy
         b. Rifampin (Rifadin/Rimactane) 600 mg PO each day (or 10 mg/kg daily; maximum, 600 mg/dose)
         c. Ethambutol (Myambutol), 15–25 mg/kg PO each day (maximum, 2.5 grams/dose), preceded by screening of color vision
            i. Note: Ethambutol (Myambutol) may cause red/green color blindness as an adverse effect, as well as changes in visual acuity.
         d. Pyrazinamide, 15–30 mg/kg in three divided doses daily (maximum, 2 grams/dose)
      2. Modification of regimen may be necessary if drug susceptibility studies demonstrate resistance to first-line drugs
         a. If isolate proves to be fully susceptible to INH and RIF, then ethambutol may be dropped
      3. Therapy is continued usually for 6–9 months (6 months for most patients, 9 months for HIV-positive and/or immunocompromised patients)
      4. Intermittent directly observed therapy may follow one of three regimens:
         a. INH + rifampin + pyrazinamide + ethambutol daily for 2 months, followed by INH + rifampin 2–3 times weekly for an additional 4 months, especially if susceptibility to INH/rifampin is noted
         b. INH + rifampin + pyrazinamide + ethambutol daily for 2 weeks, followed by the same agents 2 times weekly for 6 weeks, then INH + rifampin 2 times weekly for 4 months, if susceptibility to INH/rifampin is noted
         c. Thrice-weekly dosing of INH + rifampin + pyrazinamide + ethambutol for 24 doses (8 weeks); followed by thrice-weekly dosing of INH + rifampin for 54 doses (18 weeks)
         d. Patients with advanced HIV (CD4 counts less than 100/µl) should be treated with daily or three-times-weekly therapy in both the initial and the continuation phases.
      5. For nonadherent patients, directly observed treatment may be initiated at 3 times per week, usually after 2 weeks of observed therapy, often in hospital
   C. Prophylaxis
      1. Consider for the following patients:
         a. Asymptomatic, with a positive PPD and a normal chest x-ray
         b. Exposed to active TB who have a negative PPD
         c. Undergoing immunosuppressive therapy for other reasons
         d. HIV infected
      2. Treatment

a. INH, 300 mg PO daily, although controversy exists as to whether 6 months or up to 1 year of therapy should be given; the standard regimen consists of a duration of 9 months, which is also the preferred duration for HIV-positive patients
b. Pyridoxine, 50 mg PO daily, may be also chosen during INH therapy to prevent neuropathy

ACUTE RESPIRATORY DISTRESS SYNDROME (ARDS)/ACUTE LUNG INJURY (ALI)

I. **Etiologies: any of the numerous causes of acute systemic inflammation**
   A. Bacteremia or other severe systemic infections
   B. Massive trauma or injury, including burns and smoke inhalation
   C. Pancreatitis
   D. Shock (any cause)
   E. Cardiopulmonary bypass
   F. Increased intracranial pressure, especially after trauma or intracranial bleeding
   G. Aspiration of fluid, including gastrointestinal contents and near drowning

II. **Incidence**
   A. Annual incidence is unknown, largely owing to lack of required reporting and misunderstanding about when and how the diagnosis is made
   B. Overall incidence in any locale will be proportionate to the incidence of known causes of the syndrome itself

III. **Clinical findings**
   A. Severe respiratory distress occurring during the course of one of the inciting events
   B. Respiratory distress often requires the early institution of mechanical ventilatory assistance; refractory hypoxemia is a classic finding
   C. Symptoms:
      1. Breathlessness
      2. Agitation
      3. Confusion
      4. Obtundation as oxygen delivery and uptake by tissues falls
   D. Other manifestations include failure of other organ systems
      1. Kidneys
      2. Liver
      3. Bone marrow (reduced platelet count)
      4. Multisystem organ failure
   E. Physical findings depend on the presentation of the condition, placing the patient at risk for ARDS. Lungs often sound clearer than the chest x-ray would suggest.
   F. Laboratory/diagnostics
      1. Arterial blood gas (ABG): PaO_2/FiO_2 ratio. If less than 300, then acute lung injury; if less than 200, then acute respiratory distress syndrome (ARDS)
      2. Complete blood count with differential white count and platelet count
      3. Coagulation studies
         a. Prothrombin time
         b. Partial thromboplastin time
         c. Fibrinogen level
         d. Fibrin degradation products
      4. Renal and liver function
      5. Urinalysis
      6. Blood and urine cultures
      7. Sputum culture and Gram stain
   G. X-rays
      1. Chest x-ray—often shows evolving bilateral infiltrates (e.g., "whited out")

CHAPTER 27　　Restrictive (Inflammatory) Lung Diseases

2. Other x-rays—as indicated by the patient's presenting problems (e.g., trauma)

IV. **Treatment**
   A. Airway
      1. Assess the adequacy of ventilation and the degree of work used during spontaneous ventilation
      2. Intubate if ventilation is significantly compromised, especially if altered mentation is noted
   B. Breathing: institute mechanical ventilation
      1. If work of breathing is not being met, as evidenced by the following:
         a. Patient fatigue
         b. Elevated $PaCO_2$ (partial pressure of carbon dioxide in arterial blood)
      2. If measured, hypoxemia is not correctable with an FIO_2 (fraction of inspired oxygen) of 0.5
   C. Circulation: vigorous fluid resuscitation should be started if hypotension is present
      1. Regulated by hemodynamic parameters, especially left ventricular ejection fraction
   D. Correct the underlying etiology of the ARDS
   E. Support needed
      1. Mechanical ventilatory assistance often requires the institution of positive end-expiratory pressure
      2. Ventilatory pressures over 45 cm H_2O may require the use of:
         a. Reduced tidal volumes
         b. Pressure-cycled ventilation
         c. High-frequency oscillatory ventilation
         d. Permissive hypercapnia, with bicarbonate repletion to avoid excessive acidosis
      3. The patient should be sedated for comfort
      4. Nutritional support should be started early
         a. Use enteral route (total parenteral nutrition may be used with caution when enteral route is unavailable)
         b. Most patients require nearly twice their usual daily caloric requirements to counteract the tremendous energy expenditure used in combating ARDS

V. **Despite refinements in the provision of care for patients with ARDS, overall mortality remains at nearly 40%**

VI. **Special considerations**
   A. The risk of pulmonary barotrauma, including pneumothorax or pneumomediastinum, is high with this disorder.
   B. Sudden increases in ventilating pressure with desaturation in arterial oxygen tension indicate the need for an immediate repeat chest x-ray and for possible chest tube insertion
   C. Repeated physical and radiographic assessments of the lungs may be needed to rule out barotrauma in the mechanically ventilated patient with ARDS

IDIOPATHIC PULMONARY FIBROSIS (IPF)

I. **Etiology/general concepts**
   A. Etiology is unknown; strongly linked to cigarette smoking
   B. Prior to treatment, rule out the following:
      1. Inhalation exposure
      2. Autoimmune disorders
      3. Chronic lung infection
         a. Tuberculosis
         b. Deep fungal infection
            i. Histoplasmosis
            ii. Coccidioidomycosis

C. In patients with prior malignancy, the lymphangitic spread of tumor to the lungs should be excluded.

II. Incidence
A. Unknown; IPF is the most common cause of interstitial lung disease among elderly patients
B. More common in men than in women

III. Clinical findings
A. Symptoms
1. Progressive (slow or rapid) dyspnea
2. Cough (nonproductive)
3. Specific questioning of the patient about prior exposure to the following:
    a. Inorganic dusts
        i. Silica
        ii. Asbestos
    b. Organic dusts (e.g., in silos, where hypersensitivity pneumonia may be acquired)
    c. Fumes
        i. Chlorine
        ii. Sulfur dioxide
    d. Drugs
        i. Chemotherapeutic agents (e.g., bleomycin)
        ii. Antibiotics (e.g., nitrofurantoin and sulfa)
        iii. Gold salts (during the course of therapy for rheumatoid arthritis)
        iv. Amiodarone (for cardiac arrhythmias)
    e. Radiation to lung parenchyma
    f. Risk factors for *Pneumocystis carinii* pneumonia
        i. Immunosuppression from HIV infection
        ii. Chemotherapy for lymphoma or lymphocytic leukemia and other malignancies
        iii. Immunosuppression for organ transplantation
    g. Known chronic heart failure
B. Physical exam findings
1. Rales ("Velcro crackles") may be heard on auscultation
C. Laboratory/diagnostics
1. Changes within the lung parenchyma, especially in the lower lobes, demonstrated by chest x-ray and high-resolution CT scanning
    a. Interstitial infiltrates
    b. Nodules
    c. Cystic (or "honeycombing") changes
2. Pulmonary function testing typically demonstrates a restrictive ventilatory defect.
    a. Some patients may show a coexisting bronchoconstriction in small airways
    b. The diffusing capacity of lung for carbon monoxide is commonly reduced—a manifestation of altered ventilation and perfusion relationships within the lungs.
3. ABG analysis and pulse oximetry
    a. May demonstrate hypoxemia, typically as the disease progresses
    b. Carbon dioxide retention indicates severe disease
4. Laboratory findings generally are not helpful
    a. PPD testing should be done
    b. Prior exposure to deep fungi, including *Histoplasma capsulatum* (chicken coops in the Midwest) and *Coccidioides immitis* (dust in the Southwest desert and Central Valleys of California), may be assessed with complement fixation serologic studies for deep fungi, although prior exposure does not necessarily equate with active disease
        i. Histoplasmosis
        ii. Coccidioidomycosis

CHAPTER 27 Restrictive (Inflammatory) Lung Diseases

        iii. Blastomycosis
- 5. Obtaining tissue for diagnosis
    - a. Fiber-optic bronchoscopy with transbronchial biopsy of the lung parenchyma is safe and should be done first
    - b. Bronchoalveolar lavage to assess for inflammation and to obtain secretions for culture (e.g., acid-fast bacilli, fungi, and *Nocardia*) may be performed at the same time
    - c. Because biopsies obtained at bronchoscopy may be inadequate for diagnosis and are subject to sampling error, patients deemed healthy enough to undergo open lung biopsy should be considered for thoracoscopic lung biopsy. If further assurance is required, then the diagnosis of IPF is correct.
        - i. Obtain preoperative pulmonary function tests
- D. Vaccination: influenza and pneumococcal polysaccharide vaccine should be offered to patients with IPF, as these infections are poorly tolerated in patients with interstitial lung disease
- E. Therapy
    - 1. Corticosteroids (prednisone 1 mg/kg/day for 12 weeks)
        - a. Used for acute exacerbation, although scientific evidence/support for benefit is lacking
        - b. Many patients report subjective improvement
        - c. Far fewer demonstrate objective improvement radiographically or on pulmonary function testing
        - d. Use caution with elderly because of its significant side effects (bone demineralization, immunosuppression, and hyperglycemia)
    - 2. Alternative treatments that may be considered in selected patients include cyclophosphamide (Cytoxan), 1 mg/kg/day, or azathioprine (Imuran), 3 mg/kg/day, although data to support immunosuppressive therapy in this setting is limited.
    - 3. Noninvasive use of positive airway pressure (by mask) may be beneficial in selected patients
- F. Prognosis: IPF is usually a progressive illness, and the prognosis is often poor over time
- G. Patients with rapidly progressive or end-stage disease should be counseled on palliative care and end-of-life issues.

SARCOIDOSIS

I. Definition
- A. Characterized pathologically by the presence of non caseating granulomas and interstitial lung disease
- B. Systemic manifestations:
    - 1. Lymphadenopathy
    - 2. Cardiac involvement
    - 3. Iritis
    - 4. Cutaneous lesions
    - 5. Arthritis
    - 6. Gastrointestinal involvement
    - 7. Other organs may be involved

II. Incidence
- A. Unknown
- B. More common among females, North Americans, African Americans, and northern European Caucasians
- C. May be seen in all races
- D. Typically, the onset of symptoms is between the ages of 20 and 40 years

III. **Clinical findings**
   A. Symptoms
      1. Progressive dyspnea (slow or rapid)
      2. Nonproductive cough
   B. Physical exam findings
      1. Depends on specific organ involvement
      2. Lung examination may be normal.
      3. Rales ("Velcro crackles") may be heard on auscultation when interstitial disease (for example, fibrosis) is present
   C. Laboratory/diagnostics
      1. Chest x-ray may demonstrate the following: (The stages shown are useful in staging pulmonary involvement by sarcoidosis.)
         a. Stage 0: normal chest x-ray
         b. Stage I: bilateral hilar lymphadenopathy (BHL)
         c. Stage II: BHL plus pulmonary infiltrates
         d. Stage III: pulmonary infiltrates without BHL
         e. Stage IV: pulmonary fibrosis
      2. Pulmonary function testing typically demonstrates a restrictive ventilatory defect
         a. Some patients may show a coexisting bronchoconstriction in small airways
         b. The diffusing capacity of lung for carbon monoxide is commonly reduced—a manifestation of altered ventilation and perfusion relationships within the lungs
      3. ABG analysis and pulse oximetry
         a. May demonstrate hypoxemia, typically as the disease progresses
         b. Carbon dioxide retention indicates severe disease
      4. Laboratory findings generally are not helpful
         a. PPD testing should be done
         b. Prior exposure to deep fungi may be assessed with complement fixation serologic studies for deep fungi, although prior exposure does not necessarily equate active disease.
            i. Histoplasmosis
            ii. Coccidioidomycosis
            iii. Blastomycosis
      5. Obtaining tissue for diagnosis of pulmonary sarcoidosis
         a. Fiberoptic bronchoscopy with transbronchial biopsy of the lung parenchyma is safe and should be done first.
         b. Bronchoalveolar lavage to assess for inflammation and to obtain secretions for culture (e.g., acid-fast bacilli, fungi, and *Nocardia*) may be performed at the same time.
         c. Because biopsies obtained at bronchoscopy may be inadequate for diagnosis and are subject to sampling error, patients deemed healthy enough to undergo open lung biopsy should be considered for thoracoscopic lung biopsy if further assurance is required that the diagnosis of sarcoidosis is correct
         d. If other organs are involved, biopsy of one of those sites may be beneficial in establishing the diagnosis.
         e. If BHL is present, cervical mediastinal exploration with biopsy of a node is reasonable.
      6. Blood tests
         a. CBC
         b. Calcium (sarcoidosis is associated with hypercalcemia)
         c. Liver function tests
         d. BUN
         e. Creatinine

7. ECG
8. Urinalysis
9. PPD
10. Ophthalmologic examination

D. Therapy
  1. Corticosteroids
     a. Initial dose of prednisone includes 0.3–0.6 mg/kg ideal body weight (usually 20–40 mg/day) x 6 weeks. No formal data is available to guide maintenance dosing of oral glucocorticoids.
     b. Maintenance dose of prednisone is 0.25–0.5 mg/kg (usually 10–20 mg) per day dose. Maintenance dose is continued for at least 6–8 months, with a total treatment time of about 1 year.
     c. Many patients report subjective improvement. Proper length of therapy in patients who respond to treatment is unknown.
     d. Far fewer demonstrate objective improvement radiographically or by pulmonary function testing
     e. Use is cautioned with elderly due to significant side effects (bone demineralization, immunosuppression, and hyperglycemia)
  2. Alternative treatments that may be considered in selected patients; a variety of immunosuppressive agents have been used to treat refractory pulmonary sarcoidosis include:
     a. Cyclophosphamide (Cytoxan), 25–50 mg/day (not to exceed 150 mg/day), or
     b. Azathioprine (Imuran), 2 mg/kg or 50 mg PO daily. Due to the toxicity of cyclophosphamide, it is reserved as a "third-line" drug
  3. Methotrexate, 7.5 mg PO daily (which can be increased by 2.5 mg every two weeks with a maximum dose of 10–15 mg per week) and chloroquine (250–750 mg PO daily or every other day) also have been used alternatively in sarcoidosis.

HEART FAILURE/CARDIOGENIC PULMONARY EDEMA

I. **Etiology: numerous causes are known**
  A. Coronary artery disease with myocardial ischemia and infarction, aggravated by the following:
    1. Obesity
    2. Limited exercise
    3. Dyslipidemia
    4. Cigarette smoking
  B. Cardiac arrhythmias
    1. Tachycardia (especially)
    2. Bradycardia
  C. Hypertension
  D. Valvular dysfunction of the heart
  E. Thyroid dysfunction, including the following:
    1. Hyperthyroidism
    2. Hypothyroidism
  F. Diabetes mellitus
  G. Viral myocarditis
  H. Idiopathic cardiomyopathy
  I. Renal failure
  J. Drug therapy, especially certain chemotherapeutic agents

II. **Incidence**
  A. Heart failure is a common disorder that leads to frequent outpatient visits and inpatient hospitalizations, despite the availability of modern therapeutic interventions

B. In general, heart failure can be described in the following ways:
   1. Is progressive
   2. Eventuates in frequent hospitalizations
   3. Carries a guarded prognosis over time
III. **Clinical manifestations are related to the development of restrictive ventilatory defects within the lung parenchyma that are initially mild and later severe.**
   A. Symptoms
      1. Progression from exertional dyspnea to orthopnea and paroxysmal nocturnal dyspnea
      2. Frank respiratory failure may be noted
      3. Dry cough is commonly seen
      4. The time course of this progression may be slow or abrupt
   B. Classification is based on New York Heart Association (NYHA) functional scale
      1. NYHA 1: no limitations from ordinary activities
      2. NYHA 2: slight limitations with moderate exertion
      3. NYHA 3: marked limitation with activity and comfortable only at rest
      4. NYHA 4: patients who should be on complete rest; symptoms with any activity and occasionally at rest
   C. Physical exam findings: secondary responses lead to detectable signs of fluid retention
      1. Edema and jugular venous distention
      2. Rales
      3. Tachycardia or bradycardia
      4. Inability to tolerate lying flat in the supine position (orthopnea)
      5. Tachypnea
      6. Pleural effusions
      7. Ascites (when heart failure is advanced)
   D. Diagnosis
      1. ECG
         a. Assess for ischemia or infarction
         b. Determine cardiac rhythm
      2. Chest x-ray, looking for the following:
         a. Vascular redistribution to upper lung fields
         b. Presence of the following:
            i. Interstitial edema
            ii. Kerley B lines
         c. Pleural effusions (usually bilateral or on the right)
         d. Cardiomegaly
      3. Assessment of oxygenation to ensure adequate oxygenation of blood and to assess for carbon dioxide retention
         a. ABG analysis
         b. Pulse oximetry
      4. CBC to rule out anemia
      5. Chemistries
         a. Thyroid function: thyroid-stimulating hormone
            i. If thyroid-stimulating hormone is abnormal, perform free triiodothyronine (Free T3) and free thyroxine (Free T4) to determine true disease versus euthyroid sick state, especially in acutely ill
         b. Renal function
            i. BUN
            ii. Creatinine
         c. Liver function
         d. Electrolytes (including magnesium levels)

CHAPTER 27   Restrictive (Inflammatory) Lung Diseases

6. Cardiac enzyme evaluation, especially if recent myocardial infarction or unstable angina pectoris is suspected
7. Echocardiography to assess the following:
   a. Systolic function of the heart; rate of demise is more significant than the actual ejection fraction
   b. Valvular function
   c. Dyskinesia
      i. Global
      ii. Segmental
   d. Diastology
   e. Right heart pressures and function (right ventricular systolic pressure) to determine presence of pulmonary hypertension, either acute or chronic
8. Pulmonary function studies are not useful during acute pulmonary edema, but when the patient is stable, they have the following purposes:
   a. May help to demonstrate the presence of a restrictive ventilatory defect in early heart failure (reduced vital capacity)
   b. May help to evaluate for coexisting COPD, especially among smokers
9. Occasionally, patients with heart failure will require pulmonary artery catheterization to document the severity of the problem, especially when hypotension is present.
   a. Aggressive fluid therapy could further aggravate heart failure
   b. If needed, determination can be made of the following:
      i. Cardiac output
      ii. Cardiac index
      iii. Systemic vascular resistance
      iv. Pulmonary capillary wedge pressure
10. In general, insertion of a pulmonary artery catheter is not necessary in treating patients with heart failure.

E. Treatment
   1. Correct the cause of the heart failure, if known (especially ischemia). Nitrates may be indicated clinically; however, these may or may not be appropriate, depending on the underlying cause (arrhythmia, valvular heart disease, etc.)
      a. Sublingual nitroglycerin
      b. Nitroglycerin patches, such as Nitro-Dur 0.4 mg, applied daily
      c. Oral, long-acting nitrates, such as isosorbide
   2. Emphasize long-term priorities of improved diet (sodium restriction), weight control, and exercise
   3. Control dyslipidemia with diet, exercise, and pharmacologic therapy
   4. Supplement oxygen, usually via nasal cannula at low flow rates (e.g., 2 L/min).
      a. In frank pulmonary edema, oxygen should be supplied in higher amounts
      b. Use mask delivery PRN to adequately oxygenate the blood
   5. If the patient is unable to sustain the work of breathing during an acute episode of heart failure, attempt should be made at noninvasive positive pressure ventilation via continuous positive airway pressure (CPAP) followed by intubation and mechanical ventilatory assistance, if necessary. This will help to redistribute edema out of the lungs and back into the vascular space, as well as to offload the work of breathing and save energy.
   6. Improve contractility of the myocardium
      a. Eliminate cardiac depressants
         i. Calcium channel blockers
         ii. β-blockers (in acute decompensation)
      b. Supply additional inotropic force in acute decompensation (dobutamine and milrinone)

c. Decrease afterload with an ACE inhibitor as blood pressure tolerates
  d. Decrease preload with morphine and diuresis
  e. Use β-adrenergic antagonists to help regulate catecholamines if blood pressure and heart rate will tolerate
  f. These measures will reduce interstitial edema and ventilatory restriction, thereby improving respiratory symptoms.
  g. Aggressiveness of these measures must be proportionate to the severity of interstitial edema and the degree of respiratory distress present

BIBLIOGRAPHY

Bartlett, J. G. (2010). *Workshop on issues in the design of clinical trials for antibacterial drugs for hospital acquired pneumonia and ventilator associated pneumonia*. Chicago, IL: Univ. of Chicago Press.

Cecil, R. L., Goldman, L., & Schafer, A. I. (2012). *Goldman's Cecil medicine* (24th ed.). Philadelphia, PA: Elsevier/Saunders.

Centers for Disease Control and Prevention. (2005). Guidelines for the investigation of contacts of persons with infectious tuberculosis: Recommendations from the National Tuberculosis Controllers Association and CDC. *Morbidity and Mortality Weekly Report, 54*(RR-15), 1–37.

Emanuel, L. L. (2011). *Palliative care: Core skills and clinical competencies* (2nd ed.). Philadelphia, PA: Saunders.

Guidelines for the prevention of ventilator-associated pneumonia in adults in Ireland. (2011). Dublin: Health Protection Surveillance Centre.

Hawkins, N. M. (2010). *Heart failure and chronic obstructive pulmonary disease common partners, common problems*. Glasgow: University of Glasgow.

Kamangar, N., Royani, P., & Shorr, A. F. (2013). In S. P. Peters (Ed.), *Sarcoidosis.* Retrieved November 30, 2013, from http://www.emedicine.medscape.com/ article/301914-overview

Longo, D. L., Fauci, A., Hauser, S., Jameson, J., & Loscalzo, J. (2012). *Harrison's principles of internal medicine* (18th ed.). New York, NY: McGraw-Hill.

Mall, M. A. (2014). *Cystic fibrosis*. Sheffield: European Respiratory Society.

McPhee, S. J., Papadakis, M. A., & Rabow, M. W. (Eds.). (2013). *CURRENT medical diagnosis and treatment 2013* (52nd ed.). New York, NY: McGraw Hill/Appleton & Lange.

Murali, S. (2012). *Pulmonary hypertension*. Philadelphia, PA: Saunders/Elsevier.

Nathanson, N. (2007). *Viral pathogenesis and immunity* (2nd ed.). Amsterdam: Elsevier Academic Press.

Pneumonia Severity Index Calculator. (2003). Agency for Healthcare Research and Quality. Rockville, MD. http://pda.ahrq.gov/psicalc.as

Pokorski, M. (2013). *Neurobiology of respiration*. Dordrecht: Springer.

Weinstock, M. B., Neides, D. M., Chan, M., Schumick, D. R. (2009). *Resident's guide to ambulatory* care (6th ed.). Colombus, OH: Anadem Publishing Inc.

Yancy, C. W., Jessup, M., Bozkurt, B., Butler, J., Casey, D. E., Drazner, M. H., . . . Wilkoff, B. L. (2013). 2013 ACCF/AHA guidelines for the management of heart failure: Executive summary: A report of the American College of Cardiology Foundation/American Heart Association Task Force on practice guidelines. *Journal of the American College of Cardiology*, *62*(16), 1495–1539.

CHAPTER 28

Pulmonary Hypertension and Pulmonary Vascular Disorders

HALEY M. HOY • IVAN ROBBINS • THOMAS W. BARKLEY, JR.

PULMONARY HYPERTENSION

I. **Etiology**
   A. Increased pulmonary vascular resistance
      1. Vasoconstriction (e.g., due to hypoxemia and acidosis)
      2. Loss of vasculature (e.g., due to emphysema and lung resection)
      3. Occlusion of the pulmonary vasculature (e.g., due to pulmonary embolism [PE])
      4. Relative stenosis of the pulmonary vasculature (e.g., vasculitis)
   B. Increased pulmonary venous pressure
      1. Left ventricular failure or hypertrophy
      2. Valvular heart disease (e.g., mitral valve stenosis and aortic valve stenosis)
      3. Constrictive pericarditis
   C. Increased pulmonary blood flow (left-to-right shunt)
   D. Polycythemia (primary or secondary; e.g., from hypoxemia)
   E. Idiopathic pulmonary arterial hypertension, seen most often in young women
      1. World Health Organization (WHO) classification:
         a. WHO group I: pulmonary arterial hypertension
            i. Idiopathic pulmonary arterial hypertension
            ii. Familial pulmonary arterial hypertension
            iii. Associated pulmonary arterial hypertension: collagen vascular disease (e.g., scleroderma), congenital shunts between systemic and pulmonary circulation, portal hypertension, HIV infection, drugs, toxins, or other diseases or disorders
            iv. Associated with venous or capillary disease
         b. WHO group II: pulmonary hypertension associated with left heart disease
            i. Atrial or ventricular disease
            ii. Valvular disease (e.g., mitral stenosis)
         c. WHO group III: pulmonary hypertension associated with lung diseases and/or hypoxemia
            i. Chronic obstructive pulmonary disease (COPD), interstitial lung disease
            ii. Sleep-disordered breathing, alveolar hypoventilation
            iii. Chronic exposure to high altitude

iv. Developmental lung abnormalities
d. WHO group IV: pulmonary hypertension due to chronic thrombotic and/or embolic disease
  i. PE in the proximal or distal pulmonary arteries
  ii. Embolization of other matter, such as tumor cells or parasites
e. WHO group V: miscellaneous, hematologic, and systemic disorders
  i. Myeloproliferative disorders
  ii. Sarcoidosis
  iii. Sickle cell disease

II. **Incidence**
  A. Note: The incidence of secondary pulmonary hypertension is related to the incidence of the cause of pulmonary hypertension.

III. **Signs/symptoms**
  A. Dyspnea with exertion
  B. Those related to the cause of the pulmonary hypertension
  C. Substernal discomfort
  D. Fatigue
  E. Syncope
  F. Palpitations

IV. **Subjective/physical examination findings**
  A. Splitting of the second cardiac sound; pulmonic valve component of the second heart sound (P2) is increased in intensity
  B. Peripheral edema related to right ventricular (RV) failure
  C. Ascites
  D. RV heave
  E. Loud pulmonic valve

V. **Laboratory/diagnostics**
  A. Lab:
    1. Complete blood count: increase in hemoglobin and hematocrit if hypoxemia present
  B. Radiographs:
    1. Chest x-ray: increased size of the proximal pulmonary arteries; visible narrowing of the pulmonary arteries in the medial third of the lung (typically seen in emphysema)
  C. Cardiac: electrocardiogram, echocardiogram, and right heart catheterization
    1. Two-dimensional echocardiography is used to diagnose pulmonary hypertension
    2. Cardiac catheterization is used to confirm the diagnosis
      a. Elevated mean pulmonary artery pressure with normal pulmonary capillary wedge pressure, elevated pulmonary artery systolic pressure, and tricuspid regurgitation velocity
  D. Pulmonary function testing: to assess for obstructive and restrictive ventilatory defects
  E. Consider tests to rule out thromboembolic disorders
    1. Lower-extremity Doppler
    2. Ventilation/perfusion lung scan
    3. Computed tomography (CT)

VI. **Treatment**
  A. Treatment of underlying disorders that may contribute to hypoxemia, including the following:
    1. COPD
    2. Congestive heart failure
    3. Obstructive sleep apnea
  B. Supplemental oxygen during the night
  C. Consider anticoagulation due to increased risk for intrapulmonary thrombosis and thromboembolism.

D. If polycythemia is severe, with hematocrit above 60%, therapeutic phlebotomy should be considered to yield a hematocrit of approximately 55%. Consider adding diuretics for fluid retention
E. Pharmacologic therapy—usually started for symptomatic patients in WHO functional classes II, III, or IV if patients showed no acute vasoreactivity or did not respond well to calcium channel blockers
   1. Prostanoids
      a. Calcium channel blockers
         i. Nifedipine, 90–240 mg PO daily
         ii. Diltiazem, 240–720 mg daily
         iii. Limited role in therapy; should not be use empirically to treat pulmonary arterial hypertension in the absence of demonstrated acute vasoreactivity
         iv. May be used in WHO functional classes I-IV
         v. If improvement in functional class to class I or II is not seen, additional or alternative therapy should be instituted.
      b. Prostacyclins
         i. Epoprostenol (Flolan, Veletri)
            (a) Initiated in controlled setting/hospital
            (b) Initial: 2 ng/kg/min IV; titrate upward in increments of 2 ng/kg/min every 15 min or longer until dose-limiting effects or intolerance develops
         ii. Treprostinil (Remodulin, Tyvaso)
            (a) Initiated in controlled setting/hospital
            (b) Injection: 1.25 ng/kg/min continuous SQ or central line IV infusion; decrease to 0.625 ng/kg/min if initial dose cannot be tolerated
            (c) Oral: 3 breaths (18 mcg) via oral inhalation per treatment session, QID during waking hours approximately 4 hr apart; reduce to 1 or 2 breaths if 3 breaths is not tolerated
         iii. Iloprost (Ventavis)
            (a) Oral: 2.5 mcg inhaled; if tolerated, increase dose to 5 mcg inhaled six to nine times per day (no more than every 2 hr) during waking ts; maximum daily dose of 45 mcg
   2. Endothelin receptor antagonists
      a. Ambrisentan (Letairis)
         i. Must enroll in Letairis education and access program
         ii. 5 mg PO once daily; may increase to 10 mg once daily if 5-mg dose is tolerated
      b. Bosentan (Tracleer)
         i. Must enroll in Tracleer access program
         ii. Initial: 62.5 mg PO BID for 4 weeks
         iii. Maintenance: up to 125 mg PO BID
   3. PDE5 inhibitors
      a. Sildenafil (Revatio), 5–20 mg PO TID
      b. Tadalafil (Cialis), 40 mg PO once daily
F. Consider referral for transplantation

PULMONARY VASCULAR DISORDERS

I. **Pulmonary embolism**
   A. Definition
      1. Clot (thromboembolus) or other undissolved solid, liquid, or gaseous material that has traveled to the lung via the venous system and become lodged in the pulmonary arterial circulation, interrupting blood flow
      2. Extent of lung tissue injury is determined by the size of the embolus, which is considered massive if more than 50% of flow is obstructed

3. Accurate diagnosis is the key to reducing associated mortality
4. Death occurs as a result of RV failure
B. Etiology/incidence/predisposing factors
   1. Predisposing factors for thrombotic emboli (Virchow triad) include the following:
      a. Venous stasis: deep venous thrombosis in lower extremities and pelvis leads to 70% of pulmonary emboli
         i. Prolonged immobility or surgery involving general anesthesia longer than 30 min
         ii. Congestive heart failure
         iii. Dehydration
         iv. Obesity
         v. Advanced age
      b. Vessel wall injury (e.g., surgery, fractured hip and/or pelvis)
      c. Hypercoagulability (e.g., increased owing to estrogen supplies, malignancy)
      d. Genetic predisposition
   2. Other etiologies
      a. Fat embolism: orthopedic trauma (especially through marrow-containing bone) and surgery
      b. Air embolism (e.g., from a central line)
      c. Tumor fragments
      d. Amniotic fluid embolism
      e. Septic debris (e.g., indwelling venous access device)
C. Signs/symptoms
   1. Dyspnea, insidious or sudden in onset, is the most common symptom
   2. Apprehension, anxiety, and perception of "impending doom"
   3. Substernal discomfort
   4. Pleuritic pain with PE with infarction
   5. Hemoptysis with pulmonary infarction
   6. Syncope
D. Subjective/physical examination findings (may range from none to frank cardiovascular collapse)
   1. Tachycardia
   2. Tachypnea and dyspnea
   3. Initially elevated blood pressure
   4. Diaphoresis
   5. Chest pain (dull, central, and pleuritic with pulmonary infarction)
   6. Decreased cardiac output
   7. Hypotension and shock
   8. Signs of RV overload
      a. Jugular venous distention
      b. Increased intensity, second heart sound
   9. Peripheral phlebitis
   10. Signs of fat embolization
      a. Sudden, marked dyspnea in a susceptible patient
      b. Altered consciousness
      c. Body temperature elevation higher than 102°F
      d. Petechiae over the thorax, shoulders, and axillae
E. Laboratory/diagnostics
   1. Arterial blood gas analysis
      a. Acute respiratory alkalosis
      b. Variable degrees of hypoxemia
   2. ECG: nonspecific changes

a. Most common is sinus tachycardia; atrial fibrillation is common as well
3. Chest x-ray: normal, or with small infiltrates and/or effusion
4. Ventilation/perfusion lung scan
   a. If read as high probability for PE, treat with anticoagulants
   b. If read as indeterminate or low probability for PE, consider pulmonary angiography if clinical suspicion remains high
   c. If the chest x-ray is abnormal, or if COPD is present, lung scanning may lead to an erroneous interpretation. Consider CT angiogram
5. Pulmonary angiography remains the accepted gold standard for detecting the presence of pulmonary emboli
6. Venous Doppler studies of the lower extremities may reveal the presence of deep venous thrombosis, which requires anticoagulation, in part obviating the need for evaluation of PE.
7. Some authorities believe that spiral-cut, high-resolution CT scan of the chest reliably shows central PE

F. Management
1. These agents have the FDA labeling for pulmonary embolism:
   a. Fondaparinux (Arixtra)
      i. 5 mg SQ once daily for patients whose weight is less than 50 kg
      ii. 7.5 mg SQ once daily for patients whose weight ranges from 50–100 kg
      iii. 10 mg SQ once daily for patients whose weight exceeds 100 kg
   b. Argatroban
      i. Use weight-based dosing to achieve a partial thromboplastin time of 1.5–3 times the baseline
   c. Dabigatran (Pradaxa), 150 mg PO BID
2. Anticoagulation for venous thromboembolism
   a. Heparin may be started while confirmatory tests are being conducted
      i. Weight-based dosing
         (a) Initial bolus of 80 units/kg followed by a continuous infusion of 18 units/kg/hr
      ii. Dosage sufficient to maintain the partial thromboplastin time (PTT) at 2–2.5 times control
      iii. Some hospitals use a heparin protocol, with PTT checks every 6 hr, to guide heparin therapy.
   b. Low-molecular weight heparin (e.g., enoxaparin [Lovenox]), 1 mg/kg subcutaneously every 12 hr, is an acceptable alternative to heparin
      i. It also carries a lower risk of bleeding and of heparin-induced thrombocytopenia.
      ii. No extensive monitoring of coagulation parameters is needed
   c. Warfarin (Coumadin)
      i. Begun at the time diagnosis of PE is confirmed; usual first dose is 5–10 mg PO
      ii. Heparin is continued until therapeutic anticoagulant levels are achieved with warfarin.
      iii. Monitor the international normalized ratio (INR) after initial daily doses of Coumadin
         (a) Adequate oral anticoagulant effect is achieved when the INR is 2–2.5 for at least 2–3 days
      iv. Length of treatment: 3–6 months for the initial episode of PE; for recurrent episodes, treat for 6–12 months or longer, or consider placement of an indwelling vena cava filter to protect against massive embolization in patients with ongoing risk factors

d. Rivaroxaban (Xarelto), 15 mg PO BID with food for 21 days, followed by 20 mg PO once daily with food
      i. Is an oral Xa inhibitor in the anticoagulant family
      ii. Approved in patients with deep vein thrombosis/PE
      iii. No monitoring required (no INRs to be checked)
      iv. Must be renally dosed
      v. May cause irreversible bleeding, which is treatable only with fresh frozen plasma
3. Fibrinolytic treatment: note contraindications before instituting this therapy (see fibrinolytic therapy for myocardial infarction in Angina and Myocardial Infarction)
4. May be appropriate for massive proximal PE associated with persistent systemic hypotension and signs of right heart strain, as well as in patients with very little cardiopulmonary reserve
5. Recombinant tissue plasminogen activator (Alteplase): 100 mg as a continuous infusion over 2 hr
6. Streptokinase: 250,000 units over 30 min; then 100,000 units/hr for 24 hr
   a. Rarely used; streptokinase has been associated with increased bleeding risk (compared to alteplase), increased incidence of allergic response (compared to alteplase), and resistance to affect due to antibody formation
7. Fibrinolytic therapy: after completed, begin heparin or enoxaparin when the PTT is less than 2 times control
8. Hemodynamic support may be needed for massive emboli with hypotension
9. Surgical embolectomy: reserved for those patients with massive emboli in central pulmonary arteries in whom the clot is creating hypotension and shock
10. Inferior vena cava interruption ("umbrella" device; Greenfield filter)
    a. Indicated when the risk of further emboli is perceived to be high
    b. Indicated with an absolute risk to anticoagulation
11. Supplemental oxygen is indicated to keep oxygen saturation above 90%

II. Pulmonary vasculitis
A. Wegener granulomatosis
   1. Necrotizing granulomas of the respiratory tract (upper and lower), pulmonary microangiitis, and glomerulonephritis
   2. Associated with the following:
      a. Hemoptysis
      b. Dyspnea
      c. Cough
      d. Pulmonary infiltrates
   3. Antineutrophilic cytoplasmic antibodies are often positive.
   4. Treatment includes prednisone, 1 mg/kg per day, or cyclophosphamide (Cytoxan), 2 mg/kg/day, with reasonable chance of remission within 1 year
   5. Treatment has two components:
      a. Induction of remission with initial immunosuppressive therapy
      b. Maintenance immunosuppressive therapy for a variable period to prevent relapse
   6. Treatment is based on disease severity (mild, moderate, to severe disease)
      a. Glucocorticoids in combination with methotrexate, cyclophosphamide, or rituximab
   7. Prophylaxis against opportunistic infections (i.e., PCP/PJP) during induction therapy may be necessary
   8. When initiating glucocorticoid therapy, there is disagreement among experts as to whether therapy should begin with pulse methylprednisolone (7–15 mg/kg to a maximum dose of 500–1,000 mg/day for 3 days) in all patients or only in those with necrotizing or crescentic glomerulonephritis or more severe respiratory disease.
      a. Induction:

i. Prednisone, 1 mg/kg/day (maximum of 60–80 mg per day)
ii. Oral cyclophosphamide, 1.5–2 mg/kg per day
iii. IV cyclophosphamide, 0.5g/m² every 2 weeks for 3–6 months
iv. Rituximab, 375 mg/m² per week for 4 weeks
v. Methotrexate—not FDA labeled for this indication; trial data suggests 20–25 mg PO per week
   b. Maintenance
      i. Methotrexate, 0.3 mg/kg per week (maximum dose of 15 mg); if tolerated, the dose increases in 2.5 mg increments each week to a dose of 20–25 mg per week
      ii. Azathioprine, 2 mg/kg per day
 B. Lymphomatoid granulomatosis
   1. Systemic granulomatous angiitis involving the following:
      a. Lung
      b. Brain
      c. Skin (especially)
      d. Upper respiratory tract (rarely)
      e. Kidneys (rarely)
   2. Associated with the eventual development of lymphoma in many cases
   3. In general, treatment options for pulmonary lymphomatoid granulomatosis follow those for diffuse large B-cell lymphoma.
   4. The choice of treatment should be based upon the presence of symptoms, history of using an inciting medication, extent of extrapulmonary involvement, and careful assessment of the histopathologic grade of the lesion. When a medication is implicated, it should be stopped and the patient observed for changes in the extent of the disease.
   5. Refer to hematology oncology specialist for consultation and/or treatment
III. **Implications for geriatric patients**
 A. Heart failure with preserved ejection fraction is a commonly under-recognized cause of pulmonary hypertension in the elderly
 B. Very unlikely to be pulmonary artery hypertension; more likely to be pulmonary venous hypertension due to left ventricular systolic or diastolic failure, aortic or mitral valve disease, or left atrial non-compliance in the elderly

BIBLIOGRAPHY

Benza, R. L., Miller, D. P., Barst, R. J., Badesch, D. B., Frost, A. E., & McGoon, M. D. (2012). An evaluation of long-term survival from time of diagnosis in pulmonary arterial hypertension from the REVEAL Registry. *Chest, 142*(2), 448–456.

Bishop, B. M., Mauro, V. F., & Khouri, S. J. (2012). Practical considerations for the pharmacotherapy of pulmonary arterial hypertension. *Pharmacotherapy, 32*(9), 838–855. doi:10.1002/j.1875–9114.2012.01114.x

Boilson, B. A., Schirger, J. A., & Borlaug, B. A. (2010). Caveat medicus! Pulmonary hypertension in the elderly: A word of caution. *European Journal of Heart Failure, 12*, 89–93.

Bonderman, D., Wexberg, P., Heinzl, H., & Lang, I. M. (2012). Non-invasive algorithms for the diagnosis of pulmonary hypertension. *Thrombosis and Haemostasis, 108*(6), 1037–1041. doi:10.1160/th12–04–0239

Bossone, E., D'Andrea, A., D'Alto, M., Citro, R., Argiento, P., Ferrara, F., . . . Naeije, R. (2013). Echocardiography in pulmonary arterial hypertension: From diagnosis to prognosis. *Journal of the American Society of Echocardiography, 26*(1), 1–14. doi:10.1016/j.echo.2012.10.009

Chan, L., Kennedy, M., Woolstenhulme, J. G., Nathan, S. D., Weinstein, A. A., Connors, G., . . . Keyser, R. E. (2013). Benefits of intensive treadmill exercise training on cardiorespiratory function and quality of life in patients with pulmonary hypertension. *Chest, 143*(2), 333–343.

Charalampopoulos, A., Raphael, C., Gin-Sing, W., & Gibbs, J. S. (2012). Diagnosing and managing pulmonary hypertension. *Practitioner, 256*(1756), 21–25.

Cracowski, J. L., & Leuchte, H. H. (2012). The potential of biomarkers in pulmonary arterial hypertension. *American Journal of Cardiology, 110*(6 Suppl), 32s-38s. doi:10.1016/j.amjcard.2012.06.014

de Man, F. S., Tu, L., Handoko, M. L., Rain, S., Ruiter, G., François, C., . . . Guignabert, C. (2012). Dysregulated renin-angiotensin-aldosterone system contributes to pulmonary arterial hypertension. *American Journal of Respiratory and Critical Care Medicine, 186*(8), 780–789. doi:10.1164/rccm.201203–0411OC

Foris, V., Kovacs, G., Tscherner, M., Olschewski, A., & Olschewski, H. (2013). Biomarkers in pulmonary hypertension: What do we know? *Chest, 144*(1), 274–283. doi:10.1378/chest.12–1246

Frazier, A. A., & Burke, A. P. (2012). The imaging of pulmonary hypertension. *Seminars in Ultrasound, CT, and MR, 33*(6), 535–551. doi:10.1053/j.sult.2012.06.002

Gabler, N. B., French, B., Strom, B. L., Liu, Z., Palevsky, H. I., Taichman, D. B., . . . Halpern, S. D. (2012). Race and sex differences in response to endothelin receptor antagonists for pulmonary arterial hypertension. *Chest, 141*(1), 20–26.

Georgiopoulou, V. V., Kalogeropoulos, A. P., Borlaug, B. A., Gheorghiade, M., & Butler, J. (2013). Left ventricular dysfunction with pulmonary hypertension: Part 1: Epidemiology, pathophysiology, and definitions. *Circulation. Heart Failure, 6*(2), 344–354. doi:10.1161/circheartfailure.112.000095

Gologanu, D., Stanescu, C., & Bogdan, M. A. (2012). Pulmonary hypertension secondary to chronic obstructive pulmonary disease. *Romanian Journal of Internal Medicine, 50*(4), 259–268.

Guazzi, M., Castelvecchio, S., Bandera, F., & Menicanti, L. (2012). Right ventricular pulmonary hypertension. *Current Heart Failure Reports, 9*(4), 303–308. doi:10.1007/s11897–012–0106–8

Humbert, M., Gerry Coghlan, J., & Khanna, D. (2012). Early detection and management of pulmonary arterial hypertension. *European Respiratory Review, 21*(126), 306–312. doi:10.1183/09059180.00005112

Iwasawa, T. (2013). Diagnosis and management of pulmonary arterial hypertension using MR imaging. *Magnetic Resonance in Medical Sciences, 12*(1), 1–9.

Judge, E. P., & Gaine, S. P. (2013). Management of pulmonary arterial hypertension. *Current Opinion in Critical Care, 19*(1), 44–50. doi:10.1097/MCC.0b013e32835c5137

Lewczuk, J., Romaszkiewicz, R., Lenartowska, L., Piszko, P., Jagas, J., Nowak, M., . . . Wrabec, K. (2013). The natural history of thromboembolic pulmonary hypertension. Since when is it chronic? A proposal of an algorithm for the diagnosis and treatment. *Kardiologia Polska, 71*(5), 522–526. doi:10.5603/kp.2013.0102

Ling, Y., Johnson, M. K., Kiely, D. G., Condliffe, R., Elliot, C. A., Gibbs, J. S., . . . Peacock, A. J. (2012). Changing demographics, epidemiology, and survival of incident pulmonary arterial hypertension: Results from the pulmonary hypertension registry of the United Kingdom and Ireland. *American Journal of Respiratory and Critical Care Medicine, 186*(8), 790–796. doi:10.1164/rccm.201203–0383OC

Liu, C., Chen, J., Gao, Y., Deng, B., & Liu, K. (2013). Endothelin receptor antagonists for pulmonary arterial hypertension. *Cochrane Database of Systematic Reviews, 2*. doi:10.1002/14651858.CD004434.pub5

Malenfant, S., Margaillan, G., Loehr, J. E., Bonnet, S., & Provencher, S. (2013). The emergence of new therapeutic targets in pulmonary arterial hypertension: From now to the near future. *Expert Review of Respiratory Medicine, 7*(1), 43–55. doi:10.1586/ers.12.83

Mandel, J., & Poch, D. (2013). In the clinic. Pulmonary hypertension. *Annals of Internal Medicine, 158*(9). doi:10.7326/0003–4819–158–9–201305070–01005

Mauritz, G. J., Kind, T., Marcus, J. T., Bogaard, H. J., Postmus, P. E., Boonstra, A., . . . Vonk-Noordegraaf, A. (2012). Progressive changes in right ventricular geometric shortening and long-term survival in pulmonary arterial hypertension. *Chest, 141*(4), 935–943.

McLaughlin, V. V., Langer, A., Tan, M., Clements, P. J., Oudiz, R. J., Tapson, V. F., . . . Rubin, L. J. (2013). Contemporary trends in the diagnosis and management of pulmonary arterial hypertension: An initiative to close the care gap. *Chest, 143*(2), 324–332.

Ng, C., & Jenkins, D. P. (2013). Surgical management of chronic thromboembolic pulmonary hypertension. *British Journal of Hospital Medicine (London), 74*(1), 31–35.

Nider, V. (2013). Pulmonary arterial hypertension. Recognition is the first essential step. *Advance for NPs and PAs, 4*(5), 33–37.

O'Callaghan, D. S., & Humbert, M. (2012). A critical analysis of survival in pulmonary arterial hypertension. *European Respiratory Review, 21*(125), 218–222. doi:10.1183/09059180.00003512

Peacock, A. (2013). Pulmonary hypertension. *European Respiratory Review, 22*(127), 20–25. doi:10.1183/09059180.00006912

Poor, H. D., & Ventetuolo, C. E. (2012). Pulmonary hypertension in the intensive care unit. *Progress in Cardiovascular Diseases, 55*(2), 187–198. doi:10.1016/j.pcad.2012.07.001

Rabinovitch, M. (2012). Molecular pathogenesis of pulmonary arterial hypertension. *Journal of Clinical Investigation, 122*(12), 4306–4313. doi:10.1172/jci60658

Rajdev, A., Garan, H., & Biviano, A. (2012). Arrhythmias in pulmonary arterial hypertension. *Progress in Cardiovascular Diseases, 55*(2), 180–186. doi:10.1016/j.pcad.2012.06.002

Rubin, L. J., Simonneau, G., Badesch, D., Galie, N., Humbert, M., Keogh, A., . . . Kymes, S. (2012). The study of risk in pulmonary arterial hypertension. *European Respiratory Review, 21*(125), 234–238. doi:10.1183/09059180.00003712

Singh, G. K., Levy, P. T., Holland, M. R., & Hamvas, A. (2012). Novel methods for assessment of right heart structure and function in pulmonary hypertension. *Clinics in Perinatology, 39*(3), 685–701. doi:10.1016/j.clp.2012.06.002

Skoro-Sajer, N. (2012). Optimal use of treprostinil in pulmonary arterial hypertension: A guide to the correct use of different formulations. *Drugs, 72*(18), 2351–2363. doi:10.2165/11638260–000000000–00000

Sood, N. (2013). Managing an acutely ill patient with pulmonary arterial hypertension. *Expert Review of Respiratory Medicine, 7*(1), 77–83. doi:10.1586/ers.12.73

Stacher, E., Graham, B. B., Hunt, J. M., Gandjeva, A., Groshong, S. D., McLaughlin, V. V., . . . Tuder, R. M. (2012). Modern age pathology of pulmonary arterial hypertension. *American Journal of Respiratory and Critical Care Medicine, 186*(3), 261–272. doi:10.1164/rccm.201201–0164OC

Tackett, K. L., & Stajich, G. V. (2013). Combination pharmacotherapy in the treatment of pulmonary arterial hypertension: Continuing education article. *Journal of Pharmacy Practice, 26*(1), 18–28. doi:10.1177/0897190012466046

Thomas, M., Ciuclan, L., Hussey, M. J., & Press, N. J. (2013). Targeting the serotonin pathway for the treatment of pulmonary arterial hypertension. *Pharmacology and Therapeutics, 138*(3), 409–417. doi:10.1016/j.pharmthera.2013.02.002

Tonelli, A. R., Arelli, V., Minai, O. A., Newman, J., Bair, N., Heresi, G. A., & Dweik, R. A. (2013). Causes and circumstances of death in pulmonary arterial hypertension. *American Journal of Respiratory and Critical Care Medicine, 188*(3), 365–369. doi:10.1164/rccm.201209–1640OC

Vachiery, J. L., & Gaine, S. (2012). Challenges in the diagnosis and treatment of pulmonary arterial hypertension. *European Respiratory Review, 21*(126), 313–320. doi:10.1183/09059180.00005412

Ventetuolo, C. E., & Klinger, J. R. (2012). WHO Group 1 pulmonary arterial hypertension: Current and investigative therapies. *Progress in Cardiovascular Diseases, 55*(2), 89–103. doi:10.1016/j.pcad.2012.07.002

Voelkel, N. F., Mizuno, S., & Bogaard, H. J. (2013). The role of hypoxia in pulmonary vascular diseases: A perspective. *American Journal of Physiology. Lung Cellular and Molecular Physiology, 304*(7), L457–465. doi:10.1152/ajplung.00335.2012

Waxman, A. B. (2012). Exercise physiology and pulmonary arterial hypertension. *Progress in Cardiovascular Diseases, 55*(2), 172–179. doi:10.1016/j.pcad.2012.07.003

Waxman, A. B., & Zamanian, R. T. (2013). Pulmonary arterial hypertension: New insights into the optimal role of current and emerging prostacyclin therapies. *American Journal of Cardiology, 111*(5 Suppl), 1A-16A; quiz 17A-19A. doi:10.1016/j.amjcard.2012.12.002

Wilkins, M. R., Wharton, J., & Gladwin, M. T. (2013). Update in pulmonary vascular diseases 2012. *American Journal of Respiratory and Critical Care Medicine, 188*(1), 23–28. doi:10.1164/rccm.201303–0470UP

Wilson, S. R., Ghio, S., Scelsi, L., & Horn, E. M. (2012). Pulmonary hypertension and right ventricular dysfunction in left heart disease (Group 2 pulmonary hypertension). *Progress in Cardiovascular Diseases, 55*(2), 104–118. doi:10.1016/j.pcad.2012.07.007

Wu, W. H., Yang, L., Peng, F. H., Yao, J., Zou, L. L., Liu, D., . . . Jing, Z. C. (2013). Lower socioeconomic status is associated with worse outcomes in pulmonary arterial hypertension. *American Journal of Respiratory and Critical Care Medicine, 187*(3), 303–310. doi:10.1164/rccm.201207-1290OC

Yao, A. (2012). Recent advances and future perspectives in therapeutic strategies for pulmonary arterial hypertension. *Journal of Cardiology, 60*(5), 344–349. doi:10.1016/j.jjcc.2012.08.009

Zimner-Rapuch, S., Amet, S., Janus, N., Deray, G., & Launay-Vacher, V. (2013). Pulmonary hypertension: Use of oral drugs in patients with renal insufficiency. *Clinical Drug Investigation, 33*(1), 65–69. doi:10.1007/s40261-012-0045-x

CHAPTER 29

Chest Wall and Secondary Pleural Disorders

JENNIFER COATES • THOMAS W. BARKLEY, JR. • CHARLENE M. MYERS

DISORDERS OF THE CHEST WALL

I. **Components of the chest that may contribute to respiratory dysfunction**
   A. Spine
   B. Rib cage
   C. Costosternal margins
   D. Pleura
   E. Respiratory muscles

II. **Disorders of the spine**
   A. Congenital scoliosis
      1. The spine assumes an S-shaped curvature
      2. May induce a restrictive ventilatory defect
      3. Most often, scoliosis remains an insignificant variable, unless one of the following occurs:
         a. The curvature is severe
         b. Superimposed chest disease makes the work of breathing difficult
      4. In these instances, the risk of respiratory failure may increase.
   B. Kyphosis of the spine
      1. The spine has an accentuated dorsal curve
      2. May induce a restrictive ventilatory defect
      3. May coexist with scoliosis
      4. Can increase the risk of breathing problems in the presence of other chest diseases
      5. Acquired kyphosis
         a. Results from osteoporosis
         b. Common clinical problem resulting from vertebral collapse with pain
         c. Treatment of the pain may introduce the additional risk of ventilatory compromise
   C. Ankylosing spondylitis
      1. Chronic inflammatory disease of the joints of the axial skeleton
      2. Patient will have pain and progressive stiffening of the spine
      3. Chest expansion becomes limited as the disease progresses

III. Rib and sternal fracture and sternal dehiscence after cardiac surgery
  A. Fracture of the ribs, or even of the sternum, can occur spontaneously or as the result of trauma or surgery
  B. The instability of the chest wall, with flailing of the wall outward during inspiration and associated chest pain resulting from fractures, limits chest wall movement, especially if multiple fractures are present.
  C. Abnormal movement of the chest wall can result in hypoventilation and in poor secretion clearance
  D. Pain medication may facilitate breathing, but it can also lead to hypoventilation and ventilatory failure
  E. Milder problems theoretically can be helped with chest wall binders; however, with significant impairment of ventilation, positive pressure ventilation to stabilize the chest wall may be necessary.
  F. Sternal dehiscence following open heart surgery or surgical procedures involving the mediastinum similarly can result in respiratory compromise.

IV. Costochondral junctions
  A. Costosternal junctions may become inflamed owing to the following:
    1. Arthritis (autoimmune in origin)
       a. Rheumatoid disease
       b. Systemic lupus erythematosus
    2. Costochondritis (Tietze syndrome)
       a. Inflammation of the cartilage that connects rib to the sternum; causes pain and tenderness at costosternal joint, when taking deep breath, or upon coughing
  B. Although typically not serious, costochondritis may be confused with other more serious conditions within the chest.
  C. Costochondritis is more common in young women
  D. Tenderness over the affected area is common
  E. NSAIDs and heat are helpful in relieving the pain

PLEURAL DISORDERS

I. Pleuritis
  A. Also called pleurisy
  B. Defined as pain due to acute pleural inflammation
  C. Pain is typically localized, sharp, and fleeting and made worse by coughing, sneezing, and deep breathing.
  D. Multiple different possible etiologies, treatment depends on cause

II. Pleural effusion
  A. Increased amounts of fluid within the pleural space
    1. Transudative: due to increased hydrostatic or decreased oncotic pressure
       a. Causes include congestive heart failure, cirrhosis, and hypoalbuminemia
    2. Exudative: due to increased production of fluid due to abnormal capillary permeability or decreased lymphatic clearance from pleural space
       a. Causes include malignancy, rheumatoid arthritis, vasculitis, and lupus
    3. Empyema: infection and pus accumulation in the pleural space
    4. Hemothorax: blood in the pleural space
    5. Chylothorax: due to ruptured thoracic ducts and accumulation of chyle in the pleural space
    6. Parapneumonic effusion: exudate that accompanies an infection accumulating in the pleural space
  B. Symptoms
    1. Dyspnea
    2. Pleuritic chest pain

CHAPTER 29 Chest Wall and Secondary Pleural Disorders

C. Physical examination findings
   1. Tachypnea
   2. Dullness on percussion, with diminished or absent breath sounds over the affected area
   3. Pleural friction rub
   4. Fever, especially if the fluid is infected
D. Chest x-ray
   1. Increased amount of fluid between the visceral and the parietal pleura
   2. Layering out of the fluid on decubitus chest x-rays
   3. Loculation of fluid along the lateral chest wall (may be confirmed by ultrasonography over the affected area)
   4. Blunting of the costophrenic angles: appears as a linear shadow ascending vertically and clinging to the ribs in a meniscus pattern
      a. Lateral check x-ray: at least 75 ml of pleural fluid needed
      b. Posteroanterior chest x-ray: at least 175 ml of pleural fluid needed
      c. Lateral decubitus x-ray: amounts as small as 5 ml may blunt the costophrenic angle
E. Management
   1. Observation with or without diuresis: If risk of infection is small, and if it is likely that the effusion is due to heart failure, then the response may be assessed by doing the following:
      a. Following the effusion by serial chest x-rays
      b. Looking for a decrease in the amount of fluid over time during diuresis
   2. Thoracentesis is indicated in the following circumstances:
      a. The cause of the effusion must be evaluated for the following:
         i. Risk of infection
         ii. Malignancy
      b. The patient is dyspneic
         i. Procedure is therapeutic
         ii. Procedure can be used diagnostically when fluid is sent for laboratory evaluation
   3. Laboratory evaluation of pleural fluid
      a. Cell count and differential white blood cell count
      b. Chemistries—collect serum and pleural fluid levels of the following studies:
         i. Total protein
         ii. Glucose
         iii. Lactate dehydrogenase (LDH) levels
         iv. Amylase level
         v. A pleural exudate is an effusion that has one or more of the following:
            (a) Ratio of pleural fluid protein to serum protein greater than 0.5
            (b) Ratio of pleural fluid LDH to serum LDH greater than 0.6
            (c) Pleural fluid LDH more than two-thirds the upper limit of normal serum LDH
         vi. A transudative effusion typically has a serum glucose equal to pleural fluid glucose, and a pH between 7.40 and 7.55.
      c. Gram's stain and fluid cultures, as indicated by the patient's clinical status
         i. Bacteria (aerobic and anaerobic)
         ii. Acid-fast bacilli
         iii. Fungi
      d. Special serologic tests may be considered.
         i. Carcinoembryonic antigen in a patient with known colon cancer
         ii. CA125 in a woman with known ovarian cancer
      e. Determination of fluid pH, which tends to be low in the following situations:
         i. Empyema due to tuberculosis or anaerobic bacterial pathogens

ii. Rheumatoid involvement of the pleura
f. Pleural fluid cytologic examination to assess for metastatic cancer to the pleura
4. Further management issues:
   a. If the fluid is bloody, insertion of a chest tube is often required.
   b. Empyema requires chest tube insertion and probable surgical intervention.
      i. Antimicrobials alone are not curative when empyema is present.
      ii. All antimicrobials used should be selected on the basis of pleural fluid culture results, including antimicrobial sensitivity data.
   c. Repeated thoracentesis is an acceptable method of draining reaccumulations of malignant effusions, especially when the procedure is needed infrequently.
   d. Malignant effusions treated with chest tube drainage may also be sclerosed (creating scar tissue, in hopes of preventing recurrence).
      i. A sclerosing agent is introduced through the chest tube after drainage of the effusion is completed.
      ii. This sclerosing process is called pleurodesis.
F. Gerontologic considerations
   1. The chest wall muscle compliance decreases with age because the ribs become ossified (less flexible) and joints become stiffer.
   2. Respiratory muscle strength and endurance decrease with aging
   3. Antibiotic doses may need to be reduced in the elderly patient due to alterations in renal function or predisposition to medication side effects.
   4. The incidence of lung cancer increases with age; therefore, malignancy needs to be included in the list of pleural effusion differential diagnoses in the elderly patient.

BIBLIOGRAPHY

Girdhar, A., Shujaat, A., & Bajwa, A. (2012). Management of infectious processes of the pleural space: A review. *Pulmonary Medicine.* doi:10.1155/2012/816502

Goldman, L., & Ausiello, D. (Eds.). (2011). *Cecil textbook of medicine* (24th ed.). Philadelphia, PA: WB Saunders.

Halter, J., Ouslander, J., Tinetti, M., Studenski, S., High, K., & Asthana, S. (2009). *Hazzard's geriatric medicine and gerontology* (6th ed.). New York, NY: McGraw-Hill.

Light, R. W. (2007). *Pleural diseases*. Philadelphia, PA: Lippincott Williams & Wilkins.

Longo, D., Fauci, A. S., Kasper, D. L., Hauser, S. L., Jameson, L. J., & Loscalzo, J. (2012). *Harrison's principles of internal medicine* (18th ed.). New York, NY: McGraw-Hill.

McCance, K. L., & Huether, S. E. (Eds.). (2013). *Pathophysiology: The biologic basis for disease in adults and children.* Philadelphia, PA: Elsevier Health Sciences.

McGrath, E. E., & Anderson, P. B. (2011). Diagnosis of pleural effusion: A systematic approach. *American Journal of Critical Care, 20*(2), 119–128.

Papadakis, M. A. (2014). *Current medical diagnosis & treatment 2013*. S. J. McPhee (Ed.). New York, NY: McGraw-Hill Education Medical.

Rubenstein, W., & Talbot, Y. (2013). *Medical teaching in ambulatory care*. Toronto, ON: University of Toronto Press.

CHAPTER 30

Respiratory Failure

DAVID A. MILLER • THOMAS W. BARKLEY, JR.

DEFINITIONS AND CONCEPTS

I. **Breathing**
   A. Breathing is understood as the movement of air into and out of the lungs.
   B. Physiologically, breathing is controlled by the metabolic needs of the body (i.e., oxygen and carbon dioxide levels in the blood) as perceived by the central nervous system (chemoreceptor input).
   C. Breathing is also under voluntary control in conscious, alert individuals.

II. **Ventilation**
   A. Ventilation is the aspect of breathing that refers to the actual movement of air into and out of the lungs.
   B. Ventilation is determined by the volume of air moved (tidal volume) and by the ventilatory rate.
   C. Individuals who are alert and spontaneously breathing vary the amount of air inhaled and exhaled with each breath, as well as the respiratory rate, responding to the control of the central nervous system over the ventilatory act.
   D. Yawning and sighing are normal variations seen during the act of ventilation.

III. **Respiration**
   A. Respiration refers to the following:
      1. Actual use of oxygen at the cellular level
      2. Removal from the cellular environment of the following products:
         a. Carbon dioxide
         b. Metabolic wastes, especially metabolic acids
            i. Lactic acid
            ii. Ketoacids
   B. Cellular respiration is dependent on two variables:
      1. Perfusion of capillaries with oxygen and nutrient-laden blood in adequate amounts
         a. Cellular uptake and use of oxygen normally are independent of oxygen delivery.
      2. Venous blood flow that removes cellular metabolic wastes to the heart, lungs, and kidney
         a. For distribution to other cells, especially the following:

i. Alveoli
ii. Liver
iii. Kidneys
b. For further metabolism PRN and eventual removal from the body via these routes:
i. Expiration
ii. Stool
iii. Urine

THE EFFECTS OF AGING ON THE NEED FOR RESPIRATORY ASSISTANCE, INCLUDING INTUBATION

I. **Physiological changes**
   A. Reduced lung elasticity and increased ventilation–perfusion mismatching
   B. Reduced chest wall compliance and diaphragmatic and intercostal muscle strength
   C. Reduced clearance of airway secretions
   D. Altered responsiveness to hypoxemia and hypercarbia
II. **Effects of comorbidities**
   A. Increase the risk of respiratory failure
      1. Heart failure
      2. Chronic obstructive pulmonary disorder (COPD)
      3. Dementia
      4. Chronic inactivity
      5. Chronic kidney disease
III. **Ethical issues**
   A. Assessing for prior autonomous choices in the use of life-prolonging interventions among the elderly is essential, if possible. Family members are crucial in this regard.
   B. Patient age is not an indication to withhold ventilator assistance

VENTILATORY FAILURE

I. **Ventilatory failure refers to absent or inadequate movement of oxygen into the lungs and/or of carbon dioxide out of the lungs.**
   A. Apnea—absence of movement of respiratory gases
   B. Hypopnea—inadequate movement of respiratory gases
II. **Ventilatory failure is best assessed by measurement of the partial pressure of carbon dioxide in arterial blood ($PaCO_2$) and/or end-tidal CO_2 levels.**
III. **Causes of ventilatory failure**
   A. Ventilatory failure may be induced by overdose of medications (e.g., sedatives, hypnotics, and opioids) relative to the body's ability to continue to respond to metabolic and cellular respiratory needs while influenced by these drugs. Elderly persons are particularly susceptible to the respiratory depression associated with the use of these drugs.
      1. Unintentional overdose (e.g., iatrogenic oversedation in the presence of COPD)
      2. Intentional overdose
         a. Iatrogenic sedation with the intent to control ventilation
         b. Drug overdose with suicidal intent
   B. The ability to get oxygen into and carbon dioxide out of the lungs is impaired by acquired acute pathology related to the following:
      1. Infections of the lungs (e.g., in patients with COPD)
      2. Neuromuscular disease
         a. Myasthenia gravis in crisis
         b. Guillain-Barré syndrome
         c. Traumatic head or spinal cord injury
      3. Pulmonary edema of cardiogenic or noncardiogenic origin

RESPIRATORY FAILURE

I. **Definition**
   A. Failure of adequate oxygen delivery to cells (e.g., during hypotension)
   B. Failure of the cell's ability to use oxygen (e.g., cyanide poisoning, carbon monoxide poisoning)
II. **The term "shock" is best reserved for situations in which respiratory failure is generalized throughout the body.**
   A. The sepsis syndrome with hypotension poses risk not only to the lungs but also to critically important organs, including the kidneys, heart, liver, gut, and central nervous system.
   B. In sepsis syndrome, oxygen delivery to cells becomes pathophysiologically supply dependent. Hence,
      1. Ventilation must ensure an adequate supply of oxygen to the body.
      2. Circulation requires adequate volume support and systemic vascular resistance to ensure delivery of oxygen and nutrients to cells without overloading the ability of the heart to pump blood into the circulation.
      3. Pulmonary artery catheter monitoring may become necessary on a temporary basis for determining cardiac status and systemic vascular resistance.
      4. The amount of oxygen returning to the heart reflects the overall distribution of oxygen and nutrients to cells (mixed venous oxygen saturation [SvO_2] monitoring).
III. **The goal of treating respiratory failure is prevention of cellular ischemia and death while the cause of respiratory failure is corrected.**
   A. Control of ventilation, and oxygen and nutrient supplies, is critical
      1. Control of the airway is essential
   B. Also critical is the prevention of problems associated with mechanical ventilation.
      1. Pneumothorax
      2. Nosocomial pneumonia
      3. Indwelling catheter-related sepsis
      4. Malnutrition during the course of respiratory failure

TREATMENT

I. **Various modalities are potentially indicated**
   A. For hypoxemia when ventilation appears unlabored and sustainable
      1. Supplemental oxygen by mask
   B. For hypoxemia and hypercapnia and the patient is fully alert
      1. Supplemental oxygen via nasal prongs
      2. Consideration for bilevel positive airway pressure to keep ventilation near normal for patient
   C. For hypoxemia when ventilation is labored and/or hypercapnia is worsening
      1. Bilevel positive airway pressure
      2. Intubation and mechanical ventilation
II. **Support measures for comorbid illnesses need to be continued as indicated.**
III. **Nutritional support should be started as soon as possible to avert caloric restriction during a time of higher caloric need.**

BIBLIOGRAPHY

Brown, C. A. (2013). The decision to intubate. In D. S. Basow (Ed.), *UpToDate*. Waltham, MA: UpToDate.

Brown, C. A., & Arbelaez, C. (2013). Emergency airway management in the geriatric patient. In D. S. Basow (Ed.), *UpToDate*. Waltham, MA: UpToDate.

Centers for Medicare & Medicaid Services (CMS). (2013). *2014 ICD-10 PCS and GEMs.* Retrieved November 25, 2013, from http:///www.cms.gov/Medicare/Coding/ICD10/2014-ICD-10-PCS.html

Dirkes, S. (2011). Acute kidney injury: Not just acute renal failure anymore? *Critical Care Nurse, 3*(1), 37–49.

Goldman, L., & Shafer, A. I. (Eds.) (2012). *Goldman's Cecil medicine* (24th ed.). Philadelphia, PA: Saunders.

Longo, D. L., Kasper, D. L., Jameson, J. L., Fauci, A. S., Hauser, S. L., & Loscalzo, J. (Eds.) (2011). *Harrison's principles of internal medicine* (18th ed.). New York, NY: McGraw Hill.

Slutsky, A. S., & Ranieri, V. M. (2013). Ventilatory-induced lung injury. *New England Journal of Medicine, 369*, 2126–2136. doi:10.1056/NEJMra1208707

University of Miami Geriatric and Ethics Programs. (2013). *Geriatrics: Decision-making, autonomy, valid consent and guardianship.* Retrieved November 27, 2013, from http://www.miami.edu/index.php/ethics/projects/geriatrics_and_ethics/decision-making_autonomy_valid_consent_and_guardianship/

University of Miami Geriatric and Ethics Programs. (2013). *Geriatrics: End-of-life issues.* Retrieved November 27, 2013, from http://www.miami.edu/index.php/ethics/projects/geriatrics_and_ethics/end-of-life_issues/

CHAPTER 31

Pneumothorax

BIMBOLA AKINTADE • THOMAS W. BARKLEY, JR.

I. **Definition**
   A. The presence of air in the pleural space, resulting from perforation of the chest wall or pleura, causes the lung to collapse
   B. Types
      1. Spontaneous: disruption of the visceral pleura
         a. Air enters the pleural space from the lung
         b. Occurs in individuals with or without underlying lung disease
      2. Traumatic
         a. Open: penetrating chest trauma
            i. Parietal pleura is disrupted
            ii. Air enters the pleural space from the atmosphere
         b. Closed: blunt chest trauma
            i. The visceral pleura is disrupted
            ii. Air enters the pleural space from the lung
         c. Iatrogenic
            i. Disruption of the visceral pleura as a complication of an invasive thoracic procedure
            ii. May also occur after procedures involving the neck or the abdomen
      3. Tension
         a. As a result of a spontaneous or traumatic pneumothorax, air enters the pleural space but is unable to exit.
         b. As pressure rises in the pleural space, the lung collapses, the mediastinum shifts to the other side, and venous return to the right heart is impaired.
         c. Tension pneumothorax is a medical emergency

II. **Etiology/incidence/predisposing factors**
   A. Penetrating or blunt chest trauma
   B. Rupture of a subpleural bleb or invasion of visceral pleura by disease (e.g., necrotizing pneumonia)
   C. Intrinsic lung disease

1. Chronic obstructive pulmonary disease
2. Tuberculosis
3. Sarcoidosis
4. Pulmonary fibrosis
5. Bronchogenic carcinoma
- D. Barotrauma resulting from mechanical ventilation with increased positive end-expiratory pressure.
- E. Complication of invasive thoracic, neck, or abdominal diagnostic of therapeutic procedures
    1. Insertion of intravenous access devices
    2. Needle biopsy of liver or lung
    3. Thoracentesis

III. **Subjective/physical exam findings: depend on degree of lung collapse and mechanism involved**
- A. Possible sudden onset of dyspnea and shortness of breath
- B. Pleuritic chest pain, may be sharp and severe
- C. Apprehension and agitation

IV. **Physical examination findings: depend on degree of lung collapse and mechanism involved**
- A. Splinting and decreased inspiratory expansion of involved hemithorax
- B. Bulging of the intercostal spaces on the affected side during exhalation
- C. Decreased breath sounds and fremitus, along with a hyperresonant percussion note over the affected area
- D. Tracheal deviation toward the unaffected side
- E. Subcutaneous emphysema
- F. Possible Hamman sign (mediastinal crepitus on auscultation)
- G. In the mechanically ventilated patient with positive end-expiratory pressure, development of high peak inspiratory pressure with decreased compliance may occur.
- H. In patients with tension pneumothorax, signs of decreased cardiac output resulting from impaired venous return

V. **Laboratory/diagnostics**
- A. Arterial blood gases: mild to moderate hypoxemia and hypercapnia
- B. Chest x-ray
    1. Increased translucency confirms the degree of lung collapse
    2. Recognition of small pneumothoraces, particularly in mechanically ventilated patients, crucial to prevention of tension pneumothorax

VI. **Management**
- A. Tension pneumothorax
    1. Immediate decompression with 14- to 16-gauge needle into the second intercostal space, midclavicular line
    2. Insertion of chest tube at the fourth or fifth intercostal space midaxillary line to closed water-seal drainage
- B. Spontaneous pneumothorax: depends on size
    1. If small, give supplemental oxygen with 100% non-rebreather mask and observe
    2. If collapse is greater than 20%, insert a chest tube and connect it to a water-seal drainage
- C. Traumatic pneumothorax
    1. Prompt chest tube insertion, fourth or fifth intercostal space midaxillary line with closed chest drainage
- D. Negative pressure (application of suction to chest drainage apparatus)
    1. Use when water seal fails to re-expand the lung after 24–48 hr
    2. Use when persistent pneumothorax perpetuates hypoxemia and/or hypercapnia

BIBLIOGRAPHY

Baird, M. S., & Bethel, S. (2010). *Manual of critical care nursing: nursing interventions and collaborative management* (6th ed.). St. Louis, MO: Mosby.

Corbridge, T. C., & Singer, B. D. (2009). Basic invasive mechanical ventilation. *Southern Medical Journal, 102,* 1238–1245.

Dellinger, R. P., & Parrillo, J. E. (2013). *Critical care medicine: principles of diagnosis and management in the adult* (4th ed.). St. Louis, MO: Mosby.

Feller-Kopman, D., & Yarmus, L., (2012). Pneumothorax in the critically ill patient. *Chest, 141,* 1098–1105.

Fix, B., & Jones, J. (2009). *Critical care notes: Clinical pocket guide.* Philadelphia, PA: F.A. Davis.

Goldman, G., & Ausicello D. (2012). *Cecil textbook of medicine* (24nd ed.). Philadelphia, PA: WB Saunders.

Rakel, R. E., & Bope, E. T. (2013). *Conn's current therapy.* Philadelphia, PA: WB Saunders.

Ureden, L. D., Stacey, K. M., & Lough, M. E. (2013). *Thelan's critical care nursing: Diagnosis and management* (7th ed.). St. Louis, MO: Mosby.

Ureden, L. D., Stacey, K. M., & Lough, M. E. (2011). *Priorities in critical care nursing* (6th ed.). St. Louis, MO: Mosby.

CHAPTER 32

Lower Respiratory Tract Pathogens

DAVID A. MILLER • THOMAS W. BARKLEY, JR.

I. **Defined as pathogens found below the larynx**
   A. Note that pathogens in all parts of the lower respiratory tract are the same
   B. Recommended pharmacological treatment may require revision after the results of sputum and blood cultures are obtained (see Table 32.1)
   C. Considerations in older adults
      1. Comorbid conditions (heart failure, chronic obstructive pulmonary disease [COPD], diabetes, altered mental status, dementia, dysphagia, and cancer)
      2. Altered immunological status with aging
      3. Aspiration and residence in long-term care facilities may require broader-spectrum antibiotic coverage.
      4. More than 50% of all cases of pneumonia occur in adults older than 65 years. Comorbidity is a strong predictor of mortality from community-acquired pneumonia in the elderly, as is low body temperature, hypotension, elevation of creatinine above 1.5 mg/dl, debility, and being older than 85 years.
      5. Microbiology
         a. *Streptococcus pneumoniae* still predominates
         b. May be polymicrobial, including other bacteria and respiratory viruses
         c. Causative organisms are not identified in 60% of cases among the elderly.
         d. Antimicrobial resistance patterns in the local community and in long-term care facilities need to be reviewed, if available.
         e. Antimicrobial choices need to be addressed by these resistance patterns due to the prevalence of resistance among all bacteria responsible for pneumonia in elderly patients. This resistance is a global problem.
   D. Immunization against the pneumococcus and annual influenza vaccines is important. Pneumococcal vaccination does not guarantee pneumococcal pneumonia will be prevented by the vaccine.

CHAPTER 32   Lower Respiratory Tract Pathogens

II. Milder disease requires only narrow-spectrum antimicrobials, if any
III. Severe disease requires a combination of antimicrobials while cultures are pending.
IV. The suggestions in Table 32.1 apply to therapy that is chosen empirically while sputum and blood cultures are pending.
   A. When culture data are available, antimicrobials used should be reviewed and changed if necessary.
   B. The narrowest-spectrum antimicrobial that is reasonably expected to effectively treat the patient's lower respiratory tract infection should be used.
V. **Recall that antimicrobial therapy is intended to help clear pulmonary infection**
   A. Other pharmacological and nonpharmacological therapies should be considered as well.
   B. Examples:
      1. Supplemental oxygen
      2. Treatment of underlying COPD
      3. Hydration and nutritional support
VI. The most common causes of community-acquired pneumonia are shown in Table 32.2.
VII. Organism and treatment considerations for various pneumonias are depicted in Tables 32.4 through 32.8.
VIII. Table 32.10 lists pharmacological treatment options selected on the basis of suspected/known organisms for lower respiratory tract infection.

Table 32.1	Lower Respiratory Tract Pathogens and Treatment Considerations (Modified From Karmanger, 2013)	
Lower respiratory tract infection	**Organism**	**Recommended pharmacological treatment**
Acute tracheo-bronchitis	Viral	No therapy indicated
	Mycoplasma pneumoniae	Doxycycline, macrolides (note the risk of QT segment prolongation and torsade de points, including azithromycin)
	Chlamydia pneumoniae	Doxycycline, macrolides (note the risk of QT segment prolongation and torsade de points, including azithromycin)
	Bordetella pertussis	Macrolides (note the risk of QT segment prolongation and torsade de points, including azithromycin)
Acute bacterial exacerbation of COPD	Viral, with secondary bacterial infection	Therapy may be unnecessary
	Streptococcus pneumoniae	Consider amoxicillin, trimethoprim-sulfamethoxazole, doxycycline, second-generation cephalosporin
	Haemophilus pneumoniae	Amoxicillin preferred if susceptible. Consider fluoroquinolones, azithromycin (risk as noted above), and tetracyclines
	Moraxella catarrhalis	For severe cases, consider amoxicillin-clavulanate, clarithromycin or azithromycin (risk as noted above), oral cephalosporin, telithromycin, fluoroquinolone (with resistant *S. pneumoniae* coverage)

Table 32.1 Lower Respiratory Tract Pathogens and Treatment Considerations (Modified From Karmanger, 2013)

Lower respiratory tract infection	Organism	Recommended pharmacological treatment
Influenza	Influenza H and B (winter months)	Zanamivir (Relenza), 10 mg (two inhalations BID), or Oseltamivir (Tamiflu), 75 mg BID
	Other viral	Supportive therapy; may check for respiratory syncytial virus in elderly or immunocompromised patients, although ribavirin (Virazole) effectiveness in this setting is unknown
Pneumonia	Community-acquired	See Tables 32.4 and 32.5

Table 32.2 Pathogens in Community-Acquired Pneumonia

Typical bacterial pathogens (approx. 85%)	*Streptococcus pneumoniae* Penicillin-sensitive *S. pneumoniae* Penicillin-resistant *S. pneumoniae* *Haemophilus influenzae* Ampicillin-sensitive *H. influenzae* Ampicillin-resistant *H. influenzae* *Moraxella catarrhalis* (all strains penicillin resistant)
Atypical respiratory pathogens (approx. 15%)	*Legionella* species *Mycoplasma* species *Chlamydia pneumoniae*
Less common bacterial pathogens	*Klebsiella pneumoniae* (only in those with chronic alcoholism) *Staphylococcus aureus* (postviral, influenza setting) *Pseudomonas aeruginosa* (especially in patients with bronchiectasis)

Table 32.3 Outpatient Bacterial Pneumonia With Comorbidity in Patients 60 years or Older (Modified From Karmanger, 2013)

Organisms	*Streptococcus pneumoniae*
	Haemophilus influenzae
	Aerobic Gram-negative bacilli
	Staphylococcus aureus
	Miscellaneous:
	    Moraxella catarrhalis
	    Legionella species
	    Mycoplasma species

Therapy for Specific Comorbidity:	COPD (no recent antibiotics or oral corticosteroids, past 3 months): First choice: newer macrolides (warning regarding prolonged QT and torsade de pointes, including azithromycin) Second choice: doxycycline
	COPD (recent antibiotics or oral corticosteroids in past 3 months): First choice: respiratory fluoroquinolone Second choice: amoxicillin/clavulanate plus macrolide (warning, as above), or second-generation cephalosporin plus macrolide
	Suspected microaspiration, oral anaerobes: First choice: amoxicillin/clavulanate and/or macrolide or fourth-generation fluoroquinolone (e.g., moxifloxacin) Second choice: third-generation fluoroquinolone (e.g., levofloxacin) plus clindamycin or metronidazole

Table 32.4	Patients With Community-Acquired Bacterial Pneumonia Admitted to a Hospital (Modified From Karmanger, 2013)

Organisms:	*Streptococcus pneumoniae*
	Haemophilus influenzae
	Polymicrobial (including aerobic bacteria)
	Aerobic Gram-negative bacilli
	Legionella species
	Staphylococcus aureus
	Chlamydia pneumoniae
	Miscellaneous
	    Mycoplasma pneumoniae
	    Moraxella catarrhalis

Therapy:	First choice: respiratory fluoroquinolone Second choice: second- or third-generation cephalosporin plus macrolide

Table 32.5	Patients With Severe Community-Acquired Bacterial Pneumonia Admitted to an ICU
Organisms:	*Streptococcus pneumoniae* *Legionella* species Aerobic Gram-negative bacilli *Mycoplasma pneumoniae* Miscellaneous *Haemophilus influenzae*
Therapy:	First choice: antipseudomonal fluoroquinolone (e.g., ciprofloxacin) plus antipseudomonal β-lactam (e.g., ceftazidime, piperacillin-tazobactam, carbapenem) or aminoglycoside (e.g., gentamicin, tobramycin, amikacin) Second choice: triple therapy with antipseudomonal β-lactam plus aminoglycoside plus macrolide

Table 32.6	Patients With Mild to Moderate Hospital-Acquired Bacterial Pneumonia, No Unusual Risk Factors, and Onset at Any Time; or Patients With Severe Hospital-Acquired Pneumonia With Early Onset (Excludes Immunosuppressed Elderly Patients) (Modified From Karmanger, 2013)
Core organisms:	Enteric Gram-negative bacilli (Nonpseudomonal) *Enterobacter* species *Escherichia coli* *Klebsiella* species *Proteus* species *Serratia marcescens* *Haemophilus influenzae* Methicillin-sensitive *Staphylococcus aureus* *Streptococcus pneumoniae*
Core antibiotics:	Cephalosporin Second-generation or antipseudomonal third-generation β-lactam/β-lactamase inhibitor combination If allergic to penicillin, fluoroquinolone or clindamycin plus aztreonam

Table 32.7	Patients With Mild to Moderate Hospital-Acquired Bacterial Pneumonia With Risk Factors, Onset at Any Time (Modified From Karmanger, 2013)
Organisms:	Core organisms, plus one of the following: -Anaerobes (recent abdominal surgery, witnessed following aspiration) -*Staphylococcus aureus* (coma, head trauma, diabetes mellitus, and renal failure) -*Legionella* (high-dose steroids) -*Pseudomonas aeruginosa* (prolonged ICU stay, steroids, antibiotics, and structural lung disease)
Therapy:	Core antibiotics plus: -Clindamycin or β-lactam/β-lactamase inhibitor alone or with vancomycin (until methicillin-resistant *Staphylococcus aureus* is excluded) -Erythromycin, possibly with rifampin -Linezolid -Treat as severe hospital-acquired pneumonia (see Table 32.8)

Table 32.8	Patients With Severe Hospital-Acquired Bacterial Pneumonia With Risk Factors and Early Onset or Patients With Severe Hospital-Acquired Pneumonia and Late Onset.
Core organisms, plus the following:	*Pseudomonas aeruginosa* *Acinetobacter* species Consider methicillin-resistant *Staphylococcus aureus*
Therapy:	Aminoglycoside or ciprofloxacin plus one of the following: -Antipseudomonal penicillin -β-lactam/β-lactamase inhibitor -Ceftazidime or cefoperazone -Imipenem, possibly with vancomycin -Linezolid

Table 32.9 Select Pharmacological Treatment Options Based on Suspected/Known Organism

Organism	Drug	Recommended pharmacological treatment options
Haemophilus influenzae (β-lactamase positive)	Amoxicillin/clavulanate (Augmentin)	500 mg/125 mg PO every 8 hr or 875 mg/125 mg every 12 hr
	Cefuroxime (Ceftin)	500 mg PO BID
	Erythromycin (EES, Erythrocin, E-mycin) (significant resistance but active against most strains)	250–500 mg PO BID
	Clarithromycin (Biaxin) (significant resistance but active against most strains) (macrolide risks as noted above)	250–500 mg PO every 12 hr or extended-release 1000 mg BID for 7 days
	Azithromycin (Zithromax) (significant resistance but active against most strains) (macrolide risks as noted above)	Day 1: 500 mg PO Days 2–5: 250 mg/day PO
	Moxifloxacin (Avelox)	400 mg PO daily for 7–14 days
	Telithromycin (Ketek)	800 mg PO daily for 7–10 days
Haemophilus influenzae (β-lactamase negative)	Amoxicillin	500 mg–1 gram PO every 8 hr
	Amoxicillin/clavulanate (Augmentin)	500 mg/125 mg PO every 8 hr or 875 mg/125 mg every 12 hr
	Cefuroxime (Ceftin)	500 mg PO BID
	Erythromycin (EES, Erythrocin, E-mycin) (significant resistance but active against most strains)	250–500 mg PO BID
	Clarithromycin (Biaxin) (significant resistance but active against most strains)	250–500 mg PO every 12 hr or extended-release 1000 mg BID for 7 days
	Azithromycin (Zithromax) (significant resistance but active against most strains) (risks as noted previously)	Day 1: 500 mg PO Days 2–5: 250 mg/day PO
	Moxifloxacin (Avelox)	400 mg PO daily for 7–14 days
	Telithromycin (Ketek)	800 mg PO daily for 7–10 days
Streptococcus pneumoniae (resistant)	Amoxicillin (significant resistance, but active against most strains)	500 mg–1 gram PO every 8 hr (Note: Doses of 80 mg/kg/day may be effective against nonmeningeal, penicillin-resistant *Streptococcus pneumoniae*.)
	Moxifloxacin (Avelox)	400 mg PO daily for 7–14 days
	Telithromycin (Ketek)	800 mg PO daily for 7–10 days

Table 32.9	Select Pharmacological Treatment Options Based on Suspected/Known Organism	
Organism	**Drug**	**Recommended pharmacological treatment options**
Chlamydia pneumoniae	Azithromycin (Zithromax) (macrolide risks as noted above)	Day 1: 500 mg PO Days 2–5: 250 mg PO daily Community-acquired pneumonia: 500 mg PO/IV daily for 7–10 days
	Telithromycin (Ketek)	800 mg PO daily for 7–10 days
	Levofloxacin (Levaquin)	500 mg PO/IV daily for 7–14 days or 750 mg PO/IV daily for 5 days
	Moxifloxacin (Avelox)	400 mg PO daily
Legionella/ legionellosis	Erythromycin (EES, E-Mycin, Ery-Tab) (macrolide risks as noted above)	250 mg erythromycin stearate/base (or 400 mg ethylsuccinate) every 6 hr PO 1 hr before meals, or 500 mg every 12 hr or 333 mg PO every 8 hr; increase to 4 grams/day, depending on severity of infection; 15–20 mg/kg/day IV every 6 hr in divided doses; not to exceed 4 grams daily
	Levofloxacin (Levaquin)	500 mg PO/IV daily; adjust dose in renal disease
	Trovafloxacin (Trovan)	100–200 mg PO daily; 200 mg IV daily
	Azithromycin (Zithromax) (macrolide risks as noted above)	Day 1: 500 mg PO Days 2–5: 250 mg PO daily or 500 mg IV daily
	Clarithromycin (Biaxin) (macrolide risks as noted above)	250 mg PO BID; may increase to 500 mg PO 3 times a day or 500 mg PO every 12 hr
	Ciprofloxacin (Cipro)	250–750 mg PO every 12 hr; 200–400 mg IV every 12 hr
	Ofloxacin (Floxin)	400 mg PO/IV every 12 hr
	Sparfloxacin (Zagam)	200 mg PO daily
	Doxycycline (Vibramycin)	100 mg PO/IV every 12 hr
	Moxifloxacin (Avelox)	400 mg PO daily for 10 days
Streptococcus pneumoniae	Amoxicillin	500 mg–1 gram PO every 8 hr
	Amoxicillin/Clavulanate	500 mg/125 mg every 8 hr or 875 mg/125 mg every 12 hr
	Cefuroxime (Ceftin)	500 mg PO BID
	Erythromycin (EES, Erythrocin, E-mycin)	250–500 mg PO BID
	Clarithromycin (Biaxin)	250–500 mg PO every 12 hr or extended-release 1000 mg BID for 7 days
	Azithromycin (Zithromax)	Day 1: 500 mg PO Days 2–5: 250 mg/day PO
	Moxifloxacin (Avelox)	400 mg PO daily for 7–14 days
	Telithromycin (Ketek)	800 mg PO daily for 7–10 days

Table 32.9		Select Pharmacological Treatment Options Based on Suspected/Known Organism
Organism	Drug	Recommended pharmacological treatment options
Mycoplasma pneumoniae	Tetracycline (Sumycin)	500 mg PO BID for 1–4 weeks
	Erythromycin (EES, Erythrocin, E-mycin) (macrolide risks as noted above)	500 mg PO 4 times a day for 7–10 days
	Azithromycin (Zithromax) (macrolide risks as noted above)	Day 1: 500 mg PO Days 2–5: 250 mg/day PO
	Clarithromycin (Biaxin) (macrolide risks as noted above)	250–500 mg PO BID for 7–14 days
	Moxifloxacin (Avelox)	400 mg PO daily for 7–14 days
	Telithromycin (Ketek)	800 mg PO daily for 7–10 days
	Tetracycline (Sumycin)	500 mg PO 4 times a day
	Doxycycline (Vibramycin)	100 mg PO BID
	Erythromycin (EES) (macrolide risks as noted above)	500 mg PO/IV every 6 hr
	Clarithromycin (Biaxin) (macrolide risks as noted above)	500 mg PO BID or 1 gram PO every day 7–14 days

BIBLIOGRAPHY

Centers for Medicare & Medicaid Services. (2013). *2014 ICD-10 PCS and GEMs.* Retrieved November 25, 2013, from http:///www.cms.gov/Medicare/Coding/ICD10/2014-ICD-10-PCS.html

Food and Drug Administration. (2013). *FDA drug safety communication: Azithromycin (Zithromax or Zmax) and the risk of potentially fatal heart rhythms.* Retrieved November 25, 2013, from http://www.fda.gov/downloads/Drugs/DrugSafety/UCM343347.pdf

Garlington, W., & High, K. (2013). Evaluation of infection in the older adult. In D. S. Basow (Ed.), *UpToDate*. Waltham, MA: UpToDate.

Gilbert, D. N., Moellering, R. C., & Eliopoulos, G. M. (Eds.). (2013). *The Sanford guide to antimicrobial therapy 2013.* Sperryville, VA: Antimicrobial Therapy.

Goldman, L, & Shafer, A. I. (Eds.) (2012). *Goldman's Cecil medicine* (24th ed.). Philadelphia, PA: Saunders.

Kamanger, N. (2013). *Bacterial pneumonia. Practice essentials update.* Retrieved November 26, 2013, from http://emedicine.medscape.com/article/300157-overview

Longo, D. L., Kasper, D. L., Jameson, J. L., Fauci, A. S., Hauser, S. L., & Loscalzo, J. (Eds.). (2011). *Harrison's principles of internal medicine* (18th ed.). New York, NY: McGraw Hill.

Mandell, G. L., Bennett, J. E., & Dolin, R. (2010). *Principles and practice of infectious disease.* (7th ed.). Philadelphia, PA: Churchill Livingston.

Marrie, T. J. (2013). Epidemiology, pathogenesis, and microbiology of community-acquired pneumonia in adults. In D. S. Basow (Ed.), *UpToDate*. Waltham, MA: UpToDate.

CHAPTER 33

Obstructive Sleep Apnea

JENNIFER COATES • THOMAS W. BARKLEY, JR.

CHARACTERISTICS OF BREATHING AND SLEEP

A. Tidal volume and respiratory rate decline as a person becomes more deeply asleep. Skeletal muscle tone decreases progressively in deeper stages of sleep, with frank atony occurring during rapid eye movement sleep.
B. Peak airway resistance tends to be highest from 2:00 a.m. to 6:00 a.m. and lowest from 2:00 p.m. to 6:00 p.m.
C. Cough and shortness of breath may be aggravated during the normal sleeping period at night
D. Normal pauses in respiration are infrequent and brief, lasting 5–10 seconds. These pauses are central in origin and are not associated with physical obstruction of the oropharynx or hypopharynx.

OBSTRUCTIVE SLEEP APNEA (OSA)

I. **Etiology**
   A. Obstruction of the upper airway caused by loss of normal pharyngeal muscle tone during sleep
   B. Obstruction causes arousals and awakenings from sleep, and effective sleep time is reduced
II. **Incidence**
   A. The incidence is unknown. However, OSA and hypopnea are often under recognized in clinical practice.
   B. OSA is more commonly noted among obese individuals, but the absence of obesity does not rule out the possible existence of OSA.
   C. OSA is more common among males
III. **Clinical manifestations**
   A. The classic manifestation of significant OSA is excessive daytime sleepiness
   B. Snoring is commonly heard, although severe sleep apnea may be accompanied by quiet snoring
   C. Severe daytime sleepiness interferes with normal daytime functioning
      1. Additional attempts to "catch up" on sleep fail
      2. Driving a vehicle or operating heavy machinery may become dangerous

D. Hypoxemia during the apneic and hypopneic episodes may lead to adverse health consequences, including the following:
  1. Myocardial ischemia, infarction, arrhythmias, and heart failure
  2. Cerebral ischemia and stroke
  3. Sudden death
  4. Cardiorespiratory arrest after surgery or administration of sedatives, hypnotics, and opioids

IV. **Physical findings**
  A. Mental status reflects less than optimal alertness
  B. Obesity with fatty infiltration of the soft palate and pharyngeal wall can be found as well as a decrease in the posterior pharyngeal space; tonsillar enlargement, if present, aggravates the obstruction, as it does enlargement of the adenoids
  C. Right-sided heart failure, with peripheral edema, may be seen

V. **Diagnosis**
  A. Polysomnography (PSG), an overnight sleep study that measures airflow, muscle tone, and brain wave activity, is required
  B. The finding of more than 10 obstructive apneas/hypopneas (respiratory effort in the absence of, or significant reduction in, airflow during sleep) per hour is abnormal and justifies treatment, especially when oxygen desaturation values below 88% are documented.
  C. Oxygen desaturation measurements below 88% during sleep may require supplemental oxygen if therapy produces no improvement.

VI. **Treatment**
  A. General
    1. Avoidance of alcohol, sedatives, hypnotics, and opioids until effective therapy is begun
    2. Weight loss and maintenance, if indicated
    3. Avoidance of driving and operating heavy machinery until effective treated is provided and a significant reduction in daytime sleepiness is noted
  B. Specific
    1. Institution of nasal continuous positive airway pressure (nCPAP) or nasal bilevel positive airway pressure (nBIPAP) to stent the posterior pharynx
      a. Pressure is delivered by a mechanically driven device and is applied through a mask that is snugly and appropriately fitted over the nose or a pair of fitted nasal "pillows."
      b. A chin strap may be required to avoid pressure leaks through the mouth
      c. Humidification added to the mechanical circuitry may help prevent mucosal dryness
    2. Pressure needed to treat patients with OSA is usually between 5 and 15 cm H_2O and may be empirically chosen; however, optimal therapy is best determined by repeat PSG and titration of pressure to the level that fully alleviates obstructive events and oxygen desaturation.
    3. Follow-up to determine adherence to recommended therapies is crucial. The patient should use nCPAP during all sleeping periods.
  C. Other therapies
    1. Surgical removal of excessive tissue in the posterior pharynx if nCPAP or nBIPAP fails to alleviate excessive daytime sleepiness and to reduce the frequency of apnea and hypopnea and oxygen desaturation, as determined by follow-up PSG
      a. Uvulopalatopharyngoplasty (UPPP)
      b. Tonsillectomy and/or adenoidectomy
    2. Mandibular advancement to pull the tongue forward to create additional posterior pharyngeal space
    3. Oral devices to enhance the posterior pharyngeal space tend to be uncomfortable and, therefore, are ineffective in treating patients with OSA.

4. Tracheostomy relieves OSA promptly and was the definitive therapy before nCPAP became available. It is now reserved for those individuals with severe disease who are unable to use nCPAP or nBIPAP, or who are not candidates for surgical resection of redundant tissue.

VII. **Gerontologic considerations**
  A. The prevalence of OSA increases with age. Untreated OSA may increase the risk of metabolic syndrome or early mortality.
  B. Cognitive changes may be present in elderly patients with OSA; experts are unsure if these effects are due to hypoxia, hypersomnolence, or both. These changes may include the following:
    1. Impairments in attention
    2. Impairments in concentration
    3. Difficulty with executive functioning
    4. Working memory less
  C. Treatment with nCPAP or nBIPAP may improve cognitive functioning

BIBLIOGRAPHY

Downey, R., Gold, P. M., Rowley, J. A., & Wickramasinghe, H. (2014). Obstructive sleep apnea. *Medscape*. Retrieved from http://emedicine.medscape.com/article/295807-overview#showall

Epstein, L. J., Kristo, D., Strollo, P. J., Friedman, N., Malhotra, A., Patil, S. P., . . . Weinstein, M. D. (2009). Adult Obstructive Sleep Apnea Task Force of the American Academy of Sleep Medicine. Clinical guideline for the evaluation, management and long term care of obstructive sleep apnea in adults. *Journal of Clinical Sleep Medicine, 5*, 263–276.

Halter, J., Ouslander, J., Tinetti, M., Studenski, S., High, K., & Asthana, S. (2009, March 9). *Hazzard's geriatric medicine and gerontology* (6th ed.). New York, NY: McGraw-Hill Professional.

Kryger, M., Roth, T., & Dement, W. (2010). *Principles and practice of sleep medicine* (5th ed.). Philadelphia, PA: Elsevier.

Longo, D., Fauci, A., Kasper, D., Hauser S., Jameson, J., & Loscalzo, J. (2012). *Harrison's principles of internal medicine* (18th ed.). New York, NY: McGraw-Hill.

McPhee, S. J., & Papadakis, M. A. (2014). *Current medical diagnosis and treatment* (53rd ed.). New York, NY: McGraw Hill Lange.

Olaithe, M., & Bucks, R. S. (2013). Executive dysfunction in OSA before and after treatment. *Sleep, 36*, 1297.

Vasu, T. S., Grewal, R., Doghramji, K. (2012) Obstructive sleep apnea syndrome and perioperative complications: A systematic review of the literature. *Journal of Clinical Sleep Medicine, 8*, 199–207.

CHAPTER 34

Oxygen Supplementation

CAROL THOMPSON • THOMAS W. BARKLEY, JR. • CHARLENE M. MYERS

BASIC PRINCIPLES OF OXYGEN SUPPLEMENTATION

I. **The goal of oxygen supplementation is to increase the fraction of inspired oxygen (FIO_2).**
   A. The diffusion gradient is increased, thereby facilitating an increased partial pressure of oxygen in arterial blood (PaO_2)
II. **Supplemental oxygen supply is accessed through a wall source or a portable oxygen cylinder.**
   A. Wall oxygen is sourced from outlets fed from a large bulk tank outside the facility
      1. Supplied at a constant pressure of 50 lb per square inch (PSI)
      2. Requires only a flowmeter (Thorpe tube) for delivery
      3. Duration of flow is generally not an issue for the clinician
   B. Cylinder oxygen is sourced from portable metal cylinders of various sizes
      1. Cylinder sizes are identified in descending order by letter designations H, E, D, B, A, AA, and DD
         a. The most common cylinder for providing portable oxygen in the hospital is the E cylinder
      2. All cylinders have a pressure of 2200 PSI when full
         a. Pressure will fall as oxygen in the cylinder is used
         b. Oxygen supply should be considered unreliable at less than 500 PSI
      3. Cylinders require a regulator for reduction of pressure and control of flow
         a. Pressure is maintained at constant 50 PSI despite changing pressure within the cylinder
         b. Flow is metered by a Bourdon gauge
      4. When portable oxygen is needed, duration of flow is an important consideration (i.e., "How long will this tank last?")
         a. Duration of flow in minutes is calculated by multiplying the PSI (subtract 500 for safety buffer) by the "cylinder factor" (0.28 for an E cylinder), then dividing by liters per minute of flow. The D cylinder factor is 0.16 and M cylinder factor is 1.56.
         b. Example: [(2200 - 500) x 0.28] ÷ 4 = 119 minutes
         c. A full E cylinder that delivers 4 L per minute should safely last about 2 hr

C. Oxygen outlets, meters, gauges, and tanks are color coded (green) to distinguish them from other gases (various colors) or suction sources (white).
   1. Caution is required because neighboring Canadian standards color code oxygen as white
   2. Always read label on the cylinder
III. **Oxygen supplementation is indicated when an actual or potential deficit of global or specific tissue oxygenation is present.**
   A. Deficit may result from decreased supply of oxygen or increased demand for oxygen (or combination)
      1. Decreased supply may be due to ventilation, diffusion, or perfusion defects (or combination)
         a. Ventilation defect examples
            i. Overdose
            ii. Sedation
            iii. Flail chest
            iv. Asthma
         b. Diffusion defect examples
            i. Pneumonia
            ii. Acute respiratory distress syndrome (ARDS)
            iii. CHF
            iv. Chronic obstructive pulmonary disease (COPD)
         c. Perfusion defect examples
            i. Shock
            ii. Anemia
            iii. Hypovolemia
            iv. Stroke
            v. Angina/MI
            vi. Sickle cell crisis
      2. Increased demand may be due to exertion or hypermetabolic states.
         a. Examples of exertion
            i. Fatigue
            ii. Seizures
         b. Examples of hypermetabolism
            i. Hyperthermia
            ii. Hyperthyroidism
   B. Supplemental oxygen should be provided at the lowest FIO_2 that will abolish significant threats of real or potential tissue oxygenation deficits.
      1. Avoid FIO_2 that exceeds 0.50 for longer than 24 hr
         a. Risk for effects of oxygen toxicity
            i. Alveolar damage
            ii. Loss of surfactant
            iii. Atelectasis
      2. Anticipate risk of ventilatory suppression in patients with history of carbon dioxide retention (e.g., COPD)
         a. Avoid overcorrection of mild hypoxemia (may depress primary ventilatory stimulus), especially if unable to closely monitor
         b. Severe hypoxemia (may result in tissue damage) should be corrected with anticipation of risk for ventilatory suppression (prepare for ventilatory assistance)
   C. Assess frequently (at least daily) for need to continue supplementation
      1. Wean or discontinue supplemental oxygen as indicated by confidence for the following:
         a. PaO_2 greater than 60
         b. Oxygen saturation (SaO_2) greater than 90%
         c. Potential threat ruled out or abolished
         d. No overt distress

FACILITATION OF VENTILATION

I. **Occasionally, patients are unable to maintain spontaneous ventilation.**
   A. Examples:
      1. Impaired structure
         a. Trauma (flail chest, pneumothorax)
         b. Decreased compliance (ARDS)
         c. COPD
      2. Impaired function
         a. CNS depression (drugs, spinal cord injury [SCI])
   B. Patients require both oxygen supplementation and ventilatory assistance
II. **Airway maintenance and bag-valve-mask ventilation are the first lines of ventilatory assistance in the clinical setting.**
   A. Airway maintenance focuses on upper airway patency
      1. Primary actions to ensure patency such as proper head position and jaw thrust maneuver are well covered in basic and advanced life support courses
         a. Proper head position includes positioning to avoid aspiration of emesis
      2. Secondary actions to ensure patency consist of effective upper airway suction efforts (using Yankauer suction handle)
      3. Tertiary actions to ensure patency may include insertion of oropharyngeal airway
         a. May not be tolerated by conscious patient
         b. Proper insertion technique is needed to avoid trauma and airway compromise
         c. Insert by sliding lateral to the tongue and then rotating the tip to the posterior part of the tongue
         d. Secure and monitor closely to avoid or detect displacement and airway compromise
   B. Bag-valve-mask ventilation focuses on delivery of adequate tidal volume and FIO_2.
      1. Self-inflating bag provides reservoir for oxygen and means of delivering volume
         a. High-flow oxygen (12–15 L/minute) produces FIO_2 of near 1 (100%) in the reservoir
         b. Manual compression of the bag displaces reservoir volume into the airway through positive pressure
         c. Degree to which the bag is compressed determines volume delivered
      2. Valve prevents aspiration of expired air into the bag-reservoir during bag reinflation
      3. Sealing of the upper airway with a mask is required for positive-pressure ventilation
         a. Improper seal will result in failure to deliver volume and FIO_2
         b. Efforts to produce a seal must include maintenance of head and jaw position to avoid compromise of airway patency
         c. The "C-E grip" with thumb and forefinger (forming C) around the bag/mask junction and the third, fourth, and fifth fingers (forming E) hooked under the end of the jaw can be effective in producing a seal.
         d. Assistance provided by a second person is preferred but may be required if teeth/dentures are absent.
      4. Mouth-to-mouth ventilation should be considered "last resort" in clinical settings.
         a. Ventilation with exhaled air via mouth-to-mouth delivers decreased FIO_2 (0.16 vs 0.21) and increased carbon dioxide (CO_2) (0.05 vs greater than 0.01).
         b. Oral shielding device such as a pocket mask should be used to prevent body fluid exposure of both victim and rescuer
   C. Even well-administered mouth-to-mouth breathing delivers an FIO_2 of only 16% to 17%, compared with 21% oxygen in room air.
III. **A pocket mask device allows mouth-to-mouth ventilation without personal contact.**
   A. Some pocket masks have a port that allows administration of supplemental oxygen
   B. Pocket mask devices are eminently portable

CHAPTER **34**   **Oxygen Supplementation**

IV. Bag-valve-mask devices
  A. Bag-valve-mask devices allow administration of supplemental oxygen via a face mask and a reservoir bag
  B. Depending on oxygen flow and operator skill, high concentrations of oxygen may be administered
  C. Self-inflating bags are as follows:
   1. Versatile
   2. Can be used with or without supplemental oxygen
   3. Available in various sizes appropriate for infants, children, and adults
  D. The major complication of a bag-valve-mask device involves inflation of the stomach resulting from poor airway maintenance or high ventilation pressures.
   1. Be alert for the development of gastric distention
   2. Relieve distention through placement of a nasogastric tube
   3. Do not compress the distended stomach manually; emesis may result
  E. The mask is an essential component of the device and should be sized to the patient.
   1. A well-fitting mask with a seal that encompasses the nose and the mouth is important in ensuring adequate ventilation.
   2. The mask should be clear to allow visualization of emesis.
  F. The airway in an unconscious patient is more easily maintained with an oropharyngeal airway.
   1. The device will lift the tongue from the posterior pharynx.
   2. Oropharyngeal airways are not tolerated by patients with intact gag reflexes.
   3. A small degree of skill is required for placement of the oropharyngeal airway.
      a. Inept placement may traumatize the soft tissues of the oropharynx or may occlude the airway
      b. To safely place the airway, the following steps must be taken:
         i. Open the patient's mouth
         ii. Move the tongue aside with a tongue blade
         iii. Insert the oropharyngeal airway with the tip pointing laterally, then rotate once posterior to the tongue
  G. A nasopharyngeal airway is a soft plastic device placed through the nares that provides a passage through the posterior pharynx
   1. Lubrication with lidocaine jelly facilitates placement and enhances patient tolerance
   2. A nasopharyngeal airway is usually tolerated by a conscious patient.
   3. Nasopharyngeal airways are especially useful in the following patients:
      a. Those with orofacial trauma
      b. Those in whom the oropharynx is not accessible

V. Suction devices are an important adjunct to ventilation.
  A. Sudden cessation of ventilation may be due to airway occlusion caused by emesis or a mucous plug
  B. Accumulation of saliva and airway secretions can also cause occlusion
  C. A rigid suction device (e.g., Yankauer suction) is generally more useful than a flexible catheter for airway maintenance in the posterior pharynx.

DEVICES FOR OXYGEN SUPPLEMENTATION

I. Nasal prongs are the simplest means of delivering supplemental oxygen.
  A. Inspired room air is mixed with oxygen that has been stored in the reservoir (nasal cavity).
   1. Prongs deliver oxygen into the nasal cavity, which acts as a reservoir.
   2. Inspiratory air flow through the oropharynx creates lower pressure at the posterior nasopharynx (Bernoulli's principle), and oxygen stored in nasal cavity is drawn in via the nasopharynx.

B. FIO_2 is generally determined by liter flow of oxygen per minute (L/minute) into the reservoir (nasal cavity).
   1. Generally ordered in terms of L/minute up to maximum of 6 L/minute
   2. As a general rule, each L/minute of oxygen flow increases FIO_2 by approximately 0.04 (4%).
      a. For 2 L/minute, FIO_2 is approximately 0.28–0.32
      b. For 4 L/minute, FIO_2 is approximately 0.35–0.38
      c. For 6 L/minute, FIO_2 is approximately 0.42–0.45
   3. Oral breathing is assumed; only a patent nasal airway is required
C. Advantages
   1. Well tolerated during eating, speaking, or activity
   2. Relatively inexpensive, simple to use
D. Disadvantages
   1. Effectiveness can be sensitive to placement
      a. Prongs must be within nares to be effective
   2. May require humidification to prevent drying of nasal mucosa
      a. Always use humidification at flows greater than 3 L/minute
   3. Caution is required to prevent pressure injury at contact points over ears, cheeks, and nares

II. **Face masks can provide a higher FIO_2 than is attained with nasal prongs.**
   A. A properly functioning face mask can provide an FIO_2 level of 0.40 to almost 1 (100%).
   B. Supplemental oxygen masks do not require a tight seal to the face.
      1. Mask design assumes or prevents entrainment of room air under edge of mask
   C. Simple face masks use relatively low flow rates (5–8 L/minute).
      1. Low flow allows room air to be entrained under edge of mask on inspiration.
         a. FIO_2 is imprecise and is limited to less than 0.6 because of variable mixing with room air.
      2. Lower cost and less drying than with nasal cannula
      3. Patients may feel claustrophobic, which may interfere with eating or speaking.
   D. Venturi masks use velocity to create pressure gradient for more precise control of FIO_2 up to 0.6
      1. Oxygen is funneled through Venturi nozzle past "window" entraining room air (Bernoulli's principle) precisely to desired FIO_2
         a. Size of Venturi or window may be adjusted to produce desired FIO_2
      2. High-velocity flow into confined space of mask produces pressure greater than room air
         a. Inhaled air comes from precise FIO_2 in mask
         b. No room air pulled under edge of mask to dilute FIO_2
      3. More expensive but produces more reliable FIO_2; otherwise, same advantages and disadvantages as simple mask
   E. Non-rebreather masks use high flow rates (11–15 L/minute), reservoir bags, and valves to deliver FIO_2 near 100%
      1. High rate of flow fills large-volume reservoir bag with 100% oxygen with greater pressure than room air.
         a. Reservoir bag must be fully distended for proper function
         b. Inhaled volume comes from high-pressure reservoir bag with FIO_2 near 1
         c. High-pressure source prevents entrainment or room air under edge of mask
      2. Exhalation into mask closes one-way valve, preventing mixing with inhaled air source
         a. Exhaled air is blown out under edge of mask and is, thus, not "re-breathed."
      3. Can deliver maximal oxygen supplementation short of assisted ventilation device
      4. Expensive and bulky; otherwise, similar advantages and disadvantages as other masks

BIBLIOGRAPHY

Boyer, A., Vargas, F., Delacre, M., Saint-Léger, M., Clouzeau, B., Hilbert, G., & Gruson, D. (2011). Prognostic impact of high-flow nasal cannula oxygen supply in an ICU patient with pulmonary fibrosis complicated by acute respiratory failure. *Intensive Care Medicine, 37,* 558–559. doi: 10.1007/s00134–010–2036–9

Considine, J., Botti, M., & Thomas, S. (2012). Descriptive analysis of emergency department oxygen use in acute exacerbation of chronic obstructive pulmonary disease. *Internal Medicine Journal, 42,* e38-e47. doi:10.1111/j.1445–5994.2010.02220.x

Gerstein, N. S., Carey, M. C., Braude, D. A., Tawil, I., Persen, T. R., Deriy, L., & Anderson, M. S. (2013). Efficacy of facemask ventilation techniques in novice providers. *Journal of Clinical Anesthesia, 25,* 193–197. Retrieved from http://dx.doi.org/10.1016/j.jclinane.2012.10.009

Ehrenwerth, J., Elsenkraft, J. B., & Berry, F. M. (2013). *Anesthesia equipment: Principles and applications.* Philadelphia, PA: Saunders.

Hegde, S. & Prodhan, P. (2013). Serious air leak syndrome complicating high-flow nasal cannula therapy: A report of 3 cases. *Pediatrics, 131,* e939–944. doi:10.1542/peds.2011–3767

Hemmings, H. C., & Egan, T. D. (2013). *Pharmacology and physiology for anesthesia: Foundations and clinical applications.* Philadelphia, PA: Elsevier/Saunders.

Lee, J. H., Rehder, K. J., Williford, L., Cheifetz, I. M., & Turner, D. A. (2013). Use of high flow nasal cannula in critically ill infants, children, and adults: A critical review of the literature. *Intensive Care Medicine, 39,* 247–257. doi:10.1007/s00134–012–2743–5

Martí, S., Pajares, V., Morante, F., Ramón, M., Lara, J., Ferrer, J. & Güell, M. (2013). Are oxygen-conserving devices effective for correcting exercise hypoxemia? *Respiratory Care, 58,* 1606–1613. doi:10.4187/respcare.02260

Peel, D., Neighbour, R., & Eltringham, R. J. (2013). Evaluation of oxygen concentrators for use in countries with limited resources. *Anaesthesia, 68,* 706–712. doi:10.1111/anae.12260

Restrepo, R., D., Hirst, K. R., Wittnebel, L., & Wettstein, R. (2012). AARC clinical practice guidelines: Transcutaneous monitoring of carbon dioxide and oxygen: 2012. *Respiratory Care, 57,* 1955–1962. doi:10.4187/respcare.02011

Rice, K. L., Schmidt, M. F., Buan, J. S., Lebahn, F., & Schwarzock, T. K. (2011). Accu[Osub2] oximetry-driven oxygen-conserving device versus fixed-dose oxygen devices in stable COPD patients. *Respiratory Care, 56,* 1901–1905. doi:10.4187/respcare.01059

Ritchie, J. E., Williams, A. B., Gerard, C., & Hockey, H. (2011). Evaluation of a humidified nasal high-glow oxygen system, using oxygraph, capnography and measurement of upper airway pressures. *Anaesthesia Intensive Care, 39*(6), 1103–1110.

Schibler, A., Pham, T. M., Dunster, K. R., Foster, K., Barlow, A., Gibbons, K., & Hough, J. L. (2011). Reduced intubation rates for infants after introduction of high-flow nasal prong oxygen delivery. *Intensive Care Medicine, 37,* 847–853. doi:10.1007/s00134–011–2177–5

Urbano, J., Castillo, J., López-Herce, J., Gallardo, J. A., Solana, M. J., & Carrillo, Á. (2012). High-flow oxygen therapy: Pressure analysis in a pediatric airway model. *Respiratory Care, 57,* 721–726. doi:10.4187/respcare.01386

CHAPTER 35

Mechanical Ventilatory Support

AMITA AVADHANI • THOMAS W. BARKLEY, JR. • CHARLENE M. MYERS

INDICATIONS FOR MECHANICAL VENTILATION

I. **Inadequate intrinsic respiratory capacity to prevent or compensate for severe hypoxia and/or hypercarbia due to the following:**
   A. Neuromuscular (NM) depression or failure
      1. Drugs
         a. Opioids
         b. Sedatives
         c. NM blockers
      2. Trauma
         a. Spinal cord injury
         b. Phrenic nerve injury
      3. Disease
         a. Guillain-Barré syndrome
         b. Amyotrophic lateral sclerosis
         c. Myasthenia gravis
         d. Shock
      4. Exhaustion
         a. Status asthmaticus
         b. Sustained severe work of breathing
      5. Sustained apnea of any cause
   B. Persistent hypoxia (partial pressure of oxygen in arterial blood [PaO_2] less than 60 mmHg) and/or hypercarbia (partial pressure of carbon dioxide in arterial blood [$PaCO_2$] greater than 50 mmHg) refractory to noninvasive supplemental oxygen and/or airway maintenance (suction and position)
      1. Diffusion defects
         a. Aspiration
         b. Pulmonary edema
         c. Acute respiratory distress syndrome
         d. Chronic obstructive pulmonary disease
         e. Pneumonia

CHAPTER **35** Mechanical Ventilatory Support

   2. Ventilation defects
      a. Chronic obstructive pulmonary disease
      b. Pickwickian syndrome
      c. Flail chest
      d. Pneumothorax
      e. Atelectasis
   3. Perfusion defects
      a. Shock
      b. Pulmonary embolus
      c. Malignant arrhythmias

GENERAL PRINCIPLES OF VENTILATION

I. **Inspiratory airflow occurs as the result of a pressure gradient in which extrapulmonary pressure is greater than intrapulmonary pressure.**
   A. This can result from lowering intrapulmonary pressure to below extrapulmonary pressure or by raising extrapulmonary pressure to above intrapulmonary pressure.
      1. Normal human inspiration occurs when chest volume is expanded by contraction of the diaphragm and elevation of the ribs, creating a negative intrapulmonary pressure and drawing air into the lungs. ("People suck to breathe.")
      2. Mechanical ventilation creates positive extrapulmonary pressure generated by a device that forces air into the lungs. ("Ventilators blow to breathe.")
         a. Positive-pressure ventilation requires a sealed airway, most commonly attained by an endotracheal tube (ETT) with an inflatable cuff.
II. **Expiratory airflow occurs as the result of a pressure gradient in which intrapulmonary pressure is raised to above extrapulmonary pressure.**
   A. Normal expiration, whether inspiration is spontaneous or mechanical, relies on passive elastic recoil of lung tissue and of chest wall muscles
      1. Chest wall and abdominal musculature can actively augment passive elastic recoil
      2. Mechanical positive-pressure ventilators cannot create an expiratory pressure gradien

VARIABLES FOR MECHANICAL VENTILATORS

I. **Tidal volume refers to the volume of air entering (inhaled) or leaving (exhaled) the lungs with each breath.**
   A. When a ventilator mode uses a target tidal volume in adults, the settings should be in the range of 6–8 ml/kg ideal body weight in adults. (The goal is not to exceed the plateau pressure of 30 cm of H_2O to prevent barotrauma.)
      1. The most common practice is to approximate tidal volume within 50 ml (400, 450, 500, 550, etc.) and then to adjust the effect
      2. To avoid barotrauma, minimal effective tidal volume should be used
   B. When the target is airway pressure, tidal volume may vary with compliance
II. **Rate is the number of mechanical breaths delivered each minute**
   A. A mechanical breath cycle may be defined by a tidal volume target or by a pressure target
   B. Set ventilator rates will be adjusted to achieve pH and $PaCO_2$ goals
III. **Fraction of inspired oxygen (FIO_2) is the decimal value produced by dividing partial pressure of oxygen (PO_2) by total pressure of the mixture.**
   A. FIO_2 is most correctly expressed by a decimal value rather than a percentage
      1. FIO_2 of room air is approximately 0.21
      2. FIO_2 of 100% oxygen is 1
   B. FIO_2 settings on ventilators typically range from 0.35–1, depending on patient requirements
      1. FIO_2 that exceeds 0.5 for longer than 24 hr may result in oxygen toxicity
IV. **Inspiratory cycles vary as follows**
   A. Volume cycled: pressure limited (volume targeted)

1. A preset tidal volume is delivered unless a set pressure limit is reached, terminating the cycle.
   a. Ensures that tidal volume is not determined by compliance but has higher risk of barotrauma
B. Pressure cycled: volume limited (pressure targeted)
   1. A preset pressure is delivered unless a volume limit is reached, terminating the cycle
      a. Allows more natural tidal volume with less risk of barotrauma
      b. Rate may have to be adjusted to compensate for variable tidal volumes

V. **Positive end-expiratory pressure (PEEP) prevents the return of intrapulmonary pressure to equal extrapulmonary pressure at the end of expiration.**
   A. Effect is that of an incomplete expiration: increased functional residual volume (FRV) remains
      1. The result of increased FRV is twofold
         a. A greater number of alveoli opened for gas exchange throughout ventilatory cycle
         b. Additional alveoli opened at peak inspiration because of tidal volume "stacked" on increased functional residual volume
   B. Effect of increased alveolar ventilation is twofold
      1. Increased PaO_2 without increase in FIO_2
      2. Reduced atelectasis
   C. Risks
      1. Barotrauma due to hyperdistention and high intrapulmonary pressures
      2. Impedance of central venous return, resulting in lower cardiac output
         a. Most significant with low central venous pressure or right ventricular diastolic dysfunction
         b. Increased intracranial pressure
   D. Typical PEEP settings range from 5–10 cm H_2O
      1. "Higher" PEEP up to 10–20 cm H_2O may be used with low-compliance conditions such as acute respiratory distress syndrome

VI. **Continuous positive airway pressure (CPAP) is functionally equivalent to PEEP**
   A. CPAP is effectively PEEP without mechanically delivered inspirations (rate = 0)
   B. Patient must have independent inspiratory capability
   C. Has the same risks and benefits as PEEP

VII. **Pressure support reflects an augmentation of flow rate during spontaneous inspiration**
   A. The result is to overcome resistance to flow through ventilator circuit (valves, corrugated tubing, and narrow lumina), thus reducing spontaneous inspiratory effort or work of breathing.
   B. At higher levels of pressure, it can provide full ventilatory support

VIII. **Alarms alert the clinician to unacceptable deviations from various critical ventilator variables**
   A. High-pressure alarms when proximal airway pressures exceed set limits
      1. Secretion accumulation
      2. Patient coughing
      3. Spontaneous dyssynchrony
      4. Decreasing compliance
      5. Pneumothorax
      6. Airway occlusion
   B. Low-pressure alarms when proximal airway pressure does not reflect current ventilator function
      1. Disconnected tubing
      2. ETT cuff leak
   C. Low-volume alarms when volume returned to the ventilator is less than the set limit

1. May result from disconnecting tubing, from ETT cuff leak
2. May result from decreased patient tidal volumes (shallow breaths)
D. Low FIO_2 alarms if below set FIO_2
   1. Interruption in oxygen supply
E. Apnea alarms if no spontaneous or mechanical breath detected within set time frame
   1. Patient apnea
   2. Mechanical failure

MODES OF MECHANICAL VENTILATION

I. **Controlled mandatory ventilation**
   A. Patient receives only set tidal volume at a set rate
      1. Patient cannot add spontaneous breaths
         a. Sedation and/or NM blockade will be required to reduce anxiety and prevent interference with ventilator function
      2. Minute volume will be equal to set rate x set tidal volume

II. **Assist control ventilation**
   A. Patient will receive set tidal volume at set rate
      1. Patient can add spontaneous breaths but will receive set tidal volume with the initiation of each spontaneous breath
         a. The delivery of ventilator breaths will not be synchronized with spontaneous breaths.
         b. Sedation may be required to prevent hyperventilation (hypocarbia) and ventilator dyssynchrony.
      2. Minute volume will be equal to (set rate + spontaneous rate) x set tidal volume

III. **Intermittent mandatory ventilation (IMV)**
   A. Patient will receive set tidal volume at set rate
      1. Patient can add spontaneous breaths at own tidal volume
         a. The delivery of ventilator breaths may not be synchronized with spontaneous breaths (IMV)
         b. The delivery of ventilator breaths can be synchronized with spontaneous breaths (synchronized IMV)
      2. Minute volume will be equal to (set rate x set tidal volume) + (spontaneous rate x own tidal volume)
      3. Typically used with pressure support ventilation, which augments spontaneous breaths and minute volume

IV. **Pressure control ventilation**
   A. The patient will receive a set rate delivered up to a set pressure.
   B. The tidal volume will vary with each breath according to compliance, and minute volume may be adversely affected with poor compliance if the tidal volumes are very low.
   C. May be used with inverse ratio ventilation
      1. Inspiratory time is lengthened, and expiratory time is shortened
      2. Barotrauma risk is reduced
      3. Oxygenation may be improved

SPECIAL ASPECTS OF VENTILATOR MANAGEMENT

I. **Ventilator settings: mode, rate, tidal volume, PEEP, and FiO_2 written as: mode/FiO_2/tidal volume/rate/PEEP/PS**
   A. Example: assist control (AC) / 1 (100%) / 14 / 450 / +5 / +5
II. **Assessment**
   A. Complete physical assessment of all organ systems is warranted
   B. Particular attention to respiratory assessment is required

1. Observe for distress, cyanosis, symmetry, spontaneous/mechanical ratio, location, and placement (centimeter mark at lips) of ETT
2. Palpate for fremitus, crepitus, and subcutaneous emphysema
3. Auscultate for the following:
   a. Bilateral and equal distribution of normal breath sounds
   b. Adventitious sounds
   c. Evidence of ETT cuff leak
4. Percuss for hyperresonance

III. Airway management
A. Humidification is essential to avoid extreme drying of respiratory mucosa
   1. A heat-moisture exchanger is an "artificial nose" that traps expired moisture to humidify inspired air.
      a. Placed in ventilator tubing near ETT
   2. Cascade acts as "bubbler" to humidify oxygen before it enters the inspiratory circuit
B. ETT cuff pressure should be adequate to seal the airway but not exceed the capillary filling pressure of the tracheal mucosa.
   1. Optimal pressure can be approximated with the minimal leak technique.
      a. Use syringe to add or remove air in the cuff until very minimal air leak is auscultated
   2. More precisely, optimal cuff pressure can be obtained with the use of a bulb manometer to adjust pressure to 2–4 mmHg below average capillary filling pressure of 25–28 mmHg
      a. Be aware of conditions in which capillary filling pressures are below average
C. ETT position should not extend the distal tip beyond the level of the carina
   1. ETT 22-cm mark even with lips is a good approximation for most adults
   2. On chest x-ray, tip of ETT should be 2–4 cm above the carina
   3. Breath sounds should be audible bilaterally

IV. Suctioning
A. Suction only as necessary
B. Use small catheter with only moderate suction
C. Oxygenate pre-peri-post to maximize oxygen saturation (SaO_2)
D. Minimize or avoid the use of saline lavage to prevent iatrogenic pneumonia
E. Make no more than a three 10-second suction passes before allowing the patient to rest
F. Monitor vitals, pulse oximetry, and SpO_2
G. Perform subglottal suction to reduce risks of aspiration and ventilator-related pneumonia
H. In-line suction systems reduce risks of hypoxemia and ventilator-related pneumonia.

V. Nutrition
A. Feed early and adequately
B. Consider placement of a small-bore feeding tube beyond the pylorus to reduce risks of reflux and aspiration pneumonia

VI. Weaning from mechanical ventilation
A. The basic requirement is that the initial indication for ventilation has been improved or eliminated
B. Other factors will affect readiness to wean:
   1. Time on ventilator
   2. Psychological readiness
   3. Nutritional status
   4. Ability to clear airway (cough)
   5. Hemodynamic stability
C. Assessing readiness to wean
   1. Conduct a spontaneous breathing trial daily when the following conditions are met:
      a. FiO_2 of 0.40 or less and PEEP of 8 or less
      b. PEEP and FiO_2 less than or equal the values of previous day

c. Patient has acceptable spontaneous breathing efforts (may decrease vent rate by 50% for 5 minutes to detect effort)
d. Systolic BP of 90 mmHg or more without vasopressor support
e. No NM blocking agents or blockade (acute respiratory distress syndrome network protocol)
2. Additional factors to consider before attempting weaning:
   a. Physical ability
      i. Respiratory rate less than 30 breaths per minute
      ii. Minute ventilation less than 12 L/minute
   b. Mechanical efficiency
      i. Vital capacity 10–15 ml/kg
      ii. Negative inspiratory force greater than 20 cm H_2O
   c. Oxygenation and ventilation
      i. PaO_2 greater than 60 on FIO_2 less than 0.50
      ii. $PaCO_2$ less than 50 with pH 7.35–7.45
      iii. PEEP +5 or less with SaO_2 greater than 92%
   d. Hemodynamics
      i. Cardiac index greater than 2.3 L/min/m^2, mean arterial pressure less than 60 mmHg, heart rate less than 120 beats per minute and more than 60 beats per minute, and pulmonary capillary wedge pressure less than 18 mmHg
   e. Secretions
      i. Not copious, easily coughed to tip of ETT for suction
D. Techniques
   1. Spontaneous breathing trial for 30–120 minutes
      a. If trial is successful, patient usually will tolerate extubation
      b. If trial is not tolerated, weaning should be delayed until the next day
      c. Trials should take place daily until patient is ready to be extubated, or a different method is determined to be more effective.
   2. Alternate periods on ventilator and CPAP to condition respiratory muscles
   3. Use pressure support to minimize ventilator-induced work of breathing
E. Extubation
F. Criteria for termination of wean
   1. Opposite of readiness to wean
   2. Do early in day
   3. Patient should be rested, aware, and cooperative
   4. Have suction, O_2 device, and reintubation equipment close at hand
   5. Elevate head of bed (HOB)
   6. Suction well
   7. Extubate
   8. Monitor closely

BIBLIOGRAPHY

Bagga, S., Paluzzi, D. E., Chen, C. Y., Riggio, J. M., Nagaraja, M., Marik, P. E., & Baram, M. (2014). Improved compliance with lower tidal volumes for initial ventilation setting—using a Computerized Clinical Decision Support System. *Respiratory Care, 59*(8), 1172–1177. doi:10.4187/respcare.02223

Beaudin, A. E., Walsh, M. L., & White, M. D. (2012). Central chemoreflex ventilatory responses in humans following passive heat acclimation. *Respiratory Physiology & Neurobiology, 180*(1), 97–104. doi:10.1016/j.resp.2011.10.014

Burkhart, C. S., Dell-Kuster, S., Gamberini, M., Moeckli, A., Grapow, M., Filipovic, M., . . . Steiner, L. A. (2010). Modifiable and non-modifiable risk factors for postoperative delirium after cardiac bypass surgery with cardiopulmonary bypass. *Journal of Cardiothoracic and Vascular Anesthesia, 24*(4), 555–559. doi:10.1053/j.jvca.2010.01.003

Cairo, J. M. (2012). *Pilbeam's Mechanical Ventilation: Physiological and clinical applications* (5th ed.). St Louis, MO: Elsevier Mosby.

Carpene, N., Vagheggini, G., Panait, E., Gabbrielli, L., & Ambrosino, N. (2010). A proposal of a new model of long-term weaning: Respiratory intensive care unit and weaning center. *Respiratory Medicine, 104*(10), 1505–1511. doi:10.1016/j.rmed.2010.05.012

Carter, A., Fletcher, S. J., & Tuffin, R. (2013). The effect of inner tube placement on resistance and work of breathing through tracheostomy tubes: A bench test. *Anesthesia, 68*(3), 276–282. doi:10.1111/anae.12094

Chui, K. K., & Lusardi, M. M. (2012). Aging and activity tolerance: Implications for orthotic and prosthetic rehabilitation. In M. M. Lusardi, M. Jorge, & C. C. Nielsen (Eds.), *Orthotics and prosthetics in rehabilitation* (3rd ed., pp. 14–37). Philadelphia, PA: Elsevier Saunders.

Finucane, B. T., Tsui, B. C. H., & Santora, A. H. (2010). *Principles of airway management* (4th ed.). New York, NY: Springer.

Güldner, A., Carvalho, N. C., Pelosi, P., & Gama de Abreu, M. (2012). Biphasic PAP/airway pressure release ventilation in ALI. In M. Ferrer and P. Pelosi (Eds.), *European Respiratory Monograph 55: New developments in mechanical ventilation* (pp. 81–96). Sheffield, UK: European Respiratory Society.

Haas, C. F., & Loik, P. S. (2012). Ventilator discontinuation protocols. *Respiratory Care, 57*(10), 1649–1662. doi:10.4187/respcare.01895

Hasan, A. (2010). *Understanding mechanical ventilation: A practical handbook.* London, UK: Springer-Verlag.

Hess, D. R. (2011). Patient-ventilator interaction during noninvasive ventilation. *Respiratory Care, 56*(2), 153–167. doi:10.4187/respcare.01049

Hraiech, S., Brégeon, F., Brunel, J.-M., Rolain, J.-M., Lepidi, H., Andrieu, V., . . . Roch, A. (2012). Antibacterial efficacy of inhaled squalamine in a rat model of chronic *Pseudomonas aeruginosa* pneumonia. *Journal of Antimicrobial Chemotherapy, 67*(10), 2452–2458. doi:10.1093/jac/dks230

Kahn, A., Gnanapandithan, K., & Agarwal, R. (2011). Weaning from mechanical ventilation. In P. S. Shankar, S. Raoof, & D. Gupta (Eds.), *Textbook of pulmonary and critical care medicine, Vols. 1 and 2* (pp. 1974–1982). New Delhi: Jaypee Brothers Medical Publishers Ltd.

Krüger, W., & Ludman, A. J. (2014). *Core knowledge of critical care medicine.* New York, NY: Springer.

Marchese, S., Corrado, A., Scala, R., Corrao, S., & Ambrosino, N. (2010). Tracheostomy in patients with long-term mechanical ventilation: A survey. *Respiratory Medicine, 104*(5), 749–753. doi:10.1016/j.rmed.2010.01.003

Mittal, M. K., & Wijdicks, E. F. M. (2013). Muscular paralysis: Myasthenia gravis and Guillain-Barré syndrome. In J. E. Parrillo and R. P. Dellinger (Eds.), *Critical care medicine: Principles of diagnosis and management in the adult* (4th ed., pp. 1121–1129). Philadelphia, PA: Elsevier Saunders.

Papaioannou, V., Dragoumanis, C., & Pneumatikos, I. (2010). Biosignal analysis techniques for weaning outcome assessment. *Journal of Critical Care, 25*(1), 39–46. doi:10.1016/j.jcrc.2009.04.006

Patel, V. P., & Shapiro, J. M. (2012). Mechanical ventilation in the cardiac care unit. In E. Herzog (Ed.), *The cardiac care unit survival guide* (pp. 279–293). Philadelphia, PA: Wolters Kluwer Health/Lippincott, Williams, & Wilkins.

Petrucci, N., & De Feo, C. (2013). Lung protective ventilation strategy for the acute respiratory distress syndrome. *Cochrane Database of Systematic Reviews, 2*, CD003844. doi:10.1002/14651858.CD003844.pub4

Porteus, C., Hedrick, M. S., Hicks, J. W., Wang, T., & Milsom, W. K. (2011). Time domains of the hypoxic ventilatory response in ectothermic vertebrates. *Journal of Comparative Physiology B, 181*(3), 311–333. doi:10.1007/s00360-011-0554-6

Sessler, C. N., & Murevich, K. M. (2013). Use of sedatives, analgesics, and neuromuscular blockers. In J. E. Parrillo & R. P. Dellinger (Eds.), *Critical care medicine: Principles of diagnosis and management in the adult* (4th ed., pp. 255–271). Philadelphia, PA: Elsevier Saunders.

Skaar, D. J., & Weinert, C. G. (2011). Sedatives and hypnotics. In J.-L. Vincent, E. Abraham, F. A. Moore, P. M. Kochanek, & M. P. Fink (Eds.), *Textbook of critical care* (6th ed., pp. 1366–1373). Philadelphia, PA: Elsevier Saunders.

Stevens, J. P., & Howell, M. D. (2012). Preventing harm and improving quality in the intensive care unit. *Hospital Medicine Clinics, 1*(1), e12-e35. doi:10.1016/j.ehmc.2011.11.008

Von Dossow-Hanfstingl, V., Deja, M., Zwissler, B., & Spies, C. (2011). Postoperative management: Extracorporeal ventilatory therapy. In P. Slinger, R. S. Blank, J. Campos, E. Cohen, & K. McRae (Eds.), *Principles and practice of anesthesia for thoracic surgery* (pp. 635–648). New York, NY: Springer.

Widjicks, E. F. M. (2010). *The practice of emergency and critical care neurology*. New York, NY: Oxford University Press.

SECTION FOUR

Management of Patients with Gastrointestinal Disorders

CHAPTER 36

Peptic Ulcer Disease

ALICIA HUCKSTADT • CHARLENE M. MYERS

PEPTIC ULCER DISEASE

I. **Definition**
   A. A gastrointestinal (GI) ulcer is a loss of enteric surface epithelium that extends deep enough to penetrate the muscularis mucosae, and is usually over 5 mm in diameter.
   B. Peptic ulcer disease (PUD) refers to a chronic disorder in which the patient has a lifelong underlying tendency to develop mucosal ulcers at sites that are exposed to peptic juice (i.e., acid and pepsin).
      1. The most common locations are the duodenum and the stomach.
      2. Ulcers may also occur in the esophagus, jejunum, and ileum and at the gastroenteric anastomoses.

II. **Etiology**
   A. PUD is a common disorder with approximately 500,000 new cases diagnosed each year in the United States and 4 million causes of ulcer recurrence.
   B. *Helicobacter pylori* is present in more than 75%–90% of duodenal ulcers; it occurs at a lower rate with gastric ulcers but is found in most gastric ulcers in which nonsteroidal anti-inflammatory drugs (NSAIDs) cannot be implicated.
   C. An imbalance exists between mucosal defense mechanisms (protective factors) and mucosal damaging mechanisms (aggressive factors).
      1. Protective factors
         a. Mucosal barrier (bicarbonate and gastric mucus)
         b. Sufficient blood supply to gastric mucosa and submucosa
         c. Competent sphincters (pyloric and lower esophageal sphincter [LES]), which prevent bile salt reflux into the stomach and the esophagus
         d. Certain medications
            i. H2 blockers
            ii. Antacids
            iii. Sucralfate (Carafate)
            iv. Colloidal bismuth suspension
            v. Anticholinergics
            vi. Misoprostol (Cytotec)
            vii. Omeprazole (Prilosec)
      2. Aggressive factors
         a. *H. pylori* infection
         b. Gastric acid
         c. Pepsin
         d. Bile acids
         e. Decreased blood flow to gastric mucosa

			f. Incompetent sphincters
			g. Various medications
				i. Aspirin
				ii. NSAIDs
				iii. Glucocorticoids
				iv. Cigarette smoking
				v. Gastrinoma
				vi. Stress (especially posttraumatic)
				vii. Alcohol
				viii. Impaired proximal duodenal bicarbonate secretion

III. **Risk factors**
	A. Highly associated
		1. Smoking more than one half pack of cigarettes per day
		2. Drugs (NSAIDs)
		3. Genetics
		4. Acid hypersecretory states such as the Zollinger-Ellison syndrome (condition caused by non-insulin-secreting tumors of the pancreas, which secrete excess amounts of gastrin)
		5. Cytomegalovirus
		6. Crohn's disease
		7. Lymphoma
	B. Possibly associated with:
		1. Alcohol
		2. Corticosteroids
		3. Stress
		4. Decreased prostaglandin levels associated with aging
	C. Low association or no association with:
		1. Spices
		2. Alcohol
		3. Caffeine
		4. Acetaminophen

IV. **Types of peptic ulcers**
	A. Duodenal ulcers
		1. Ulcers occur five times more in the duodenum
		2. In all, 90%–95% occur in the first portion of the duodenum.
		3. Duodenal ulcers are four times more common than gastric ulcers.
		4. Duodenal ulcers have 10% lifetime prevalence for men and 5% for women.
		5. New cases have declined over the last 30 years
		6. The most common age range is 30–55 years
	B. Gastric ulcers
		1. They are most commonly seen in the lesser curvature of the stomach near the incisura angularis.
		2. New cases are increasingly likely because of widespread NSAIDs and aspirin use
		3. Gastric ulcers are three to four times more prevalent than duodenal ulcers in NSAID users.
		4. The peak age of incidence is 55–70 years (rare before age 40)

V. **Subjective/physical exam findings**
	A. Duodenal ulcers
		1. Epigastric pain ("gnawing," "aching," and "hunger-like") occurs 1–3 hr after eating. The pain is rhythmic and periodic.
		2. Nocturnal pain that awakens a patient from sleep
		3. Usually relieved by antacid or food ingestion
		4. Heartburn (suggests reflux disease)
		5. Epigastric tenderness: usually midline or right of midline
	B. Gastric ulcers
		1. Epigastric pain similar to that associated with duodenal ulcers and also rhythmic and periodic
		2. Pain is not usually relieved by food
		3. Food may precipitate symptoms
		4. Nausea and anorexia

C. Often unremarkable
D. The most common exam finding is epigastric tenderness to palpation.
    1. At or to the left of the midline with gastric ulcer
    2. Located 1 inch or farther to the right of midline with duodenal ulcer
E. Signs and symptoms of shock from acute or chronic blood loss
F. Nausea and vomiting if the pyloric channel is obstructed
G. Boardlike abdomen and rebound tenderness in the event of perforation
H. Hematemesis or melena if the ulcer is bleeding

VI. Laboratory/diagnostics

A. Laboratory findings do not play a major role in diagnosing PUD but may assist the clinician in defining an underlying disorder or complication
B. Laboratory studies are typically normal in uncomplicated disease
C. For detection of *H. pylori*, the following tests are performed:
    1. Histopathology (endoscopic biopsy)—gold standard
    2. Urea breath test
        a. Positive test implies active infection
        b. More expensive than serum and fecal tests
        c. Proton pump inhibitors (PPIs) may cause false-negative results and should be withheld for at least 7–14 days before testing is done.
    3. Serum *H. pylori* antibody test
        a. Positive test does not necessarily imply an active infection; it may reflect previous infection
        b. Lower sensitivity (85%) and specificity (79%) than fecal antigen or urea breath (both have 95% sensitivity and specificity)
    4. Fecal antigen for *H. pylori*
        a. Detects active infection by measuring fecal excretion of *H. pylori* antigens
        b. Good test to use to assess whether treatment has been successful
        c. PPIs may cause false-negative results and should be withheld for at least 7–14 days before testing is done
D. Complete blood count may indicate anemia due to acute or possibly chronic blood loss
E. Leukocytosis suggests ulcer penetration or perforation
F. Elevated serum amylase level with severe epigastric pain suggests possible ulcer penetration into the pancreas
G. Fasting serum gastrin levels to identify the Zollinger-Ellison syndrome
H. Upper GI barium studies
    1. For uncomplicated dyspepsia
    2. Those diagnosed with gastric ulcers should undergo endoscopy after 8–12 weeks of treatment to distinguish benign from malignant ulcers.
I. Endoscopy
    1. Procedure of choice for diagnosis of duodenal and gastric ulcers
    2. Identifies superficial and very small ulcers
    3. Biopsy may be performed
    4. Electrocautery of any bleeding ulcers can be carried out
    5. Gastric pH can be measured in suspected gastrinoma
    6. Esophagitis, gastritis, or duodenitis can be diagnosed
    7. *H. pylori* can be detected
    8. Higher cost than barium studies

VII. Complications of PUD

A. GI bleeding (20% of cases)
    1. Clinical manifestations
        a. Hematemesis
        b. Melena
        c. Hematochezia
        d. "Coffee ground" emesis
    2. Physical examination
        a. Pallor
        b. Tachycardia
        c. Hypotension

d. Diaphoresis
3. Laboratory findings
   a. Decreased hematocrit due to bleeding or hemodilution from IV fluids
   b. Blood urea nitrogen may rise owing to absorption of blood nitrogen from the small intestine and as a result of prerenal azotemia.
4. Diagnostics: endoscopy after the patient has stabilized
5. Management
   a. In approximately 80% of cases, bleeding stops spontaneously within a few hours after admission to the hospital.
   b. IV hydration with normal saline
   c. Blood transfusion as required
   d. Continuous IV infusion of H_2 blockers at a dose adequate to maintain gastric pH greater than 4
   e. Vasopressin (Pitressin) and IV octreotide (Sandostatin) should not be used for bleeding ulcers
   f. Surgery if bleeding persists

B. Perforation (5%–10% of cases)
   1. Subjective data
      a. Severe abdominal pain
      b. Epigastric pain that radiates to back or right upper quadrant
   2. Physical examination
      a. Ill appearance
      b. Boardlike abdomen
      c. Severe epigastric tenderness
      d. Absent bowel sounds
      e. Knee-to-chest position
      f. Patient may have symptoms of hypovolemia, fever
   3. Laboratory findings
      a. Leukocytosis is almost always present
      b. Amylase levels may be mildly elevated
   4. Diagnostics
      a. Abdominal x-rays may reveal free air in the peritoneal cavity
      b. Upper GI radiography with water-soluble contrast may be useful
      c. Barium studies are contraindicated
   5. Therapy
      a. Surgery
      b. Patients who are considered poor candidates for surgery or who present more than 24 hr after perforation and are stable, may be followed closely while on IV fluids, nasogastric suction, and broad-spectrum antibiotics
      c. If their condition deteriorates, they should be taken to surgery

C. Gastric outlet obstruction (2% of cases)
   1. Caused by edema or narrowing of the pylorus or duodenal bulb
   2. Subjective findings:
      a. Early satiety
      b. Nausea
      c. Vomiting of undigested food
      d. Epigastric pain unrelieved by food or antacids
      e. Weight loss
   3. Physical examination findings:
      a. "Succussion splash" may be audible on physical examination and is caused by large amounts of air and fluid in the stomach
      b. Nasogastric aspiration may return a large amount (more than 200 ml) of foul-smelling fluid
   4. Diagnostics
      a. Upper GI endoscopy should be performed after 24–72 hr to determine the source of obstruction
      b. At 72 hr, all patients should be given the saline load test, accomplished by instilling 750 ml of normal saline into the stomach and checking the residual in 30 minutes.

CHAPTER 36 Peptic Ulcer Disease

      c. Residual volume greater than 400 ml is considered positive
      d. Patient should remain on nasogastric suction for 5–7 additional days
  5. Laboratory: metabolic alkalosis and hypokalemia may be present
  6. Therapy:
      a. Normal saline IV infusion with potassium chloride, if patient has an electrolyte imbalance due to vomiting and poor digestion (i.e., 1 liter normal saline with 40 mEq potassium chloride per liter at 100 ml/hour, titrated up or down according to the patient's condition)
          i. For example, someone who is dehydrated with an increased heart rate, decreased urinary output, and decreased central venous pressure/pulmonary capillary wedge pressure may require more fluids.
          ii. By comparison, those with a history of heart failure or who have signs and symptoms of cardiac overload (e.g., crackles, jugular venous distention, or edema) may require less fluid.
      b. IV H_2 blockers
          i. Ranitidine (Zantac), 50 mg every 6–8 hr up to 150 mg/day
          ii. Famotidine (Pepcid), 20 mg at bedtime or BID
          iii. Cimetidine (Tagamet), 400 mg at bedtime or BID
          iv. Nizatidine (Axid), 300 mg at bedtime
      c. Nasogastric decompression
      d. Total parenteral nutrition for the severely malnourished
  7. Surgery: traditional
  8. Upper GI endoscopy with dilatation of the obstruction has proven successful

VIII. Medical therapy for PUD
  A. Acid-antisecretory agents
    1. Acid-antisecretory agents (H_2-receptor antagonists): Although these drugs are effective, proton pump inhibitors (PPIs) are now preferred for those with known PUD because of their ease of use and superior efficacy.
      a. Decrease gastric acid secretion by blocking histamine H_2 receptors on parietal cells
      b. Effectively inhibit nocturnal acid output but not as effective at inhibiting meal-stimulated acid secretion
      c. Agents:
          i. Ranitidine (Zantac)
          ii. Famotidine (Pepcid)
          iii. Nizatidine (Axid)
          iv. Cimetidine (Tagamet): rarely used today because it inhibits hepatic cytochrome P-450 metabolism, which raises serum concentrations of theophylline, warfarin, lidocaine, and phenytoin and may cause gynecomastia or impotence, among other interactions
      d. Dosages:
          i. Ranitidine, 150 mg PO BID or 300 mg at bedtime
          ii. Nizatidine, 150 mg PO BID or 300 mg at bedtime
          iii. Famotidine, 20 mg PO BID or 40 mg at bedtime
          iv. Cimetidine, 300 mg PO QID or 800 mg at bedtime
      e. Symptom relief usually occurs within 2 weeks
      f. Healing of duodenal ulcers is usually attained within 6 weeks of initiation of therapy
      g. Gastric ulcer healing is delayed by 2–4 weeks compared with duodenal ulcers, but the duration of therapy of 8 weeks is sufficient.
    2. PPIs
      a. Suppress gastric acid secretion by inhibition of the hydrogen/potassium adenosine triphosphate ($H+K+$-ATPase) enzyme system at the secretory surface of the gastric parietal cell
      b. Indications for treatment of the following:
          i. Duodenal ulcers
          ii. Severe erosive esophagitis
          iii. Poorly responsive gastroesophageal reflux disease

c. Agents: each of the following PPIs, when given once daily, results in healing of greater than 90% of duodenal ulcers after 4 weeks and 90% of gastric ulcers after 8 weeks
      i. Omeprazole (Prilosec), 20 mg PO daily (duodenal ulcer) or 40 mg PO daily (gastric ulcer)
      ii. Lansoprazole (Prevacid), 15 mg PO daily (duodenal ulcer) or 30 mg PO daily (gastric ulcer)
      iii. Rabeprazole (Aciphex), 20 mg PO daily (duodenal ulcer)
      iv. Pantoprazole (Protonix), 40–80 mg PO daily (duodenal/gastric ulcer)
      v. Esomeprazole (Nexium), 20 mg PO daily (duodenal ulcer) or 20–40 mg PO daily (gastric ulcer)
      vi. Dexlansoprazole (Dexilant), 30 mg PO daily (duodenal ulcer) or 3060 mg PO daily (gastric ulcer)
   d. Should be administered 30 minutes before meals
   e. PPIs are remarkably safe in short-term therapy. Serum gastrin levels may rise by more than 500 pg/ml in 10% of patients given long-term therapy; therefore, serum gastrin levels should be checked after 6 months of therapy, and treatment should be terminated or decreased if levels rise to above 500 pg/ml.
      i. Long-term use may decrease vitamin B12, iron, and calcium absorption, and may cause enteric infections (including *Clostridium difficile*), hip fracture, or pneumonia.
B. Agents that enhance mucosal defenses:
   1. Sucralfate
      a. Forms a protective barrier against acid, bile, and pepsin
      b. May cause constipation
      c. May bind some medications; therefore, doses should be separated by at least 2 hr. Requires dosage adjustment in renal impairment, as it may cause aluminum toxicity.
      d. Associated with decreased incidence of nosocomial pneumonia in some studies
      e. Requires an acidic environment; therefore, antacids, PPIs, and H2 blockers should be avoided
      f. One gram four times a day has the same efficacy as H2 blockers in the treatment of duodenal ulcers (6–8 weeks' duration)
      g. Efficacy against gastric ulcers is less firmly established
      h. Maintenance dose: 1 gram BID
   2. Prostaglandin analog (misoprostol [Cytotec])
      a. Promotes ulcer healing by stimulating mucous and bicarbonate secretion and by modestly inhibiting acid secretion
      b. Used solely as a prophylactic agent in the prevention of NSAID-induced ulcers rather than for treatment of active ulcers
         i. With the advent of PPIs and cyclooxygenase-2-selective NSAIDs, misoprostol is now used less for this indication
      c. High incidence of diarrhea
      d. May stimulate contractions in pregnant patients and may induce abortion
      e. Initial dose: 100 mcg four times a day with food; increased to 200 mcg four times a day if well tolerated
   3. Antacids
      a. No longer used as first-line agents; commonly used, as required, to supplement other antiulcer therapies owing to rapid relief of symptoms
      b. Low-dose aluminum- and magnesium-containing antacids promote ulcer healing by stimulating gastric mucosal defenses, rather than neutralizing gastric acidity.
      c. Dosage: 30 ml 1–3 hr after meals and at bedtime
      d. High dosages are associated with diarrhea, hypermagnesemia, and hypophosphatemia
C. *H. pylori* eradication therapy
   1. Combination drug therapy is necessary to achieve adequate rates of eradication and to decrease failures due to antibiotic resistance
   2. Combination therapy consists of two antibiotics, plus a PPI with or without bismuth.
   3. Regimens using PPIs include the following:

a. Omeprazole, 20 mg
b. Rabeprazole, 20 mg
c. Lansoprazole, 30 mg
d. Pantoprazole, 40 mg
e. Esomeprazole, 40 mg
f. All PPIs are given BID, except for esomeprazole, which is given once daily
g. Examples:
   i. Metronidazole + omeprazole + clarithromycin (MOC)
      (a) Metronidazole (Flagyl) (if allergic to penicillin), 500 mg BID with meals
      (b) Omeprazole, 20 mg BID before meals (may use PPI of choice)
      (c) Clarithromycin (Biaxin), 500 mg BID with meals for 7 days
      (d) Instruct patient that Flagyl should not be taken with alcohol or vinegar
   ii. Amoxicillin + omeprazole + clarithromycin (AOC)
      (a) Amoxicillin (Amoxil), 1 gram BID with meals
      (b) Omeprazole, 20 mg BID before meals (may use PPI of choice)
      (c) Clarithromycin (Biaxin), 500 mg BID with meals for 7 days
      (d) Preferred for those whose disease is resistant to metronidazole
   iii. Metronidazole + omeprazole + amoxicillin (MOA)
      (a) Metronidazole 500 mg BID with meals
      (b) Omeprazole, 20 mg BID before meals (may use PPI of choice)
      (c) Amoxicillin, 1 gram BID with meals for 7–14 days
4. Regimens that use bismuth compounds:
   a. Require four times a day dosing and have a greater number of adverse effects than PPI regimens
   b. BMT:
      i. Bismuth subsalicylate, 2 tablets four times a day
      ii. Metronidazole, 250 mg four times a day
      iii. Tetracycline (Tetracyn), 500 mg four times a day
      iv. All pills are taken with meals and at bedtime
   c. BMT + Omeprazole (above regimen with the following):
      i. Omeprazole, 20 mg BID before meals for 7 days
5. A 5-day treatment regimen with three antibiotics (amoxicillin, 1 gram BID; clarithromycin, 250 mg BID; and metronidazole, 400 mg BID), plus either lansoprazole, 30 mg BID; or ranitidine, 300 mg BID is an effective, cost-saving option for patients older than 55 years who have no history of PUD. This regimen may be cost-effective; however, efficacy needs to be further evaluated.
6. Antiulcer therapy is recommended for 3–7 weeks after the treatment regimens described previously to ensure symptom relief and ulcer healing.
   a. Duodenal ulcers: omeprazole, 40 mg daily, or lansoprazole, 30 mg daily, should be continued for 7 additional weeks.
   b. H2 blockers or sucralfate can be given for 6–8 weeks
   c. Testing for confirmation of eradication; typically recommended for:
      i. Any patient with an *H. pylori* associated ulcer
      ii. Patients with persistent dyspeptic symptoms, despite test-and-treat strategy
      iii. Patients with *H. pylori* associated MALT lymphoma
      iv. Patients who have undergone resection of early gastric cancer
D. Surgery for refractory ulcers is rarely performed today. If needed, methods include selective vagotomy for duodenal ulcer or ulcer removal with antrectomy, or hemigastrectomy without vagotomy for gastric ulcers.

IX. **Suggested follow-up**
A. Duodenal ulcer: no further evaluation is necessary if the patient is symptom-free after 8 weeks of therapy
B. Gastric ulcer: repeat endoscopy should be performed 4–6 weeks after therapy is completed
   1. Completely healed ulcers require no follow-up
   2. Partially healed ulcers

a. If greater than 50% healing occurs and findings are negative for carcinoma, 6 weeks of additional therapy is required, followed by reevaluation.
b. If healing is greater than 59% but findings are positive for carcinoma, surgical intervention is required.
c. Less than 50% healing requires surgery

GASTROESOPHAGEAL REFLUX DISEASE (GERD)

I. **Definition**
   A. Chronic condition in which gastric contents enter into and remain within the lower esophagus because of impaired esophageal function
   B. GERD is a symptomatic clinical condition or histologic alteration that results from episodes of gastroesophageal reflux that may produce inflammation of the esophagus (reflux esophagitis).

II. **Etiology**
   A. Anatomic factors
      1. Hypotensive LES pressures
      2. Hiatal hernia
         a. Decreased esophageal clearance of gastric contents: severity depends on length of contact time between the gastric contents and the esophagus
         b. Composition and volume of refluxate: the combination of acid, pepsin, and bile produces a potent refluxate that may cause damage to the esophagus; acidic gastric fluid (pH less than 4.0) is extremely caustic to the mucosa
         c. Delayed gastric emptying (due to gastroparesis or partial gastric outlet obstruction) may contribute to gastroesophageal reflux by producing an increase in gastric volume that may increase the frequency and amount of fluid that is refluxed.

III. **Incidence**
   A. Affects 20% of U.S. adults with at least weekly episodes, 10% have daily symptoms
   B. Contributing factors
      1. Dietary
         a. Caffeinated food and/or drinks
            i. Coffee
            ii. Tea
            iii. Cola
            iv. Chocolate
         b. Esophageal irritants
            i. Citrus fruits
            ii. Vinegar
            iii. Spicy foods
            iv. Tomatoes
         c. Excessive fluids with meals
         d. Large meals
         e. Fatty meals
         f. Meals within 2–3 hr of bedtime
         g. Lower esophageal sphincter relaxants
            i. Onions
            ii. Garlic
            iii. Mint
            iv. Alcoholic beverages
         h. Lying down immediately after eating
      2. Non-dietary
         a. Anxiety
         b. Obesity
         c. Pregnancy
         d. Tight-fitting clothing
         e. Smoking
      3. Pharmacologic agents
         a. α-adrenergic antagonists

b. Anticholinergics
c. Antihistamines
d. Aspirin
e. Benzodiazepines
f. Calcium channel blockers
g. β-adrenergic agonists
h. Cholecystokinin
i. Levodopa
j. Nitrates
k. NSAIDs
l. Opioids
m. Progestins
n. Prostaglandins
o. Secretin
p. Somatostatin
q. Theophylline
r. Tricyclic antidepressants
s. Transdermal nicotine

IV. **Signs/symptoms**
A. Hallmark symptom: heartburn (pyrosis)
1. Described as substernal sensation of warmth or burning that may radiate to the neck, throat, and/or back
2. Generally associated with large meals; occurs 30–60 minutes after eating
3. Often aggravated by the supine position and bending over
B. Regurgitation
C. Water brash (hypersalivation)
D. Dysphagia (difficulty swallowing)
E. Odynophagia (pain on swallowing)
F. Hemorrhage
G. Belching
H. Early satiety
I. Atypical symptoms
1. Pulmonary symptoms
a. Recurrent pneumonia
b. Bronchospasm
2. Chest pain
3. Cough
4. Hoarseness
5. Hiccups
6. Sore throat
7. Nighttime choking
8. Halitosis

V. **Laboratory/diagnostics**
A. Clinical history, including presenting symptoms and associated risk factors, is the most useful tool in the diagnosis of GERD.
B. Barium swallow is the simplest, least expensive test but is also the least sensitive. Useful as a screening tool to accomplish the following:
1. To rule out the following complications:
a. Inflammation
b. Ulcers
c. Strictures
2. To evaluate the following:
a. Dysphagia
b. Odynophagia
c. Significant weight loss
d. Occult blood loss

C. Endoscopy is an excellent study for the diagnosis and evaluation of reflux esophagitis and other complications of GERD (strictures and Barrett esophagus). During endoscopy:
   1. Biopsy specimens can be obtained
   2. Strictures can be dilated
D. The Bernstein test is an intraesophageal acid perfusion study that can be used to confirm that the patient's symptoms are acid related.
   1. The test requires an alternating infusion of 0.1 N hydrochloric acid and normal saline into the esophagus.
   2. With reflux esophagitis, symptoms of heartburn occur with infusion of acid but not with infusion of saline.
E. The most specific and sensitive diagnostic test used to detect the presence of abnormal acid reflux is 24-hour ambulatory pH monitoring.
   1. This test remains the gold standard for many practitioners.
   2. It is performed by passing a small electrode pH probe intranasally and placing it approximately 5 cm above the LES.
   3. The frequency and severity of reflux can be determined with this study.
F. Esophageal manometry measures esophageal pressure
   1. Identifies abnormalities of the LES
   2. Identifies esophageal muscle contraction abnormalities

VI. Management
   A. Phase 1 treatment modalities
      1. Elevate head of the bed 4–6 inches (increases esophageal clearance)
      2. Avoid vigorous exercise 2–3 hr before bedtime
      3. Avoid large, high-fat meals and eating 2–3 hr before bedtime (decreases gastric volume)
      4. Avoid foods that may decrease LES pressure
         a. Fats
         b. Chocolate
         c. Alcohol
         d. Peppermint
         e. Spearmint
      5. Avoid foods that have an irritant effect directly on the esophageal mucosa
         a. Spicy foods
         b. Citrus juice
         c. Tomato juice
         d. Coffee
      6. Add protein-rich meals to the diet (to augment LES pressure)
      7. Reduce weight (to reduce symptoms)
      8. Eliminate smoking, if applicable (to decrease spontaneous esophageal sphincter relaxation)
      9. Avoid alcohol (to increase amplitude of the LES and peristaltic waves and the frequency of contractions)
      10. Avoid tight-fitting clothes
      11. Eliminate exacerbating medications (see Contributing Factors of GERD, above)
      12. Use antacids and alginic acid PRN
         a. After meals and at bedtime, 80–100 mEq of neutralizing activity (usually 30 ml/8–10 tablets)
            i. Chooz
            ii. Gaviscon
            iii. Gelusil
            iv. Gelusil II
            v. Maalox Plus
            vi. Maalox TC
            vii. Mylanta
            viii. Mylanta II
            ix. Riopan
            x. Tums
         b. Liquid and tablet form are preferred.

13. Try over-the-counter H$_2$ blockers
    a. Famotidine, 10 mg up to BID
    b. Ranitidine, 50–100 mg up to BID
    c. Cimetidine, 200 mg up to BID
B. Phase 2 treatment modalities
    1. Continue the nonpharmacologic therapies. Weight loss is recommended for GERD patients who are overweight or have had recent weight gain. Head of bed elevation and avoidance of meals 2–3 hrs before bedtime recommended for patients with nocturnal GERD.
C. Phase 3 treatment modalities
    1. Inadequate response after 2–4 weeks of phase 2 management necessitates progression to phase 3
    2. Increase the dose of the initial drug
    3. The initial course of therapy is usually 8–12 weeks. Long-term therapy may be necessary to maintain remission in some patients who relapse.
        a. Omeprazole (Prilosec), 20 mg PO daily
        b. Lansoprazole (Prevacid), 15–30 mg PO daily
        c. Rabeprazole (Aciphex), 20 mg PO daily
        d. Pantoprazole (Protonix), 40 mg PO daily
        e. Esomeprazole (Nexium), 20 mg PO daily
        f. Dexlansoprazole (Dexilant), 30 mg PO daily
            i. PPI therapy should be initiated at once a day dosing
            ii. For patients with partial response to once daily therapy, BID dosing should be considered.
            iii. Non-responders to PPI should be referred for evaluation.
D. Step-up versus step-down theory in management
    1. Step up: begins with lifestyle modifications and use of over-the-counter medications. Medication may be stepped up to other drugs if symptoms are not resolved.
    2. Step down: begins with a PPI, the most effective treatment, and then is reduced to a lower dosage or a less effective drug (this does not work in patients with severe esophagitis)
E. Phase 4 treatment modalities
    1. Surgical intervention
        a. Reserved for those in whom medical management has failed or complications have developed
        b. Indications include the following:
            i. Reflux-related pulmonary disease
            ii. Persistent ulcerative esophagitis
            iii. Recurrent esophageal strictures
            iv. Large hiatal hernia
        c. The Nissen fundoplication procedure has a cure rate of approximately 90%.
        d. Stretta procedure
            i. Involves application of radiofrequency energy into the LES in an outpatient setting
            ii. Indicated by a prolonged history of GERD with stable or worsening symptoms after use of PPIs

BIBLIOGRAPHY

Bredenoord, A. J., Pandolfino, J. E., & Smout, P. M. (2013). Gastro-esophageal reflux disease. *Lancet, 381*, 1933–1942.

DiMarino, M. C. (2014). Drug treatment of gastric acidity. *Merck Manuals.* Retrieved from http://www.merckmanuals.com/professional/gastrointestinal_disorders/gastritis_and_peptic_ulcer_disease/drug_treatment_of_gastric_acidity.html

Dunphy, L. M., Winland-Brown, J. E., Porter, B. O., & Thomas, D. J. (2011). Abdominal problems. *Primary care: The art and science of advanced practice care nursing* (3rd ed.). Philadelphia, PA: FA Davis.

Laine, L., & Jensen, D. M. (2012). Management of patients with ulcer bleeding. *American Journal of Gastroenterology, 107*, 345–360. doi:10.1038/ajg.2011.480

CHAPTER 37

Liver Disease

MICHALYN D. PELPHREY • CHARLENE M. MYERS

MAJOR LIVER DISEASES

I. **Hepatitis**
   A. Definition: Hepatitis refers to an inflammation of the liver that can be caused by many drugs and toxic agents, as well as viruses. Hepatitis A, C, D, E, and G are all RNA viruses. Hepatitis B is the only DNA virus. All types of hepatitis produce similar illnesses.
   B. Viral hepatitis
      1. Hepatitis A virus (HAV)
         a. Etiology
            i. Usually, it is spread by fecal–oral route, including contaminated food sources, water, and shellfish; spread by parenteral route is rare
            ii. Spread is enhanced by crowding and by poor sanitation.
            iii. Maximum infectivity occurs 2 weeks before clinical illness.
            iv. Blood and stool are infectious during a 2- to 6-week incubation period.
            v. Mortality rate is low, and fulminant hepatitis A is uncommon
         b. Laboratory/diagnostics
            i. Immunoglobulin IgM anti-HAV: excellent diagnostic test
            ii. First laboratory test ordered with acute illness with increased alanine transaminase (ALT) and aspartate transaminase (AST)
            iii. IgM occurs during the first week of clinical disease
            iv. IgM disappears after 3–6 months
               (a) Positive interpretation: HAV infection within the preceding 6 months
               (b) Negative interpretation: no HAV infection within the preceding 12 months
            v. IgG anti-HAV—presence of IgG
               (a) Indicates previous exposure and noninfectivity
               (b) Confers lifelong immunity
            vi. Negative interpretation: no previous HAV infection
         c. Medical management
            i. Supportive
               (a) Consists of bed rest until jaundice resolves
               (b) No heavy lifting, straining, or activity
            ii. High-calorie diet
               (a) Small, frequent meals with supplements

(b) High carbohydrates
(c) Low proteins
(d) No fatty foods
iii. Potentially hepatotoxic medications should be avoided
iv. Restriction of alcohol
v. Most patients do not require hospitalization
vi. If patients show signs of encephalopathy or severe coagulopathy, fulminant hepatic failure should be suspected, and hospitalization is necessary.
vii. Administer antiemetics to decrease nausea and vomiting
d. Vaccinations
i. Hepatitis A: In the United States, two vaccines are available: Havrix and VAQTA. Both consist of inactivated HAV.
ii. Hepatitis A vaccination is recommended for all children aged 1 year, for persons who are at increased risk for infection, for persons who are at increased risk for complications from hepatitis A, and for any person wishing to obtain immunity.
2. Hepatitis B virus (HBV)
a. Etiology
i. HBV: blood-borne virus that is present in saliva, semen, and vaginal secretions
ii. Transmission
(a) Sex
(b) Contaminated blood and blood products
(c) Parenteral drug abuse
(d) Perinatal
(e) Body piercing
(f) Tattooing
(g) Recreational cocaine
iii. Approximately 350 million people are chronically infected worldwide
iv. 15%–40% of carriers of HBV are likely to develop serious hepatic sequela in their lifetime
v. Coinfection, superinfection, or chronic infection with hepatitis D virus markedly increases mortality and morbidity.
b. Diagnosis
i. Hepatitis B surface antigen or hepatitis B core antigen (HBsAg or anti-HBc IgM [IgM antibody to hepatitis B core antigen]). HBsAg is often detected in patients with acute HBV infection and is detectable in the serum of patients with active viral replication. Anti-HBc IgM can facilitate differentiation of acute from chronic HBV.
ii. Total hepatitis B core antibody (anti-HBc) is very useful as a serologic marker of acute hepatitis during a gap when patients have cleared HBsAg, but anti-HBs (antibody to hepatitis B surface antigen) cannot be detected. It also indicates past exposure or infection with hepatitis B.
iii. Hepatitis B surface antibody (anti-HBs) appears after clearance of HBsAg and/or after successful hepatitis vaccination.
iv. The appearance of anti-HBs and disappearance of HBsAg indicate the following:
(a) Recovery from HBV
(b) Noninfectivity
(c) Protection from recurrent infection
v. Hepatitis B e-antigen (HBeAg) found during acute or chronic infection. Presence indicates viral replication with high level of HBV.
vi. Hepatitis B e-antibody (HBeAb) produced by immune system temporarily during acute HBV infection or during or after a burst in replication. Conversion from e-antigen to e-antibody is a predictor of long-term clearance of HBV in patients being treated with antiviral therapy and indicates lower viral HBV.

- c. Medical management
  - i. The treatment of chronic hepatitis B is indicated if the risk of liver-related morbidity and mortality in 5–10 years and the likelihood of achieving viral suppression are high.
  - ii. Treatment not indicated if the risk of liver-related morbidity or mortality in the next
    20 years and the likelihood of achieving viral suppression are low
  - iii. Many considerations such as safety and efficacy of treatment, risks of resistance, and cost should be given when picking antiviral therapy agent for chronic HBV treatment. The following are approved agents:
    - (a) Peginterferon α: 180 mcg SQ once a week for 48 weeks; has many side effects; efficacy is limited to a small percentage of selected patients
    - (b) Lamivudine: 100 mg PO daily; not preferred due to resistance; adjust dose for renal impairment
    - (c) Adefovir: 10 mg PO daily; adjust dose for renal impairment; less potent than other agents and linked to increasing rate of antiviral resistance; best used as a
      second-line drug following the first year of therapy
    - (d) Entecavir: 0.5–1 mg PO daily; adjust dose for renal impairment
    - (e) Telbivudine: 600 mg PO daily; adjust dose for renal impairment; not preferred due to resistance
    - (f) Tenofovir: 300 mg PO daily
    - (g) Peginterferon, entecavir, or tenofovir are the first-line drugs recommended for treatment of hepatitis B.
  - iv. Can be complicated by cirrhosis or hepatocellular carcinoma leading for need for liver transplant
- d. Vaccination
  - i. Hepatitis B vaccine (Hep B) contains HBsAg, the primary antigenic protein in the viral envelope.
  - ii. Promotes synthesis of specific antibodies directed against HBV
  - iii. Marketed under the trade names Recombivax HB and Engerix B
    - (a) These vaccines are made from a viral component rather than from a live virus; therefore, they cannot cause disease.
    - (b) All vaccines should be administered in three doses. Once the first dose has been given, the second dose is given 1 month (or longer) later; the third dose is given in 6 months.
  - iv. In 2001, the FDA approved a new vaccine directed against both hepatitis A and hepatitis B. This agent, marketed as Twinrix, is approved for use in adults, adolescents, and children between the ages of 1 and 18 years.
  - v. Postexposure prophylaxis with immune globulin can be used to prevent HBV infection and subsequent development of liver disease
3. Hepatitis C virus (HCV/non-A non-B virus)
   - a. Etiology
     - i. HCV: blood-borne virus
     - ii. Most common chronic blood-borne infection in the United States
     - iii. Approximately 3.2 million people are chronically infected
     - iv. Risk of sexual and perinatal transmission is small
     - v. Of those infected, 70%–85% develop chronic HCV infection
     - vi. Approximately 70%–90% of HCV infection from former or current IVDU
     - vii. Majority of people infected may not be aware of infection because most people are asymptomatic
     - viii. Six genotypes with several subtypes have been identified. Genotypes 2 and 3 are more sensitive to antiviral treatment. Genotype 1, which is the most common in the United States, is more difficult to treat.

CHAPTER 37   Liver Disease

- b. Diagnosis
    - i. Anti-HCV (anti-HCV antibody)
        - (a) First-line test when diagnosis is suspected
        - (b) Highly sensitive—if negative, infection is unlikely
        - (c) Specificity depends on the situation—if positive in a person with risk factors and elevated liver enzymes, specificity is high
        - (d) Positive anti-HCV—hepatitis C infection is present until it is proven otherwise
    - ii. Most recombinant immunoblot assay—positive patients are infectious, and a polymerase chain reaction can be used to confirm HCV infection
        - (a) Gold standard for confirmation of infection
        - (b) Detects actual virus, not antibodies
        - (c) Differentiates prior exposure from current viremia
- c. Medical management
    - i. In patients with chronic hepatitis C, standard of care therapy has been the use of peginterferon and ribavirin. It is administered for 48 weeks for HCV genotypes 1, 4, 5, and 6 and for 24 weeks for HCV genotypes 2 and 3. Sustained viral response is achieved when HCV polymerase chain reaction is negative at 6 months after the completion of treatment. This is considered a virological cure for HCV. Sustained virological response (SVR) is achieved in 40%–50% of genotype 1 patients. SVR is achieved in 80%–90% of genotype 2 and 3 patients. Depending on the patient's weight, dosing varies as follows:
        - (a) 66–80 kg: peginterferon alfa-2b 1.5 mcg/kg/week SQ with ribavirin 400 mg PO BID for 48 weeks for genotype 1 or 24 weeks for genotypes 2 and 3
        - (b) 81–105 kg: peginterferon alfa-2b 1.5 mcg/kg/week SQ with ribavirin 600 mg PO BID for 48 weeks for genotype 1 or 24 weeks for genotypes 2 and 3
        - (c) Over 105 kg: peginterferon alfa-2b 1.5 mcg/kg/week SQ with ribavirin 600 mg PO in the morning and 800 mg PO in the evening for 48 weeks for genotype 1 or 24 weeks for genotypes 2 and 3
    - ii. The American Association for the Study of Liver Diseases recommends the addition of protease inhibitors Boceprevir or Telaprevir to markedly improve SVR rates in genotype 1 patients.
        - (a) Boceprevir 800 mg PO with food three times a day OR telaprevir 750 mg PO with food (not low-fat) three times per day (every 7–9 hr) in combination with peginterferon alfa and ribavirin
        - (b) At this time, boceprevir and telaprevir should not be used to treat patients with genotype 2 or 3 HCV infections.
    - iii. Newly approved medications are due to be released. These medications have had such promising results during study that it is believed that it will now be possible to cure most people of hepatitis C infection in the very near future.
    - iv. It is estimated that between 15% and 20% of patients with chronic HCV develop cirrhosis within 20 years of disease onset, which may lead to need for liver transplant
    - v. HCV cirrhosis patients have 2%–8% annual risk of developing hepatocellular carcinoma
- d. Vaccination/screening
    - i. Hepatitis C: no vaccination for active or passive immunity available
    - ii. New CDC recommendation for an age-based screening strategy consisting of one-time testing for HCV for those at highest risk, including everyone born between 1945 and 1965

4. Hepatitis D virus (delta agent)

a. An uncommon incomplete RNA virus that causes hepatitis only when accompanied by HBV infection
b. Combined infection has a worse prognosis than HBV alone, along with an increased incidence of fulminant hepatitis
c. There is no vaccination or specific treatment for the hepatitis D virus, but it can be prevented with HBV vaccination.
5. Hepatitis E virus (enterically transmitted or epidemic non-A non-B virus)
   a. An acute infection, does not lead to chronic infection, and rare in the United States
   b. Ingestion of fecal matter, even in microscopic amounts; usually associated with contaminated water supply in countries with poor sanitation
   c. Incubation period is 2–9 weeks (the mean is 6 weeks)
   d. Clinical disease is similar to HAV, except it is more severe
   e. Mortality rate is 1%–2% in general population and 10%–20% in pregnant women—significantly higher than HAV
   f. No current approved vaccination
6. Hepatitis G virus (HGV)
   a. Uncertain what role, if any, it plays in etiology of liver disease
   b. A recently identified virus that is transmitted percutaneously and may cause mild acute hepatitis and chronic viremia lasting as long as 9 years
   c. Detected in 50% of intravenous drug abusers and in 20% of hemophiliac patients
   d. Diagnostic tests are not currently available
7. Viral hepatitis risk factors
   a. Health care providers/other occupational risks; positive needlestick
   b. Hemodialysis patients
   c. Recipients of blood and/or blood products
   d. Intravenous drug users
   e. Sexually active men who have sex with men or those with multiple heterosexual partners
   f. Household exposure
   g. Intimate exposure
   h. Persons in underdeveloped countries
   i. Body piercing
   j. Tattooing
8. Viral hepatitis subjective findings (extremely variable)
   a. Prodromal phase
      i. Malaise, myalgia, arthralgia, and easy fatigue
      ii. Upper respiratory symptoms (nasal discharge and pharyngitis)
      iii. Anorexia, nausea, and vomiting are common.
      iv. Diarrhea or constipation may occur.
      v. Aversion to smoking (HBV)
      vi. Skin rashes, arthritis, or serum sickness may be seen early in HBV.
      vii. Fever usually less than 103.1°F (39.5°C) (more common in HAV)
      viii. Mild, constant abdominal pain in the right upper quadrant or epigastrium that is often aggravated by exertion
   b. Icteric phase
      i. Clinical jaundice occurs after 5–10 days but may occur at the same time as the initial symptoms
      ii. Most patients never develop clinical icterus
      iii. Intensification of prodromal symptoms usually occurs with the onset of jaundice; this is generally followed by progressive improvement
      iv. Dark urine/clay-colored stools
      v. Patient may be asymptomatic
9. Viral hepatitis physical findings
   a. Jaundice

CHAPTER 37   Liver Disease

      b. Tender hepatomegaly
      c. Splenomegaly
      d. Posterior cervical lymphadenopathy (rare)
      e. Rash (HBV)
      f. Arthritis (rare)
      g. Examination findings may be normal
   10. Laboratory/diagnostics
      a. WBC count is normal or may be low
      b. Urinalysis—proteinuria is common; bilirubinuria may occur before jaundice
      c. Greatly increased ALT and AST levels (greater than 500 IU/L; normal, 0–35 IU/L)
      d. Increased bilirubin and alkaline phosphatase levels; may remain elevated after ALT and AST have normalized
      e. Prothrombin time (PT) and glucose level are usually normal; increased PT or decreased glucose level indicates severe liver damage
C. Autoimmune hepatitis (AIH)
   1. Etiology
      a. Generally unresolving inflammation of liver of unknown cause
      b. Working model for pathogenesis postulates environmental triggers, failure of immune tolerance mechanisms and a genetic predisposition together lead to a t cell-mediated immune attack of the liver
      c. Symptoms range from asymptomatic or similar to viral hepatitis symptoms
   2. Laboratory/diagnostics
      a. Based on histologic abnormalities, abnormal levels of serum globulins and presence of one or more autoantibodies
      b. Women are more frequently affected than men
      c. Abnormal serum aminotransferases, especially with lower or normal alkaline phosphatase
      d. Serum globulin or IGG greater than one and a half times normal
      e. Positive ANA, SMA, or LKM 1 antibodies at titers greater than 1:80
      f. In patients with negative conventional autoantibodies in whom AIH is suspected, other serological markers including at least anti-SLA and atypical p-ANCA should be tested.
      g. Diagnosis of AIH should be considered in all patients with acute or chronic hepatitis of undetermined cause
   3. Medical treatment
      a. Prednisone monotherapy
         i. Induction therapy: 50–60 mg PO daily
         ii. Maintenance therapy: 5–20 mg PO daily
      b. Prednisone and azathioprine
         i. Induction therapy:
            (a) Prednisone 30 mg PO daily
            (b) Azathioprine 50 mg PO daily
         ii. Maintenance therapy:
            (a) Prednisone 5–10 mg PO daily
            (b) Azathioprine 50 mg PO daily
      c. Conventional therapy is continued until remission, treatment failure, incomplete response, or drug toxicity.
      d. May lead to liver transplant in both the acute and chronic settings
D. Nonalcoholic steatohepatitis
   1. Etiology

a. Nonalcoholic fatty liver disease (NAFLD) occurs where there is evidence of hepatic steatosis by either imaging or histology and there are no other causes for secondary hepatic fat such as significant alcohol consumption, medication, or hereditary disorders that could be cause. There is a presence of steatosis with no evidence of hepatocellular injury in the form of ballooning of hepatocytes.
b. Nonalcoholic steatohepatitis (NASH) is steatosis with inflammation, with hepatocyte injury or ballooning without fibrosis.
c. Obesity, diabetes, and dyslipidemia are associated risk factors
2. Laboratory/diagnostics
   a. When evaluating those with suspected NAFLD, it is important to exclude competing etiologies for steatosis or other common liver diseases.
   b. Serum aminotransferase levels and imaging such as ultrasound, CT scan, or MRI can be used as initial screening but are not reliable in determining steatohepatitis or fibrosis.
   c. Liver biopsy may need to be performed to determine if hepatic inflammation or fibrosis is present.
   d. A validated scoring system called the "NAFLD fibrosis score" is now being used to predict advanced fibrosis.
      i. A score less than negative 1.455: 90% sensitivity and 60% specificity of excluding advanced fibrosis
      ii. A score greater than 0.676 has a 67% sensitivity and 97% specificity of identifying the presence of advanced fibrosis
3. Treatment
   a. Lifestyle intervention
      i. Weight loss
      ii. Exercises
   b. Medications
      i. Vitamin E, 800 IU/day, has been shown to improve liver histology in nondiabetic adults with biopsy proven NASH.
      ii. There have been some studies that pioglitazone and rosiglitazone have shown improvement in liver histology for NASH patients; however, these have not been established as a recommendation.
   c. Bariatric surgery
      i. Premature to consider as an established option for specific treatment of NASH but is not contraindicated if otherwise eligible for the surgery
   d. May lead to cirrhosis and need for liver transplantation

II. Primary biliary cirrhosis

A. Etiology
  1. Primary biliary cirrhosis (PBC) is often considered a model autoimmune disease because of its hallmark serologic signature or antimitochondrial antibody and specific bile duct pathology.
     a. Antimitochondrial antibody positive in 90%–95% of patients
     b. A unique feature of PBC is the high degree of involvement of the small intrahepatic bile ducts
  2. Thought to be a combination of environmental triggers and genetic predisposition
  3. Cholestatic disease with progressive course, which can extend over many decades
B. Laboratory/diagnostics
  1. Abnormal liver tests, including alkaline phosphatase, mild elevation of ALT and AST, and present and increased immunoglobulins
  2. In patients without cirrhosis, the degree of elevation of alkaline phosphatase is strongly related to the severity of ductopenia and inflammation.
  3. Hyperbilirubinemia also reflects the severity of ductopenia and biliary necrosis.
  4. Histologic evidence of nonsuppurative destructive cholangitis and destruction of interlobular bile ducts

C. Treatment
1. The only approved drug to treat PBC is ursodiol (ursodeoxycholic acid [UDCA]), 13–15 mg/kg/day
2. May lead to need for liver transplantation

III. **Primary sclerosing cholangitis**
A. Etiology
1. Chronic cholestatic liver disease characterized by inflammation and fibrosis of both intrahepatic and extrahepatic bile ducts leading to multifocal bile duct strictures
2. Likely immune-mediated and progressive disorder usually leading to cirrhosis
B. Diagnosis
1. Made with patients that have cholestatic biochemical profile (elevated alkaline phosphatase and AST/ALT) and cholangiography by either magnetic resonance cholangiopancreatography or endoscopic retrograde cholangiopancreatography showing characteristic bile duct changes with multifocal strictures and segmental dilations
2. Patients often asymptomatic and diagnosis is made incidentally
3. Episodes of cholangitis are very uncommon at presentation.
4. Approximately 60%–80% of patients with primary sclerosing cholangitis (PSC) also have either Crohn disease or ulcerative colitis as well
5. Endoscopic retrograde cholangiopancreatography is the gold standard for diagnosing PSC, but magnetic resonance cholangiopancreatography can also be used.
6. Patients with PSC are at increased risk for developing cholangiocarcinoma. The estimated
ten-year cumulative risk of developing cholangiocarcinoma is approximately 7%–9%.
C. Treatment
1. The endoscopic management of strictures to relieve biliary obstruction is the major treatment for PSC.
2. Patients with symptoms from dominant stricture such as cholangitis, jaundice, pruritus, and worsening liver function are appropriate for endoscopic management.
3. The only long-term effective treatment for PSC is liver transplantation.

IV. **Hereditary hemochromatosis**
A. Etiology
1. Most common genetic disorder in Caucasians; most prevalent in northern European origin, particularly Nordic or Celtic ancestry
2. Genetic predisposition increases the inappropriate absorption of dietary iron that can lead to cirrhosis, hepatocellular carcinoma, diabetes, and heart disease
B. Diagnosis
1. Diagnosis is based on increased iron stores demonstrated by elevated ferritin levels and increased hepatic iron content. Hemochromatosis gene detection can further define the diagnosis. C282y homozygotes account for 80%–85% of typical patients with hereditary hemochromatosis.
2. Phenotypic expression does not always lead to severe iron overload and the accompanied organ damage and clinical manifestations of hemochromatosis. Three stages of progression of hemochromatosis have been identified.
   a. Stage 1—patients with the genetic disorder, with no increase in iron stores
   b. Stage 2—patients with the genetic disorder, with evidence of iron overload, with no evidence of tissue or organ damage
   c. Stage 3—those who have the genetic disorder with iron overload and deposition to the degree that tissue and organ damage occurs
C. Treatment/screening
1. Those with iron overload should undergo therapeutic phlebotomy weekly as tolerated. Goal is target ferritin level of 50–100 µg/L.
2. Vitamin C and iron supplements should be avoided
3. Dietary restrictions are unnecessary

4. Those with cirrhosis should be screened for hepatocellular carcinoma. There is an annual incidence of 3%–4% risk of developing hepatocellular carcinoma with hemochromatosis cirrhosis
5. Family screening is recommended for patients with hereditary hemochromatosis for all first-degree relatives with iron studies, ferritin, and hemochromatosis gene mutation analysis.

V. Alcoholic liver disease
A. Etiology
1. It is the most common cause of cirrhosis and accounts for 40% of deaths from cirrhosis in the United States.
2. It is estimated that more than 7.4% of Americans meet the Diagnostic and Statistical Manual of Mental Disorders, Fourth Edition criteria for the diagnosis of alcohol abuse and or dependence in 1994.
3. The amount of alcohol is the most important risk factor; however, amount consumed and liver disease are not clearly linear
   a. Compared with men, women have been shown to be twice as sensitive to alcohol-mediated hepatotoxicity and may require less alcohol intake to lead to severe liver disease.
   b. Drinking outside meal times has been reported to increase the risk of alcoholic liver disease (ALD).
   c. Binge drinking (drinking five drinks for men and four drinks for women) in one sitting also increases the risk of ALD.
4. Obesity has been associated with the increased risk of ALD.
5. Genetic factors also predispose people to alcoholism and ALD.

B. Diagnosis
1. Diagnosis is based on history of significant alcohol intake, clinical evidence of liver disease, and supporting laboratory abnormalities
2. Denial and underreporting of alcohol intake make it a difficult diagnosis
3. Various questionnaires have been developed—CAGE, MAST, and AUDIT
4. No single laboratory definitely establishes ALD
5. In approximately 70% of patients, the AST/ALT ratio is higher than 2—suggestive of ALD
6. Alcoholic hepatitis has high mortality rate. Maddrey's discriminant function (MDF) is a prognostic score to stratify the severity of illness.
   a. MDF = 4.6 × patients PT − control PT plus total bilirubin
   b. Patients that score greater than or equal to 32 have 1 month mortality as high as 30%–50%

C. Treatment
1. Abstinence is the most important treatment for ALD
2. Alcoholic hepatitis treatment
   a. Assess and treat for nutritional deficiencies
   b. Severe MDF score greater than 32 should be considered for a 4-week course of prednisone 40 mg/day for 28 days
   c. Prednisolone may be preferred over prednisone because prednisone requires a conversion to the active prednisolone in the liver, a process that may be impaired in alcoholic hepatitis.
   d. If steroids are contraindicated, pentoxifylline, 400 mg TID for 4 weeks, can be used in patients with severe alcoholic hepatitis.
3. ALD is the second most common indication for liver transplant for chronic liver disease in the Western World.

VI. Wilson disease
A. Etiology
1. A familial autosomal recessive disease that, if not treated, may be lethal. It may manifest with neurologic symptoms accompanied by chronic liver disease leading to cirrhosis.

2. It is caused by the absence of a gene, which is expressed mainly in hepatocytes and functions with the transmembrane transport of copper within hepatocytes, which leads to the decreased excretion of copper into bile. Decreased excretion results in copper accumulation and injury.
3. Eventually, the copper is released in the bloodstream and deposited in the brain, kidneys, and cornea.
4. Wilson disease should be considered in any individual between the ages of 3 and 55 years with liver abnormalities of uncertain cause.

B. Diagnosis
1. Abnormal aminotransferase generally abnormal
2. Ceruloplasmin that is significantly low, less than 50 mg/L, should be taken as a strong evidence of Wilson disease
3. A 24-hr urinary copper should be obtained on all patients with suspicion of Wilson disease. Findings greater than 40 µg may indicate Wilson disease.
4. Liver biopsy for the measurement of hepatic copper content remains the best evidence of Wilson disease. Content greater than 250 µg/gram dry weight is indicative of Wilson disease.
5. Wilson disease should be suspected in any patient presenting with acute hepatic failure with Coombs-negative intravascular hemolysis, modest elevation in AST and ALT or low alkaline phosphatase, and a ratio of alkaline phosphatase to bilirubin of less than 2.

C. Treatment
1. Pharmacological therapy available
   a. D-Penicillamine general chelator
      i. Initial therapy: 750–1500 mg PO daily resulting in an initial 24 hr cupriuresis of over
         2 mg/day; optimal dose is based on urinary copper excretion and free copper serum
      ii. Maintenance therapy: up to 2000 mg/day; dosing based on urinary copper excretion and free copper in serum
   b. Pyridoxine 25 mg PO daily may be given to prevent pyridoxal phosphate deficiency
   c. Trientine-general chelator 750–1250 mg/day PO in 2–4 divided doses, may be increased to a maximum of 2 grams/day
   d. Zinc, 50 mg PO 3 times a day; blocks intestinal absorption of copper
2. Patients should avoid intake of food and water high in copper
3. Liver transplant is the only option for those with decompensated cirrhosis or those who present with acute liver failure (ALF) unresponsive to medical therapy.
4. Treatment is lifelong, unless liver transplant is performed
5. All first-degree relatives of patients diagnosed with Wilson disease should be screened.

VII. **Fulminant liver failure/acute liver failure (ALF)**
A. Definition
1. ALF is a rare but catastrophic illness that results from sudden, marked impairment of liver cell function. Acute onset of liver disease occurs with coagulopathy, and with no previous history of liver disease. Hepatic encephalopathy develops within 8 weeks of onset of illness. It is referred to as "fulminant hepatic failure."

B. Etiology
1. Viral hepatitis (A, B, C, D, or E)
2. Hepatitis caused by other viruses (cytomegalovirus; herpes viruses 1, 2, and 6; and Epstein-Barr virus)
3. Drug-induced injury (e.g., acetaminophen)
4. Toxins (e.g., Amanita phalloides mushrooms and organic solvents)
5. Metabolic disorders
6. Vascular events (e.g., heatstroke)
7. Miscellaneous disorders (e.g., Wilson disease, AIH, and liver tumor)
8. Estimated 2,000 cases in United States per year

9. High morbidity and mortality
C. Clinical manifestations/diagnosis
   1. Initial signs are vague and include the following:
      a. Weakness
      b. Fatigue
      c. Loss of appetite
      d. Weight loss
      e. Abdominal discomfort
      f. Nausea and vomiting
      g. Change in bowel pattern
   2. Patients with ALF should be hospitalized and monitored frequently in ICU.
   3. Transplant center should be contacted and plans for transfer should be initiated early in the evaluation process. Early transfer is important as the patient's condition may deteriorate very rapidly.
   4. Initial lab evaluation should be extensive to try to determine the etiology
      a. Chemistries, ABG, lactate, toxicology screen, acetaminophen level, viral hepatitis serologies, ceruloplasmin, autoimmune markers, HIV, amylase, lipase, and PT/international normalized ratio (INR)
D. Specific etiology management
   1. Acetaminophen toxicity
      a. If ingestion is within 4 hr, give activated charcoal (1 gm/kg orally)
      b. Begin N-acetylcysteine in any suspected or possible acetaminophen toxicity (140 mg/kg PO or nasogastrically, diluted in 5% solution, followed by 70 mg/kg every 4 hr × 17 doses or intravenous dose of 150 mg/kg in 5% dextrose over 15 min with 50 mg/kg given over 4 hr, followed by 100 mg/kg over 16 hr)
   2. Viral hepatitis
      a. Supportive care for viral hepatitis A and E; no virus-specific treatment is available
      b. Acute hepatitis B should be treated with one of the hepatitis B antiviral agents
   3. Wilson disease
      a. Should obtain ceruloplasmin, urinary copper level, and slit lamp exam for Kayser–Fleischer rings
      b. A high bilirubin-to-alkaline phosphatase ratio greater than 2.0 is a reliable indicator for Wilson disease.
   4. Acute fatty liver of pregnancy/HELLP syndrome
      a. Triad of jaundice, coagulopathy, and low platelets along with features of preeclampsia are indicators of HELLP.
      b. Steatosis on imaging
      c. Can have intrahepatic hemorrhage or hepatic rupture requiring emergent intervention
      d. Prompt delivery of baby critical in good outcome
   5. If etiology remains unclear, liver biopsy may be appropriate, but the risk/benefit ratio has to be weighed due to likely coagulopathy.
E. ICU management
   1. Cerebral edema and intracranial hypertension are the most critical complications to monitor. If cerebral edema is identified, measures to decrease ICP must be done.
      a. Hyperventilation
      b. Hypertonic sodium chloride
      c. Mannitol
      d. Barbiturates if other measures fail
   2. In cases of grade III or IV encephalopathy
      a. Intubate for airway protection
      b. CT scan of the head to evaluate for cerebral edema
      c. ICP monitoring recommended

CHAPTER **37** Liver Disease

  3. Hemodynamics and renal failure
     a. Fluid resuscitation with normal saline for hypotension
     b. Dialysis if needed for renal failure
     c. Vasopressor such as norepinephrine for volume refractory hypotension
     d. Goal to keep MAP greater than 75 and CPP 60–80 mmHg
     e. Monitor closely for acidosis and hypoglycemia
  F. Clinical predictors for poor prognosis in ALF
     1. King's College criteria—prognostic model for poor prognosis—only an indicator not absolute
        a. Acetaminophen-induced ALF is considered for liver transplant in case of the following:
           i. pH less than 7.3 or lactate greater than 3 after fluid resuscitation
           ii. Presence of grade 3 or 4 encephalopathy
           iii. INR greater than 6.5
           iv. Creatinine greater than 3.4
        b. Nonacetaminophen ALF—consider liver transplant if the following criteria are met:
           i. INR greater than 6.5 and encephalopathy present at all or any three of following:
              (a) Age less than 10 or greater than 40 years
              (b) Jaundice for greater than 7 days before encephalopathy
              (c) Bilirubin greater than 17 mg/dl
              (d) Unfavorable etiology such as Wilson disease, idiosyncratic drug reaction, and seronegative hepatitis
     2. Model for End-stage Liver Disease (MELD)—prognostic model used to determine severity of liver disease by using patient's laboratory values and the following formula:

        $$\text{MELD} = 3.8 \times \log_e(\text{serum bilirubin [mg/dl]})$$
        $$+ 11.2 \times \log_e(\text{INR})$$
        $$+ 9.6 \times \log_e(\text{serum creatinine [mg/dl]})$$
        $$+ 6.4$$

        a. Primarily used to prioritize patients on waitlist for liver transplantation based on liver disease severity and short-term mortality risk; can potentially be used to predict mortality rate for patients with acute alcoholic hepatitis and variceal hemorrhage

VIII. **Chronic liver disease sequela and management**
  A. Can lead to multiorgan failure
  B. Reduced liver metabolic processes
  C. Impaired bile formation and flow
  D. Increased incidence of infection
  E. Cardiac
     1. Hyperdynamic circulation
     2. Portal hypertension
     3. Arrhythmias
     4. Edema
     5. Activity intolerance
  F. Dermatologic
     1. Jaundice
     2. Spider angiomas
     3. Pruritus
  G. Fluid and electrolytes
     1. Ascites
     2. Water retention
     3. Decreased vascular volume
     4. Hypokalemia
     5. Hyponatremia (hemodilution)
     6. Hypernatremia

7. Hypoglycemia
8. Hypoalbuminemia
H. Gastrointestinal
   1. Abdominal discomfort
   2. Decreased appetite
   3. Diarrhea
   4. GI bleeding
   5. Varices
   6. Malnutrition
   7. Nausea and vomiting
I. Hematologic
   1. Anemia
   2. Impaired coagulation
   3. Disseminated intravascular coagulopathy
J. Immune system
   1. Increased risk for infection, which may lead to sepsis
K. Neurologic
   1. Hepatic encephalopathy
L. Respiratory
   1. Dyspnea
   2. Hyperventilation
   3. Hypoxemia
M. Renal
   1. Renal failure (hepatorenal syndrome)—patients in end-stage liver disease may develop any of the following:
      a. Azotemia
      b. Oliguria
      c. Hyponatremia
      d. Low urinary sodium levels
      e. Hypotension
N. Laboratory findings/diagnostics
   1. Bilirubin—elevated (normal, 1 mg/dl)
   2. Albumin—decreased (normal, 3.5–5.5 grams/dl)
   3. PT—prolonged; high prognostic value in acute liver injury (normal, 10–12 seconds)
   4. Partial thromboplastin time—prolonged (normal, 25–41 seconds)
   5. Liver enzyme level assessment is not the same as a liver function test; liver enzyme levels assess the presence of dysfunction but do not actually determine how well the liver is working
   6. Liver enzymes can be classified into two major types:
      a. Aminotransaminases
         i. AST (formerly SGOT)—elevated (normal, 0–40 U/L)
         ii. ALT (formerly SGPT)—greater specificity for liver disease
         iii. In most liver diseases, AST increase is less than that of ALT
            (a) AST/ALT ratio, less than 1
            (b) Normal ALT, 0–35 U/L
      b. Phosphatases
         i. Alkaline phosphatase—normal, 30–120 U/L
         ii. Gamma-glutamyltranspeptidase—normal, 0–30 U/L
            (a) These liver enzymes are released during cellular injury and are no longer released when hepatocytes begin to heal.
            (b) If injury is severe enough to cause necrosis, these enzymes are initially very high and then decline because no additional enzymes are available for release.

7. Ammonia—elevated (normal, 10–80 µg/dl)

O. Management
1. Hepatic encephalopathy
   a. Administer lactulose (Cephulac), 15–30 ml every 3–4 hr (orally or nasogastrically) until the patient produces three to four loose stools daily
   b. Gut cleansing with enemas might also be used
   c. Limit protein to lean proteins
   d. Rifaximin, 550 mg BID, recommended for those not controlled or tolerating lactulose therapy
2. Monitor for hypoglycemia.
   a. Intravenous infusion of 10% glucose
   b. Rate depends on blood glucose level
   c. May start at 50–100 ml/hr and is titrated depending on glucose levels
   d. Glucose intravenous push 50% if needed
3. Coagulopathy
   a. Vitamin K, 10 mg subcutaneously daily for 3 days, if PT is greater than 14 seconds and INR is greater than 2
   b. Fresh frozen plasma
4. Hyponatremia
   a. Free water restriction
   b. Less than 1000–1500 ml of water per day for those with a serum sodium level lower than 125 mEq/L
   c. Hold diuretics
5. Hypokalemia: potassium chloride replacement
6. Variceal bleeding: Refer to Gastrointestinal Bleeding chapter
7. Ascites
   a. Low-sodium diet—2 grams daily
   b. Fluid restriction—1000–1500 ml daily for those with a serum sodium level less than 125 mEq/L
   c. Diuretic therapy
      i. Spironolactone, 100 mg/day in divided doses to 400 mg maximum
      ii. Furosemide (Lasix), 20–40 mg/day
      iii. Goal is to reduce weight 1 lb/day in those with ascites and 2 lb/day in those with ascites and edema
      iv. Dose may have to be increased for this weight loss to be achieved
   d. For those with tense ascites, paracentesis may be necessary to drain 3–6 L for comfort and to decrease the risk for respiratory complications.
      i. Administer albumin 6–8 grams for each liter removed, to protect intravascular volume
      ii. The need for colloid replacement to prevent effective hypovolemia after LVP remains controversial; it is likely unnecessary for paracentesis of 5 L or less.
      iii. Dextran may be rarely used as well
8. Intravenous bicarbonate may be necessary for severe acidosis in which there is too much acid in the body fluids. Bicarbonate prevents the pH of blood from becoming too acidic.
9. Monitor BUN/serum creatinine (Cr) for elevation. Dialysis may be necessary
10. Closely monitor respiratory and hemodynamic status. Vasopressors and intubation may be necessary
11. Avoid hepatotoxic substances
12. Cholestyramine for pruritis management
    a. Initial therapy: 4 grams PO once or BID
    b. Maintenance therapy: 8–16 grams PO daily in 2 or more divided doses; max dose should not exceed 24 grams daily

13. Colestipol, 2 grams PO every day or every 12 hr (tablets) OR 5 grams PO every day (granules) in water or juice, may be helpful for those with pruritus as well
14. When symptoms become unmanageable, transplantation should be considered.

BIBLIOGRAPHY

Ahmed, F. (2013). What about us? Recent advances in the treatment of chronic hepatitis C threaten to leave some parts of the world behind. *Journal of Viral Hepatitis, 20*(5), 367–368.

Bacon, B. R., Adams, P. C., Kowdley, K. V., Powell, L. W., & Tavill, A. S. (2011). *Diagnosis and management of hemochromatosis: 2011 practice guideline by the American Association for the Study of Liver Disease.* Retrieved from http://www.aasld.org/practiceguidelines/Documents/Bookmarked%20Practice%20Guidelines/Hemochromatosis%202011.pdf

Bride, G. M. (2013). *Clinical guidelines for advanced practice nursing: an interdisciplinary approach* (2nd ed.). Burlington, MA: Jones & Bartlett Learning.

Centers for Disease Control and Prevention. (2009). *Viral hepatitis A fact sheet*. Retrieved May 15, 2007, from www.cdc.gov/ncidod/diseases/hepatitis/a/fact.htm

Centers for Disease Control and Prevention. (2009). *Viral hepatitis B fact sheet*. Retrieved May 15, 2007, from www.cdc.gov/ncidod/diseases/hepatitis/b/fact.htm

Centers for Disease Control and Prevention. (2012). *Hepatitis B FAQs for health professionals*. Retrieved December 1, 2013, from http://www.cdc.gov/hepatitis/HBV/HBVfaq.htm

Centers for Disease Control and Prevention. (2012). *Hepatitis E FAQs for health professionals.* Retrieved December 1, 2013, from http://www.cdc.gov/hepatitis/HEV/HEVfaq.htm

Centers for Disease Control and Prevention. (2013). *Hepatitis A FAQs for health professionals.* Retrieved December 1, 2013, from http://www.cdc.gov/hepatitis/HAV/HAVfaq.htm

Centers for Disease Control and Prevention. (2013). *Hepatitis C FAQs for health professionals.* Retrieved December 1, 2013, from http://www.cdc.gov/hepatitis/HCV/HCVfaq.htm

Centers for Disease Control and Prevention. (2013). *Hepatitis D.* Retrieved December 1, 2013, from http://www.cdc.gov/hepatitis/HDV/index.htm

Centers for Disease Control and Prevention. (2013, July 16). *Vaccine recommendations of the ACIP.* Retrieved September 29, 2014, from http://www.cdc.gov/vaccines/hcp/acip-recs/vacc-specific/hepb.html

Chalasani, N., Younossi, Z., Lavine, J. E., Diehl, A. M., Brunt, E. M., Cusi, K., . . . Sanyal, A. J. (2012). *The diagnosis and management of the non-alcoholic fatty liver disease: Practice guideline by the American Association for the Study of Liver Disease, American College of Gastroenterology, and the American Gastroenterological Association.* Retrieved from http://www.aasld.org/practiceguidelines/Documents/NonalcoholicFattyLiverDisease2012_25762_ftp.pdf

Chapman, R., Fevery, J., Kalloo, A., Nagorney, D. M., Boberg, K. M., Shneider, B., & Gores, G. J. (2010). Diagnosis and management of primary sclerosing cholangitis. *AASLD practice guidelines.* Retrieved from http://www.aasld.org/practiceguidelines/Documents/Practice%20Guidelines/PSC_2-2010.pdf

Desai, M. C. (2013). *Successful strategies for the discovery of antiviral drugs*. Cambridge: Royal Society of Chemistry.

DiPiro, J. T. (2014). *Pharmacotherapy: A pathophysiologic approach* (9th ed.). New York, NY: McGraw-Hill.

Friedman, L. S. (2012). *Handbook of liver disease* (3rd ed.). Philadelphia, PA: Elsevier/Saunders.

Ghany, M. G., Nelson, D. R., Strader, D. B., Thomas, D. L., & Seeff, L. B. (2011). An update on treatment of genotype I chronic hepatitis C virus infection: *Practice guideline by the American Association for the Study of Liver Disease.* Retrieved from http://www.aasld.org/practiceguidelines/Documents/AASLDUpdateTreatmentGenotype1HCV11113.pdf

Greenberger, N. J. (2012). Current diagnosis & treatment gastroenterology, hepatology, & endoscopy (2nd ed.). New York: McGraw-Hill Medical.

Lange, C. (2013). O144: Vitamin D deficiency and hepatitis C. *Journal of Viral Hepatitis, 20,* 8–9.

Lee, M. (2012). Adherence with use of oral agents in the treatment of chronic hepatitis B. *Current Hepatitis Reports, 11*(2), 70–74.

Lee, W. M., Larson, A. M., & Stravitz, R. T. (2011). *AASLD position paper: The management of acute liver failure* (update 2011). Retrieved from http://www.aasld.org/practiceguidelines/Documents/AcuteLiverFailureUpdate2011.pdf

Lehne, R. A. (2010). *Study guide, pharmacology for nursing care* (7th ed.). St. Louis, MO: Saunders/Elsevier.

Lindor, K. D., Gershwin, M. E., Poupon, R., Kaplan, M., Bergasa, N. V., & Heathcote, E. J. (2009). Primary biliary cirrhosis. *AASLD practice guidelines.* Retrieved from http://www.aasld.org/practiceguidelines/Documents/Bookmarked%20Practice%20Guidelines/PrimaryBillaryCirrhosis7–2009.pdf

Lok, A. S., & McMahon, B. J. (2009). Chronic hepatitis B: Update 2009. *AASLD practice guidelines.* Retrieved from http://www.aasld.org/practiceguidelines/Documents/Bookmarked%20Practice%20Guidelines/Chronic_Hep_B_Update_2009%208_24_2009.pdf

Manns, M. P., Czaja, A. J., Gorham, J. D., Krawitt, E. L., Vergani, G. M., Vergani, D., & Vierling, J. M. (2010). Diagnosis and management of autoimmune hepatitis. *AASLD practice guidelines.* Retrieved from http://www.aasld.org/practiceguidelines/Documents/AIH2010.pdf

Mann, S. J. (2012). *Hypertension and you: Old drugs, new drugs, and the right drugs for your high blood pressure.* Lanham, Md.: Rowman & Littlefield Publishers.

McCaughan, G. W. (2012). *Advanced therapy for hepatitis C.* Chichester, West Sussex: Blackwell.

McPhee, S. J., & Papadakis, M. A. (2011). *Current medical diagnosis & treatment 2011* (50th ed.). New York, NY: McGraw-Hill Medical.

O'Shea, R. S., Dasarathy, S., & McCullough, A. J. (2010). Alcoholic liver disease. *AASLD practice guidelines.* Retrieved from http://www.aasld.org/practiceguidelines/Documents/Bookmarked%20Practice%20Guidelines/AlcoholicLiverDisease1–2010.pdf

Pagana, K. D., & Pagana, T. J. (2010). *Mosby's manual of diagnostic and laboratory tests* (4th ed.). St. Louis, MO: Mosby/Elsevier.

Roberts, E. A., & Schilsky, M. I. (2008). Diagnosis and treatment of Wilson disease: An update. *AASLD practice guidelines.* Retrieved from http://www.aasld.org/practiceguidelines/Documents/Bookmarked%20Practice%20Guidelines/Diagnosis%20and%20Treatment%20of%20Wilson%20Disease.pdf

Runyon, B. A. (2013). Management of adult patients with ascites due to cirrhosis: Update 2012. *AASLD practice guideline.* Retrieved from http://www.aasld.org/practiceguidelines/Documents/ascitesupdate2013.pdf

Schiff, E. R. (2012). *Schiff's diseases of the liver* (11th ed.). Chichester, West Sussex, UK: John Wiley & Sons.

Symposium, C. F. (2009). *Interferon.* Hoboken: John Wiley & Sons.

Wells, B. G. (2009). *Pharmacotherapy handbook* (7th ed.). New York, NY: McGraw-Hill Medical Pub. Division.

CHAPTER 38

Biliary Dysfunction

MICHALYN PELPHREY • CHARLENE M. MYERS

CHOLECYSTITIS

I. **Definition**
   A. Inflammation of the gallbladder, acute or chronic, associated with gallstones (cholelithiasis) in more than 90% of cases
II. **Etiology/contributing factors/risk factors**
   A. Gallstones
      1. Gallstones become impacted within the cystic duct
      2. Inflammation occurs behind the obstruction
      3. Gallstones are the most common form of gallbladder disease
      4. Most stones are formed from cholesterol
   B. Acalculous cholecystitis
      1. 5% of cases
      2. Should be considered with unexplained fever 2–4 weeks after surgery or any stressful situation
         a. Multiple trauma
         b. Critical illness with a prolonged period of poor oral intake
   C. Bacteria/infectious agents, especially in patients with AIDS (cytomegalovirus, *Cryptosporidium*)
   D. Neoplasms (primary or metastatic)
   E. Strictures of the common bile duct
   F. Ischemia
   G. Torsion (twisting of cystic duct)
   H. Possible contributing factors:
      1. Obesity
      2. Pregnancy
      3. Sedentary lifestyle
      4. Low-fiber diets
   I. Risk factors:
      1. Female
      2. Advanced age

3. Rapid weight loss
4. Fad diets
5. High levels of cholesterol

III. **Signs/symptoms**
  A. Can be present for years without causing symptoms
    1. When symptoms do develop, they often present similarly to indigestion (i.e., bloating, gassiness, and abdominal discomfort).
  B. A stone may become lodged, causing biliary colic
    1. Sudden onset
    2. Intense epigastric or right upper quadrant pain that may radiate to the shoulder or back (infrascapular region)
    3. Often associated with a full or fatty meal
  C. Nausea and vomiting
    1. Occurs in approximately 70% of cases
    2. Vomiting offers some relief for many patients
  D. Feeling of abdominal fullness
  E. Anorexia (inability to finish an average-sized meal)
  F. Dyspepsia
  G. Recurrent episodes of biliary colic lasting longer than 12 hr

IV. **Subjective/physical exam findings**
  A. Elevated body temperature
  B. Local tenderness that is almost always accompanied by muscle guarding and rebound pain
  C. Positive Murphy's sign (deep pain on inspiration while fingers are placed under the right rib cage)
  D. Palpable gallbladder in 5% of cases
  E. Jaundice in 20% of cases
  F. Right upper quadrant pain, tenderness, guarding, fever, and leukocytosis that continues or progresses after 2–3 days indicates severe inflammation and possible gangrene, empyema, or perforation

V. **Laboratory/diagnostics**
  A. Mild leukocytosis: white blood cell (WBC) count, 12,000–20,000/mcl
  B. Serum bilirubin mildly increased (greater than 4 mg/dl)
  C. Increased levels of the following:
    1. Alanine transaminase (normal, 1–35 units/L)
    2. Aspartate transaminase (normal, 0–35 units/L)
    3. Lactate dehydrogenase (LDH) (normal, 50–150 units/L)
    4. Alkaline phosphatase (normal, 30–120 units/L)
  D. Amylase level (normal, 0–130 units/L)
    1. Elevated
    2. If greater than 500 units, concomitant pancreatitis should be suspected
  E. Electrocardiogram
    1. Normal
    2. Electrocardiogram is important to rule out myocardial infarction as the cause of symptoms
  F. Chest x-ray to rule out pneumonia
  G. Flat plate of the abdomen may show radiopaque gallstones (20% of cases)
  H. Hepato-iminodiacetic acid scan to visualize cystic duct obstruction
    1. A positive test consists of nonvisualization of the gallbladder after 4 hr
    2. This test is reliable if bilirubin is less than 5 mg/dl
  I. Ultrasound: best study for diagnosing gallstones; dilated gallbladder with a thickened gallbladder wall, pericholecystic fluid, and sonographic Murphy's sign are seen in patients with acute cholecystitis

J. Endoscopic retrograde cholangiopancreatography (ERCP)
   1. Can be used to diagnose stones in the gallbladder if noninvasive studies have been found negative
   2. Gives information on the status of biliary and pancreatic ducts
K. Tokyo Guidelines for diagnostic criteria and severity assessment
   1. Diagnostic criteria for acute cholecystitis
      a. Local signs of inflammation—Murphy's sign, right upper quadrant mass/pain/tenderness
      b. Systemic signs of inflammation—fever, elevated CRP, elevated WBC
      c. Imaging findings characteristics of acute cholecystitis
         i. Definite diagnosis—one item in a and one in b are positive
         ii. Item c confirms the diagnosis when acute cholecystitis is suspected clinically
   2. Severity assessment
      a. Mild (grade I) acute cholecystitis—no findings of organ dysfunction and mild disease in the gallbladder
      b. Moderate (grade II) acute cholecystitis—accompanied by any one of the following:
         i. Elevated WBC greater than 18,000
         ii. Palpable tender mass in right upper quadrant
         iii. Duration of complaints greater than 72 hr
         iv. Marked local inflammation (gangrenous cholecystitis, emphysematous cholecystitis, abcess)
      c. Severe (grade III) acute cholecystitis
         i. Accompanied by dysfunctions of organ systems (hypotension, decreased level of consciousness, renal dysfunction, PaO_2/FiO_2 ration less than 300, hepatic dysfunction, hematological dysfunction)

VI. Treatment
A. Nothing by mouth (NPO) or low-fat, low-volume meals
B. If NPO, nasogastric tube to low wall suction
C. IV fluids
   1. To maintain intravascular volume and electrolytes, 5% dextrose in 0.45 normal saline (NS), 125 ml/hr
   2. Note signs of dehydration, and increase fluids PRN
      a. Tachycardia
      b. Hypotension
      c. Decreased urinary output
D. Pain can be controlled with antispasmodics, NSAIDs, and if necessary, some opiate analgesics (morphine, hydromorphone [Dilaudid])
E. IV antibiotics
   1. Typically, a third-generation cephalosporin (e.g., cefazolin, cefuroxime, ceftriaxone) with the addition of metronidazole (1 gram IV loading dose, followed by 500 mg IV every 6 hr) in mild-to-moderate cases of community-acquired acute cholecystitis
   2. Piperacillin/tazobactam (3.375 grams IV every 6 hr or 4.5 grams IV every 8 hr)
   3. Ampicillin/sulbactam (3 grams IV every 6 hr)
   4. Meropenem (1 gram IV every 8 hr)
   5. For more severe cases, use imipenem/cilastatin (500 mg IV every 6 hr)
F. Antispasmodics and antiemetics

G. Surgery consultation: Early laparoscopic cholecystectomy is considered the treatment of choice for most patients. In randomized trials and meta-analysis, early treatment has been associated with shorter hospitalization. When laparoscopic cholecystectomy is performed in patients with moderate to severe cholecystitis, it should be performed by a highly experienced surgeon. If anatomical identification is difficult, the surgery should be converted to open cholecystectomy.
   1. In those with severe cholecystitis, initial conservative management with antibiotics is recommended with the use of cholecystostomy, PRN.
H. ERCP with sphincterotomy and extraction of stones can be performed along with cholecystectomy for patients with a stone in the common bile duct (choledocholithiasis).
I. Gallstones that are primarily composed of cholesterol and are smaller than 2 cm in diameter can be treated by pharmacologic dissolution, which should not be used as a primary treatment in acute cholecystitis but can be used as a measure in chronic cholecystitis
   1. Ursodiol/ursodeoxycholic acid (10–15 mg/kg/day) for 12–24 months
      a. Monitor every 6 months with an ultrasound scan of the gallbladder
      b. Recurrence rate has been found to be high after discontinuation of the medication
   2. Non-overweight patients who have stones that are radiolucent, small, lacking in calcification, few in number, and floating may benefit from chenodeoxycholic acid/chenodiol, which blocks hepatic synthesis of cholesterol, and ursodeoxycholic acid/ursodiol, which blocks intestinal uptake.
      a. Chenodeoxycholic acid/chenodiol 250 mg PO, BID for the first 2 weeks; increase the dose by 250 mg/day each week until a range of 13−16 mg/kg/day in 2 divided doses or until the maximum tolerated dose is reached
   3. Contact dissolution by instillation of methyl tert-butyl ether percutaneously into the gallbladder

ACUTE PANCREATITIS

I. **Definition**
   A. Acute, inflammatory autodigestive process of the pancreas
II. **Etiology**
   A. Acute biliary tract disease (e.g., gallstones)
   B. Alcoholism and acute intoxication
   C. Smoking
   D. Hypertriglyceridemia
   E. Hypercalcemia
   F. Autoimmune pancreatitis
   G. Hereditary pancreatitis
   H. Sphincter of Oddi dysfunction
   I. Pancreatic divisum
   J. Traumatic pancreatitis
   K. Infectious causes (e.g., mumps, cytomegalovirus, *Mycobacterium* avium-intracellulare complex)
   L. Idiopathic pancreatitis
   M. Hypoperfusion induced pancreatitis
   N. ERCP
   O. Medications
      1. Azathioprine (Imuran)
      2. Sulfonamides
      3. Thiazide diuretics
      4. Estrogen
      5. Furosemide (Lasix)
      6. Corticosteroids

7. Tetracycline
8. Valproic acid
9. Metronidazole
10. L-asparaginase
11. Methyldopa
12. Pentamidine
13. Ethacrynic acid
14. Procainamide
15. Sulindac
16. Nitrofurantoin
17. Angiotensin-converting-enzyme (ACE) inhibitors
18. Danazol
19. Cimetidine
20. Diphenoxylate
21. Piroxicam
22. Gold
23. Ranitidine
24. Sulfasalazine
25. Isoniazid
26. Acetaminophen
27. Cisplatin
28. Opiates
29. Erythromycin

III. **Signs/symptoms**
   A. Epigastric abdominal pain
      1. May radiate to the back or to the right or the left
      2. Usually
         a. Has an abrupt onset
         b. Is steady and severe
         c. Is worsened by walking or lying supine
      3. May be alleviated by
         a. Knee-to-chest position
         b. Leaning forward
         c. Sitting
   B. Nausea and vomiting
   C. In severe attacks
      1. Weakness
      2. Sweating
      3. Anxiety
   D. Epigastric tenderness and guarding
   E. Absent or hypoactive bowel sounds, distention (resulting from ileus)
   F. Fever
   G. Tachycardia, hypotension, cool/pale skin (due to decreased intravascular volume)
   H. Tachypnea, decreased breath sounds (caused by pleural effusion)
   I. Jaundice
   J. Steatorrhea
   K. If hypocalcemic
      1. Chvostek sign and/or
      2. Trousseau sign
   L. Ascites
   M. Crackles if pleural effusion is present
   N. Right upper quadrant mass may be palpated

CHAPTER **38** Biliary Dysfunction

O. If intra-abdominal bleeding is present (hemorrhagic pancreatitis)
   1. Flank discoloration (Grey Turner's sign) and/or
   2. Umbilical discoloration (Cullen's sign)

IV. **Laboratory/diagnostics**
   A. Elevated serum amylase and lipase levels
      1. Serum lipase remains elevated longer than serum amylase and is more specific
      2. Isoamylase is preferred by some clinicians as the initial test for reducing the risk of erroneously diagnosing pancreatitis by excluding occasional cases of salivary hyperamylasemia.
      3. The recommended cutoff for diagnosis is amylase three times above normal range or less than three times with abdominal pain typical of pancreatitis with CT scan to confirm diagnosis.
      4. Normal amylase does not rule out pancreatitis
   B. Elevated urine amylase level
   C. Elevated serum trypsin levels, which are diagnostic of pancreatitis in the absence of renal failure, are the most accurate indicators of the disease. Measurements are obtained by radioimmunoassay; however, this test is not readily available in most laboratories.
   D. For those patients who present to the emergency department with acute abdominal pain and a high degree of suspicion for pancreatitis, a negative dipstick for urinary trypsinogen-2 is useful to rule out acute pancreatitis.
   E. Leukocytosis (10,000–30,000/μl)
   F. Hematocrit may be elevated initially owing to hemoconcentration; decreased hematocrit may suggest hemorrhage or disseminated intravascular coagulopathy
   G. Hyperglycemia (in severe disease) with islet cell damage
   H. Elevated BUN concentration (usually resulting from dehydration)
   I. AST and LDH levels may be elevated as the result of tissue necrosis
   J. Bilirubin and alkaline phosphatase levels may be increased as a result of common bile duct obstruction.
   K. Hypocalcemia (less than 7 mg/dl) in severe disease (due to saponification of fat)
   L. Hypokalemia may be present because of associated vomiting; hyperkalemia may occur as the result of acidosis or renal insufficiency
   M. Low albumin
   N. Elevated C-reactive protein concentration after 48 hr suggests the development of pancreatic necrosis
   O. Monitor arterial blood gases for hypoxemia (due to acute respiratory distress syndrome, atelectasis, or pleural effusion) and acidosis (due to lactic acidosis, respiratory acidosis, or renal insufficiency)
   P. Abdominal plain film may show the following:
      1. A sentinel loop (ileus)
      2. Pancreatic calcifications
      3. Gallstones
   Q. Abdominal ultrasonography for detecting gallstones and pancreatic pseudocysts
   R. Contrast-enhanced CT scan is superior to ultrasound in defining the extent of pancreatitis and in diagnosing pseudocysts, necrosis, and fistulas
   S. ERCP may be indicated for some patients but should not be performed during acute stages of the disease
   T. Magnetic resonance imaging/cholangiopancreatography (MRI/MRCP) has several advantages over CT scan, including the evaluation of biliary tract and the pancreatic duct, and is free of radiation risk. MRI can assess the severity of acute pancreatitis by detecting the extent of necrosis and fluid collections like a CT scan but better allows definition of solid debris within collections. There is a magnetic resonance severity index that corresponds well with the Ranson score.

V. **Management**
   A. IV hydration to maintain intravascular volume
      1. Fluid therapy is the cornerstone of management of acute pancreatitis
      2. Note: remember that hypovolemia and shock are major causes of death early in the disease process. Patients may have sequestered up to 12 L of fluid on presentation of symptoms. It is imperative that the practitioner closely monitor fluid status and make fluid replacement a high priority when treating acute pancreatitis.
      3. Lactated Ringer or NS solution with 20 mEq KCl/L at 75–100 ml/hr
      4. Increase PRN to maintain adequate blood pressure (BP) (try to keep systolic blood pressure [SBP] higher than 100 mmHg and mean arterial pressure [MAP] higher than 60 mmHg), urinary output (try to keep more than 30 ml/hr), heart rate (try to keep less than 100 beats per minute), and pulmonary capillary wedge pressure (PCWP)/central venous pressure (try to keep PCWP between 11 and 14 mmHg). These are reasonable goals, but they should be individualized for each patient.
      5. Fresh frozen plasma and albumin may also be infused
      6. Patients with acute hemorrhagic pancreatitis may need red blood cells in addition to fluid therapy to restore vascular volume.
      7. Those patients who fail to respond to fluid therapy alone may need vasoactive agents (e.g., dopamine and dobutamine) to support BP.
   B. Pain control
      1. Morphine (Morphine sulfate, 2–10 mg IV every 4 hr, PRN), hydromorphone (Dilaudid, 0.5–1.5 mg IV or SQ, every 4 hr, PRN), and fentanyl (25–75 mcg IV/SQ, every 2 hr, PRN) are reasonable alternatives to meperidine and are more desirable due to adverse effects associated with meperidine
   C. Antibiotics—not used prophylactically
      1. For patients who have evidence of the following:
         a. Septicemia
         b. Pancreatic abscess
         c. Inflammation caused by biliary stones
      2. Should be broad-spectrum agents (e.g., imipenem-cilastatin [Primaxin], 250–500 mg every 6–8 hr)
      3. Prophylactic antibiotics not recommended, regardless of type or severity
      4. Infected necrosis should be suspected in patients with pancreatic or extrapancreatic necrosis who deteriorate (clinical instability, sepsis, increased WBC, fevers) or fail to improve after 7–10 days of hospitalization.
      5. If empiric antibiotics initiated, antibiotics that penetrate pancreatic necrosis should be used.
         a. Carbapenems or quinolones plus metronidazole (500 mg IV every 8 hr)
   D. NPO until clinical improvement, then the following:
      1. Supplements
      2. Small, frequent meals
         a. Low cholesterol
         b. High protein
         c. Low fat
         d. Bland
   E. Nasogastric tube for ileus or vomiting
   F. Monitor calcium levels and replace PRN
   G. Monitor pulmonary function
   H. Enteral nutrition may be necessary
      1. Has shown significant reduction in mortality and multiorgan failure, operative interventions and systemic infections compared to parenteral nutrition

2. Pancreatic stimulation is overcome by feeding via nasojejunal tube delivering tube feeds beyond the ligament of Tritz into jejunum
  I. Insulin may be needed in cases of hyperglycemia
  J. Surgery in selected cases
     1. Gallstones
     2. Perforated peptic ulcer
     3. Need for excision or drainage
  K. If pancreatitis is caused by biliary obstruction, stent placement via ERCP may be used to decrease the likelihood of recurrent episodes.
VI. **Prognosis**
  A. The Ranson criteria have identified criteria for predicting the prognosis of patients with acute pancreatitis. The number of prognostic signs present within the first 48 hr after admission helps to determine the patient's chances of morbidity and mortality.
     1. Fewer than three risk factors: approximately 1% mortality rate
     2. Three to four risk factors: 16% mortality
     3. Five to six risk factors: 40% mortality
     4. More than seven risk factors: close to 100% mortality
     5. Prognostic signs at admission or diagnosis
        a. Older than age 55 (older than age 70 for gallstones)
        b. WBC count greater than 16,000/mcl
        c. Blood glucose higher than 200 mg/dl
        d. LDH greater than 350 international units/L
        e. AST greater than 250 international units/L
     6. Prognostic signs during initial 48 hr
        a. Hematocrit drops by more than 10 ml/dl
        b. BUN increases by more than 5 mg/dl
        c. Calcium level declines by 8 mg/dl
        d. Arterial oxygen pressure declines by 60 mmHg
        e. Base deficit exceeds 4 mEq/L
        f. Estimated fluid sequestration exceeds 6,000 ml
  B. APACHE II predicts the severity of acute pancreatitis
     1. Twelve physiological parameters and additional points for age and underlying medical conditions (rectal temperature, MAP, heart rate, respiration rate, FIO_2, arterial pH, serum sodium, serum potassium, serum creatinine, hematocrit, and WBC)
     2. It can be applied at time of admission and daily to assess progression on disease.
     3. A score of 8 or more points predicts 11%–18% mortality
  C. BISAP score
     1. The variables are as follows:
        a. Blood urea nitrogen level greater than 25 mg/dl
        b. Impaired mental status
        c. Systemic inflammatory response syndrome
        d. Age older than 60 years
        e. Pleural effusion
     2. Each score is worth 1 point. There is a steady increase in the risk of mortality with the increasing number of points.
        a. 0 points: mortality rate of 0.1%
        b. 1 point: mortality rate of 0.4%
        c. 2 points: mortality rate of 1.6%
        d. 3 points: mortality rate of 3.6%
        e. 4 points: mortality rate of 7.4%
        f. 5 points: mortality rate of 9.5%

BIBLIOGRAPHY

Banks, P. A., Bollen, T. L., Dervenis, C., . . . Vege, S. S. (2012) Classification of Acute Pancreatitis. *Gut, 62*, 101–111. Retrieved from http://gut.bmj.com/content/62/1/102.short

Chauhan, S., & Forsmark, C. E. (2010). Pain management in chronic pancreatitis: A treatment algorithm. *Best Practice and Research Clinical Gastroenterology, 24*, 323–335.

Ferri, F. F. (2011). *Practical guide to the care of the medical patient* (8th ed.). St. Louis, MO: Mosby.

Fujikawa, T., Tada, S., Abe, T., Yoshimoto, Y., Maekawa, H., Shimoike, N., & Tanaka, A. (2012). Is early laparoscopic cholecystectomy feasible for acute cholecystitis for the elderly? *Journal of Gastroenterology and Hepatology Research, 1*(10).

Greenberger, N. J., & Sharma, P. (2014) Update in gastroenterology and hepatology. *Annals of Internal Medicine, 161*, 205–209.

Greenberger, N. J., & Paumgartner, G. (2011). Diseases of the gallbladder and bile ducts. In D. L. Kasper, E. Braunwald, A. S. Fauci, S. Hauser, D. Longo, & J. L. Jameson (Eds.), *Harrison's principles of internal medicine* (18th ed.). New York, NY: McGraw-Hill.

Greenberger, N., Blumberg, R., & Burakoff, R. (2011). *Current diagnosis and treatment, gastroenterology, hepatology & endoscopy* (2nd ed.). New York, NY: McGraw Hill.

Gurusamy, K., Samraj, K., Gluud, C., Wilson, E., & Davidson, B. R. (2010). Meta-analysis of randomized controlled trials on the safety and effectiveness of early versus delayed laparoscopic cholecystectomy for acute cholecystitis. *British Journal of Surgery, 97*, 141–150.

Hawkins, J., & Roberto-Nichols, D. M. (2011). *Guidelines for nurse practitioners in gynecologic settings* (10th ed.). New York, NY: Springer.

Imrey, P. B., & Law, R. (2012). Antibiotic prophylaxis for severe acute pancreatitis. *American Journal of Surgery, 203*, 556–557.

Krumberger, J. M., & Hammer, B. (2012). Gastrointestinal alterations. In M. L. Sole, D. Klein, & M. Moseley (Eds.), *Introduction to critical care nursing* (6th ed.). Philadelphia, PA: WB Saunders.

McPhee, S. J., Papadakis, M. A., & Tierney, L. M. (Eds.). (2014). *Current medical diagnosis and treatment* (46th ed.). New York, NY: McGraw Hill/Appleton & Lange.

Muniraj, T., Gajendran, M., Thiruvengadam, S., Raghuram, K., Rao, S., & Devaraj, P. (2012). Acute pancreatitis. *Disease-a-Month, 58*, 98–144. Retrieved from http://dx.doi.org/10.1016/j.disamonth.2012.01.005

Nikfarjam, M., Niumsawatt, V., & Christophi, C. (2011). Outcomes of contemporary management of gangrenous and non-gangrenous acute cholecystitis. *HPB (Oxford), 13*, 551–558.

Sitaramin, S., & Friedman, L. S. (2012). *Essentials of gastroenterology*. Hoboken, NJ: Wiley-Blackwell.

Stefanidis, D., Richardson, W. S., Chang, L., Earle, D. B., & Fanelli, R. D. (2009). The role of diagnostic laparoscopy for acute abdominal conditions: An evidence based review. *Surgical Endoscopy, 23*, 16–23.

Tenner, S., Baillie, J., DeWitt, J., & Vege, S. S. (2013). American College of Gastroenterology Guideline: Management of acute pancreatitis. *American Journal of Gastroenterology, 108*, 1400–1415.

Wiseman, J. T., Sharuk, M. N., Singla, A., Cahan, M., Litwin, D. E., . . . Shah, S. A. (2010). Surgical management of acute cholecystitis at a tertiary care center in the modern era. *Archives of Surgery, 145*, 439–444.

Wittau, M., Mayer, B., Scheele, J., Henne-Bruns, D., Dellinger, E. P., & Isenmann, R. (2011). Systematic review and meta-analysis of antibiotic prophylaxis in severe acute pancreatitis. *Scandinavian Journal of Gastroenterology, 46*, 261–270.

CHAPTER 39

Inflammatory Gastrointestinal Disorders

LISA A. JOHNSON • CHARLENE M. MYERS

DIVERTICULITIS

I. **Definition**
   A. Perforation of a colonic diverticulum; can either be a localized microperforation (most common) or a macroperforation with abscess formation or generalized peritonitis
   B. Fifty percent of people older than 50 years have diverticulosis; 10%–25% of those with diverticulosis develop diverticulitis

II. **Etiology**
   A. Not clearly proven
   B. Low-fiber diet believed to be the leading cause in Western societies
   C. Weakness and defects in the colon wall

III. **Subjective/physical examination findings**
   A. Lower left quadrant pain (mild to moderate) and fever are the main clinical features
   B. Patients with free perforation present with more generalized pain and peritoneal signs
   C. Constipation is common and may alternate with diarrhea
   D. Fever and abdominal tenderness, guarding, palpable mass, spasms, and rebound tenderness indicate inflammation due to abscess
   E. Nausea and vomiting
   F. Bowel sounds are usually hypoactive
   G. Dysuria and frequency may be present

IV. **Laboratory/diagnostics**
   A. Leukocytosis is common, although those with mild diverticulitis may have a normal white blood cell count
   B. Elevated procalcitonin level, erythrocyte sedimentation rate, and C-reactive protein are caused by inflammation
   C. CT scan of the abdomen is obtained to look for evidence of diverticulitis, to determine its severity, and to exclude abscess or fistula formation
   D. Presence of colonic diverticula with colonic wall thickening, pericolic fat inflammation (streaking), abscess formation, or extraluminal air, all suggest varying levels of diverticulitis
   E. Barium enema may reveal strictures, obstruction, masses, or fistulas, but it should not be used in acute stages because it may cause free perforation

F. Flexible sigmoidoscopy may show inflamed mucosa but should be avoided during the acute phase. Patients should wait 4–6 weeks before having invasive examination of colon.

V. **Management**
   A. Outpatient:
      1. Patients with mild symptoms and no peritoneal signs can be managed as an outpatient.
      2. Oral antibiotics, clear liquids to 48- to 72-hour advancement to low-fiber (residue) diet as tolerated. Avoid laxatives. Most patients improve in 2–3 days.
      3. In patients with acute uncomplicated diverticulitis, antibiotic treatment duration is 7–10 days, depending upon resolution of symptoms.
         a. Ciprofloxacin (Cipro), 500 mg PO two times a day; or levofloxacin (Levaquin), 500 mg PO daily plus metronidazole (Flagyl), 500 mg PO every 8 hr
         b. Amoxicillin (Amoxil) and clavulanate, 500 mg PO three times a day; or 875 mg PO two times a day
   B. Inpatient:
      1. IV antibiotics, bowel rest, +/−TPN, and nasogastric tube (NGT) if ileus is present
      2. Antibiotic options (duration 7–10days; switch to oral after 5 days if patient improved):
         a. Fluoroquinolone (ciprofloxacin 400 mg IV every 12 hr or levofloxacin 500 mg IV QD) + metronidazole 500 mg IV every 8 hr
         b. Third or fourth generation cephalosporin (i.e. cefotaxime, ceftriaxone, or cefepime) + metronidazole 500 mg IV every 8 hr
         c. Piperacillin-tazobactam (Zosyn), 3.375 grams IV every 6 hr; or 4.5 grams IV every 8 hr
         d. Ticarcillin-clavulanate (Timentin), 3.1 grams IV every 6 hr
         e. Immunocompromised patients: imipenem 500 mg IV every 6 hr
   C. Surgical considerations:
      1. Severe disease or failure to respond to treatment within 72 hr requires surgical consultation
      2. Emergency surgical consultation is necessary for those patients who have an abscess, an obstruction, free air, or peritonitis; these conditions require surgery

INFLAMMATORY BOWEL DISEASE

I. **Ulcerative colitis**
   A. Definition
      1. Idiopathic inflammatory condition involving the mucosal surface of the colon; characterized by erosions with bleeding and friability
   B. Subjective/physical examination findings
      1. Bloody diarrhea is the cardinal sign
      2. Fecal urgency, tenesmus, and abdominal cramping
      3. Weight loss, malnutrition, anemia, and fever can occur
      4. Assessment of disease activity (Table 39.1)
   C. Laboratory/diagnostics
      1. See Table 39.1
      2. Leukocytosis during inflammation
      3. Anemia
      4. Electrolyte abnormalities (hypokalemia)
      5. Causes elevated values on liver function tests (if hepatobiliary disease is present)
      6. Stool cultures to rule out infectious colitis
      7. Sigmoidoscopy/colonoscopy with biopsy determines the extent of disease and provides histologic confirmation. Crohn's disease that only affects the colon can be difficult to determine as it may appear as ulcerative colitis.
      8. Plain abdominal x-rays exclude dilatation and are helpful in the determination of disease state
      9. Colonoscopy and barium enema should not be performed in an acute attack due to risk of perforation

CHAPTER 39 Inflammatory Gastrointestinal Disorders

Table 39.1	Assessment of disease activity in ulcerative colitis		
	Mild	**Moderate**	**Severe**
Albumin	Normal	3–3.5 grams/dl	Less than 3.0 grams/dl
Erythrocyte sedimentation rate	Less than 20 mm/hr or normal	20–30 mm/hr	More than 30 mm/hr
Heart rate (beats/minute)	Less than 90	90–100	Higher than 100
Hematocrit	Normal	30–40 mg/dl	Less than 30 mg/dl
Stool, #/day	Fewer than four	Four to six	More than six (bloody)
Temperature	Normal	99°F to 100°F	Above 100°F
Weight loss	None	1% to 10%	Greater than 10%

D. Management
   1. See table 39.2
   2. Mild/moderate active distal disease
      a. First-line therapy: oral or topical (enema/suppository) aminosalicylates or topical corticosteroids. Derivatives of 5-acetylsalicylic acid (5-ASA; sulfasalazine, mesalamine, balsalazide, and olsalazine) are currently available and result in symptomatic improvement in 50%–75% of patients
      b. Patients refractory to oral aminosalicylates or topical steroids may respond to mesalamine enemas
      c. Patients refractory to all of the above agents in maximal doses or who are systemically ill, may require treatment with oral prednisone in doses up to 40–60 mg per day or infliximab with an induction regimen of 5 mg/kg at weeks 0, 2, and 6
   3. Mild/moderate active extensive disease
      a. Sulfasalazine (Azulfidine) is the cornerstone of drug therapy for mild to moderate cases of ulcerative colitis, although it is associated with a greater number of adverse effects.
      b. First-line therapy: oral sulfasalazine or an alternate aminosalicylate at dose equivalent to
         4.8 grams/day of mesalamine
      c. For active disease, dosage should be 4 grams/day, 2 grams daily for maintaining remission
      d. It should be initiated at 500 mg/day and increased every few days up to 4–6 grams/day for the therapeutic dose
      e. Because sulfasalazine inhibits folate absorption, folate supplementation is recommended
      f. Patients with sulfa allergies should avoid this drug
      g. Consider combined oral and topical therapy for patients with distal disease
      h. Patients with mild to moderate disease who do not improve in 2–3 weeks with 5-ASA therapy should be given additional corticosteroid therapy.
         i. Topical hydrocortisone foam or enemas (80–100 mg once or BID) or 5-ASA enemas
            (4 grams once daily) may be tried first.
         ii. If therapy fails after 2 weeks, systemic steroid therapy should be initiated. Prednisone (40 mg QD) and methylprednisolone (Medrol) are the most commonly used. The patient should be tapered off steroids slowly after 2 weeks at a rate of decrease of no more than 5 mg/week.
      i. Patients refractory to oral corticosteroids can be treated with azathioprine (2–2.5 mg/kg/day) or 6-mercaptopurine (1–1.5 mg/kg/day); can be used in combination with aminosalicylates

j. Infliximab is an effective treatment for patients who are steroid refractory or steroid dependent despite adequate doses of a thiopurine, or who are intolerant of these medications
4. Severe disease
   a. Patients with severe symptoms refractory to oral/topical aminosalicylates or corticosteroids should be treated with a 7–10 day course of IV corticosteroids (300 mg hydrocortisone or 48 mg methylprednisolone equivalent/day).
   b. Patients refractory to IV corticosteroids are candidates for IV cyclosporine (4 mg/kg/day)
   c. Infliximab may also be effective in avoiding colectomy in patients failing intravenous steroids but its long-term efficacy is unknown in this setting
   d. Patients refractory to above are candidates for colectomy
   e. Patients with toxic megacolon should undergo bowel decompression, treatment with broad-spectrum antibiotics, and possibly colectomy
5. Problems of hypersensitivity and intolerance have been reported with sulfasalazine. New forms have been developed (e.g., mesalamine [Asacol], 1.2–1.6 grams; mesalamine [Pentasa], 1 gram four times a day; balsalazide [Colazal], 2.25 grams three times a day for active disease [three 750-mg capsules three times a day]).
6. Mesalamine suppositories, 500 mg BID for 3–12 weeks, are beneficial for patients with ulcerative proctitis
7. Patients with disease beyond the rectum but not beyond the descending colon may benefit from mesalamine enemas (4 grams daily)
8. Immunomodulators
   a. Maintenance of remission; acute flares unresponsive to steroids
   b. Agents: 6-mercaptopurine (Purinethol), azathioprine (Imuran), cyclosporine (Neoral), methotrexate (Trexall)
   c. Azathioprine (Imuran) has been shown to be effective in preventing relapse of ulcerative colitis for periods of up to 2 years
9. For severe cases of ulcerative colitis, hospitalization is required because the patient's condition may deteriorate rapidly.
   a. Nothing by mouth (NPO)—total parenteral nutrition may be necessary for those with poor nutritional status
   b. Avoid opioids and anticholinergics
   c. Administer IV resuscitation and blood products PRN (hematocrit less than 25%–28%)
   d. Monitor and correct electrolyte imbalances
   e. Plain abdominal x-ray (to detect toxic megacolon)
   f. Stool samples (to detect infectious disease)
   g. Surgery consultation
   h. Methylprednisolone (Solu-Medrol), 40–60 mg IV daily
10. Surgical indications include the following (25% of patients will require surgery):
    a. Toxic megacolon
    b. Fulminant colitis
    c. Perforation
    d. Hemorrhage
    e. High-grade dysplasia
    f. Carcinoma
    g. Refractory disease requiring high-dose steroids
11. Toxic megacolon
    a. Develops in less than 2% of patients; rapid disease progression with fever, dehydration, and transfusions for anemia
    b. Antibiotics (cover for gram-negative bacteria and anaerobes), NGT, and serial plain abdominal films to monitor for perforation

c. Surgery within 72 hr if failure to respond to medical management

II. **Crohn's disease**
   A. Definition
      1. Transmural process that can result in mucosal inflammation and ulceration, stricturing, fistula development, and abscess formation
      2. Patients may present with a combination of the following: chronic inflammation, intestinal obstruction, fistula formation, and abscess formation
      3. Patients with colonic disease are at risk for developing colon cancer, lymphoma, and small bowel adenocarcinoma
   B. Management
      1. Drug therapy
         a. Initial management with 5-aminosalicylic acid agents (mesalamine, 2.4–4.8 grams/day, or Pentasa, 4 grams/day orally)
         b. Corticosteroids for active disease with prednisone or methylprednisolone with long course and slow taper; flares common during tapering of steroids
         c. Immunomodulating drugs: azathioprine, mercaptopurine, or methotrexate used in two-thirds of patients who with Crohn's disease who have not responded to corticosteroids
         d. Anti–tumor necrosis factor therapies: infliximab, adalimumab, and certolizumab injections/infusions for refractory disease
      2. Mild/moderate active distal disease
         a. First-line therapy for ileal, ileocolonic or colonic disease: oral aminosalicylate
         b. Metronidazole (Flagyl®) 10–20 mg/kg/day may be used in patients not responding to oral aminosalicylates
         c. Ciprofloxacin (Cipro®) 1 gram/day is considered as effective as mesalamine (generally second-line)
         d. Oral budesonide may be considered as first-line treatment.
      3. Moderate-severe disease
         a. Corticosteroids (prednisone 40–60 mg/day or budesonide 9 mg/day) until resolution of symptoms
         b. Anti TNF monoclonal antibodies (infliximab, adalimumab, and certolizumab pegol) are effective in the treatment of moderate to severely active CD in patients who have not responded despite complete and adequate therapy with a corticosteroid or an immunosuppressive agent
      4. Severe/fulminant disease
         a. Severe symptoms despite oral corticosteroid or anti-TNF monoclonal antibodies therapy
         b. Assess need for surgical intervention (mass, obstruction, abscess)
         c. Administer IV corticosteroids (40–60 mg prednisone equivalent)
         d. Possibly use IV cyclosporine (5–7.5 mg/kg/day) or methotrexate (25 mg SQ/IM weekly) if IV steroids fail
      5. Maintenance
         a. No role for long-term corticosteroid use
         b. Azathioprine (2–3 mg/kg/day)/6-mercaptopurine (1.5 mg/kg/day) or infliximab 5 mg/kg at
            0, 2, and 6 weeks, then every 8 weeks thereafter are appropriate as first-line therapies
         c. Diet: well-balanced; may need supplemental enteral therapy or TPN for short-term management in active disease with significant weight loss

Table. 39.2 Agents Used in the Treatment of IBD

Drug Class	Agent	MOA	Adverse Effects	Comments
Aminosalicylates (5-ASA)	Sulfasalazine (Azulfidine®) **Non-sulfa containing:** Mesalamine (Asacol®) Mesalamine (Pentasa®) Olsalazine (Dipentum®) Balsalazide (Colazal®)	Sulfasalazine is cleaved by gut bacteria in the colon to sulfapyridine and mesalamine (5-ASA). The active moiety (5-ASA) imparts a topical anti-inflammatory effect on the diseased bowel.	Sulfasalazine: nausea, vomiting, diarrhea, anorexia, and hypersensitivity reactions **Non-sulfa 5-ASA:** Generally better tolerated than sulfasalazine. Nausea, vomiting, HA, alopecia, anorexia, and folate malabsorption	Used for both induction and maintenance of remission Efficacy (less active in CD affecting small intestine due to colonic activation of drug) and toxicity are dose related Dosage adjustment required for renal dysfunction Mesalamine available as enema & suppository
Corticosteroids	Prednisone (Deltasone®) Budesonide (Entocort EC®) Hydrocortisone (Solu-Cortef®) Methylprednisolone (Solu-Medrol®)	Anti-inflammatory	Nausea, vomiting, weight gain, water retention, gastritis, psychosis, adrenal suppression, glucose intolerance, osteoporosis (with long-term use)	Work quickly to suppress acute flares **NO role for maintenance therapy** **Avoid chronic use** Budesonide approximately 15 times more potent than prednisone Available as IV, oral & enema
Immunomodulators	6-mercaptopurine (Purinethol®) Azathioprine (Imuran®) Methotrexate Cyclosporine (Sandimmune®) Tacrolimus (Prograf®)	Inhibits immune response	Pancreatitis, bone marrow suppression, nausea, diarrhea, rash, hepatotoxicity	May provide steroid sparing effect Indicated only for maintenance Drug interactions: cyclosporine, methotrexate, tacrolimus Limited data available for tacrolimus dosage
Anti-TNF Monoclonal Antibodies	infliximab (Remicade), adalimumab (Humira), certolizumab (Cimzia)	Neutralizes tumor necrosis factor (TNF) and alters immune response	Most common adverse effects are infusion-related reactions: fever, chills, pruritus, urticaria, chest pain, hypotension, hypertension, dyspnea	Serious infections including sepsis and disseminated tuberculosis have been reported. A tuberculin skin test is recommended prior to initiating therapy Indicated only for Crohn's disease Very expensive

PERITONITIS

I. **Definition**
   A. Acute inflammation of the visceral and parietal peritoneum
II. **Etiology**
   A. Primary—spontaneous bacterial peritonitis (SBP) of ascitic fluid as a complication of cirrhotic ascites
      1. For SBP prophylaxis in patients with cirrhosis and ascites, norfloxacin 400 mg oral daily is recommended. Oral ciprofloxacin has been associated with a higher rate of quinolone-resistant organisms, and should be avoided. Although trimethoprim-sulfamethoxazole may also be indicated for prophylaxis, studies are conflicted as to its effectiveness in comparison to norfloxacin.
      2. Most cases of SBP are caused by transmigration of bacteria through the bowel wall; enteric Gram-negative bacilli are common pathogens (70%).
      3. *Klebsiella*, *Pneumococcus*, and *Enterococcus* are common as well
   B. Secondary peritonitis; peritonitis with a surgically amenable source
      1. Often polymicrobial infection
      2. Abdominal trauma/penetrating wounds
      3. Perforation resulting from appendicitis, colitis, peptic ulcer disease, diverticulitis, pancreatitis, and cholecystitis
III. **Subjective/physical examination findings**
   A. SBP: fever and abdominal pain with often a change in mental status due to hepatic encephalopathy
   B. Secondary peritonitis
      1. Acute abdominal pain, exacerbated by motion, variable location of abdominal pain
      2. High fever
      3. Nausea and vomiting
      4. Constipation
      5. Abdominal examination:
         a. Distention
         b. Rebound tenderness
         c. Generalized rigidity
         d. Decreased bowel sounds
         e. Hyperresonance to percussion
      6. Ascites
      7. Dyspnea, tachypnea
      8. Dehydration (hypotension, tachycardia)
IV. **Laboratory/diagnostics**
   A. For SBP, ascitic fluid analysis will reveal the following:
      1. Protein concentration less than 1 gram/dl
      2. Polymorphonuclear cell count greater than 250/mm; this is the most sensitive and specific test for SBP if the count is higher than 500/mm
      3. Bacteria present on Gram's stain
      4. Lactic acid level greater than 32 mg/dl
      5. Glucose concentration higher than 50 mg/dl
      6. Lactate dehydrogenase level less than 225 mU/ml
   B. The secondary peritonitis ascitic fluid analysis will reveal the following:
      1. Leukocyte count greater than 10,000/mm
      2. Lactate dehydrogenase greater than 225 mU/ml
      3. Protein levels greater than 1 gram/dl
      4. Glucose less than 50 mg/dl
      5. Presence of multiorganisms on Gram's stain or culture
   C. Blood cultures—positive in 25% of patients
   D. Leukocytosis—more pronounced in secondary peritonitis

E. Elevated BUN levels
F. Hemoconcentration (increased hematocrit)
G. Metabolic and respiratory acidosis
H. Elevated amylase levels
I. Abdominal x-ray
   1. Free air in peritoneal cavity
   2. Dilatation of large or small bowel
J. Chest x-ray—elevated diaphragm
K. CT scan and ultrasound
   1. Ascites
   2. Intra-abdominal mass

V. **Management**
   A. See table 39.2
   B. SBP: antibiotic therapy—third-generation cephalosporin
      1. Cefotaxime (Claforan), 2 grams IV every 8 hr
      2. Ceftriaxone (Rocephin), 2 grams IV every 24 hr
      3. Ampicillin 1–2 grams every 6 hr plus gentamicin dosed to achieve peak of 8–10, and trough of less than 1.5
      4. Levofloxacin 750 mg IV every 24 hr can be used for patients with penicillin allergy.
      5. Fluoroquinolones should not be used in a patient who had been receiving a fluoroquinolone for SBP prophylaxis because the infecting organism may be resistant to fluoroquinolones
      6. Traditionally, 10 days of therapy is recommended, although recent studies suggest that 5 days is sufficient.
   C. Secondary peritonitis
      1. Operative management is indicated to eliminate the source of contamination, to reduce bacterial load, and to prevent recurrence.
      2. Empiric antimicrobial coverage to include gram-negative aerobes, enteric streptococci, and anaerobes
         a. Cefotaxime 2 grams IV every 8 hr + metronidazole 500 mg IV every 8 hr
         b. Duration of antibiotics, 7+ days
      3. Monitor blood and bacterial cultures for antibiotic management
      4. IV fluid resuscitation; NPO and possible NGT placement
      5. Monitor vital signs, urinary output, and consider need for respiratory support

APPENDICITIS

I. **Definition**
   A. Acute inflammation of the vermiform appendix caused by obstruction of the appendiceal lumen by
      1. Fecaliths (most common)
      2. Inflammation
      3. Foreign body
      4. Intestinal worms
      5. Strictures
      6. Tumors
   B. Gangrene and perforation can develop if appendicitis is not treated within 36 hr
   C. Appendicitis is the most common intra-abdominal infection treated by surgeons, 250,000 appendectomies per year.

II. **Clinical manifestations**
   A. Abdominal pain
      1. Periumbilical pain initially, then right lower quadrant pain (McBurney's point)
      2. Rovsing's sign: referral of pain to the right quadrant with palpation of the lower left quadrant
      3. Psoas sign: pain with active extension of the right hip

4. Obturator sign: pain with internal rotation of the right hip
B. Anorexia
C. Nausea with or without vomiting
D. Constipation—urge to defecate, although some report diarrhea
E. Low-grade fever (high fever suggests possible perforation or another diagnosis)
F. Motionless, with right thigh drawn up
G. Guarding of the right lower quadrant

III. **Laboratory/diagnostics**
A. Moderate leukocytosis—10,000–20,000 in 75% of cases
B. Urinalysis
  1. Elevated specific gravity
  2. Hematuria
  3. Pyuria
  4. Albuminuria
C. Ultrasound is 98% accurate in diagnosing appendicitis, provided that the appendix can be visualized
D. CT scan to detect the following:
  1. Perforation
  2. Periappendiceal abscess
E. History and clinical findings are the cornerstones of diagnosis

IV. **Management**
A. See table 39.2
B. Prompt surgical intervention with appendectomy is the mainstay of treatment
C. IV fluids: correct fluid and electrolyte imbalances as indicated
D. Cefoxitin [Mefoxin], 1–2 grams, every 6–8 hr IV, cefotetan [Cefotan]
E. Gangrenous or perforated appendicitis
  1. Mild-to-moderate severity (perforated or abscessed appendicitis and other infections of mild-to-moderate severity)
     a. Single agent:
        i. Cefoxitin, 2 grams IV every 6 hr
        ii. Ertapenem, 1 gram IV every 24 hr
        iii. Moxifloxacin, 400 mg IV every 24 hr
        iv. Ticarcillin-clavulanic acid, 3.1 grams IV every 6 hr
     b. Combination therapy: one of the following drugs in combination with metronidazole,
        500 mg IV every 8 hr
        i. Cefazolin, 1–2 grams IV every 8 hr
        ii. Cefuroxime, 1.5 grams every 8 hr
        iii. Ceftriaxone, 1–2 grams IV every 12–24 hr
        iv. Cefotaxime, 1–2 grams IV every 6–8 hr
        v. Ciprofloxacin, 400 mg every 12 hr
        vi. Levofloxacin, 750 mg every 24 hr
  2. High risk or severity (severe physiologic disturbance, advanced age, or immunocompromised state)
     a. Single agent:
        i. Imipenem-cilastatin, 500 mg every 6 hr
        ii. Meropenem, 1 gram every 8 hr
        iii. Doripenem, 500 mg every 8 hr
        iv. Piperacillin-tazobactam, 3.375 grams every 6 hr
     b. Combination therapy: one of the following drugs in combinations with metronidazole, 500 mg IV every 8 hr
        i. Cefepime, 2 grams IV every 12 hr

ii. Ceftazidime, 2 grams IV every 8 hr
iii. Ciprofloxacin, 400 mg every 12 hr
iv. Levofloxacin, 750 mg every 24 hr
3. Regardless of the initial empiric regimen, the therapeutic regimen should be narrowed/adjusted once culture and susceptibility results are available.
4. Continue antibiotics for 7 days after surgery
F. Pain management after diagnosis is made, and surgery is scheduled
1. Hydromorphone (Dilaudid), 1 mg IV/SQ, every 4 hr PRN for pain, or
2. Morphine sulfate, 1–2 mg IV every 4 hr PRN for pain

BIBLIOGRAPHY

Longo, D., Fauci, A., Kasper, D., Hauser, S., Jameson, J., & Loscalzo, J. (2012). *Harrison's principles of internal medicine* (18th ed.). New York, NY: McGraw-Hill.

Halter, J. B., Ouslander, J. G., Tinetti, M. E., Studenski, S., High, K. P., & Asthana, S. (2009). *Hazzard's geriatric medicine and gerontology* (6th ed.). New York, NY: McGraw-Hill.

McPhee, S. J., & Papadakis, M. A. (2014). In M. W. Rabow (Eds.), *Gastrointestinal disorders: Medical diagnosis and treatment.* New York, NY: McGraw-Hill.

Auwaerter, P. G., Barltett, J. G., Pham, P., & Hsu, A. J. (Eds.). (2014). *The Johns Hopkins POC-IT ABX Guide.* Baltimore, MD: John Hopkins University.

U.S. Department of Health and Human Services, National Institues of Health: National Institutes of Diabetes and Digestive and Kidney Diseases. (2011). *Ulcerative colitis.* NIH Publication No. 12–1597. Retrieved November 13, 2013, from http://digestive.niddk.nih.gov/ddiseases/pubs/colitis/

CHAPTER 40

Anatomic Intestinal Disorders

CATHERINE FUNG • CHARLENE M. MYERS

SMALL BOWEL OBSTRUCTION

I. **Definition**
   A. Blockage of the lumen of the intestine that prevents normal functioning and results in distention and tremendous losses of fluid into the gut
   B. Necrosis with toxicity and possible perforation may occur with strangulation

II. **Etiology**
   A. Adhesions—most common
   B. Hernias—external and internal
   C. Volvulus—twisting of the bowel on itself, causing obstruction
   D. Strictures—due to:
      1. Crohn's disease—intestinal fibrosis occurs as a result of chronic transmural inflammation causing stricture that usually leads to obstruction.
      2. Radiation
      3. Ischemia
   E. Hematomas—related to:
      1. Trauma
      2. Anticoagulants
   F. Intussusception—slipping of one part of an intestine into another part just below it
   G. Feces (impaction)
   H. Tumors
   I. Foreign bodies

III. **Pathophysiology**
   A. The intestine proximal to the obstruction fills up with gas and fluid. This fluid is not absorbed by the intestines, causing the bowels to distend.
   B. Intestinal distention causes vomiting, which leads to more loss of fluid and electrolytes.
   C. The obstruction causes the intestine to reverse its mechanism of absorbing fluids in the gut to secreting more fluid from the intravascular space to the obstructed lumen, causing further bowel distention.

D. Dehydration commences as more fluids and electrolytes are lost into the obstructed intestinal lumen. Metabolic alkalosis, hypokalemia, and hypochloremia may result from dehydration due to fluid loss and vomiting.
E. Low intestinal blood flow occurs as the intestinal luminal pressure increases. Strangulated bowel obstruction can occur, which is a condition of intestinal ischemia, necrosis, and perforation.
F. Stasis of intestinal contents leads to overgrowth of aerobic and anaerobic bacteria proximal to the site of bowel obstruction

IV. **Clinical manifestations**
   A. Cramping periumbilical pain initially occurs sporadically, lasting seconds to minutes
   B. The pain becomes constant and diffuses as distention develops.
   C. High or proximal bowel obstruction
      1. Variable upper abdominal pain
      2. Profuse vomiting
   D. Middle or distal small bowel obstruction (SBO)
      1. Cramping, colicky, periumbilical, or diffuse pain
      2. Distention
      3. Episodic vomiting
   E. The more distal the obstruction, the greater the distention
      1. More vomiting of feculent contents
      2. Increase in nasogastric output
   F. Obstipation (extreme constipation) develops in complete obstruction.
   G. Partial obstruction—watery, possibly mucous, diarrhea
   H. Mild tenderness
   I. High-pitched "tinkling" bowel sounds and peristaltic rushes are noted early on auscultation; these sounds may be absent later
   J. Visible peristalsis may be present
   K. Signs and symptoms of dehydration
      1. Orthostatic hypotension
      2. Oliguria
      3. Elevated temperature
      4. Tachycardia

V. **Diagnostics/laboratory findings**
   A. Leukocytosis may be present
   B. Hemoconcentration—elevated hemoglobin and hematocrit
   C. Electrolyte imbalances—metabolic alkalosis due to vomiting and lack of oral intake, metabolic acidosis due to gastrointestinal bicarbonate loss, and tissue hypoperfusion due to hypovolemia
   D. Hypokalemia—the most common electrolyte imbalance
   E. Blood urea nitrogen/creatinine may be elevated due to renal hypoperfusion

VI. **Imaging**
   A. Supine and upright abdominal x-rays
      1. Ladder-like pattern of dilated bowel with air-fluid levels
      2. Little or no air in the colon or rectum with complete obstruction
      3. Thickening or "thumbprinting" of the intestinal wall with strangulation
      4. Pneumatosis in the wall of the intestines, or portal venous gas, are ominous signs and suggest urgent surgical intervention
   B. Transabdominal ultrasonography
      1. Noninvasive, radiation-free method
      2. Well tolerated by patients with acute abdominal symptoms
      3. Accurate and highly specific in the diagnosis of SBO
      4. Dilated loops of bowel filled with fluids with or without peristalsis are readily seen.

5. Not commonly the first choice in the initial workup
  C. Barium radiography confirms the diagnosis if there is uncertainty.
     1. Oral administration of about 100 ml of Gastrografin or barium followed by plain abdominal x-ray. If the contrast reaches the cecum within 24 hr, it is 95% likely there is a partial SBO. Otherwise, it should be considered a complete obstruction, and surgical intervention must be considered.
  D. Small bowel follow-through using barium can evaluate an SBO caused by Crohn's disease by identifying a tight stricture in the terminal ileum.
  E. CT scan is superior in identifying the cause of the SBO (such as internal hernia, Crohn's disease, mass, and ischemia) or signs of intestinal compromise such as ischemia, necrosis, pneumatosis, or pneumoperitoneum.
     1. Shows abdomen in cross section to uniquely diagnose
     2. Used to decide the level and cause of obstruction when undetermined by x-ray
     3. Superior to ultrasound and x-ray, with 94% accuracy in diagnosing SBO
     4. Reveals dilated loops of bowel proximal to the obstruction and decompressed or collapsed bowel distally
  F. Multidetector CT scan assists in diagnosing SBO due to matted adhesions or single adhesive band; more sensitive than the standard CT
  G. Small bowel feces sign
     1. Found in CT scan of 50% of patients and common in high-grade obstruction. It is not a useful finding in SBO by itself.
     2. Solid material containing gas bubbles found in a segment of dilated bowel
     3. Be careful not to mistake feces in the cecum for SBO at the ileocecal valve
  H. Whirl sign
     1. Found in CT scan of SBO
     2. A "swirl" of mesenteric fat and soft tissue attenuation with loops of intestine adjacent to the surrounding intestinal vessels
  I. A key diagnostic sign is finding a discrete transition point between dilated SBO and collapsed, nondistended SBO; this localizes the point of obstruction.

VII. **Management**
  A. Nil per os (NPO; nothing by mouth) — bowel rest
  B. Rapid intravenous fluids and electrolyte replacement with isotonic solution with potassium provided there is adequate kidney function. Total parenteral nutrition (TPN) and nutritional support/dietary consult may be considered to provide adequate nutrition for partial bowel obstruction and recuperation after complete bowel obstruction.
  C. Nasogastric tube (NGT) to low wall suction—for nasogastric bowel decompression and to prevent aspiration from vomiting
  D. Foley catheter to accurately monitor intake and output
  E. Obtain blood cultures, complete blood count (CBC), comprehensive metabolic panel (CMP), arterial blood gas (ABG) test, serum lactate, and amylase/lipase, in addition to diagnostic imaging
  F. Initiate antibiotics for patients with suspected perforation or small bowel obstruction in setting of diverticulitis (e.g., cefoxitin [Mefoxin] piggyback, 2 grams IV every 6 hr , cefotetan [Cofotan],
     2 grams IV every 12 hr). There is no role for antimicrobial therapy in uncomplicated small bowel obstruction.
  G. Partial obstructions usually resolve spontaneously within a few days
  H. Surgical consultation is indicated for complete obstruction or for partial obstruction that fails to improve with traditional treatment
  I. Laparoscopic adhesiolysis for SBO due to adhesions

LARGE BOWEL OBSTRUCTION

I. **Definition**
   A. Large bowel (intestinal) obstruction occurs when there is a blockage in the large bowel that prevents food from passing through. The blockage cuts off blood supply to the bowel and a part of it dies. When this happens, the pressure causes a leak that spreads bacteria into the body or blood (translocation).

II. **Etiology/Predisposing Factors**
   A. Cancers of the:
      1. Colon (primary cause)
      2. Stomach
      3. Ovary
      4. Lung
      5. Breast
   B. Abdominal surgery
   C. Abdominal radiation

III. **Signs and symptoms**
   A. A history of bowel movements, flatus, obstipation, and associated symptoms should be obtained. Complaints in patients with LBO may include the following:
      1. Abdominal distention
      2. Nausea and vomiting
      3. Crampy abdominal pain
   B. Other symptoms that may be diagnostically significant include the following:
      1. Abrupt onset of symptoms (suggestive of an acute obstructive event)
      2. Chronic constipation, long-term cathartic use, and straining at stools (suggestive of diverticulitis or carcinoma)
      3. Changes in stool caliber (strongly suggestive of carcinoma)
      4. Recurrent left lower quadrant abdominal pain over several years (suggestive of diverticulitis, a diverticular stricture, or similar problems)

IV. **Physical Exam Findings**
   A. Although a complete physical examination is necessary, the examination should place special emphasis on the following key areas:
      1. Abdomen (inspection, auscultation, percussion, and palpation—evaluate bowel sounds, tenderness, rigidity, guarding, and any mass or fullness
      2. Inguinal and femoral regions—in particular, look for a possible incarcerated hernia
      3. Rectum—assess anal patency (in a neonate), contents of anal vault, and stool consistency; perform fecal occult blood testing as appropriate

V. **Laboratory/Diagnostics**
   A. The following laboratory studies may be helpful:
      1. Complete blood count (CBC)
      2. Hematocrit
      3. Prothrombin time (PT)
      4. Type and crossmatch
      5. Serum chemistries
      6. Serum lactate (if bowel ischemia is a consideration)
      7. Urinalysis
      8. Stool guaiac test
   B. Imaging modalities that may be considered are as follows:
      1. Plain radiography (flat and upright)
         a. Upright chest: useful screen for free air which would suggest perforation and ileus rather than obstruction. The absence of free air does not exclude perforation (this finding may be absent in half of all perforations).
         b. Flat and upright abdominal film: can help distinguish severe constipation from bowel obstruction. Plain films may also help localize the site of obstruction (large vs. small bowel).

c. Sigmoid or cecal volvulus may have a kidney-bean appearance on the abdominal films
d. Intramural air is an ominous sign that suggests colonic ischemia
2. Contrast radiography with enema
3. Computed tomography (CT)—this is the imaging modality of choice if a colonic obstruction is clinically suspected; contrast-enhanced CT can help distinguish between partial and complete obstruction, ileus, and small-bowel obstruction

VI. **Management**
A. Initial therapy in patients with suspected large-bowel obstruction (LBO) includes volume resuscitation, appropriate preoperative broad-spectrum antibiotics, and timely surgical consultation
B. A nasogastric tube should be considered for patients with severe colonic distention and vomiting. The patient's intravascular volume is usually depleted, and early intravenous fluid (IVF) resuscitation with isotonic saline or Ringer lactate solution is necessary.
C. Surgical intervention is frequently indicated, depending on the cause of the obstruction. Closed loop obstructions, bowel ischemia, and volvulus are surgical emergencies.

MESENTERIC ISCHEMIA

I. **Definition**
A. Mesenteric ischemia results when the bloodstream fails to carry sufficient amounts of oxygen and other nutrients to meet intestinal needs.
B. Ischemia may be related to an artery occluded by an embolus or thrombus, or no physical occlusion may be present.

II. **Etiology**
A. Acute arterial occlusion—occurs on patients who are older than 60 years of age; 3:1 male to female ratio
  1. Embolism—cardiac embolization causes 40%–50% of the cases
    a. Atrial fibrillation/flutter
    b. Valvular disease
    c. Atrial thrombus
  2. Thrombus—thrombus formation; a link has been found between prothrombin gene 20210G/A mutation and thrombosis of digestive vessels
    a. Arterial thrombus—may occur on atheromatous plaque
    b. Spontaneously (in women on oral contraceptives)
    c. Surgical accidents
    d. Abdominal trauma
    e. Tumors
B. Mesenteric venous thrombosis—patients tend to be younger (50s–60s)
  1. Primary coagulopathies (anti-thrombin III deficiency, protein C, protein S deficiencies)
  2. Hematologic prothrombotic conditions (polycythemia vera, hyperfibrinogenemia)
  3. Disseminated intravascular coagulopathy
  4. Liver cirrhosis with portal hypertension
  5. Congestive heart failure
  6. Low-flow states (abdominal trauma, intra-abdominal infections, systemic hypotension)
  7. Pancreatitis
C. Nonocclusive mesenteric vascular disease or nonocclusive mesenteric ischemia is more common than the preceding conditions and is related to low-flow conditions and mesenteric vasoconstrictive states. The mesenteric flow is slowed down, not by an obstructive mechanism, but by arterial spasm due to pharmacotherapy or physiologic response to shock, sepsis, or cardiac dysfunction.
  1. Congestive heart failure
  2. Aortic stenosis
  3. Shock
  4. Cardiac arrhythmias

5. Vasoconstrictor drugs
III. **Clinical manifestations**
   A. Severe cramping and generalized or periumbilical abdominal pain that is out of proportion to the clinical exam presentation
   B. Early in the course of the disorder, no abnormalities are found on examination. Diagnosis requires a high index of suspicion.
   C. Possible rectal bleeding with colonic ischemia
   D. Hypotension and abdominal distention suggest infarction
IV. **Laboratory/diagnostic findings**
   A. Leukocytosis
   B. Lactic acidosis—in the late stages, suggests infarction
   C. Creatine kinase
   D. Duplex ultrasound—shows bowel spasm and vessel occlusion in the early stages; reveals fluid-filled intestinal lumen and decreased or absent peristalsis in the late stages.
   E. CT angiography—reveals an emboli, thrombi, or stenosis in the lumen of the vessel in the early stage; reveals site of infarct, ileus, and bowel thinning in the late stage.
   F. Mesenteric arteriography (digital subtraction angiography [DSA])—useful in locating vascular occlusion
   G. Barium contrast radiography—"thumbprinting" or thickening of the intestinal wall in late stages
   H. Contrast-enhanced magnetic resonance angiography has sensitivity and specificity approaching those of DSA in the detection of mesenteric ischemia
   I. CT scan imaging has evolved over several years; findings include focal or segmental bowel wall thickening, submucosal edema or hemorrhage, pneumatosis, and portal venous gas
   J. Contrast-enhanced CT detects acute mesenteric ischemia
   K. Helical CT has improved image quality and scanning times and can be used to detect nonvascular visceral abnormalities
   L. Biphasic mesenteric multidetector CT angiography (similar to CT arteriography)—efficient diagnostic tool for accurate and timely discovery of mesenteric ischemic changes
V. **Management**
   A. Occlusive disease
      1. NPO
      2. Transcatheter administration of papaverine infusion, 30–60 mg/hr within 24–48 hr
      3. Embolectomy or bypass of the occluded vessel to prevent infarction. Abdominal exploration and open surgical revascularization.
      4. If infarction has occurred, resection of that part of the bowel should be performed.
      5. Fluids and supportive care
      6. TPN may be needed and may be continued indefinitely if a large portion of the bowel is resected.
   B. Nonocclusive disease
      1. Correct hypovolemia
      2. Supportive care for heart failure, pancreatitis, or other underlying conditions
      3. Remove vasoconstricting agents and digoxin
   C. The goals are to restore intestinal perfusion, reverse ischemia, and prevent infarction.
   D. If vasopressors are required, β-adrenergic agonists, such as low-dopamine and dobutamine, are preferred.
   E. NGT for decompression
   F. Foley catheter for accurate intake and output measurement
   G. Begin antibiotic coverage before surgery if peritonitis is suspected (broad spectrum for Gram-negative bacteria and anaerobes).
      1. Imipenem-cilastatin, 500 mg IV every 6 hr
      2. Meropenem, 1 gram IV every 8 hr
      3. Doripenem, 500 mg IV every 8 hr
      4. Piperacillin-tazobactam, 3.375 grams IV every 6 hr

5. Cefepime, 2 grams IV every 8 hr plus metronidazole, 500 mg IV every 8 hr
6. Ceftazidime, 2 grams IV every 8 hr plus metronidazole, 500 mg IV every 8 hr

H. Vasodilator drugs can also be administered via an intra-arterial catheter placed during angiography.
   1. Papaverine (Paverine, Pavabid) infusion, 30–60 mg/hr
   2. Vasodilator prostaglandins
I. Pain control with opioids such as morphine or hydromorphone (Dilaudid)
J. Stent placement for stenosis or occlusions have been effective as an adjunct therapy
K. Angioplasty or surgical revascularization is the primary method of treatment for chronic mesenteric ischemia.
L. Systemic anticoagulation is warranted in venous thrombotic event of the bowels that are inoperable; heparin therapy is the common choice of treatment.

BIBLIOGRAPHY

Adler, G., Parczewski, M., Czerska, E., Loniewska, B., Kaczmarczyk, M., Gumprecht, J., . . . Ciechanowicz, A. (2010). An age-related decrease in factor V Leiden frequency among Polish subjects. *Journal of Applied Genetics, 51*(3), 337–341.

Aschoff, A. J., Stuber, G., Becker, B. W., Hoffman, M. H. K., Schmitz, B. L., Schelzig, H., . . . Jaeckle, T. (2009). Evaluation of acute mesenteric ischemia: Accuracy of biphasic mesenteric multidetector CT angiography. *Abdominal Imaging, 34*, 345–357. doi:10.1007/s00261–008–9392–8

Baumgart, D. (2012). *Crohn's disease and ulcerative colitis from epidemiology and immunobiology to a rational diagnostic and therapeutic approach.* New York, NY: Springer.

Brott, T. G., Hobson, R. W., Howard, G., Roubin, G. S., Clark, W. M., Brooks, W., . . . Meschia, J. F. (2010). Stenting versus endarterectomy for treatment of carotid-artery stenosis. *The New England Journal of Medicine, 363*, 11–23.

Carr, J. C. (2012). *Magnetic resonance angiography principles and applications.* New York, NY: Springer.

Dayton, M. T., Dempsey, D. T., Larson, G. M., & Posner, A. R. (2012). New paradigms in the treatment of small bowel obstruction. *Current Problems in Surgery, 49*(11), 642–717. doi:1067/j.cpsurg.2012.06.005

Ferri, F. (2014). *Ferri's practical guide* (9th ed.). London, UK: Elsevier Health Sciences.

Harrison, T. R. (2012). *Harrison's manual of medicine* (18th ed.). New York, NY: McGraw-Hill Medical.

Krupp, M. A. (2011). *Current medical diagnosis & treatment.* New York, NY: McGraw-Hill.

Mason, V. (2014). *Nurse practitioner's guide on how to start an independent practice.* Quanah, TX: Quanah Publishing.

Ravipati, M., Katragadda, S., Go, B., & Zarling, E. J. (2011, August). Acute mesenteric ischemia: Diagnostic challenge in clinical practice. *Practical Gastroenterology*, 35–43. Retrieved from http://www.practicalgastro.com/ pdf/August11/RavipatiArticle.pdf

Reginelli, A., Gebovese, E. A., Cappabianca, S., Iacobellis, F., Beritto, D., Fonio, P., . . . Grassi, R. (2013). Intestinal ischemia: US-CT findings correlations [Supplement 1]. *Critical Ultrasound Journal, 3*, 1–11. Retrieved from http://www.criticalultrasoundjournal.com/content/pdf/2036–7902–5–S1-S7.pdf

Rubin, G. D., & Rofsky, N. M. (2009). *CT and MR angiography: Comprehensive vascular assessment.* Philadelphia, PA: Wolters Kluwer Health/Lippincott Williams & Wilkins.

Sarac, T. P., Altinel, O., Kashyap, V., Bena, J., Lyden, S., Sruvastava, S., . . . Clair, D. (2008). Endovascular treatment of stenotic and occluded visceral arteries for chronic mesenteric ischemia. *Journal of Vascular Surgery, 47*, 485–491. doi:10.1016/j.jvs.2007.11.046

Silva, A. C., Pimenta, M., & Guimaraes, L. S. (2009). Small bowel obstruction: What to look for. *Radiographics, 29*, 423–439. doi:10.1148/rg.292085514

Sise, M. J. (2014). Acute mesenteric ischemia. *Surgical Clinics of North America, 94*(1), 165–181.

Skinner, H. B. (2014). *Current diagnosis & treatment in orthopedics* (5th ed.). New York, NY: McGraw-Hill Medical.

CHAPTER 41

Gastrointestinal Bleeding

NICOLE A. PEREZ • CHARLENE M. MYERS

ESOPHAGEAL VARICES

I. **Definition**
   A. Dilated submucosal veins that may develop in patients with underlying portal hypertension that can result in severe GI bleeding
   B. Varices can rupture at any moment and become a medical emergency.
   C. Three of ten patients will die from the initial hemorrhage
   D. Overall mortality reaches nearly 60% because rebleeding claims the lives of another 3 of 10 patients

II. **Etiology**
   A. Cirrhosis—most common
   B. Portal venous pressure of at least 12 mmHg is needed for varices to bleed (normal pressure, 2–6 mmHg)
   C. Bleeding from esophageal varices usually occurs in the distal 5 cm of the esophagus and in the upper portion of the stomach.
   D. Aspirin, used alone or in combination with other nonsteroidal anti-inflammatory drugs, has been associated with a first variceal bleeding episode in patients with cirrhosis.

III. **Clinical manifestations**
   A. Hematemesis
   B. Melena
   C. Hematochezia (indicates massive bleed, more than 1,000 ml)
   D. Abdominal discomfort
   E. Signs and symptoms of hypovolemia or shock

IV. **Laboratory/diagnostics**
   A. Esophagogastroduodenoscopy (EGD) is the gold standard for the diagnosis of esophageal varices
   B. Complete blood count (CBC)
      1. Hemoglobin/hematocrit is normal, then decreases because of volume resuscitation
      2. WBC count elevates as a result of the body's attempt to restore homeostasis
      3. Platelet count increases then decreases because of attempts to restore homeostasis and finally reflects true blood loss

C. Coagulation panel
   1. Prolonged prothrombin time (PT) and partial thromboplastin time (PTT) as well as increased INR due to decreased synthetic activity of liver
D. Electrolyte panel, liver function test, and arterial blood gas
   1. K+: decreases as a result of emesis, then may increase due to acute kidney injury from hypovolemia
   2. Na++: decreases, then increases as a result of hemoconcentration/fluid resuscitation
   3. Ca++: normal or decreased
   4. Hyperglycemia: stress response
   5. BUN/Creatinine ratio: elevated because of poor perfusion to the kidneys
   6. Lactate levels: elevated (lactic acidosis related to anaerobic metabolism)
   7. Aspartate aminotransferase (AST)/alanine aminotransferase (ALT) ratio and bilirubin level are usually abnormal in patients with underlying chronic liver disease
   8. Albumin: usually low due to several reasons such as poor synthetic function of liver and poor nutrition in such patients
   9. Arterial blood gases: respiratory alkalosis/metabolic acidosis
E. Barium studies: can be performed to define the presence of peptic ulcers, bleeding sites, tumors, and inflammation

V. **Management**
A. Emergency resuscitation
   1. Insert two large-bore (16-gauge) intravenous lines, and establish central venous pressure (CVP) line access
   2. Laboratory/diagnostics: blood type and cross match, PT/PTT/INR, complete blood count (CBC), electrolyte panel, lactate, renal, and liver function tests
   3. Infuse crystalloids/colloid/blood products (lactated Ringer solution or normal saline) for treatment of hypotension until blood products can be administered. (Note: Overzealous hydration increases portal pressure and can exacerbate or cause rebleeding of varices.)
      a. Maintain
         i. Systolic blood pressure higher than 110 mmHg,
         ii. CVP 10 mmHg or less, and
         iii. Pulmonary capillary wedge pressure 8 mmHg or less (if pulmonary artery catheter is in place)
      b. Administer fresh frozen plasma for elevated international normalized ratio (INR)
      c. Administer platelets or cryoprecipitate depending on platelets or fibrinogen levels, respectively
   4. Administer oxygen at 5–10 L/min
   5. Insert a Foley catheter
   6. Nothing by mouth (NPO)—insert nasogastric tube (NGT)
      a. However, NGT insertion is contraindicated during active hematemesis.
   7. Consult a surgeon and a gastroenterologist
B. 60%–80% of patients stop bleeding spontaneously; however, without therapy, more than half rebleed within 1 week
C. Emergency endoscopy
   1. Endoscopic band ligation—most effective
   2. Sclerotherapy with the use of agents such as ethanolamine or tetradecyl sulfate or band ligation
D. Octreotide (Sandostatin), 50 mcg IV bolus, followed by 3–5 days of continuous infusion of 50 mcg/hr, works similarly to vasopressin, has better adverse effect profile, and is better at controlling variceal hemorrhage
E. Vasopressin—vasoconstrictor that decreases portal pressures by reducing splanchnic flow (successful in only 50% of cases)
   1. Dose: 0.2–0.4 units/min to a maximum of 0.8 units/min
   2. Taper down over 24 hr after the bleeding is controlled

3. Monitor for vasopressin-induced adverse effects
   a. Chest pain
   b. Sweating
   c. Skin pallor
4. Rarely used in U.S. for acute variceal hemorrhage management, due to adverse effect profile and greater benefit of octreotide
5. Requires addition of nitroglycerin 40–400 mcg/min, titrated to maintain SBP over 90. Vasopressin should never be used without a nitrate

F. May replete with vitamin K, IM or IV, due low liver stores in cirrhosis (important for clotting factors II, VII, IX, and X; and proteins C and S)

G. Lactulose, 30 mL PO/NG BID for patients with severe liver disease, to prevent encephalopathy (titrate to 2–3 stools/day)

H. Balloon tamponade may be necessary to control bleeding
   1. Sengstaken-Blakemore tube (three ports) or
   2. Minnesota tube (four ports)
      a. Normal inflation pressure is 20–45 mmHg
      b. Inflation pressures must be continually monitored
      c. Balloons should be deflated every 8–12 hr
   3. The esophageal balloon must be deflated before the gastric tube is removed to prevent tube displacement upward and occlusion of the airway
      a. Keep scissors at the bedside
      b. Possible complications:
         i. Gastric balloon rupture—occlusion of airway
         ii. Esophageal rupture—characterized by severe back pain
         iii. Ulcerations of the esophageal or gastric mucosa

VI. Prevention of rebleeding
A. Routine follow-up with endoscopy
B. β-blockers
   1. Propanolol (Inderal), 20 mg PO BID or nadolol (Corgard), 40 mg PO daily
   2. Adjusted to the maximal tolerated dose
      a. Increased gradually until heart rate falls by 25% or reaches 55 beats per minute
   3. Used frequently in combination with sclerotherapy
C. Transjugular intrahepatic portosystemic stent (TIPS)—for patients with recurrent bleeds despite the therapies listed previously
D. Portosystemic shunt—usually reserved for patients for whom β-blockers have failed or for those who are noncompliant (TIPS is used more commonly than portosystemic shunt)
E. Liver transplantation

VII. Prevention of first episode of variceal bleeding
A. A high mortality rate is associated with variceal hemorrhage
B. All patients with cirrhosis should undergo diagnostic endoscopy to locate any varices that may be present.
C. Banding prophylactically has been noted to decrease the incidence of first-time bleeding
D. Nonselective β-blockers (i.e., propanolol)
E. Sclerotherapy in patients who have never had a bleed results in increased mortality compared with those treated with a placebo or with β-blockers and, therefore, is not recommended.

UPPER GASTROINTESTINAL BLEEDING

I. Definition
A. Acute upper gastrointestinal bleeding refers to loss of blood within the intraluminal gastrointestinal tract from any location between the upper esophagus and the duodenum at the ligament of Treitz.
B. Patient history is very important in determination of the time of onset of bleeding, severity, and possible causes

II. Etiology
A. Peptic ulcer disease (PUD)
B. Esophageal and gastric varices as a result of portal hypertension
C. Mallory-Weiss tear
D. Vascular abnormalities
E. Neoplasm
F. Gastric or duodenal erosion
G. Aortoenteric fistula
H. Dieulafoy vascular malformation—submucosal artery usually located in the proximal stomach abnormally close to the mucosa that causes erosion of the epithelium and may result in massive upper tract bleeding
I. Hematobilia—blood in the bile or bile ducts
J. Ménétrier disease
   1. Gastritis of unknown cause
   2. Marked by excessive proliferation of stomach mucosal folds

III. Clinical manifestations
A. Abdominal discomfort
B. Hematemesis presenting as bright red vomitus or "coffee grounds" emesis
C. Melena, in most cases evidenced by 50–100 mL of blood in the upper gastrointestinal (UGI) tract; hematochezia in massive UGI bleeds (more than 1,000 ml)
D. Signs and symptoms of hypovolemic shock, such as hypotension and tachycardia, are present in severe cases or with acute loss (e.g., more than 40% blood volume).
E. Orthostatic changes are noted in patients with a loss of 20% or more of blood volume.
F. Skin pallor
G. Spider angiomas, palmar erythema, caput medusae, and icterus suggest chronic liver disease
H. NGT aspirate—bright red blood indicates active bleeding and is associated with a higher mortality than melena

IV. Laboratory/diagnostics
A. Blood type and cross match for at least 4 units of packed red blood cells
B. Hemoglobin and hematocrit poorly reflect degree and severity of blood loss
C. PT/PTT/INR, platelet count, electrolytes, BUN/creatinine, and liver enzymes
D. ECG in the elderly and in patients with coronary artery disease (CAD) may indicate ischemia related to severe anemia
E. Barium studies are of little value
F. Endoscopy is both diagnostic and therapeutic. Endoscopic evaluation of the UGI tract should be considered in asymptomatic patients who present with a high suspicion for liver cirrhosis and esophageal varices who have a positive fecal occult blood test.
G. Capsule endoscopy: small camera ingested to examine entire length of small bowel. Provides direct visualization of the mucosa and sends images to the computer to be reviewed. Intervention cannot be provided by this method.
H. Nuclear bleeding scan and angiography

V. Management
A. Rapid clinical evaluation and assessment of hemodynamic status (i.e., airway, breathing, and circulation [ABCs])
B. Endotracheal intubation may be indicated
C. Consult with a gastroenterologist and a surgeon
D. Patients with significant blood loss
   1. Insert two large-bore intravenous lines (16-gauge) or a central line for fluid resuscitation
   2. Blood transfusions for high-risk patients are made on a case-by-case basis with the goal to adequately oxygenate end organs and tissues
      a. Keep hematocrit above 30%
      b. Young/healthy patients: maintain hematocrit above 20%
   3. Patients with coagulopathies (elevated INR): 1–2 units fresh frozen plasma and 2.5–10 mg vitamin K IM or IV

4. Low platelet counts: transfuse platelets
E. NGT placement—tap water gastric lavage
   1. If aspirate does not clear after 2–3 L, continued active bleeding is assumed
   2. More urgent resuscitation and endoscopic interventions are indicated
F. Endoscopy—should be considered in all patients with UGI bleeding
   1. Should be performed as an emergency procedure in a patient with active hemorrhage after stabilization
   2. Active, self-limiting bleeds: perform within 24 hr, unless one of the following occurs:
      a. Portal hypertension or aortoenteric fistula is suspected
      b. Bleeding recurs after initial stabilization
   3. Patients with chronic blood loss may undergo elective endoscopy.
   4. Treatment options include the following:
      a. Thermal coagulation (i.e., cauterization)
      b. Injection therapy with epinephrine or sclerosant
      c. Band ligation
G. Acute pharmacologic therapies
   1. IV proton pump inhibitors
      a. Pantoprazole (Protonix) or esomeprazole (Nexium), 80 mg IV bolus, followed by continuous infusion of 8 mg/hr
H. Endoscopic therapy
   a. Band ligation
   b. Sclerotherapy
   c. Laser therapy
   d. Clips
I. Balloon tamponade
J. Surgery is indicated for the following:
   1. Severe bleeding or rebleeding in which two endoscopic treatments have failed;
   2. Massive exsanguinating hemorrhage in which resuscitative efforts have failed;
   3. When more than 6–8 units of blood were needed during the first 24-hr period;
   4. Slow, continuous bleeding that lasts longer than 48 hr; and
   5. Nonsurgical patients, consult an interventional radiologist for arteriography/embolization
K. Intra-arterial embolization or vasopressin (thermal ablation)—performed by interventional radiologists and rarely used; associated with severe adverse effects
L. TIPS
M. Supportive care
N. Antibiotic prophylaxis
   1. Significantly reduces bacterial infections and may reduce all-cause mortality, bacterial infection mortality, rebleeding events, and hospitalization length
   2. Short term (7 day maximum) antibiotic prophylaxis should be instituted in any patient with cirrhosis and GI hemorrhage.
      a. Norfloxacin (Noroxin), 400 mg PO twice a day or ciprofloxacin (Cipro) IV (in patients whom oral administration is not possible)
   3. Patients with advanced cirrhosis, particularly in areas with high resistance to quinolone organisms
      a. Ceftriaxone (Rocephin), 1 gram/day

LOWER GASTROINTESTINAL BLEEDING

I. Definition
   A. Bleeding that originates below the ligament of Treitz, for example, in the small intestine or colon
   B. Up to 10% of patients who present with hematochezia have a UGI source of bleeding (e.g., PUD)
II. Etiology
   A. Diverticulosis (40% of patients)

B. Vascular ectasias
   1. Painless bleeding ranging from acute hematochezia to chronic occult blood loss
   2. Most common in patients older than 70 years or in patients with chronic renal failure
C. Neoplasms
   1. Benign or malignant
   2. Usually manifest by chronic, occult blood loss
   3. Sometimes evidenced by periodic hematochezia
   4. Occasionally manifests by massive lower tract bleeding
D. Inflammatory bowel disease (i.e., ulcerative colitis)
   1. Abdominal pain
   2. Tenesmus
      a. Spasmodic contraction of the anal sphincter
      b. Pain
      c. Persistent desire to empty the bowel, with involuntary ineffectual straining efforts
   3. Urgency
E. Anorectal disease
   1. Small amounts of bright red blood on the toilet tissue, streaking in the stool, or dripping into the toilet
   2. Rarely results in significant blood loss
   3. Painless bleeding is indicative of internal hemorrhoids
   4. Painful bleeding may indicate anal fissure
F. Ischemic colitis
   1. Seen in the elderly who have a history of atherosclerosis
   2. Results in hematochezia or bloody diarrhea
   3. Usually associated with pain and cramps
G. Others
   1. Radiation-induced colitis
   2. Infectious colitis
      a. *Shigella* spp.
      b. *Campylobacter* spp.
      c. *Escherichia coli*
   3. Other systemic conditions (rare)

III. **Clinical manifestations**
   A. Most patients with lower gastrointestinal bleeding present with hematochezia; although occasionally, melena will be present in bleeding from the upper small intestine.
   B. Chronic blood loss
      1. Skin pallor
      2. Tachycardia
      3. Postural hypotension
   C. Acute blood loss
      1. Altered mental status
      2. Hypotension
      3. Shock
      4. Gross evidence of rectal blood loss
   D. Rule out vaginal and urethral bleeding in females

IV. **Laboratory/diagnostics**
   A. Rule out UGI source by placing an NGT
   B. CBC
      1. Anemia—when blood loss has been subacute or chronic
      2. CBC may be normal in acute and massive bleeds because of hemoconcentration.
   C. Serum iron, total iron-binding capacity, and ferritin help to confirm iron deficiency when the patient is anemic and GI blood loss is suspected.
   D. Fecal occult blood test in stable patients whose GI blood loss is questionable
   E. Anoscopy and sigmoidoscopy

F. Colonoscopy should be performed in all patients with significant lower gastrointestinal bleeding within 6–24 hr after admission to the hospital after the colon has been cleansed.
G. Arteriography or technetium-99m (^{99m}Tc)–labeled red blood cell scintigraphy
H. Small intestine push enteroscopy is used in recurrent bleeding of unknown origin; consists of a long, small-diameter endoscope that may reach to the distal jejunum
I. Capsule imaging may help in the identification of distal small intestinal bleeds.

V. **Management**
   A. Resuscitate hemodynamically compromised patients
      1. Place two large-bore (16-gauge) intravenous lines and/or pulmonary artery catheter
      2. Administer lactated Ringer solution or normal saline and/or blood products
      3. Monitor heart rate, blood pressure, mean arterial pressure, and pulmonary capillary wedge pressure/CVP
      4. Titrate infusion rate to maintain perfusion
   B. Discontinue aspirin and all nonsteroidal anti-inflammatory drugs; treat the cause of the bleeding
   C. IV proton pump inhibitor (treatment of choice)
      1. Pantoprazole (Protonix) or esomeprazole (Nexium), 80 mg IV bolus, followed by continuous infusion of 8 mg/hr
   D. Blood type and cross match for 4 units of packed red blood cells
   E. Colonoscopic therapies—Electrocoagulation is useful in the treatment of patients with vascular ectasia of the colon.
   F. Angiographic techniques
      1. Intra-arterial vasopressin
      2. Embolization
   G. Endoscopic hemostatic therapy
   H. Surgery
      1. Depends on the nature and location of the bleeding
      2. Usually a segmental or subtotal colectomy is indicated

BIBLIOGRAPHY

Alford, K. F. (2012). Gastrointestinal alterations. In M. L. Sole, D. Klein, & M. Moseley (Eds.), *Introduction to critical care nursing* (6th ed., pp. 312–315). Philadelphia, PA: WB Saunders.

Barkun, A. N., Bardou, M., Kuipers, E. J., Sung, J., Hunt, R. H., Martel, M., . . . Sinclair, P. (2010). International consensus recommendations on the management of patients with nonvariceal upper gastrointestinal bleeding. *Annals of Internal Medicine, 152*(2), 101–113.

Chavez-Tapia, N. C., Barrientos-Gutierrez, T., Tellez-Avila, F. I., Soares-Weiser, K., & Uribe, M. (2010). Antibiotic prophylaxis for cirrhotic patients with upper gastrointestinal bleeding. *Cochrane Database of Systematic Reviews, 9*, CD002907. doi:10.1002/14651858.CD002907.pub2

Chen, Y.-I., & Peter, G. (2012). Prevention and management of gastroesophageal varices in cirrhosis. *International Journal of Hepatology*, 1–6.

Ferri, F. F. (2010). *Practical guide to the care of the medical patient* (8th ed.). Philadelphia, PA: Mosby Elsevier.

Ferlitsch, A., Schoefl, R., Puespoek, A., Miehsler, M., Schoeniger-Hekele, M., Hofer, H., Gangl, A., & Homoncik, M. (2010). Effect of virtual endoscopy simulator training on performance of upper gastrointestinal endoscopy in patients: A randomized controlled trial. *Endoscopy, 42*(12), 1049–1056.

Garcia-Tsao, G., & Bosch, J. (2010). Management of varices and variceal hemorrhage in cirrhosis. *The New England Journal of Medicine, 362*, 823–832.

Inadomi, J. M., Bhattacharya, R., Dominitz, J. A., & Hwang, Ho J. (2013). In T. Yamada (Ed.), *Yamada's handbook of gastroenterology* (3rd ed.). Hoboken, NJ: Wiley-Blackwell.

Kappelman, M. D., Palmer, L., Boyle, B. M., & Rubin, D. T. (2010). Quality of care in inflammatory bowel disease: A review and discussion. *Inflammatory Bowel Diseases, 16*(1), 125–133.

SECTION FIVE

Management of Patients with Genitourinary Disorders

CHAPTER 42

Urinary Tract Infections

MICHELE H. TALLEY • CHARLENE M. MYERS

URINARY TRACT INFECTIONS

I. **Definition**
   A. Presence of a significant number of pathogenic organisms in the urine with the potential to invade tissues of the urinary tract and adjacent structures, including the bladder, urethra, prostate, renal parenchyma (kidneys), and collecting system
   B. Causes inflammation in the urinary epithelium
   C. Associated with a positive urine culture: more than 100,000 colonies in asymptomatic patients and between 100 and 10,000 colonies in symptomatic patients
   D. Classified as lower urinary tract (bladder and urethra) and upper urinary tract (kidney and ureters)
   E. Defined as uncomplicated (occurs in normal working urinary tract) versus complicated (occurs with defects in urinary tract or in individuals with other health problems)

II. **Etiology/incidence**
   A. Urinary tract infection (UTI) is more common in women than in men.
   B. UTIs are the most common bacterial infection in the elderly, and nursing home patients are more likely to have resistant pathogens compared with others of the same age.
   C. Common uropathogens
      1. *Escherichia coli* is the most common causative organism (64.5% of cases)
      2. *Staphylococcus aureus* (6% of cases)
      3. *Proteus mirabilis* (4.7% of cases)
      4. *Klebsiella saprophyticus* (4.3% of cases)
      5. *Enterococcus faecalis* (3.6% of cases)
      6. *Proteus vulgaris* (2.7% of cases)
      7. *Pseudomonas aeruginosa* (2.4% of cases)
      8. *Enterobacter* spp. (1.9% of cases)
      9. *Staphylococcus epidermidis* (1.8% of cases)
      10. *Providencia* spp. (1.7% of cases)
      11. High risk for those patients who are critically ill
      12. Elderly patients have gender-associated differences in UTIs
         a. Elderly women most often have *E. coli*

b. Elderly men are likely to have *P. mirabilis* but may also have *Enterococcus* spp. or coagulase-negative staphylococci
c. The following organisms are also commonly found in the elderly: *Klebsiella pneumoniae, Serratia* spp., *Citrobacter* spp., *Enterobacter, Morganella morganii,* and *P. aeruginosa*
d. *Providencia* spp. UTI is found in institutionalized patients
e. Elderly patients with diabetes often have group B streptococcal UTIs
13. Catheter-associated UTI is caused by a biofilm (a layer of uropathogens living along the catheter); the best strategy to prevent these infections is to avoid catheterization when possible and remove urinary catheters as soon as possible once they are no longer medically necessary.
a. *Candida* spp. are common fungal causes of UTIs
D. Risk factors for both genders:
1. Diabetes mellitus
2. Urinary instrumentation and catheterization
3. Obstruction of normal flow of urine due to calculi, tumors, and urethral strictures
4. Neurogenic bladder disease resulting from stroke, multiple sclerosis, and spinal cord injury
5. Vesicoureteral reflux
E. Contributing factors in women:
1. Short urethra
2. Sexual intercourse
3. Use of a spermicide
4. Pregnancy
5. Previous UTI
6. New sexual partner (within the past year)
7. History of UTI in first-degree female relative
F. Contributing factors in men:
1. Prostatic enlargement, resulting in urine residual
2. Prostatitis
3. Lack of circumcision
4. Homosexuality
5. Having a sexual partner with vaginal colonization by uropathogens
6. HIV infection

III. **Signs/symptoms**
A. Lower urinary tract (cystitis/urethritis/prostatitis)
1. Dysuria
2. Urinary frequency
3. Urgency
4. Suprapubic pain
5. Hematuria with bacteriuria
6. Malodorous urine
7. Incontinence
8. Fever and chills are uncommon but may be present
9. No flank or costovertebral pain
B. Upper urinary tract (pyelonephritis, renal abscess)
1. Flank pain or costovertebral-angle tenderness
2. Fever (temperature higher than 38°F)
3. Hematuria
4. Nausea and vomiting
5. Mental status changes (in elderly patients)
6. Malaise

CHAPTER 42 Urinary Tract Infections

7. Shaking chills (rigors)
8. Tachypnea (related to fever)
9. Tachycardia (related to fever)
10. If symptoms last for longer than 3 days, abscess formation should be considered.

IV. **Laboratory/diagnostics**
   A. Urine culture and sensitivity testing: The detection of bacteria in the culture is considered the diagnostic gold standard. Culture results are not available until 24 hr after collection. Point-of-care testing aids in early detection.
   B. Point-of-care testing includes urinalysis and urine dipstick tests
      1. Clean-catch urinalysis (diagnose UTI with positive nitrite or leukocyte esterase positive test; may also diagnose UTI with blood in urine)
      2. Urine microscopy
         a. Pyuria: presence of more than 10 leukocytes/ml
         b. Bacteriuria: more than 100,000 bacteria/ml; indicates active infection
         c. Bacterial counts of 10,000–100,000/ml may also indicate infection, especially if accompanied by pyuria.
         d. In urine specimens obtained by suprapubic aspiration or in-and-out catheterization, bacterial colony counts of 100–10,000/ml indicate infection
         e. Occasional erythrocytes, white cell casts, and mild proteinuria may be present in acute pyelonephritis
         f. Elevated erythrocyte sedimentation rate in pyelonephritis
      3. Leukocyte esterase dipstick test: positive (purple in 60 seconds)—signifies pyuria or white blood cells (WBCs) in the urine
         a. False positives may occur with kidney stones, tumors, urethritis, and poor collection techniques
         b. False negatives may occur with uncomplicated or early UTIs
      4. Nitrate dipstick test: positive for protein, blood, nitrates (pink in 30 seconds)—may be false negative in uncomplicated UTI, with diuretics early in the course of UTI, with inadequate levels of dietary nitrates, or in the presence of bacteria that do not produce nitrate reductase, such as *Staphylococcus saprophyticus*, *Enterococcus*, and *Pseudomonas*
   C. CBC: leukocytosis with a left shift in acute pyelonephritis
   D. Blood culture may be indicated for suspected pyelonephritis or sepsis.
   E. If sexually transmitted infections are suspected, order *Neisseria gonorrhoeae* (GC) culture and chlamydia test.
   F. To rule out obstruction, calculi, and papillary necrosis in men with UTIs and in women with recurrent UTIs, consider the following:
      1. X-ray voiding cystourethrography
      2. Computed tomography (CT) scan of the abdomen and pelvis: with and without contrast
      3. Ultrasound: pelvis (urethra)
      4. Magnetic resonance imaging of the pelvis: with and/or without contrast

V. **Management**
   A. Acute cystitis
      1. First-line therapy
         a. Single-dose regimen: fosfomycin trometamol (Monurol), 3-gram sachet in a single dose
         b. Three-day regimen (preferred over single-dose regimen due to high relapse rates related to single-dose regimen) to 7-day regimen
            i. Sulfonamides: trimethoprim-sulfamethoxazole (TMP-SMZ) (Bactrim DS), 160 mg/800 mg BID PO for 3 days (can be ineffective in many patients because of the emergence of resistant organisms)
            ii. Sulfonamides: trimethoprim, 100 mg BID PO for 3 days
               (a) Prescription should be informed by local antimicrobial resistance patterns

iii. Urinary antiseptics: nitrofurantoin (Macrobid), 100 mg PO BID for 5 days with meals, use with caution in elderly patients
   2. Second-line therapy
      a. Quinolones: ciprofloxacin (Cipro), 250 mg BID PO for 3 days; levofloxacin, 250–500 mg once daily PO for 3 days
      b. β-lactams (e.g., amoxicillin-clavulanate, cefdinir, cefaclor, and cefpodoxime proxetil) for
         3–7 days
         i. Appropriate choice for therapy when other recommended agents cannot be used due to inferior efficacy and more adverse effects, compared with other UTI antimicrobials
B. Uncomplicated upper UTI
   1. Outpatient therapy
      a. Quinolones: ciprofloxacin, 500 mg BID PO or 1 gram (extended release) once daily PO for
         7 days (may consider giving an initial IV 400 mg dose with the oral dose); levofloxacin,
         750 mg once daily PO for 5 days
         i. If fluoroquinolone resistance exceeds 10%, consider giving initial 1 gram ceftriaxone IV or a consolidated 24 hr dose of an aminoglycoside
      b. Sulfonamides: TMP-SMZ, 160 mg/800 mg BID PO for 14 days (if susceptibility is known; if susceptibility is unknown, consider giving initial IV 1 gram ceftriaxone or a consolidated 24-hr dose of an aminoglycoside)
      c. Oral β-lactams for 10–14 days (less effective than fluoroquinolones)
   2. Inpatient therapy
      a. Cefotaxime or ceftriaxone IV
      b. Fluoroquinolone IV (depending on local resistance prevalence for severe or anaphylactic PCN allergic patients)
      c. Aminoglycoside IV with or without ampicillin IV
C. Catheter-associated UTI
   1. If the microorganism is bacterial, treat with an antibiotic for 7–14 days
   2. If candiduria, treat with fluconazole, 200–400 mg/day for 14 days
D. Special considerations
   1. Patients with acute bacterial pyelonephritis
      a. Should be hospitalized
         i. Surgery may be necessary when a structural abnormality or a large stone is blocking the urinary tract.
      b. Inpatient therapy
         i. First-line therapy for complicated polynephritis and nosocomial/hospital-acquired UTI
            (a) Aminoglycosides: gentamicin or tobramycin
               1. Not to be used as monotherapy for pyelonephritis
               2. Doses are individualized and based on normal renal function with defined peak levels of 5–10 mg/L and trough levels less than 2
               3. Aminoglycosides are to be avoided in patients with pre-existing renal disease. Patients with normal renal functions may use a daily dose of 15 mg/kg (Hartford nomogram).
            (b) Penicillins: ampicillin, 1 gram every 4–6 hr IV (should cover *Enterococcus* if Gram-positive cocci present on culture or Gram stain)
            (c) Cephalosporins: cefazolin, 1–2 grams every 8 hr IV; not routinely used for empiric therapy
         ii. Others to consider (based on susceptibility and patient allergies)

- (a) Sulfonamides: TMP/SMX, 160/800 mg every 12 hr IV
- (b) Aminoglycosides: amikacin (reserved for highly resistant organisms), 15 mg/kg/day IV in patients whose renal function meets criteria, individualized to achieve peak of 20–30 mg/L and trough levels less than 10
- (c) Antipseudomonal penicillins: piperacillin, 3 grams every 4 hr IV
- (d) Penicillin-β-lactamase inhibitor combinations: piperacillin/tazobactam, 4 grams/500 mg every 8 hr IV
- (e) Cephalosporins: cefotaxime, 1–2 grams every 8 hr IV; ceftriaxone, 1–2 grams every 24 hr IV; cefepime, 2 grams every 12 hr IV; or ceftazidime, 0.5–2 grams every 8 hr IV. Doses are individualized and based on obesity and pre-existence of pulmonary infections.
- (f) Miscellaneous antibiotic class: aztreonam, 1–2 grams every 6 hr IV (although has limited use, active for Gram-negative bacteria including *P. aeruginosa*; good for those with nosocomial infection when aminoglycosides are contraindicated or when patient penicillin sensitive); imipenem/cilastatin, 500 mg every 6 hr IV (covers broad spectrum of bacteria: Gram-positive, Gram-negative, and anaerobic; active against *Enterococci* and *P. aeruginosa* and resistant organisms; can cause *Candida* superinfection); or vancomycin, 500 mg every 6 hr or 1 gram every 12 hr IV (evaluate renal function)
- (g) Quinolones: ciprofloxacin, 200–400 mg every 12 hr IV, or levofloxacin, 500 mg daily IV

    2. Pregnant women
        a. Quinolones cannot be given during pregnancy
        b. Sulfonamides cannot be given near the time of delivery; cephalexin is a reasonable choice

E. Treatment for discomfort
    1. Phenazopyridine hydrochloride (Pyridium), 200 mg PO 3 times a day for 2 days, may be added for discomfort associated with irritation
F. Aseptic techniques are essential if indwelling catheters are required.
    1. Modification of catheter material to confer antimicrobial activity may play an important part in the prevention of catheter-related infection
    2. Silver-impregnated catheters have been shown to effectively reduce the number of catheter-related infections; silver has antimicrobial activity against both Gram-positive and Gram-negative bacteria
G. Behavioral modifications
    1. Recommend abstinence or reduction in sexual activity
    2. Discuss means of contraception other than the use of spermicides as they alter the normal flora of the vagina, thus promoting the colonization of uropathogens
    3. May suggest the following: increase water intake, decrease carbonated drink intake, not delaying urination, and wiping front to back after defecating
H. Consider prophylaxis in patients with recurrent lower UTI
    1. Prophylactic antibiotic selection made on basis of community-resistance patterns, side effects, and cost
    2. Postcoital antimicrobial prophylaxis: single dose of antimicrobial drug as soon as possible after intercourse
        a. Urinary antiseptics: nitrofurantoin, 50–100 mg PO
        b. Sulfonamides: TMP-SMX, 40 mg/200 mg PO or 80 mg/400 mg PO
        c. Sulfonamides: TMP, 100 mg PO
        d. Cephalosporins: cephalexin, 250 mg PO
    3. Continuous prophylaxis with antimicrobial

a. Urinary antiseptics: nitrofurantoin, 50–100 mg PO at bedtime
b. Sulfonamides: TMP-SMX, 40 mg/200 mg PO at bedtime
c. Sulfonamides: TMP, 100 mg PO at bedtime
d. Cephalosporins: cephalexin, 125–250 mg PO at bedtime
e. No conclusive evidence supports selection of a particular drug, dosage, duration or schedule of treatment. However, 6 months of treatment, followed by observation for reinfection after discontinuing prophylaxis, has been recommended.
4. Prophylactic antibiotic selection may reduce the risk of recurrent UTIs in female patients with two episodes of infection in the previous year.
    a. Antibiotic selection should be informed by community resistance patters, side effects, and local costs.
I. No need to repeat urinalysis with culture and sensitivity tests after therapy in uncomplicated cystitis and pyelonephritis; must repeat in pregnant women
J. Emphasize compliance with medication and follow-up

BIBLIOGRAPHY

Baron, E. J., Miller, J. M., Weinstein, M. P., Richter, S. S., Gilligan, P. H., Thompson, R. B., . . . Pritt, B. S. (2013). A guide to utilization of the microbiology laboratory for diagnosis of infectious diseases: 2013 recommendations by the Infectious Diseases Society of America (IDSA) and the American Society for Microbiology (ASM). *Clinical Infectious Diseases, 57*(4), e22-e121.

Giesen, L. G., Cousins, G., Dimitrov, B. D., van de Laar, F. A., & Fahey, T. (2010). Predicting acute uncomplicated urinary tract infection in women: A systematic review of the diagnostic accuracy of symptoms and signs. *BMC Family Practice, 11*, 78–92.

Glass, A. S., Kovshilovskaya, B., & Breyer, B. N. (2012). Sexually transmitted infection and long-term risk of lower urinary tract symptoms. *European Urological Review, 7*(1), 133–136.

Gupta, K., Hooten, T., Naber, K. G., Wullt, B., Colgan, R., Miller, L. G., . . . European Society for Microbiology and Infectious Diseases. (2011). International clinical practice guidelines for the treatment of acute uncomplicated cystitis and pyelonephritis in women: A 2010 update by the Infectious Diseases Society of America and the European Society for Microbiology and Infectious Diseases. *Clinical Infectious Diseases, 52*(5), e103-e120.

Halter, J. B., Ouslander, J. G., Tinetti, M. E., Studenski, S., High, K., & Asthana, S. (Eds.). (2009). *Hazzard's geriatric medicine and gerontology* (6th ed.). New York, NY: McGraw-Hill.

Hooten, T. M. (2012). Uncomplicated urinary tract infection. *NEJM, 366*(11), 1028–1037.

Hooten, T. M., Bradley, S. F., Cardenas, D. D., Colgan, R., Geerlings, S. E., Rice, J. C., . . . Infectious Diseases Society of America. (2010). Diagnosis, prevention, and treatment of catheter-associated urinary tract infection in adults: 2009 international clinical practice guidelines from the Infectious Diseases Society of America. *Clinical Infectious Disease, 50*(5), 625–663.

Kodner, C. M., & Gupton, E. K. (2010). Recurrent urinary tract infections in women: Diagnosis and management. *American Family Physician, 82*(6), 638–643. Retrieved from http://www.aafp.org/afp/2010/0915/p638.pdf.

Lazarus, E., Casalino, D. D., Remer, E. M., Arellano, R. S., Bishoff, J. T., Coursey, C. A., . . . Expert Panel on Urologic Imaging. (2011). *ACR appropriateness criteria recurrent lower urinary tract infection in women.* [online publication]. Reston, VA: American College of Radiology (ACR).

Linhares, I., Raposo, T., Rodrigues, A., & Almeida, A. (2013). Frequency and antimicrobial resistance patterns of bacteria implicated in community urinary tract infections: A ten-year surveillance study (2000–2009). *BMC Infectious Diseases, 13*(19), 1–14. doi:10.1186/1471–2334–13–19

Longo, D. L., Fauci, A. S., Kasper, D. L., Hauser, S., Jameson, J., & Loscalzo, J. (Eds.). (2012). *Harrison's principles of internal medicine* (18th ed.). New York, NY: McGraw-Hill.

Marinosci, F., Zizzo, A., Coppola, A., Rodano, L., Laudisio, R., & Antonelli Incalzi, R. (2013). Carbapenem resistance and mortality in institutionalized elderly with urinary tract infection. *JAMDA, 14*(7), 513–517.

CHAPTER 43

Acute Kidney Injury and Chronic Kidney Disease

STEVEN W. BRANHAM • CHARLENE M. MYERS

PRIMARY KIDNEY REGULATION OF PHYSIOLOGIC FUNCTIONS:

I. **Acid–base status**
II. **Maintain water balance**
III. **Electrolyte balance**
IV. **Hormone production and metabolism**
V. **Gluconeogenesis in fasting states**
VI. **Various regulatory functions are lost at different states of disease progression. In early disease, the onset is often insidious.**

ACUTE KIDNEY INJURY

I. **Acute kidney injury and chronic kidney disease in perspective**
   A. Acute kidney injury (AKI) is an abrupt loss of kidney function while chronic kidney disease (CKD) can develop over months to years. In both states, the degree of dysfunction is related to cause and comorbid factors.
   B. In AKI, recovery is often attained with medical management, while in CKD, progression is delayed by medical management.
   C. Both conditions may require dialysis based on the degree of dysfunction if conservative measures fail.
   D. AKI in the presence of CKD requires aggressive management to prevent permanent progression of CKD.
   E. Although recovery typically occurs in AKI, the condition is associated with a lifetime risk of developing CKD.

II. **Definition**
   A. An acute loss of renal function typically occurring within 24–48 hr
   B. Overall incidence is 3/1,000 with approximately 5/100,000 requiring dialysis for short-term management
   C. AKI accounts for 5%–7% of hospital admissions and 30% of intensive care unit admissions, which are associated with higher mortality
   D. Increased cost, increased length of stay, and increased in/out-of-hospital mortality are associated with AKI

Table 43.1	RIFLE Method for Acute Kidney Infection	
RIFLE class	**GFR rate reduction**	**Urine output reduction**
Risk	Increase serum creatine × 1.5 or decrease of GFR greater than 25% from baseline	UO less than 0.5 ml/kg/hr for 6 hr
Injury	Increase serum creatine × 2 or decrease of GFR greater than 50% from baseline	UO less than 0.5 ml/kg/hr for 12 hr
Failure	Increase serum creatine × 1.5 or decrease of GFR greater than 25% from baseline	UO less than 0.3 ml/kg/hr for 12 hr or anuria for 12 hr
Loss	Complete loss of renal function for greater than 4 weeks	
End-stage kidney disease	Need for RRT for greater than 3 months	

    E. AKI progresses from the inability to excrete metabolic waste products, such as urea nitrogen and creatinine, to the inability to maintain proper fluid and electrolyte balance.
        1. Typically, acute increases in serum creatinine levels from baseline (i.e., an increase of at least 0.5 mg/dl) occur. AKI can progress to complete renal failure when serum creatinine level increases by at least 0.5 mg/dl/day and urine output is less than 400 ml/day (oliguria).
    F. Generally, AKI resolves within three months of onset
    G. There are age and comorbidity factors that are related to an increase in occurrence regardless of etiology of AKI. Even with full recovery from AKI, an episode increases the lifetime risk of development of CKD with the exact mechanisms and specific etiology yet unknown.
    H. Two major methods are used to identify AKI
        1. The Acute Dialysis Quality Initiative group developed a stratification method based on abrupt onset of renal impairment, loss, and the need for renal replacement therapy (RRT) coupled with duration (see Table 43.1)
        2. A second widely accepted classification method is based on the global etiology of injury to the kidney consisting of prerenal, intrarenal, and postrenal causation.
III. **Risk, injury, failure, loss, end-stage kidney disease stratification method for AKI (RIFLE) (see table 43.1)**
IV. **Etiology classification method prerenal, intrarenal, and postrenal (prerenal and postrenal have the greatest incidence of recovery and not progressing to end-stage kidney disease where RRT is required)**
    A. Prerenal (60%–70% of cases)
        1. Characterized by diminished renal perfusion resulting from a decrease in blood supply to the kidneys
            a. No nephron damage is present
        2. Causes
            a. Intravascular volume depletion (absolute decrease in blood volume)
                i. Hemorrhage
                ii. Gastrointestinal losses (e.g., diarrhea, vomiting, and large amount of nasogastric tube aspirate)
                iii. Urinary losses (e.g., diabetes insipidus and use of diuretics)
                iv. Skin losses (third spacing, large surface area burns, and/or wounds)
            b. Vasodilatory states (relative decrease in blood volume)
                i. Sepsis
                ii. Anaphylaxis
                iii. Drugs
                    (a) Angiotensin-converting enzyme (ACE) inhibitors, which may inhibit intrinsic renal autoregulation
                    (b) Nonsteroidal anti-inflammatory drugs (NSAIDs), which may decrease renal blood flow

c. Decreased cardiac output (relative decrease in blood volume)
    i. Congestive heart failure
    ii. Myocardial infarction
    iii. Cardiogenic shock
d. Arterial occlusion/vasoconstrictive states (catecholamines)
e. Uncontrolled hypertension/atherosclerosis
f. Liver disease (advanced hepatic disease that may cause hepatic renal syndrome due to vasoconstriction in the kidneys)

3. Results in increased tubular sodium and water reabsorption (in an attempt at reexpansion of circulating blood volume)
    a. Oliguria
    b. Decreased urine sodium (less than 20 mEq/L)
    c. High urine osmolality (higher than 500 mOsm/L)
    d. Urine-specific gravity: increased (higher than 1.020)
4. Decreased distal tubular flow may cause increased urea absorption and decreased potassium secretion with marginal effect on creatinine
5. BUN-to-creatinine ratio increased (20:1)
6. Ratio of urine-to-plasma (U/P) levels of creatinine greater than 40
7. Fraction excretion of sodium is a very sensitive test
    a. Formula:

$$\frac{U_{Na} \times P_{Cr}}{P_{Na} \times U_{Cr}} \times 100$$

Note. U_{Na} = urine sodium; U_{Cr} = urine creatinine; P_{Na} = plasma sodium; P_{Cr} = plasma creatinine

    b. Less than 1% = prerenal
    c. Greater than 1% = intrinsic
    d. Greater than 2%–4% = postrenal
8. Increased renal "threshold" for plasma ions: increased bicarbonate (HCO_3^-) generation leads to contraction alkalosis
9. Increased uric acid reabsorption: hyperuricemia
10. Increased antidiuretic hormone secretion: increased water reabsorption; urinary osmolality greater than serum osmolality
11. Hyponatremia with free water loading until volume is restored
12. Urinary sediment: hyaline casts

B. Intrarenal (intrinsic) (25%–40% of cases)
1. Abrupt decrease in glomerular filtration rate (GFR) due to tubular cell damage that results from renal ischemia or nephrotoxic injury
2. Acute tubular necrosis—accounts for most hospital-associated cases of intrinsic acute renal failure (ARF) around 50%
    a. Ischemic
        i. Decreased cardiac output
        ii. Prolonged hypotension
        iii. Volume depletion
        iv. Catecholamines
        v. Volume shift
        vi. Liver disease ("hepatorenal syndrome")
    b. Nephrotoxic
        i. Endogenous (e.g., hemoglobinuria [hemolysis], myoglobinuria [rhabdomyolysis], hyperuricemia, and multiple myeloma)

ii. Exogenous (e.g., aminoglycosides, contrast media, ethylene glycol, amphotericin B, cyclosporine, antineoplastics such as cisplatin, and heavy metals)
iii. Drug-induced treatment principles
   (a) The ideal methods stop the offending agent
   (b) If discontinuing the drug is not an option, then the drug needs to be renally dosed based on creatinine clearance, which is based on specific drug recommendations and renal clearance rates.
iv. Treatment and prevention of contrast-related kidney injury
   (a) Fluid administration (high-level evidence)
      1. IV administration of fluids has not been proven superior over oral fluids in preventing contrast-related injury.
      2. Hydration is key to the likelihood of AKI prevention, but other factors such as concomitant heart failure must be considered when assessing volume status and adequacy of volume status
      3. Optimal prevention starts with oral or IV replacement prior to dye loading (1 L) and should continue for 24 hr
      4. Postcontrast fluids are administered to attain a urine output volume of 300 ml/hr (if no comorbid conditions and does not develop fluid overload symptoms)
      5. When IV methods are selected, 0.45% normal saline is frequently selected as the sodium content most closely approximates urine sodium output assisting in the prevention acute iatrogenic hypernatremia, which can occur when 0.9% normal saline is used at these rates.
   (b) Adjunctive prevention methods (limited or no proof of outcome difference)
      1. IV/oral administration of N-acetylcysteine, 600 mg every 12 hr for 48–72 hr (before and after contrast) has been used to prevent contrast-induced injury but has not been shown to be superior to fluid alone
         a. When N-acetylcysteine is used, it is typically given before and after contrast to decrease in the incidence of dye-induced nephrotoxicity.
   (c) The administration of sodium bicarbonate has also been used but has limited advantage over fluid administration and should be reserved in cases when acidosis is present.
   (d) In diabetic patients receiving metformin or combinations containing the drug should be withheld for 48 hr prior to the dye load (based on risk benefit of the need for the test in light of the potential for kidney damage).
      1. If at all possible, an alternate test should be used or noncontrast imaging if the drug has been dosed in the prior 24-hr period. In patients who present to the hospital and need to withhold nephrotoxic drugs, these medications should be considered.
3. Acute tubulointerstitial nephritis accounts for 10%–15% of cases of intrinsic renal failure. This is caused by the following:
   a. Bacterial pyelonephritis: infectious causes may include streptococcal infection, leptospirosis, cytomegalovirus, histoplasmosis, and Rocky Mountain spotted fever
   b. More than 70% of cases are related to drug-induced hypersensitivity to the following:
      i. Penicillins
      ii. Cephalosporins
      iii. Sulfonamides and sulfonamide-containing diuretics
      iv. NSAIDs
      v. Rifampin
      vi. Phenytoin

CHAPTER 43 Acute Kidney Injury and Chronic Kidney Disease

      vii. Allopurinol
- c. Immunologic disorders—more commonly associated with glomerulonephritis, but may also be associated with:
  - i. Systemic lupus erythematosus (SLE)
  - ii. Sjögren syndrome
  - iii. Sarcoidosis
  - iv. Cryoglobulinemia
- d. Idiopathic conditions

4. Urinalysis: urinary sediment, with the following:
   a. Renal tubular epithelial cells
   b. Cellular debris
   c. Pigmented granular casts
   d. Renal tubular cell casts
   e. "Muddy brown" coarse granular casts (Table 43.2)
5. Urine volume
   a. Anuria: less than 100 ml/24 hr
   b. Oliguria: 100–400 ml/24 hr
   c. Nonoliguria: greater than 400 ml/24 hr
   d. Polyuria: greater than 6 L/24 hr
6. Urine osmolality: isotonic (350 mOsm or less)
7. Urine-specific gravity: fixed (1.0008–1.012)
8. Urine Na greater than 20 mEq/L
9. FENA would be greater than 1%
10. BUN-to-creatinine ratio: less than 20:1
11. Low serum Na (less than 135 mEq)
12. Proteinuria may be seen, particularly in NSAID-induced interstitial nephritis, but is usually modest
13. Other clinical findings may include fever (greater than 80%), rash (25%–50%), arthralgias, and peripheral blood eosinophilia

C. Postrenal (5%–10% of cases)
   1. Associated with conditions that cause the obstruction of urinary flow and consequently a decrease in GFR
   2. Mechanical
      a. Calculi
      b. Tumors (prostate cancer, cervical cancer)
      c. Urethral strictures
      d. Benign prostatic hyperplasia
      e. Blood clots
      f. Occluded Foley catheter
   3. Functional
      a. Neurogenic bladder
      b. Diabetic neuropathy
      c. Spinal cord disease
   4. Urine volume may fluctuate between anuria and polyuria.
   5. Urine osmolality: isotonic (less than 350 mOsm) (initially may be high)
   6. Urine-specific gravity: fixed (1.0008–1.012)
   7. Urine Na: greater than 40 mEq/L (initially may be low—variable)
   8. FENa: variable
   9. Urinary sediment
      a. Normal or red cells
      b. White cells
      c. Crystals
   10. BUN-to-creatinine ratio: greater than 20:1

11. In-and-out catheter may reveal increased postvoid residual volume, and renal ultrasound may demonstrate hydronephrosis
12. Plain film X-ray (kidney, ureter, and bladder) of the abdomen will document the presence of two kidneys and will provide a check for kidney stones (Table 43.3)
13. Computed tomography scan or magnetic resonance imaging may also reveal obstruction
14. Retrograde urography may be used to obtain information on the ureters and the lower urinary tract
15. Renal biopsy with special immune stains and electron microscopy may assist in determining the cause of renal failure
16. Therapy may include catheter drainage, urethral stents, and percutaneous nephrostomy

V. Management

A. Therapy for ARF is aimed at:
   1. Treating the underlying cause
   2. Correcting fluid, electrolyte, and uremic abnormalities
   3. Preventing complications, including nutritional deficiencies (Figure 43.1)
B. Adjust intake to output on the basis of fluid status. Take the use of diuretics into consideration because more often, patients are overloaded, especially if they are oliguric or anuric.
C. The volume-depleted patient is usually resuscitated with saline.
D. Furosemide (Lasix) is used to convert oliguric to nonoliguric ARF but has no outcome difference
   1. Furosemide, given IV every 6 hr, is the initial treatment for volume overload
      a. The initial dose can be 20–100 mg (this depends on whether the patient takes Lasix regularly)
   2. If the response is not adequate within 1 hr, the dose is doubled. This process is repeated until adequate urine output is achieved, but higher doses are associated with tinnitus and temporary deafness.
   3. A continuous Lasix drip may be used but has not proven superior over intermittent dosing in AKI. Diuretic use in AKI has not been shown to change the outcome, and should be used to manage physiologic needs, such as water balance.
E. Maximize cardiac function and maintain optimal blood pressure for renal perfusion
F. Discontinue offending drugs
G. If benign prostatic hyperplasia is known or suspected, avoid the use of sympathomimetic medications (often found in over the counter decongestants).
H. Use may precipitate acute outlet obstruction and lead to post renal obstruction
I. ARF is a catabolic state; therefore, patients can become nutritionally deficient. Total caloric intake should be 30–45 kcal/kg/day, most of which should come from a combination of carbohydrate and lipids. In patients who are not receiving dialysis, protein should be restricted to 0.6 grams/kg/day. In patients who are receiving dialysis, protein intake should be 1–1.5 grams/kg/day.
J. Monitor for complications
   1. Electrolyte imbalances

   a. Hyperkalemia
      i. Sodium polystyrene sulfonate (Kayexalate) adds 1 mEq Na+ for each 1 mEq K+ removed via the gastrointestinal tract
      ii. Administer 15–30 grams of sodium polystyrene sulfonate mixed with 100 ml of 20% sorbitol or as an enema (50 grams in 50 ml or 70% sorbitol and 150 ml of tap water)
      iii. IV administration of calcium (10 ml of a 10% solution of calcium gluconate) is cardioprotective and temporarily reverses the neuromuscular effects of hyperkalemia.
      iv. Potassium can also be temporarily shifted into the intracellular compartment with the use of IV insulin (10 units) and glucose (25 grams), inhaled β agonist, or IV sodium bicarbonate (150 mEq in 1 L of D5W)

Table 43.2	Urine abnormalities in renal failure			
	Prerenal	**Postrenal (acute)**	**Intrinsic renal (acute)**	**Intrinsic renal (chronic)**
Urine volume	Decreased	Absent-to-wide fluctuation	Oliguric or nonoliguric	1000 ml^3 until end stage
Urine creatinine	Increased (U/P Cr ± 40)	Decreased (U/P Cr ± 20)	Decreased (U/P Cr less than 20)	Decreased (U/P Cr less than 20)
Osmolarity	Increased (±400 mOsm/kg)	Less than 350 mOsm/kg	Less than 350 mOsm/kg	Less than 350 mOsm/kg
Degree of proteinuria	Minimum	Absent	Varies with cause of renal failure: modest with ATN; nephrotic range common with acute glomerulopathies, usually less than 2 grams/24 hr with interstitial disease[a]	Varies with cause of renal disease (from 1–2 grams/day to nephrotic range)
Urinary sediment	Negative, or may have occasional hyaline cast	Negative, or hematuria with stones or papillary necrosis; pyuria with infectious prostate disease	ATN: muddy brown interstitial nephritis: lymphocytes, eosinophils (in stained preparations), and WBC casts; RPGN: RBC casts; nephrosis oval fat bodies	Broad casts with variable renal "residual" acute findings

Note: [a] Except NSAID-induced allergic interstitial nephritis with concomitant "nil disease." U/P = urine/plasma; Cr = creatinine; ATN = acute tubular necrosis; mOsm = milliosmole; RBC = red blood cells; WBC = white blood cells; RPGN = rapidly progressing glomerulonephritis; NSAID = non-steroidal anti-inflammatory drug. Adapted from F.F. Ferri's *Practical Guide to the Care of the Medical Patient Eighth Edition*, 2011. Copyright 2011 by Mosby Inc. Used with permission.

Table 43.3	Serum and radiographic abnormalities in renal failure			
	Prerenal	**Postrenal (acute)**	**Intrinsic renal (acute)**	**Intrinsic renal (chronic)**
BUN	Increased 10:1 greater than Cr	Increased by 20–40/day	Increased by 20–40/day	Stable; increase varies with protein intake
Serum creatinine	Normal/moderate increase	Increased by 2–4/day	Increased by 2–4/day	Stable increase (production equals excretion)
Serum potassium	Normal/moderate increase	Increase varies with urinary volume	Large increase (particularly when patient is oliguric); even larger increase with rhabdomyolysis	Normal until end stage, unless tubular dysfunction (type 4 RTA)
Serum phosphorus	Normal/moderate increase	Moderate increase	Increased	Becomes significantly elevated when serum creatinine surpasses 3 mg/dl
Serum calcium	Normal	Normal/decreased with PO$_4^{3-}$	Decreased (poor correlation with duration of renal failure)	Usually decreased
Renal size by ultrasound FENA	Normal/increased by less than 1	Increased and with dilated calyces less than 1 to greater than 1	Normal/increased greater than 1	Decreased and with ultrasound echogenicity greater than 1

Note: BUN = blood urea nitrogen; Cr = creatinine; RTA = renal tubular acidosis; PO$_4^{3-}$ = phosphate; FENA = fractional excretion of sodium. Adapted from F.F. Ferri's *Practical Guide to the Care of the Medical Patient*, Eighth Edition, 2011. Copyright 2011 by Mosby Inc. Used with permission.

v. Dialysis is the definitive treatment in patients with significantly elevated potassium levels and renal failure
- b. Hypernatremia
- c. Hyponatremia
- d. Hypocalcemia
- e. Metabolic acidosis
  - i. Acidosis is treated IV or orally with sodium bicarbonate when serum HCO_3 is less than 15 mEq/L, or pH is lower than 7.2
- f. Hypermagnesemia
- g. Hyperphosphatemia
2. Volume overload: pulmonary edema
3. Uremia: pericarditis
4. Infection
5. Gastrointestinal bleeding

K. Anticipate the need for dialysis. Between 20% and 60% of patients need short-term dialysis, particularly when BUN exceeds 100 mg/dl and serum creatinine exceeds 5–10 mg/dl.
1. Intravascular volume overload: pulmonary edema
2. Hyperkalemia
3. Acidosis/alkalosis
4. Uremia (symptomatic syndrome resulting from increase in nitrogenous wastes [azotemia])
   - a. Central nervous system disturbances
   - b. Gastrointestinal indications (nausea, vomiting, and anorexia)
   - c. Level of azotemia (elevation of waste products): BUN 100–200 mg/dl
5. Specific drug/toxin

L. Renally adjust dose all medications: assume that GFR is less than 10 ml/minute (normal, 80–120 ml/minute)

M. Adjust diet: low protein/Na/K

VI. RRT options in AKI and CKD

A. Hemodialysis
1. Intermittent (most common for chronic management)
   - a. Requires specialized staff
   - b. Useful in removing selected drugs in acute toxic states
   - c. Typically requires adequate mean arterial pressure to attain flow rates for clearance (normally at least 60 mmHg)
2. Continuous (similar creatine clearance to intermittent dialysis)
   - a. Continuous arterial renal replacement therapy
     - i. Requires arterial access and adequate mean blood pressure preferably at 60 mmHg
   - b. Continuous veno venous hemodialysis
     - i. Uses an external pump for flow rates so blood pressure requirements are lessened
     - ii. Both can be performed by trained intensive care unit nurses
     - iii. Benefits over intermittent dialysis have not been proven to reduce course, duration, outcome, or mortality in ARF even when the onset of treatment is started early
     - iv. Use in ARF should be based on the need for fluid removal and correction of electrolyte imbalance when conventional medical management fails
     - v. Choice should be made based on patient need, availability of services, and physiologic stability required by other replacement methods
     - vi. Some form of dialysis is indicated if fluid uremic symptoms develop, such as encephalopathy or pericarditis

B. Peritoneal dialysis
1. Useful for long-term use

CHAPTER 43 Acute Kidney Injury and Chronic Kidney Disease

2. Improved quality of life for patient over conventional dialysis methods
3. Does not provide creatinine clearance rates at the level of other RRT methods, which may limit usefulness
4. High risk for catheter site and intra-abdominal (peritoneal) infections
5. Does not provide adequate creatinine clearance rates required in catabolic states such as major surgery, burns, or sepsis, which may require conversion to an alternate RRT method during the acute state until baseline physiological state is restored

C. Renal transplantation
1. Most cost-effective with the benefit realized at about 1½–2 years posttransplant
2. Improved quality of life and functioning over chronic dialysis use
3. Limited by organ availability
4. Lifetime burden of immunosuppression use and the associated consequences

CHRONIC KIDNEY DISEASE

I. **Definition**
   A. Progressive azotemia over weeks, months, or years
      1. GFR 60 ml/minute or less for longer than 3 months, with or without kidney damage
   B. Isosthenuria is common
   C. Hypertension is common in most patients
   D. Ultrasound studies show evidence of bilateral small kidneys
   E. X-rays show evidence of renal osteodystrophy

II. **Etiology**
   A. Glomerular disease
   B. Polycystic kidney disease
   C. Hypertensive nephropathy
   D. Diabetic nephropathy
   E. Tubulointerstitial nephritis or necrosis
   F. Obstructive nephropathies
   G. Renal artery stenosis

III. **Stages based on the National Kidney Foundation Disease outcome quality initiative advisory board (recommended by the Center for Medicare Services to document renal damage–related complexity of care)**
   A. The progression of CKD occurs in five stages.
   B. Each stage reflects an increasing loss of nephrons

   1. Stage I
      a. GFR greater than 90 ml/minute
      b. Kidney damage with normal or increased GFR
   2. Stage II
      a. GFR 60–89 ml/minute
      b. Kidney damage with mild or decreased GFR
   3. Stage III
      a. GFR 30–59 ml/minute
      b. Moderate decrease in GFR with moderate complications
   4. Stage IV
      a. GFR 15–29 ml/minute
      b. Severe decrease in GFR with severe complications
   5. Stage V (kidney failure)
      a. End-stage renal disease
      b. GFR less than 15 ml/minute or dialysis
      c. Uremia and cardiovascular disease
      d. Monitor GFR. Normal is 80–120 ml/minute.
      e. Formula for calculation:
      f. Renal replacement is instituted when GFR falls to between 5 and 10 ml/minute.

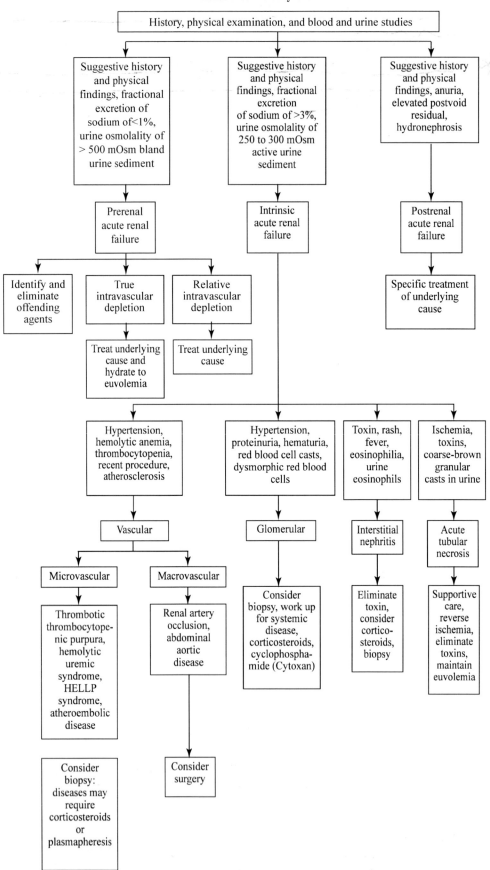

Figure 43.1. HELLP syndrome = abbreviation of symptoms associated with obstetric complication of pre-eclampsia: hemolysis, elevated liver enzymes, low platelet count; mOsm = milliosmole. Adapted from "Acute Renal Failure," by M. Agrawal and R. Swartz, 2000, Am Fam Physician, 61 (7), pp. 2077–2088. Copyright 2000 by the American Academy of Family Physicians. Used with permission.

g. Creatinine clearance is used by many practitioners as a more accurate method of estimating GFR
   i. Age and gender dependent
   ii. Normal
      (a) Males: 97–137 ml/minute/1.73 m^2
      (b) Females: 88–128 ml/minute/1.73 m^2
h. Cystatin C is a proteinase inhibitor that is not freely filtered by the glomerulus. It is felt to potentially be a better marker of renal function than creatine but is not widely available.

IV. Signs/symptoms
A. General
   1. Fatigue
   2. Weakness
B. Skin
   1. Pruritus
   2. Easy bruising
   3. Pallor, ecchymosis
   4. Excoriations
   5. Edema
   6. Xerosis
   7. Sallow complexion (ill, yellow appearing, jaundice if liver disease is present)
   8. Pale conjunctiva
   9. Reversible hair loss, nail changes
C. Ear, nose, and throat
   1. Metallic taste in the mouth
   2. Epistaxis
   3. Urinous breath
D. Pulmonary
   1. Shortness of breath
   2. Rales
   3. Pleural effusion
E. Cardiovascular
   1. Dyspnea on exertion
   2. Retrosternal pain on inspiration and pericardial friction rub caused by pericarditis related to uremia
   3. Hypertension caused by volume overload
   4. Cardiomegaly
F. Gastrointestinal
   1. Anorexia
   2. Nausea and vomiting
   3. Hiccups
G. Genitourinary
   1. Impotence
   2. Nocturia
   3. Iso-osmolar urine: Urine has an osmolarity similar to plasma osmolality despite variations in fluid intake; this indicates marked impairment in renal concentrating ability.
H. Neurologic
   1. Irritability
   2. Inability to concentrate
   3. Decreased libido
   4. Stupor
   5. Asterixis
   6. Myoclonus/hyperreflexia

7. Peripheral neuropathy associated with diabetes, if present
8. Restless leg syndrome/loss of vibratory sense
9. Seizures (rare)
   I. Anemia due to erythropoietin deficiency
V. **Management of common problems in CKD**
   A. Fluid overload
      1. Monitor weight, standing blood pressure, urine Na+ excretion, creatinine clearance (CrCl), and serum creatinine
      2. Decrease Na+ and fluid intake
      3. Diuretics
         a. Furosemide (Lasix), 20–80 mg/day initially
            i. Up to 600 mg/day; using too much of this drug may lead to side effects such as confusion, dehydration, and muscle cramps due to water and salt/mineral loss
            ii. Doses up to 1 gram/day have been used in congestive heart failure and renal failure
            iii. Continuous infusions of 100 mg/hr have been utilized
            iv. Remains effective when GFR is less than 25 ml/minute
         b. Other agents that may be used include the following but have not been proven to be more effective than furosemide:
            i. Metolazone (Zaroxolyn), 2.5–20 mg PO daily, in combination with loop diuretic only
            ii. Chlorothiazide (Diuril), 500 mg IV daily, in combination with loop diuretic only
            iii. Bumetanide (Bumex), 0.5–2 mg once daily (may repeat at 4- to 5-hour intervals, if needed, to a maximum of 10 mg/day). Continuous infusions of up to 2 mg/hr have been utilized.
            iv. Torsemide (Demadex), 10–20 mg once daily PO/IV (may increase up to 200 mg/day PRN)
   B. Hypertension
      1. Determine the patient's optimal Na+ and H_2O intact. Excess Na+/H_2O increases the level of hypertension
      2. Antihypertensive agents that maintain renal blood flow and reduce glomerular pressure and proteinuria are preferred
      3. If proteinuria is present, ACE inhibitors and calcium channel blockers may be superior to conventional treatment in decreasing proteinuria and reducing glomerular hypertension.
      4. Antihypertensives: Goal blood pressure for patients with chronic renal failure (CRF) is less than 140/80 mmHg; for those with proteinuria greater than 1–2 grams, it is less than 125/75 mmHg.
         a. ACE inhibitors
         b. Angiotensin II receptor blockers (if serum K+ and GFR permit)
         c. Calcium channel blockers
         d. Direct vasodilators
            i. Hydralazine (Apresoline)
            ii. Minoxidil (Loniten)
         e. Peripheral α blockers
            i. Doxazosin mesylate (Cardura)
            ii. Prazosin (Minipress)
         f. β blockers
            i. Propranolol (Inderal)
         g. Central α blockers
            i. Clonidine hydrochloride (Catapres)
   C. Protein catabolism

CHAPTER 43   Acute Kidney Injury and Chronic Kidney Disease

1. Limit protein intake (less than 8 grams/kg/day): The level of restriction may be increased to 0.6–0.8 grams/kg/day if restriction proves beneficial. Protein limitation is controversial as it has not shown to change the outcome of progress on CKD. It may lessen the need for dialysis times and frequency. Protein-related kidney disorders occur relatively late in CKD at GFRs of about 30. Protein restriction, if used, should be reserved for late Stage III, IV, and end-stage renal disease stage when protein abnormalities occur.
2. Provide adequate calories
3. Avoid stresses of trauma, infection, and immobilization, if possible
4. Physical activity should be moderate
5. Thyroid hormone, steroids, and tetracycline increase catabolism and must be avoided
6. Anabolic agents may help some patients avoid a negative nitrogen balance (help stimulate erythropoiesis)
   a. Fluoxymesterone (Halotestin)
   b. Nandrolone decanoate (Deca-Durabolin)

D. Acidosis: alkalizing agents are indicated when plasma HCO_3 is less than 20 mEq/L
   1. $NaHCO_3$—1 gram + 13 mEq Na; generally used in emergencies because it may cause volume overload related to Na+
   2. Sodium citrate (Shohl solution, Bicitra): 1 mEq/ml of Na+
   3. Sodium and potassium citrate and citric acid (Polycitra): monitor K+ levels, and avoid in patients with hyperkalemia

E. Hyperkalemia
   1. Avoid foods and medications high in K+
   2. Avoid hypercatabolic states
   3. Medical emergency if K+ is greater than 7 mEq/L
      a. Administer hypertonic glucose, insulin, and HCO_3
      b. Calcium gluconate or calcium chloride IV to modify myocardial irritability
      c. Correct acidosis
      d. Administer K+ ion exchange resins to remove excess potassium ions
         i. Kayexalate, 30–60 grams/day (each gram of Kayexalate resin binds with 1 mEq of K+ and subsequently releases 1 mEq of Na+)
      e. Hemodialysis
      f. Monitor ECG for flat P waves, peaked T waves, PR interval greater than 0.20 seconds, QRS complex greater than 0.10 second, and bradycardia

F. Hyperphosphatemia (choose one or more from the following; the phosphorous level should be kept below 4.6 mg/dl):
   1. Restrict phosphorus to 800–1000 mg/day
      a. Limit foods such as colas, eggs, dairy products, and meat
   2. GFR less than 20–30 ml/minute usually requires phosphate-binding agents
   3. Calcium carbonate, 650 mg three times a day
      a. Phosphate-binding agent
      b. Prevents aluminum toxicity
   4. Sevelamer (Renvela), 800–3200 mg three times a day with meals
   5. Lanthanum (Fosrenol), 1500–3000 mg per day in divided doses with meals
   6. Calcium acetate, 667 mg (two to six tablets) three times a day, with meals
   7. Aluminium hydroxide is an effective phosphate binder that can be used in the acute setting for serum phosphorous levels greater than 7 mg/dl; however, long-term use should be avoided because it can cause osteomalacia and neurologic complications. Limit duration to 3 days to avoid aluminum toxicity.
   8. Hemodialysis

G. Hypocalcemia
   1. Maintain phosphorous level at less than 6 mg/dl
   2. Calcium carbonate supplements
   3. 1,25-OH_2 vitamin D in extreme cases

- H. Hypermagnesemia: avoid Mg++ containing laxatives/antacids
- I. Anemia
    1. Iron
    2. Vitamin supplements PRN
    3. Erythropoietin weekly injections; 50–100 units/kg IV/SQ three times a week; more dosing has a black box warning for increased cardiovascular disease risks
        a. Recommended for patients on hemodialysis
- J. Neurologic problems
    1. Anticonvulsants
        a. Phenytoin
        b. Phenobarbital
    2. Sedatives
        a. Haloperidol
        b. Diphenhydramine
- K. Renal osteodystrophy
    1. Prevent acidosis, hypocalcemia, hyperphosphatemia; control hyperparathyroidism
    2. Correct low Ca (less than 6.5 mg/dl)
        a. Administer calcium supplement, such as calcium carbonate and calcium gluconate, 1–2 grams/day
        b. Titrate as necessary to control serum phosphate and calcium levels
    3. Correct high phosphorous levels (higher than 5 mg/dl). Administer phosphate binders.
    4. Correct acidosis (HCO_3 less than 15 mEq/dl). Administer $NaHCO_3$, 2–5 mEq/kg, as a 4- to 8-hr infusion (for emergency situations), or 650 mg PO three times a day, and titrate PRN.
    5. Administer vitamin D if Ca stays below 6 mg/dl (calcitrol, paricalcitol), bone pain is a problem, alkaline phosphatase levels increase, and X-rays reveal evidence of osteomalacia.
    6. Identify and treat secondary hyperparathyroidism, which is triggered by low calcium levels
        a. Limit foods high in phosphorus
        b. Administer phosphate binders (Tums, Oscal) with meals
        c. Sevelamer hydrochloride (Renagel) is currently being used and is believed to have many advantages over calcium-based phosphate binders, although it is more expensive
        d. Calcitrol or paricalcitol

VI. **RRT options**
- A. Hemodialysis
- B. Peritoneal dialysis
- C. Renal transplantation

MODIFICATION OF DRUG DOSAGES

I. **Types of drugs**
- A. Type A: eliminated entirely by the kidney
- B. Type B: eliminated entirely by extrarenal mechanism
- C. Type C: eliminated by renal and extrarenal mechanisms

II. **Decreased renal function results in the following:**
- A. Abnormal excretion rates
- B. Abnormal metabolism rates of certain drugs
- C. Abnormal sensitivity to certain drugs

III. **Before administering any drug to a patient in renal failure, consider the following:**
- A. Does this drug depend on the kidney for excretion?
- B. Does an excess blood level affect the kidney or cause nephrotoxicity?
- C. Does the effect of the drug alter electrolyte imbalance?
- D. Is the patient susceptible to the drug because of kidney disease?

IV. Modification of drug doses:
   A. Serum creatinine is greater than 10 mg/ml; renal function is 15% of normal: major modification is needed
   B. Serum creatinine is 3–10 mg/ml; renal function is 15%–20% of normal: modest changes are needed

BIBLIOGRAPHY

Acute kidney injury. (2013). *Nursing Standard, 28*(4), 21–21.

BET 3: RIFLE criteria versus acute kidney injury network (AKIN) criteria for prognosis of acute renal failure. (2011). *Emergency Medicine Journal, 28*(10), 900–901.

Bouchard, J., Soroko, S. B., Chertow, G. M., Himmelfarb, J., Ikizler, T. A., Paganini, E. P., & Mehta, R. L. (2009). Fluid accumulation, survival and recovery of kidney function in critically ill patients with acute kidney injury. *Kidney International, 76*(4), 422–427. doi:10.1038/ki.2009.159

Brar, S. S., Hiremath, S., Dangas, G., Mehran, R., Brar, S. K., & Leon, M. B. (2009). Sodium bicarbonate for the prevention of contrast induced-acute kidney injury: A systematic review and meta-analysis. *Clinical Journal of the American Society of Nephrology, 4*(10), 1584–1592. doi:10.2215/CJN.03120509; 10.2215/CJN.03120509

Cavalier, E., Delanaye, P., Vranken, L., Bekaert, A. C., Carlisi, A., Chapelle, J. P., & Souberbielle, J. C. (2012). Interpretation of serum PTH concentrations with different kits in dialysis patients according to the KDIGO guidelines: Importance of the reference (normal) values. *Nephrology, Dialysis, Transplantation, 27*(5), 1950–1956. doi:10.1093/ndt/gfr535; 10.1093/ndt/gfr535

Chao, C. T., Wu, V. C., Lai, C. F., Shiao, C. C., Huang, T. M., Wu, P. C., & Wu, K. D. (2012). Advanced age affects the outcome-predictive power of RIFLE classification in geriatric patients with acute kidney injury. *Kidney International, 82*(8), 920–927. doi:10.1038/ki.2012.237

Chawla, L. S., & Kimmel, P. L. (2012). Acute kidney injury and chronic kidney disease: An integrated clinical syndrome. *Kidney International, 82*(5), 516–524. doi:10.1038/ki.2012.208

Cheung, C. M., Ponnusamy, A., & Anderton, J. G. (2008). Management of acute renal failure in the elderly patient: A clinician's guide. *Drugs and Aging, 25*(6), 455–476.

Chronopoulos, A., Rosner, M. H., Cruz, D. N., & Ronco, C. (2010). Acute kidney injury in elderly intensive care patients: A review. *Intensive Care Medicine, 36*(9), 1454–1464. doi:10.1007/s00134–010–1957–7

Coyne, D. W. (2013). Anemia management in dialysis: Why the FDA and CMS have it right (and how KDIGO got it wrong). *Nephrology News and Issues, 27*(2), 16, 18, 20.

Faubel, S. (2013). Have we reached the limit of mortality benefit with our approach to renal replacement therapy in acute kidney injury? *American Journal of Kidney Diseases, 62*(6), 1030–033. doi:10.1053/j.ajkd.2013.09.004; 10.1053/j.ajkd.2013.09.004

Ferri, F. F. (2011). *Practical guide to the care of the medical patient* (8th ed.). Philadelphia, PA: Mosby Elsevier.

Fuchs, L., Lee, J., Novack, V., Baumfeld, Y., Scott, D., Celi, L., ... Talmor, D. (2013). Severity of acute kidney injury and two-year outcomes in critically ill patients. *Chest, 144*(3), 866–875. doi:10.1378/chest.12–2967

Gocze, I., Wohlgemuth, W. A., Schlitt, H. J., & Jung, E. M. (2013). Contrast-enhanced ultrasonography for bedside imaging in subclinical acute kidney injury. *Intensive Care Medicine, 40*(3). doi:10.1007/s00134–013–3152–0

Hoste, E. A., Doom, S., De Waele, J., Delrue, L. J., Defreyne, L., Benoit, D. D., & Decruyenaere, J. (2011). Epidemiology of contrast-associated acute kidney injury in ICU patients: A retrospective cohort analysis. *Intensive Care Medicine, 37*(12), 1921–1931.

Joannidis, M., Metnitz, B., Bauer, P., Schusterschitz, N., Moreno, R., Druml, W., & Metnitz, P. G. (2009). Acute kidney injury in critically ill patients classified by AKIN versus RIFLE using the SAPS 3 database. *Intensive Care Medicine, 35*(10), 1692–1702. doi:10.1007/s00134–009–1530–4

Jorgensen, A., L. (2013). Contrast-induced nephropathy: Pathophysiology and preventive strategies. *Critical Care Nurse, 33*(1), 37–47. doi:10.4037/ccn2013680

Kellum, J. A., Lameire, N., & for the KDIGO AKI Guideline Work Group. (2013). Diagnosis, evaluation, and management of acute kidney injury: A KDIGO summary (Part 1). *Critical Care (London, England), 17*(1), 204. doi:10.1186/cc11454

Kovacevic, B., Ignjatovic, M., Zivaljevic, V., Cuk, V., Scepanovic, M., Petrovic, Z., & Paunovic, I. (2012). Parathyroidectomy for the attainment of NKF-K/DOQI and KDIGO recommended values for bone and mineral metabolism in dialysis patients with uncontrollable secondary hyperparathyroidism. *Langenbeck's Archives of Surgery, 397*(3), 413–420. doi:10.1007/s00423–011–0901–9; 10.1007/s00423–011–0901–9

Koyner, J. L. (2012). Assessment and diagnosis of renal dysfunction in the ICU. *Chest, 141*(6), 1584–1594. doi:10.1378/chest.11–1513

Lamb, E. J., Levey, A. S., & Stevens, P. E. (2013). The kidney disease improving global outcomes (KDIGO) guideline update for chronic kidney disease: Evolution not revolution. *Clinical Chemistry, 59*(3), 462–465. doi:10.1373/clinchem.2012.184259

London, G., Coyne, D., Hruska, K., Malluche, H. H., & Martin, K. J. (2010). The new kidney disease: Improving global outcomes (KDIGO) guidelines—Expert clinical focus on bone and vascular calcification. *Clinical Nephrology, 74*(6), 423–432.

Mårtensson, J., Martling, C. R., & Bell, M. (2012). Novel biomarkers of acute kidney injury and failure: Clinical applicability. *British Journal of Anaesthesia, 109*(6), 843–850. doi:10.1093/bja/aes357

Matzke, G. R., Aronoff, G. R., Atkinson, A. J., Jr., Bennett, W. M., Decker, B. S., Eckardt, K. U., & Murray, P. (2011). Drug dosing consideration in patients with acute and chronic kidney disease-A clinical update from kidney disease: Improving global outcomes (KDIGO). *Kidney International, 80*(11), 1122–1137. doi:10.1038/ki.2011.322; 10.1038/ki.2011.322

Li, P. K. T., Burdmann, E. A., & Mehta, R., L. (2013). Acute kidney injury: Global health alert. *Internet Journal of Nephrology, 8*(1), 1–1.

Sankarasubbaiyan, S., Janardan, J., D., & Kaur, P. (2013). Outcomes and characteristics of intermittent hemodialysis for acute kidney injury in an intensive care unit. *Indian Journal of Nephrology, 23*(1), 30–33. doi:10.4103/0971–4065.107193

Scharman, E. J., & Troutman, W. G. (2013). Prevention of kidney injury following rhabdomyolysis: A systematic review. *Annals of Pharmacotherapy, 47*(1), 90–105. doi:10.1345/aph.1R215

Serpa Neto, A., Veelo, D. P., Peireira, V. G., de Assuncao, M. S., Manetta, J. A., Esposito, D. C., & Schultz, M. J. (2013). Fluid resuscitation with hydroxyethyl starches in patients with sepsis is associated with an increased incidence of acute kidney injury and use of renal replacement therapy: A systematic review and meta-analysis of the literature. *Journal of Critical Care, 29*(1). doi:10.1016/j.jcrc.2013.09.031

Shavit, L., Korenfeld, R., Lifschitz, M., Butnaru, A., & Slotki, I. (2009). Sodium bicarbonate versus sodium chloride and oral *N*-acetylcysteine for the prevention of contrast-induced nephropathy in advanced chronic kidney disease. *Journal of Interventional Cardiology, 22*(6), 556–563. doi:10.1111/j.1540–8183.2009.00500.x

Singbartl, K., & Kellum, J. A. (2012). AKI in the ICU: Definition, epidemiology, risk stratification, and outcomes. *Kidney International, 81*(9), 819–825. doi:10.1038/ki.2011.339

tevens, P. E., Levin, A., & Kidney Disease: Improving Global Outcomes Chronic Kidney Disease Guideline Development Work Group Members. (2013). Evaluation and management of chronic kidney disease: Synopsis of the kidney disease: Improving global outcomes 2012 clinical practice guideline. *Annals of Internal Medicine, 158*(11), 825–830. doi:10.7326/0003–4819–158–11–201306040–00007

Strachan, J. M., & DeVile, M. P. (2012). Contrast-induced acute kidney injury: What is the prevalence of prevention protocols? *Intensive Care Medicine, 38*(5), 915–915. doi:10.1007/s00134–012–2479–2

Zimmerman, J., L., & Shen, M., C. (2013). Rhabdomyolysis. *Chest, 144*(3), 1058–1065. doi:10.1378/chest.12–2016

CHAPTER 44

Benign Prostatic Hyperplasia

JENNIFER J. ROBERG • CHARLENE M. MYERS

I. **Definition**
   A. Benign prostatic hyperplasia (BPH) is the enlargement of the prostate gland, a condition commonly seen in men older than 50 years of age.
   B. Progressive condition that can cause obstruction of the urethra with interference in urine flow
   C. Hyperplastic process that results from an increase in cell numbers
II. **Etiology/incidence**
   A. Incidence is age related
      1. Men ages 41–50 years: 20%
      2. Men ages 51–60 years: 50%
      3. Men older than 80 years of age: more than 90%
   B. Exact cause is unknown
   C. May be a response of the prostate gland to androgen hormones over time
   D. Dietary fat may play a role
III. **Clinical manifestations**
   A. Irritative symptoms—consequence of bladder dysfunction
      1. Frequency
      2. Dysuria
      3. Urgency
      4. Nocturia
      5. Incontinence
   B. Obstructive symptoms
      1. Hesitancy
      2. Straining
      3. Starting and stopping
      4. Dribbling
      5. Retention
      6. Decreased force and caliber of stream
      7. Sensation of incomplete bladder emptying
      8. Double voiding (urinating a second time within 2 hr)
   C. Focal or uniform enlargement
      1. On digital rectal examination, the prostate may be enlarged. Size does not correlate with severity of symptoms or with degree of obstruction.

2. The prostate should feel smooth and rubbery
3. Focal enlargement, nodularity, or extreme hardness may represent malignancy; further investigation is indicated
   a. Transrectal ultrasound
   b. Biopsy
D. Palpable bladder consistent with urinary retention

IV. Laboratory findings
A. Urinalysis
   1. Pyuria suggests infection
   2. Hematuria may be a sign of malignancy
B. Urine culture to rule out urinary tract infection (UTI) if irritative symptoms are present
C. BUN/creatinine to assess for renal insufficiency
D. Prostate-specific antigen (PSA)
   1. Considered optional, yet most practitioners include it in the initial evaluation
   2. Levels suggestive of prostate cancer
      a. Between 4 ng/ml and 10 ng/ml suggest a risk of approximately 25%
      b. Above 10 ng/ml suggest a risk of more than 50%
      c. Below 4 ng/ml does not guarantee that the patient does not have cancer
   3. Because an overlap is seen between levels in BPH and in prostate cancer, its use is controversial
   4. Other causes of elevated PSA include:
      a. Prostate cancer
      b. Bacterial prostatitis
      c. UTI
E. Transrectal ultrasound with a palpable nodule or elevated PSA

V. Management
A. Mild symptoms
   1. Patient may recover spontaneously over time ("watchful waiting")
   2. Avoid medications that can worsen symptoms
      a. Decongestants, diuretics, and other sympathomimetics (act on α receptors to enhance prostate muscle tone, which increases dynamic obstruction)
      b. Anticholinergics (antihistamines), bowel antispasmodics, tricyclic antidepressants, opiates, and antipsychotics; these decrease bladder muscle contraction, thus increasing urine retention
B. Mild to moderate symptoms
   1. Alpha (α) blockers, the preferred agents for BPH, relax muscle fibers in the prostate gland and capsule and in the internal urethral sphincter, thereby facilitating emptying of the bladder. No effect on blood pressure for the following agents:
      a. Terazosin (Hytrin), 1 mg at bedtime, increasing up to 10 mg at bedtime as necessary or tolerated
      b. Prazosin (Minipress), 1–5 mg PO BID
      c. Doxazosin (Cardura), 1–8 mg daily
      d. Hypotension and dizziness are the most commonly reported adverse effects.
      e. Combination therapy: tamsulosin (Flomax) (α1a blockade), 0.4 or 0.8 mg daily; alfuzosin (Uroxatral) 10 mg once daily; silodosin (Rapaflo), 8 mg once daily with a meal
   2. Hormonal manipulation
      a. Finasteride (Proscar), 5 mg/day
         i. Blocks conversion of testosterone to dihydrotestosterone
         ii. Works on the epithelial component of the prostate, resulting in reduction in the size of the gland and improvement in symptoms
         iii. Six months of therapy is required for maximal effect
      b. Dutasteride (Avodart), 0.5 mg once a day
      c. Estrogens, antiandrogens, or gonadotropin-releasing hormone (GnRH) may be used, but only if finasteride is not tolerated because of adverse effects
   3. Combination of α blockers and hormonal manipulation
   4. Phytotherapy
      a. Use of plants or plant extracts for medicinal purposes
      b. Several plant extracts have become popular:
         i. Saw palmetto berry

ii. Bark of *Pygeum africanum*
iii. Roots of *Echinacea purpurea* and *Hypoxis rooperi*
iv. Pollen extract
v. Leaves of the trembling poplar
vi. Rye
vii. Common or stinging nettle
viii. Pumpkin/squash
   c. Herbal remedies sold as "dietary supplements"
   d. Safety and efficacy have not been evaluated by the FDA or any regulatory agency
   e. No requirement for proof of efficacy/safety prior to marketing
5. Safety and efficacy has not been evaluated by the FDA or any regulatory agency. Avoid medications that increase obstructive symptoms (as noted previously)

C. Severe symptoms
  1. Surgery may be necessary if significant urinary symptoms exist
  2. Types of surgeries:
     a. Transurethral resection of the prostate (TURP)
        i. Low mortality (1%) but moderate morbidity (18%)
        ii. Should bring improvement in the signs and symptoms of BPH
        iii. Repeat resection is needed in less than 10% of cases
        iv. Retrograde ejaculation may occur after the procedure has been performed
        v. Uncommon complications
           (a) Bladder neck contracture
           (b) Urethral stricture disease
           (c) Incontinence
     b. Open simple prostatectomy
     c. Transurethral incision of the prostate (TUIP)
        i. No tissue is resected
        ii. Antegrade ejaculation is usually maintained
        iii. Can usually be performed as an outpatient procedure
        iv. May benefit patients with BPH associated with smaller glands, especially younger men

D. The following options offer promise but few long-term data on their effectiveness have been gathered.
  1. Laser therapy
     a. Two primary energy sources of lasers have been used: neodymium: yttrium-aluminum-garnet (Nd:YAG) and holmium:YAG.
     b. Transurethral laser-induced prostatectomy (TULIP) is performed under transrectal ultrasound guidance.
     c. Advantages
        i. Minimal blood loss
        ii. Rare occurrence of transurethral resection syndrome
        iii. Ability of clinicians to treat patients on anticoagulation therapy
        iv. Outpatient therapy
     d. Disadvantages
        i. Lack of tissue for pathologic evaluation
        ii. Longer postoperative catheterization time
        iii. More frequent irritative voiding complaints
        iv. Expense of laser fibers and generators
  2. Transurethral needle ablation of the prostate (TUNA)
     a. A special catheter is passed into the urethra, and then interstitial radiofrequency needles are deployed from the end of the catheter to pierce the mucosa of the prostatic urethra.
     b. Tissue is heated by radiofrequencies; this results in coagulative necrosis. Improvement in voiding has been reported
  3. Transurethral electrovaporization of the prostate
     a. High current densities result in heat vaporization of tissue, which creates a cavity in the prostatic urethra
     b. Long-term comparative data versus other procedures are needed
  4. Transurethral microwave therapy (TUMT) (hyperthermia)

a. Microwave hyperthermia is commonly delivered via transurethral catheter
b. Long-term follow-up with large randomized trials is needed
5. Urethral stents may be used for patients who are not candidates for standard surgery
a. Can be performed under local anesthesia
b. Preferred to chronic catheterization or suprapubic cystostomy

VI. Gerontological considerations
1. Physiologic changes
    a. Diminished kidney mass, blood flow, and glomerular filtration rate (10% per decade after the age of 30 years)
    b. Kidneys are the primary route of elimination of most drugs or their metabolites
    c. Assessment of the estimated glomerular filtration rate (eGFR) or creatinine clearance is often required to adjust drug therapy
    d. Determine renal function through glomerular filtration rate by calculating the creatinine clearance in the elderly, using the Cockcroft-Gault equation
        i. Males:
            (a) Creatinine clearance (ml/min) = [(140 minus age in years) × (body weight in kg)]/ [72 × (serum creatinine in mg/dl)]
        ii. Females: multiply the calculated value by 85% (0.85)
        iii. Normal creatinine clearance values in adults:
            (a) Males less than 40 years = 107–139 ml/min, or 1.8–2.3 ml/second
            (b) Females less than 40 years = 87–107 ml/min, or 1.5–1.8 ml/second
            (c) Creatinine clearance values usually decrease as one ages (e.g., decrease by 6.5 ml/min for every 10 years after the age of 20)
    e. Reduced bladder elasticity, muscle tone, and capacity
    f. Increased postvoid residual and nocturnal urine production
    g. Male reproductive system changes
        i. Prostate enlargement with risk of BPH
        ii. Decreased testosterone level leads to increased estrogen-to-androgen ratio
        iii. Decreased sperm motility; fertility reduced but extant
        iv. Increased incidence of gynecomastia
    h. Sexual function
        i. Slowed arousal-increased time to achieve erection
        ii. Erection less firm, shorter lasting
        iii. Delayed ejaculation and decreased forcefulness at ejaculation
        iv. Longer interval to achieving subsequent erection
    i. Prostate
        i. By fourth decade of life, stromal fibrous elements and glandular tissue hypertrophy, stimulated by dihydrotestosterone (DHT, the active androgen within the prostate); hyperplastic nodules enlarge in size, ultimately leading to urethral obstruction
2. Clinical implications
    a. History
        i. Many men are overly sensitive about complaints of the male genitourinary system; men are often not inclined to initiate discussion and seek help; important to take active role in screening with an approach that is open, trustworthy, and nonjudgmental.
        ii. Sexual function remains important to many men, even at 80 years of age and older
        iii. Lack of an available partner, poor health, erectile dysfunction, medication adverse effects, and lack of desire are the main reasons men do not continue to have sex.
        iv. Acute and chronic alcohol use can lead to impotence in men
        v. Nocturia is reported in 66% of patients over 65 years of age due to impaired ability to concentrate urine, reduced in bladder capacity or BPH-frequent cause of insomnia
    b. Physical
        i. Digital rectal exam is almost universally dreaded by men; provide privacy, allow for dignity
    c. Assessment
        i. In men diagnosed with BPH, periodic evaluation for prostate cancer must continue.
    d. Treatment
        i. A man may not want treatment for BPH because of fear of erectile dysfunction

3. Possible findings/results
    a. Decreased drug clearance and increased risk of:
        i. Adverse drug reactions
        ii. Nephrotoxicity
        iii. Renal complications
        iv. Volume/fluid overload (especially in heart failure patients)
        v. Hyponatremia and dehydration (especially in patients taking thiazide diuretics)
        vi. Hypernatremia (especially in patients with fever)
        vii. Hyperkalemia (especially in patients taking potassium-sparing diuretics)
        viii. Metabolic acidosis
        ix. Urinary urgency
        x. Incontinence
        xi. UTIs
        xii. Polyuria at night
        xiii. Falls

BIBLIOGRAPHY

American Cancer Society. (2014). *Prostate cancer*. Retrieved from http://www.cancer.org/cancer/prostatecancer/

Barry, M. J. (2009). Decision support in the treatment of prostate conditions. In A. Edwards & G. Elwyn (Eds.), *Shared Decision-Making in Health Care: Achieving Evidence-Based Patient Choice* (2nd ed.). New York, NY: Oxford University Press.

Deters, L. A., Costabile, R. A., Leveillee, R. J., Moore, C. R., & Patel, V. R. (2014). *Benign prostatic hypertrophy*. Retrieved from http://emedicine.medscape.com/article/437359-overview

Dowling-Castronovo, A., & Bradway, C. (2012). Urinary incontinence. In M. Boltz, E. Capuezuti, T. Fulmer, & D. Zwicker (Eds.), *Evidence-based geriatric nursing protocols for best practice* (4th ed., pp. 363–387). New York, NY: Springer Publishing Company.

Emberton, M. (2010). Medical treatment of benign prostatic hyperplasia: Physician and patient preferences and satisfaction. *International Journal of Clinical Practice, 64*(10), 1425–1435.

Filson, C., Hollingsworth, J., Clemens, J., & Wei, J. (2013). The efficacy and safety of combined therapy with α-blockers and anticholinergics for men with benign prostatic hyperplasia: A meta-analysis. *Journal of Urology, 190*(6), 2153–2160.

Gardiner, S. (2005). Need to know BPH. *Pulse, 65*, 34–37.

Kennedy-Malone, L., Fletcher, K. R., Martin-Plank, L. (2014). *Advanced Practice Nursing in the Care of Older Adults*. Philadelphia, PA: FA Davis.

Kigure, T., Nakata, K., Yuri, Y., Harada, T., Miyagata, S., Fujieda, N., . . . Etori, K. (2012). Microwave thermal therapy in the treatment of benign prostatic hyperplasia and prostate cancer. *Journal of Microwave Surgery, 30*, 239–245.

Lourenco, T., Shaw, M., Fraser, C., MacLennan, G., N'Dow, J., & Pickard, R. (2010). The clinical effectiveness of transurethral incision of the prostate: A systematic review of randomised controlled trials. *World Journal of Urology, 28*, 23–32.

Lee, A. G., Choi, Y. H., Cho, S. Y., & Cho, I. R. (2012). A prospective study of reducing unnecessary prostate biopsy in patients with high serum prostate-specific antigen with consideration of prostatic inflammation. *Korean Journal of Urology, 53*(1), 50–53.

Lerma, E. V. (2009). Anatomic and physiologic changes of the aging kidney. *Clinics in Geriatric Medicine, 25*(3), 325–329.

McPhee, S. J., Papadakis, M. A., & Rabow, M. W. (Eds.). (2014). *Current medical diagnosis and treatment 2014*. New York, NY: McGraw-Hill.

McVary, K. T., Roerhborn, C. G., Alvins, A. L., Barry, M. J., Bruskewitz, R. C., Donnel, R. F., . . . Wei, J. T. (2011). Update on AUA guideline on the management of benign prostatic hyperplasia. *The Journal of Urology, 185*(5), 1793–1803.

Miller, M. (2009). Disorders of fluid balance. In S. Studenski, K. P. High, & S. Asthana (Eds.), *Hazzard's geriatric medicine and gerontology* (6th ed., pp. 1047–1058). New York, NY: McGraw-Hill.

Neelima, D., & Bhagwat, D. (2011). Benign prostatic hyperplasia: An overview of existing treatment. *Indian Journal of Pharmacology, 43*(1), 6–12.

Paolone, D. R. (2010). Benign prostatic hyperplasia. *Clinics in geriatric medicine, 26*(2), 223–239.

Parsons, J. K., & Im, R. (2009). Alcohol consumption is associated with a decreased risk of benign prostatic hyperplasia. *Journal of Urology, 182*(4), 1463–68.

Péquignot, R., Belmin, J., Chauvelier, S., Gaubert, J. Y., Konrat, C., Duron, E., & Hanon, O. (2009). Renal function in older hospital patients is more accurately estimated using the Cockcroft-Gault formula than the modification diet in renal disease formula. *Journal of the American Geriatrics Society, 57*(9), 1638–1643. doi:10.1111/j.1532–5415.2009.02385.x

Shrivastava, A., & Gupta, V. B. (2012). Various treatment options for benign prostatic hyperplasia: A current update. *Journal of Midlife Health, 3*(1), 10–19.

Uphold, C., & Graham, M. (2013). *Clinical guidelines in family practice* (5th ed.). Gainesville, FL: Barmarrae Books, Inc.

Zhang, N., & Zhang, X. (2013). Controversy of the prostate-specific antigen test era: Should prostate cancer be detected and treated in all patients? *Chinese Medical Journal, 126*(15), 2803–2804.

CHAPTER 45

Renal Artery Stenosis

MICHELE H. TALLEY • CHARLENE M. MYERS

I. **Definition**
   A. Renal artery stenosis (RAS) is defined as a stenosis or narrowing in the lumen of the main renal artery or in its proximal branches.
   B. RAS is a progressive disease in which vascular supply is interrupted and perfusion to the kidney may lead to gradual loss of renal function due to ischemia and eventual death of the organ.
   C. RAS is sometimes referred to as ischemic nephropathy (defined as decreased glomerular filtration rate [GFR] due to hemodynamically significant RAS).

II. **Pathophysiology**
   A. Reduced blood flow through the renal artery causes the kidney to release increased amounts of the hormone, renin
   B. Renin, a powerful blood pressure regulator, initiates a series of chemical events that result in hypertension.
   C. Renal vascular hypertension can be very severe and difficult to control.
   D. The kidney with RAS suffers from decreased blood flow and often shrinks (atrophies). This process is called "ischemic nephropathy."
   E. The other kidney is at risk for the development of damage caused by hypertension.
   F. Hypertensive nephrosclerosis often develops
   G. Persistently elevated blood pressures in this non-stenotic kidney may cause progressive scarring (sclerosis) leading to progressive loss of filtering function in this kidney as well.
   H. Compensatory contralateral hypertrophy may temporarily maintain renal function
   I. Unilateral RAS and bilateral RAS can ultimately lead to chronic kidney disease.

III. **Etiology**
   A. Atherosclerosis
   B. Fibromuscular dysplasia
   C. Dissection
   D. Vasculitis (e.g., Takayasu arteritis)
   E. Thromboembolic disease
   F. Renal artery coarctation

G. Extrinsic compression
H. Radiation injury
I. Renal artery aneurysm

IV. **Types of RAS**
   A. Fibromuscular dysplasia
      1. Accounts for less than 10% of RAS
      2. Due to an abnormality in the muscular lining of the renal artery
      3. Occurs in ages 25–50 years in mostly women, compared to men
      4. Familial tendency
   B. Atherosclerosis
      1. Leads to more than 90% of all cases of RAS
      2. Most RAS is caused by atherosclerosis, or "hardening of the arteries." Atherosclerosis is the buildup of cholesterol deposits, or plaque, in the lining of the arteries.
   C. Renovascular disease

V. **Signs/symptoms**
   A. Usually asymptomatic until stenosis is severe
   B. Symptoms are as follows:
      1. Increase or decrease in urination
      2. Edema
      3. Drowsiness
      4. Generalized itching
      5. Dry skin
      6. Headaches
      7. Weight loss
      8. Appetite loss
      9. Nausea
      10. Vomiting
      11. Sleep problems
      12. Discolored skin
      13. Muscle cramping
   C. RAS should be considered in the following circumstances:
      1. Onset of hypertension (usually sudden) at younger than 30 years or older than age 55
      2. Hypertension that was well controlled has become difficult to treat (despite using three or more different blood pressure control medications)
      3. Malignant, accelerated, or resistant hypertension
      4. No family history of hypertension
      5. Unexplained heart failure or "flash" pulmonary edema
      6. Asymmetric (differently sized and shaped) kidneys on ultrasound
      7. Epigastric or renal artery bruits (upon auscultation or ultrasound)
      8. Atherosclerotic disease of the aorta or peripheral arteries
      9. A decline in estimated GFR by greater than 30% from baseline renal function after initiation of angiotensin converting enzyme (ACE-I) inhibitors or angiotensin receptor blockers (ARBs)
      10. Metabolic acidosis

VI. **Laboratory/diagnostics**
   A. Noninvasive tests: ultrasonography (US), computed tomography (CT) angiography, magnetic resonance angiography (MRA), captopril renal scintigraphy, and captopril test
      1. Doppler US may be used for initial diagnostic screening; however, if the stenosis is critical (greater than 80%–90%) when using Doppler US or MRI, an invasive diagnostic test may be required.
      2. CT angiography of the renal arteries: noninvasive and allows for 3D viewing of vessels
         a. Less specific than MRA but may be used in patients in whom MRA is contraindicated
         b. Risk of contrast-induced nephropathy is present
      3. MRA can provide a functional assessment of blood flow to the kidney and kidney function.

a. Does not require use of radiation or iodinated contrast; uses gadolinium-based contrast medium and must be avoided in those with moderate- to end-stage renal failure
   b. Cannot use MRI/A in those with implanted devices
B. Invasive renal angiography: the most direct measure of hemodynamic or functional significance of a stenosis is differential pressure across the stenosis.
   1. Intra-arterial digital subtraction angiography is the definitive diagnostic test—currently, it is the gold standard. Renal artery differential pressure (RADP) can be measured during catheterization before percutaneous transluminal angioplasty (PTA), and this measurement can be used to guide treatment.
      a. A mean RADP of at least 10 mmHg or a peak RADP of at least 20 mmHg is considered significant; proceeding to PTA with either of these measurements is beneficial.
      b. The risk of contrast-induced nephropathy is present but volume of contrast needed may be controlled.
C. Renal vein renin sampling, peripheral renin levels, and captopril renal scintigraphy are not generally recommended due to low specificity and sensitivity.

VII. **Management**
   A. Treatment and control of blood pressure and renal perfusion
      1. Lifestyle changes
         a. Exercise
         b. Healthy body weight
         c. Healthy diet (low fat, low protein, low sodium, and high fiber)
         d. Smoking cessation
      2. Medical management
         a. Optimize medical therapy for glycemic, blood pressure, and cholesterol management, as defined by current evidence-based guidelines and recommended therapy
         b. Medications (ACE inhibitors and ARBs have been shown to slow the progression of kidney disease); caution is necessary, as when ACE inhibitors or ARBs are used, further decline in GFR may occur in patients with RAS. Renin-angiotensin-aldosterone system (RAAS) blockade, statins, and antiplatelet therapy (i.e., aspirin) are the cornerstone for clinical management of atherosclerotic disease, including RAS. An important feature in the treatment of patients with atherosclerotic RAS is the reduction of serum lipids and cholesterol that are contributing to atherosclerosis in the renal artery and in the kidney itself.
         c. Blood pressure lowering medications, ACE inhibitors, and ARBs have been effective in slowing the progression of kidney disease (see table 45.1 for ACE inhibitor/ARB regimens).
            i. ACE inhibitors and ARBs can cause acute renal failure; patients should have their kidney function checked within 2 weeks after starting medication.
            ii. Many individuals require two or more medications to lower BP to recommended goals. In addition to an ACE inhibitor or ARB, a diuretic, β blocker, or calcium channel blocker may be needed (See Hypertension chapter for regimens of BP-lowering agents).
         d. Management of glycemia: see Diabetes Mellitus chapter
         e. Management of atherosclerotic disease: see Coronary Artery Disease/Hyperlipidemia and Peripheral Vascular Disease chapters
      3. All patients should be assessed for coronary artery disease
      4. Minimally invasive procedures to restore blood flow to the kidneys via revascularization. Revascularization is recommended by the American Heart Association when the renal artery is reduced more than 60% of its diameter. Associated risks include hemorrhage and contrast-induced nephropathy.

      a. Percutaneous transluminal angioplasty (PTA)
          i. Risks include renal artery dissection, rupture, thrombosis, and embolism
      b. PTA with stent placement
      c. Thrombolysis (in the event of acute thrombosis)
      d. Radioablation of renal nerves
5. Surgical procedures
      a. Renal artery bypass/reconstruction
      b. Endarterectomy
      c. Other considerations: all patients with atherosclerotic RAS should be assessed for coronary artery disease; most patients should receive an ACE inhibitor or an ARB and a statin. The latter not only reduces cardiac risk but also may induce regression of RAS. An important feature in the treatment of patients with atherosclerotic RAS is the reduction of serum lipids and cholesterol that are contributing to atherosclerosis in the renal artery and in the kidney itself
6. Regular medical prophylaxis may effectively prevent stone recurrence in patients with a history of recurrence, calcium oxalate dihydrate stones, hypercalciuria, or hyperuricuria
      a. Dietary advice for all patients
      b. Renal leak hypercalciuria: 50 mg HCTZ PO daily and 5 grams potassium citrate powder PO 3 times a day after meals
      c. Absorptive stones
      d. Uric acid and calcium oxalate calculi with hyperuricuria or gouty diathesis: 100 mg allopurinol PO twice daily, as well as potassium citrate
      e. Infected stones: potassium citrate and appropriate antibiotics
      f. Cost effectiveness, patient compliance, and gastrointestinal upset may limit patient acceptability and clinical use of medical prophylaxis

Table 45.1	ACE Inhibitors and Angiotensin Receptor Blockers for Renal Artery Stenosis	
	Agent	Usual Dose/Frequency
ACE Inhibitors	Benazepril (lotensin®)	10–40 mg PO DAILY
	Captopril (capoten®)	12.5–100 mg PO BID or TID
	Enalapril (vasotec®)	5–40 mg PO DAILY or BID
	Fosinopril (monopril®)	10–40 mg PO DAILY
	Lisinopril (zestril®)	5–40 mg PO DAILY
	Moexipril (univasc®)	7.5–30 mg PO DAILY
	Perindopril (aceon®)	4–8 mg PO DAILY
	Quinapril (accupril®)	10–80 mg PO DAILY
	Ramipril (altace®)	2.5–20 mg PO DAILY
	Trandolapril (mavik®)	1–4 mg PO DAILY
Angiotensin II Receptor Antagonists	Azilsartan (edarbi®)	40–80 mg PO DAILY
	Candesartan (atacand®)	8–32 mg PO DAILY
	Eprosartan mesylate (teveten®)	400–800 mg PO DAILY or BID
	Irbesartan (avapro®)	75–300 mg PO DAILY
	Losartan (cozaar®)	25–100 mg PO DAILY
	Olmesartan (benicar®)	20–40 PO DAILY
	Telmisartan (micardis®)	20–80 mg PO DAILY
	Valsartan (diovan®)	40–320 mg PO DAILY or BID
	Azilsartan (edarbi®)	40–80 mg PO DAILY

BIBLIOGRAPHY

Academy of Nutrition and Dietetics. (2010). *Recommendations summary: CKD: Assessment of medical health/history 2010*. Evidence Analysis Library. Retrieved September 24, 2014, from http://www.andeal.org/template.cfm?template=guide_summary&key=2595

Anderson, J. L., Halperin, J. L., Albert, N., Bozkurt, B., Brindis, R. G., Curtis, L. H., . . . Shen, W.-K. (2013). Management of patients with peripheral artery disease (compilation of 2005 and 2011 ACCF/AHA guideline recommendations): A report of the American College of Cardiology Foundation/American Heart Association Task Force on Practice Guidelines. *Journal of the American College of Cardiology, 61*(14), 1555–1570. doi:10.1016/j.jacc.2013.01.004

Colyer, W. R., Eltahawy, E., & Cooper, C. J. (2011). Renal artery stenosis: Optimizing diagnosis and treatment. *Progress in Cardiovascular Diseases, 54*(1), 29–35. doi:10.1016/j.pcad.2011.02.007

Creager, M. A., Belkin, M., Bluth, E. I., Casey, D. E., Chaturvedi, S., Dake, M. D., . . . Ziffer, J. A. (2012). 2012 ACCF/AHA/ACR/SCAI/SIR/STS/SVM/SVN/SVS key data elements and definitions for peripheral atherosclerotic vascular disease: A report of the American College of Cardiology Foundation/American Heart Association Task Force on clinical data standards (writing committee to develop clinical data standards for peripheral atherosclerotic vascular disease). *Circulation, 125*(2), 395–467. doi:10.1161/CIR.0b013e31823299a1

Lao, D., Parasher, P. S., Cho, K. C., & Yeghiazarians, Y. (2011). Atherosclerotic renal artery stenosis—diagnosis and treatment. *Mayo Clinic Proceedings, 86*(7), 649–657. doi:10.4065/mcp.2011.0181

Longo, D. L., Fauci, A. S., Kasper, D. L., Hauser, S., Jameson, J., & Loscalzo, J. (Eds.). (2012). *Harrison's principles of internal medicine* (18th ed.). New York, NY: McGraw-Hill.

Madder, R. D., Hickman, L., Crimmins, G. M., Puri, M., Marinescu, V., McCullough, P. A., . . . Safian, R. D. (2011). Validity of estimated glomerular filtration rates for assessment of baseline and serial renal function in patients with atherosclerotic renal artery stenosis: Implications for clinical trials of renal revascularization. *Circulation: Cardiovascular Interventions, 4*(3), 219–225. doi:10.1161/CIRCINTERVENTIONS.110.960971

National Institute of Diabetes and Digestive and Kidney Diseases. (2014). *Renal artery stenosis*. National Kidney and Urologic Diseases Information (NKUDIC). Retrieved December 2, 2013, from http://kidney.niddk.nih.gov/kudiseases/pubs/renalarterystenosis/index.aspx

National Institute of Neurological Disorders and Stroke. (2011). *Fibromuscular dysplasia information page*. Retrieved December 2, 2013, from http://www.ninds.nih.gov/disorders/fibromuscular_dysplasia/fibromuscular_dysplasia.htm

Plouin, P. F., & Bax, L. (2010). Diagnosis and treatment of renal artery stenosis. *Nature Reviews Nephrology, 6*(3), 151–159. doi:10.1038/nrneph.2009.230

Rooke, T. W., Hirsch, A. T., Misra, S., Sidawy, A. N., Beckman, J. A., Findeiss, L. K., . . . Zierler, R. E. (2011). 2011 ACCF/AHA focused update on the guideline for the management of patients with peripheral artery disease (updating the 2005 guideline): A report of the American College of Cardiology Foundation/American Heart Association Task Force on Practice Guidelines. *Journal of the American College of Cardiology, 58*(19), 2020–2045. doi:10.1016/j.jacc.2011.08.023

Vasbinder, G. B., Nelemans, P. J., Kessels, A. G., Kroon, A. A., de Leeuw, P. W., & van Engelshoven, J. M. (2001). Diagnosis of renal artery stenosis. *Annals of Internal Medicine, 135*(6), S38.

CHAPTER 46

Nephrolithiasis

MARLA COUTURE • CHARLENE M. MYERS

RENAL CALCULI–NEPHROLITHIASIS

I. **Definition**
   A. Condition in which one or more stones are present in the pelvis, in the calyces of the kidney, or in the ureter
   B. Calculi may be composed of calcium oxalate or calcium phosphate (two most common). Can also be composed of uric acid, struvite, or cystine

II. **Etiology**
   A. Approximately 10% of the population will develop urinary calculi during their lifetime.
      1. More common in men
      2. Usual age of onset is in the 30s
      3. Approximately 35%–50% of patients will have a recurrence within 5 years
   B. Dehydration: occurs more frequently in hot, arid environments
   C. Life stress
   D. Supersaturation of urine with stone-forming salts
   E. Dietary factors
      1. Low fluid intake
      2. High sodium intake
      3. High animal protein intake
      4. High fructose intake
      5. Low dietary calcium intake
         a. Can cause oxalate levels to rise
      6. Overload of calcium supplement intake
   F. Decreased or absent stone inhibitors in the urine (e.g., citrate, magnesium, and pyrophosphate)

III. **Risk factors**
   A. Gender/age
   B. Family history
   C. Geography
   D. Genetic predisposition
   E. Preexisting medical conditions

1. Primary hyperparathyroidism
2. Obesity
3. Diabetes
4. Intestinal malabsorption
5. Inflammatory bowel disease
6. Sarcoidosis
7. Gout

F. Postsurgical comorbidities
1. Small bowel resection
2. Gastric bypass
3. Colectomy

G. Sleeping position
1. Correlation between sleep posture and unilateral renal stone formation

H. Immobility
I. Low citrate levels
J. Urinary tract infections
K. Oxidative stress
1. Stone formation linked to production of reactive oxygen species
2. Oxidative stress linked to idiopathic calcium oxalate nephrolithiasis

L. Drugs associated with stone formation:
1. Triamterene (Dyrenium)
2. Steroids
3. Vitamin D supplements
4. Carbonic anhydrous inhibitors
5. Indinavir (Crixivan): protease inhibitor
6. Colchicine
7. Chemotherapy agents

M. Dietary influences
1. Decreased renal acid excretion, a precursor of uric acid, leads to hyperuricosuria and decreases calcium oxalate solubility
2. Sodium ingestion: increases Na excretion, which increases Ca excretion and Ca mobilization from bone
3. Foods high in oxalate: increases urinary oxalate excretion (e.g., nuts, chocolate, dark green leafy vegetables, rhubarb, beets, and okra)

N. High urine pH level is the main risk factor for calcium oxalate and calcium phosphate

IV. **Types**

A. Calcium stones constitute 80% of renal calculi
B. Hypercalciuric calcium nephrolithiasis
1. Can be caused by absorptive, resorptive, and renal disorders
2. Absorptive (types I, II, and III)
a. Caused by increased absorption of calcium at the level of the small bowel (i.e., jejunum)
b. Treatment is focused on decreasing bowel absorption of calcium
c. Type I is independent of calcium intake. Urine calcium is increased on a regular or even a low-calcium diet.
d. Type II is diet-dependent. Dramatically decreasing dietary calcium may decrease hypercalciuria.
e. Type III results from a renal phosphate leak that causes increased vitamin D synthesis and increased small bowel absorption of calcium
  i. Inhibits vitamin D synthesis but not intestinal absorption
3. Resorptive
a. Because of hyperparathyroidism

b. Hypercalcemia, hypophosphatemia, and elevated levels of parathyroid hormones are present
c. Surgical resection of the adenoma, which leads to hyperparathyroidism, cures the disease and the stones
4. Renal leak
   a. Renal tubules are unable to reabsorb filtered calcium efficiently, and hypercalciuria occurs
C. Hyperuricosuric calcium nephrolithiasis
   1. Caused by dietary excess or uric acid metabolic defects
   2. In contrast to uric acid calculi, these patients will maintain a urinary pH level higher than 5.5
D. Hyperoxaluric calcium nephrolithiasis
   1. Due to primary intestinal disorders
   2. Patients usually have a history of chronic diarrhea, often with inflammatory bowel disease or steatorrhea.
   3. Calcium is unavailable to bind to oxalate, which is then freely and rapidly absorbed; this significantly promotes stone formation.
   4. Increased fluid intake must be emphasized.
E. Hypocitraturic calcium nephrolithiasis
   1. May result from chronic diarrhea, type I renal tubular acidosis, or chronic or aggressive thiazide diuretic treatment; may also be idiopathic
   2. Citrate appears to bind to calcium in solution, thereby decreasing available calcium for stone formation.
F. Uric acid calculi
   1. Frequently have urinary pH levels lower than 5.5 (average urinary pH level is 5.85)
   2. Increasing the pH to levels higher than 6.5 can dramatically increase solubility and can dissolve large stones
G. Struvite calculi
   1. Magnesium-ammonium-phosphate stones
   2. Commonly seen in women with recurrent urinary tract infections; most stones are large and cause obstruction and bleeding
   3. Radiodense
   4. Urinary pH level is high (greater than 7–7.5) = alkalotic
   5. Caused by urease-producing organisms (*Proteus* spp., *Haemophilus* spp., *Klebsiella* spp., and *Ureaplasma urealyticum*)
   6. Stones are soft and amenable to percutaneous nephrolithotomy or extracorporeal shock wave lithotripsy.
   7. Treatment requires eradicating the infection with antibiotics and the above interventional techniques
H. Cystine calculi
   1. Result of abnormal excretion of cystine, ornithine, lysine, and arginine
   2. Cystine is the only amino acid that becomes insoluble in urine
   3. Difficult to manage

V. Clinical manifestations
A. Acute flank pain (i.e., colic-like)
   1. If flank pain increases in intensity and radiates downward to the groin, this indicates that the stone has passed to the lower third of the ureter.
B. Testicular pain
C. Pain not relieved by position
D. Nausea and vomiting
E. Costovertebral angle tenderness

F. Frequency, urgency, and dysuria suggest that the stone is located in the portion of the ureter within the bladder wall
G. Oliguria and acute renal failure may occur when both collecting systems are obstructed by stones
H. Hematuria

VI. Radiologic studies/laboratory findings
A. Noncontrast helical CT has proven to be the gold standard radiographic test for diagnosing nephrolithiasis.
B. Plain films of the abdomen will reveal opaque calculi
C. Renal ultrasound (involves no radiation, but less sensitive to detecting stones)
D. An excretory or retrograde pyelogram permits the exact definition of stones and reveals the presence or absence of obstruction.
E. Urinalysis reveals blood
F. Increased white blood cell count
G. Twenty-four-hour urine collection for calcium, uric acid, phosphate, oxalate, and citrate excretion is generally reserved for those with recurrent stones
H. Urine culture: positive for urease-producing organisms
I. Serum chemistries should include calcium, electrolytes, phosphate, and uric acid.

VII. Management
A. Relieve pain, nausea, and vomiting
  1. Randomized trials note parenteral nonsteroidal anti-inflammatory drugs are as effective as narcotics for treatment of renal colic (ketorolac). Avoid use in patients with renal dysfunction, as it may lower kidney blood flow and glomerular filtration.
  2. Opioids (hydromorphone) or combination analgesics (hydrocodone/acetaminophen) may be necessary when pain is unrelieved by nonsteroidal anti-inflammatory drugs.
  3. Antiemetics (ondansetron)
B. To hasten stone passage, induce high urine flow with oral intake of at least 2–3 L of fluids per 24 hr to ensure a urine output of at least 2 L per day
C. Urethral stones of up to 10 mm and eligible for observation may be offered medical expulsive therapy.
D. Medications
  1. Antispasmodics relax the smooth muscle of the ureters and have been shown to hasten stone passage by 5–7 days.
     a. α blockers
        i. Doxazosin (Cardura), 4 mg PO daily
        ii. Tamsulosin (Flomax), 0.4 mg PO daily
     b. Calcium channel blockers
        i. Nifedipine (Procardia XL), 30 mg PO daily
  2. Medications and supplements for specific type:
     a. Type I absorptive hypercalciuria: thiazide therapy
        i. Decreases renal excretion of calcium
        ii. Increases bone density by 1% per year
        iii. Has limited long-term use (less than 5 years)
     b. Type II absorptive hypercalciuria: no specific medical therapy is available
     c. Renal hypercalciuria: hydrochlorothiazides (HCTZs) are effective as long-term therapy
     d. Hyperuricemia: purine dietary restrictions or allopurinol, or both
     e. Hyperoxaluria: oral calcium supplements should be given with meals if diarrhea or steatorrhea cannot be effectively reduced
     f. Hypocitraturia: potassium citrate supplements (20 mEq 3 times a day) are usually effective

g. Uric acid calculi: potassium citrate (liquid, crystals, or tablets—10 mEq), two tablets PO 3 or 4 times a day
   i. Fluid intake is less important; decrease protein intake
   ii. Many patients with uric acid calculi have gout
      (a) If hyperuricemia is present, allopurinol (Zyloprim) should be initiated at 300 mg/day
      (b) Doses greater than 300 mg should be divided and given BID
h. Struvite calculi: acetohydroxamic acid is an effective urease inhibitor; however, it is poorly tolerated because of gastrointestinal adverse effects
i. Cystine calculi:
   i. Increase fluid intake
   ii. Alkalinize the urine to pH greater than 7.5 and less than 8
   iii. Administer penicillamine (Cuprimine) or α-mercaptopropionylglycine (tiopronin) MPG

E. Shock wave lithotripsy and ureteroscopy
  1. Useful alternatives in treating the majority of stones
F. For larger, nonstandard stones greater than 10 mm
  1. Percutaneous antegrade ureteroscopy
  2. Laparoscopic techniques
  3. Open surgery
G. After removal, the goal is stone prevention. (see table 46.1)
  1. Recurrence rate is approximately 20%–50%
  2. Regular medical prophylaxis may effectively prevent stone recurrence in patients with a history of recurrence, calcium oxalate dihydrate stones, hypercalciuria, or hyperuricuria. (see Table 46.1)
     a. Cost effectiveness, patient compliance, and gastrointestinal upset may limit patient acceptability and clinical use of medical prophylaxis

Table 46.1	Prevention of Kidney Stones		
Type	Dietary Modifications*	Treatment	Rationale/Comments
ALL	Adequate fluid intake (make sure patient has more than 2 L of fluids/24 hr)	Promote low-glycemic diet Promote a healthy diet and exercise	
Hypercalciuria Calcium oxalate	Avoid foods high in salt (canned or processed foods, cheese, pickles, dried meats); do not add salt to food Reduce animal protein (meat, eggs) Calcium supplements if not getting enough calcium through diet Avoid foods high in oxalate (beans, spinach, rhubarb, chocolate, wheat, nuts, berries)	Thiazide diuretics: Hydrochlorothiazide 25–50 mg PO daily Potassium citrate 10–20 mEq PO TID with meals Calcium citrate 250–500 mg PO TID with meals	Increases the urinary excretion of calcium Raise the citrate and pH of urine Raise the citrate and pH of urine; bind urinary oxalate

Table 46.1	Prevention of Kidney Stones		
Type	**Dietary Modifications***	**Treatment**	**Rationale/Comments**
Calcium phosphate	Avoid foods high in salt (canned or processed foods, cheese, pickles, dried meats); do not add salt to food reduce animal protein (meat, eggs) Calcium supplements if not getting enough calcium through diet Reduce phosphate intake Decrease intake of dairy products, legumes, chocolate and nuts by about one-third	Cranberry juice: at least 16 oz per day	Acidify urine
Uric acid stones	Decrease protein intake Limiting animal protein (red meat, fish, and shellfish) Reduce or eliminate alcohol intake	Allopurinol 300 mg PO daily (adjust dose for renal dysfunction) potassium citrate 10–20 mEq PO TID with meals	Decreases uric acid in the blood and urine Raise the citrate and pH of urine
Cystine stones	Decrease methionine (sulfur) intake Avoid dairy products, eggs, legumes, greens	**Tiopronin (Thiola)** 800 mg/day ORALLY in 3 divided doses Potassium citrate 10–20 mEq PO TID with meals Penicillamine (Cuprimine) 2 grams PO daily; range 1–4 grams/day	Decreases cystine in the urine Raise the citrate and pH of urine Lowers cystine concentrations and the prevents formation of cystine calculi in the urine
Struvite stones	Avoid supplemental magnesium	Antibiotics Acetohydroxamic acid **(Lithostat)** 15 mg/kg/day PO TID; MAX 1.5 grams/day	Eliminate infection Consider surgical intervention, especially for stones greater than 10 mm or if there is evidence of ongoing obstruction or infection

Note. More information can be found in the National Kidney and Urologic Diseases Information Clearinghouse fact sheet Diet for Kidney Stone Prevention at: http://kidney.niddk.nih.gov/kudiseases/pubs/kidneystonediet/index.aspx

BIBLIOGRAPHY

Asplin, J. R., Coe, F. L., & Favus, M. J. (2011). Nephrolithiasis. In D. L. Kasper, E. Braunwald, S. Hauser, D. Longo, J. L. Jameson, & A. S. Fauci (Eds.), *Harrison's principles of internal medicine* (18th ed.). New York, NY: McGraw-Hill.

Coe, F. L., Evan, A., & Worcester, E. (2008). Kidney stone disease. *Journal of Clinical Investigation, 115*(10), 2598–2608.

Fink, H. A., Wilt, T. J., Eidman, K. E., Garimella, P. S., MacDonald, R., Rutks, I. R., . . . Monga, M. (2013). Medical management to prevent recurrent nephrolithiasis in adults: A systematic review for an American College of Physicians clinical guideline. *Annals of Internal Medicine, 158*(7), 535–543.

Frassetto, L., & Kohlstadt, I. (2011). Treatment and prevention of kidney stones: An update. *American Family Physician, 84*(11), 1234–1242.

Hall, P. M. (2009). Nephrolithiasis: Treatment, causes, and prevention. *Cleveland Clinic Journal of Medicine, 76*(10), 583–591.

Khan, S. R. (2011). Is oxidative stress, a link between nephrolithiasis and obesity, hypertension, diabetes, chronic kidney disease, metabolic syndrome? *Urological Research, 40*(2), 95–112.

Marchini, G. S., Ortiz-Alvarado, O., Miyaoka, R., Kriedgberg, C., Moeding, A., Stessman, M., & Monga, M. (2013). Patient-centered medical therapy for nephrolithiasis. *Urology, 81*(3), 511–516.

McCance, K. L., Huether, S. E., Brashers, V. L., & Rote, N. S. (2013). *Pathophysiology: The biologic basis for disease in adults and children* (7th ed.). Maryland Heights, MD: Mosby.

National Kidney and Urologic Diseases Information Clearinghouse. (2013). *Kidney stones in adults*. In F. L. Coe (Ed.). Retrieved from http://kidney.niddk.nih.gov/kudiseases/pubs/stonesadults/#acknowledgments

Orson, W. M., Pearle, M. S., & Sakhaee, K. (2011). Pharmacotherapy of urolithiasis: Evidence from clinical trials. *Kidney International, 79*(4), 385–392.

Phillips, E., Kieley, S., Johnson, E. B., & Monga, M. (2009). Emergency room management of ureteral calculi: Current practices. *Journal of Endourology, 23*(6), 1021–1024.

Phipps, S., Tolley, D. A., Young, J. G., & Keeley, F. X., Jr. (2010). The management of ureteric stones. *Annals of the Royal College of Surgeons of England, 92*(5), 368–372.

APPENDIX

Appendix A	ICD-9 Codes	
Chapter	**Condition/Topic**	**ICD-9 Code**
Section 1. Management of Patients with Neurological Disorders		
Cerebrovascular Accidents: Brain Attack	Hemorrhagic stroke	431
	Ischemic stroke	434.91
	Stroke/brain attack	434.91
	Transient ischemic attack	436
Structural Abnormalities	Aneurysm	442.9
	Hydrocephalus	331.4
Peripheral Neuropathies	Guillain-Barre syndrome	357.0
	Myasthenia gravis	358.00
Neurologic Trauma	Head trauma/traumatic brain injury	959.01
	Spinal cord trauma	952.9
Central Nervous System Disorders	Cerebral abscess	324.0
	Encephalitis	323.9
	Encephalopathy	348.30
	Meningitis	322.9
Seizure Disorders	Seizure disorders	780.39
Dementia	Dementia	290.8
Multiple sclerosis	Multiple sclerosis	340
Parkinson's Disease	Parkinson's disease	332.0
Amyotrophic Lateral Sclerosis	Amyotrophic lateral sclerosis	335.20
Section 2. Management of Patients with Cardiovascular Disorders		
Cardiovascular Assessment	Cardiovascular disorders	306.2
Hypertension	Hypertension	401.9
Coronary Artery Disease and Hyperlipidemia	Coronary artery disease	414.00
	Hyperlipidemia	272.4
Angina and Myocardial Infarction	Angina	413.9
	Myocardial infarction	410.9
Adjunct Equipment/Devices		
Peripheral Vascular Disease	Deep vein thrombosis	453.8
	Occlusive arterial disease	444.22
	Peripheral vascular disease	443.9
	Thromboangiitis obliterans (Buerger's disease)	443.1
	Venous disease	459.9
Inflammatory Cardiac Diseases	Endocarditis	424.90
	Pericarditis	423.9
Heart Failure	Heart failure	428.9

Appendix A	ICD-9 Codes	
Chapter	**Condition/Topic**	**ICD-9 Code**
Valvular Disease	Aortic regurgitation	424.1
	Aortic stenosis	424.1
	Mitral regurgitation	424.0
	Mitral stenosis	394.0
	Mitral valve prolapse	424.0
	Valvular disease	459.9
Cardiomyopathy	Cardiomyopathy	425.4
Arrhythmias	Agonal rhythm	427.89
	Asystole	427.5
	Atrial fibrillation	427.31
	Atrial flutter	427.32
	Cardiac rhythms/arrhythmias	427.9
	First-degree AV block	426.11
	Idioventricular rhythm	426.89
	Junctional/nodal	427.89
	Premature atrial contractions	427.61
	Premature ventricular contractions	427.69
	Pulseless electrical activity	427.89
	Second-degree block (Mobitz type I) (Wenckebach)	426.13
	Second-degree block (Mobitz type II)	426.12
	Sinus arrhythmia	427.9
	Sinus bradycardia	427.89
	Sinus tachycardia	427.89
	Supraventricular tachycardia	427.89
	Third-degree AV block (complete heart block)	426.0
	Ventricular fibrillation	427.41
	Ventricular tachycardia	427.1
Section 3. Management of Pulmonary Disorders		
Diagnostic Concepts of Oxygenation and Ventilation	Respiratory measurement	89.38
Measures of Oxygen and Ventilation	Respiratory measurement	89.38
The Chest X-Ray	Congestive heart failure	428.0
	Emphysema	492.8
	Pericardial effusions	423.9
	Pneumonia	486
	Pulmonary nodules (also called coin lesions)	793.1
Pulmonary Function Testing	Abnormal results of pulmonary function studies	794.2
Obstructive (Ventilatory) Lung Diseases	Asthma	493.9
	Bronchiectasis	494.0
	Chronic bronchitis	491.9
	Chronic obstructive pulmonary disease	496
	Emphysema	492.8
	Obstructive airway lesions	519.8

Appendix A	ICD-9 Codes	
Chapter	**Condition/Topic**	**ICD-9 Code**
Restrictive (Inflammatory) Lung Diseases	Acute lung injury	861.20
	Acute respiratory distress syndrome	518.5
	Cardiogenic pulmonary edema	514
	Congestive heart failure	428.0
	Idiopathic pulmonary fibrosis	515
	Pneumonia	486
	Pulmonary edema	514
	Restrictive (inflammatory) lung diseases	518.89
	Sarcoidosis	135
	Tuberculosis	011.90
Pulmonary Hypertension and Pulmonary Vascular Disorders	Pulmonary hypertension	416.0
Chest Wall and Secondary Pleural Disorders	Pleural disorders	511.0
	Chest wall disorders	306.2
Respiratory Failure	Acute respiratory failure	518.81
	Chronic respiratory failure	518.83
	Shock	785.50
Pneumothorax	Pneumothorax	512.8
Lower Respiratory Tract Pathogens	Acute tracheobronchitis	466.0
	Chronic obstructive pulmonary disease	496
	Pneumonia, community-acquired	486
Obstructive Sleep Apnea	Obstructive sleep apnea	327.23
Oxygen Supplementation	Dependence on supplemental oxygen	V46.2
Mechanical Ventilatory Support	Dependence on respiratory ventilator	V46.11
Section 4. Management of Patients with Gastrointestinal Disorders		
Peptic Ulcer Disease	Gastroesophageal reflux disease	530.81
	Peptic ulcer disease	533.9
Liver Disease	Hepatic failure	572.8
	Hepatitis	573.3
Biliary Dysfunction	Acute pancreatitis	577.0
	Cholecystitis	575.10
Inflammatory Gastrointestinal Disorders	Appendicitis	541
	Diverticulitis	562.11
	Peritonitis	567.9
	Ulcerative colitis	556.9
Anatomic Intestinal Disorders	Mesenteric ischemia	557.9
	Small-bowel obstruction	560.9
Gastrointestinal Bleeding	Esophageal varices	456.1
	Lower gastrointestinal bleeding	578.9
	Upper gastrointestinal bleeding	578.9

Appendix

Appendix A — ICD-9 Codes

Chapter	Condition/Topic	ICD-9 Code
Section 5. Management of Patients with Genitourinary Disorders		
Urinary Tract Infections	Urinary tract infections	599.0
Renal Insufficiency and Failure	Acute renal failure	584.9
	Chronic renal failure	585.9
Benign Prostatic Hyperplasia	Benign prostatic hypertrophy	600.00
Renal Artery Stenosis	Renal artery stenosis	440.1
Nephrolithiasis	Renal calculi-nephrolithiasis	592.0
Section 6. Management of Patients with Endocrine Disorders		
Diabetes Mellitus	Diabetes mellitus	250.00
	Type 1 diabetes mellitus	250.01
	Type 2 diabetes mellitus	250.02
Diabetic Emergencies	Diabetic ketoacidosis	250.30
	Hyperosmolar hyperglycemic non-ketosis	250.20
	Hypoglycemia	251.2
Thyroid Disease	Hyperthyroidism (thyrotoxicosis)	242.90
	Hypothyroidism (myxedema coma)	244.9
	Thyroid storm (thyrotoxic crisis)	242.91
Cushing's Syndrome	Cushing's syndrome	255.0
Primary Adrenocortical Insufficiency (Addison Disease) & Adrenal Crisis	Addison disease	359.5
	Addisonian crisis	255.41
	Primary adrenocortical insufficiency	255.41
Pheochromocytoma	Pheochromocytoma	194.0
Syndrome of Inappropriate Antidiuretic Hormone	Syndrome of inappropriate antidiuretic hormone	253.6
Diabetes Insipidus	Diabetes insipidus	253.5
Section 7. Management of Musculoskeletal Disorders		
Arthritis	Gout	274.9
	Osteoarthritis	715.9
	Rheumatoid arthritis	714.0
Subluxations and Dislocations	Dislocation of ankle	718.37
	Dislocation of shoulder	718.31
	Dislocation of hand	718.34
	Dislocation of hip	835
	Dislocation of shoulder joint	831
	Subluxation of unspecified scapula	831.09
	Subluxation of wrist and hand	833
Soft Tissue Injury	Disorders of soft tissue	729.90
	Soft tissue disorder related to use, overuse, and pressure	729.90
Fractures	Closed fracture	924.8
	Open fracture	924.8
	Stress fracture	733.95
Compartment syndrome	Compartment syndrome	958.8

Appendix A	ICD-9 Codes	
Chapter	**Condition/Topic**	**ICD-9 Code**
Back Pain Syndromes	Herniated disk	722.2
	Low back pain	724.2
Section 8. Management of Patients with Hematologic Disorders		
Anemias	Anemia of chronic disease (ACD)	285.29
	Anemias	285.9
	Folic acid deficiency	281.2
	Iron deficiency	280.9
	Pernicious anemia	281.0
	Thalassemia	282.49
	Vitamin B12 deficiency	281.1
Sickle Cell Disease/Crisis	Sickle cell disease/crisis	282.60
Coagulopathies	Disseminated intravascular coagulation	286.6
	Heparin-induced thrombocytopenia	287.4
	Idiopathic thrombocytopenic purpura	287.3
Section 9. Management of Patients with Oncologic Disorders		
Leukemias	Acute lymphocytic leukemia	204.0
	Acute myelogenous leukemia	205.0
	Chronic lymphocytic leukemia	204.1
	Chronic myelogenous leukemia	205.1
Lymphoma	Hodgkin's disease	201.9
	Lymphoma	202.8
	Non-Hodgkin's lymphoma	202.8
Other Common Cancers	Bladder cancer	188.9
	Breast cancer	174.9
	Cervical cancer	180.0
	Colorectal cancer	154.0
	Endometrial cancer	182.0
	Lung cancer	162.9
	Ovarian cancer	183.0
	Prostate cancer	185
Section 10. Management of Patients with Immunologic Disorders		
HIV/AIDS and Opportunistic Infections	Contact with or exposure to viral diseases	V01.79
	HIV infection	042
	Immunodeficiency	279.3
Autoimmune Diseases	Giant cell arteritis	446.5
	Systemic lupus erythematosus	710.0
Section 11. Management of Patients with Miscellaneous Health Problems		
Integumentary Disorders	Cellulitis	682.9
	Dermatitis medicamentosa (drug eruption)	693.0
	Herpes zoster (shingles)	053.9
	Integumentary disorders	709.9

Appendix A	ICD-9 Codes	
Chapter	**Condition/Topic**	**ICD-9 Code**
Ectopic Pregnancy and STIs	*Chlamydia trachomatis* infection	079.98
	Ectopic pregnancy	633.90
	Gonorrhea	098.0
	Herpes	054.9
	Pelvic inflammatory disease (PID salpingitis)	614.9
	Syphilis	097.9
Eye, Ear, Nose, and Throat Disorders	Allergic rhinitis	477.9
	Bell's palsy	351.0
	Central and branch retinal artery obstruction	362.30
	Conjunctivitis	372.30
	Corneal abrasion	918.1
	Diabetic retinopathy	362.01
	Epiglottitis	464.30
	Epistaxis	784.7
	Glaucoma	365.9
	Otitis externa	380.10
	Otitis media	382.9
	Pharyngitis	462.0
	Retinal detachment	361.9
	Sinusitis	473.9
	Temporomandibular joint disorder	524.60
	Trigeminal neuralgia (tic douloureux)	350.1
	Vertigo	780.4
Headache	Headache	784.0
Section 12. Common Problems in Acute Care		
Fever	Fever	780.6
Pain	Acute pain	338.11
	Chronic pain	338.29
	Neoplasm related pain	338.3
	Unspecified pain	780.96
Psychosocial Problems in Acute Care	Anxiety	300.00
	Delirium	780.09
	Depression	311
	Substance abuse	305.90
	Psychosis	293.81
	Violence	300.9
Management of the Patient in Shock	Anaphylactic shock	995.0
	Cardiogenic shock	785.51
	Hypovolemic shock	785.59
	Septic shock	785.52
	Shock	785.50
Nutritional Considerations	Encounter for screening for nutritional disorder	V77.99
	Nutritional deficiency	269.9

Appendix A: ICD-9 Codes

Chapter	Condition/Topic	ICD-9 Code
Fluid, Electrolyte, and Acid-Base Imbalances	Acid-base disorders	276.4
	Hypercalcemia	275.42
	Hyperkalemia	276.7
	Hypermagnesemia	275.2
	Hypernatremia	276.0
	Hyperphosphatemia	275.3
	Hypocalcemia	275.41
	Hypokalemia	276.8
	Hypomagnesemia	275.2
	Hyponatremia	276.1
	Hypophosphatemia	275.3
	Metabolic acidosis	276.2
	Metabolic alkalosis	276.3
	Respiratory acidosis	276.2
	Respiratory alkalosis	276.3
Poisoning and Drug Toxicities	Acetaminophen toxicity	965.4
	Alcohol (ethanol) toxicity	980.0
	Antiarrhythmic drug overdose	972.0
	Anticoagulant overdose	964.2
	Antidepressant toxicity	969.0
	Antipsychotic toxicity	969.3
	Barbiturate overdose	967.0
	Benzodiazepine overdose	969.4
	Beta-blocker overdose	972.0
	Calcium channel blocker overdose	972.0
	Carbon monoxide poisoning	986
	Digoxin toxicity	972.1
	Lithium toxicity	985.8
	Organophosphate (insecticide) poisoning	989.3
	Salicylate toxicity	976.4
	Stimulant toxicity	970.9
	Theophylline toxicity	974.1
Wound Management	Pressure ulcer	707.0
	Type 1 diabetes mellitus with foot ulcer	250.81
	Type 2 diabetes mellitus with foot ulcer	250.80

Appendix A	ICD-9 Codes	
Chapter	**Condition/Topic**	**ICD-9 Code**
Infections	Cellulitis	682.9
	Clostridium difficile colitis	008.45
	Dysentery	009.0
	Endocarditis	424.90
	Meningitis	322.9
	Neutropenia	288.0
	Nosocomial and ventilator-associated pneumonia	507.0
	Nosocomial bacteremia	790.7
	Nosocomial urinary tract infection	599.0
	Pharyngitis	462
	Pneumonia	486
	Simple diarrhea	787.91
	Sinusitis	473.9
	Skin and soft tissue furunculosis	680.9
	Sepsis	995.91
	Urinary tract infection	599.0
Trauma Considerations	Angina	413.9
	Aortic rupture	441.5
	Cardiac tamponade	423.9
	Collapsed lung	518.0
	Flail chest	807.4
	Lacerated liver	864.05
	Myocardial infarction	410.8
	Penetrating eye trauma	871.7
	Renal injuries	866.00
	Rib fractures	807.0
	Ruptured spleen	289.59
Solid Organ Transplantation	Complication of transplanted intestine	996.87
	Complication of transplanted kidney	996.81
	Complication of transplanted liver	996.82
	Complication of transplanted lung	996.84
	Complication of transplanted pancreas	996.86
	Heart transplantation	V50.0
	Intestinal transplantation	V42.84
	Kidney transplantation	V42.0
	Lung transplantation	V42.6
	Pancreas transplantation	V42.83
Burns	Burns	949.0
Hospital Admission Considerations		
Managing the Surgical Patient	Pre-operative examination	V72.84
Section 13. Health Promotion		
Guidelines for Health Promotion and Screening	Screening for unspecified condition	V82.9

Appendix A	ICD-9 Codes	
Chapter	**Condition/Topic**	**ICD-9 Code**
Major Causes of Mortality in the U.S.	Alzheimer's disease	331.0
	Cerebrovascular diseases	437.0
	Chronic lower respiratory diseases	519.9
	Diabetes mellitus	250.00
	Diseases of the heart	414.9
	Influenza	487.1
	Nephritic syndrome	581.9
	Nephritis	583.9
	Nephrosis	581.9
	Pneumonia	486
	Septicemia	638, 995.9
Immunization Recommendations	Diptheria	V03.5
	Hepatitis A	V05.3
	Hepatitis B	V05.3
	Influenza	V04.81
	Measles	V04.2
	Mumps	V04.6
	Polio	V04.0
	Rabies	V04.5
	Rubella	V04.3
	Smallpox	V04.1
	Tetanus	V03.7
	Varicella	V05.4

Note. Appendix A. International Classification of Diseases (2010). ICD9data.com: The Web's free 2015 medical coding reference [Data file]. Retrieved from icd9data.com

Appendix B — ICD-10 Codes

Chapter	Condition/Topic	ICD-10 Code
Section 1. Management of Patients with Neurological Disorders		
Cerebrovascular Accidents: Brain Attack	Nontraumatic intracerebral hemorrhage	I61.9
	Transient ischemic attack	G45.9
	Unspecified sequela of cerebrovascular accident	I69.90
Structural Abnormalities	Cerebral aneurysm	I67.1
	Malignant neoplasm of brain	C71
	Obstructive hydrocephalus	G91.1
Peripheral Neuropathies	Guillain-Barre syndrome	G61.0
	Myasthenia gravis	G70.0
Neurologic Trauma	Other specified injuries of head, initial encounter	S09.8XXA
	Unspecified injury of head, initial encounter	S09.90XA
	Unspecified injury to sacral spinal cord, initial encounter	S34.139A
	Unspecified injury to unspecified level of cervical spinal cord, initial encounter	S14.109A
	Unspecified injury to unspecified level of lumbar spinal cord, initial encounter	S34.109A
	Unspecified injury to unspecified level of thoracic spinal cord, initial encounter	S24.109A
Central Nervous System Disorders	Encephalitis and encephalomyelitis	G04.90
	Encephalopathy	G93.40
	Intracranial abscess and granuloma	G06.0
	Meningitis	G03.9
	Meningococcus, meningococcal	A39.0
Seizure Disorders	Seizure disorders	R56.9
Dementia	Dementia without behavioral disturbance	F03.90
Multiple sclerosis	Multiple sclerosis	G35
Parkinson's Disease	Parkinson's disease	G20
Amyotrophic Lateral Sclerosis	Amyotrophic lateral sclerosis	G12.21
Section 2. Management of Patients with Cardiovascular Disorders		
Cardiovascular Assessment	Abnormalities of heartbeat	R00
	Cardiac murmurs	R01
Hypertension	Essential hypertension	I10
	Other secondary hypertension	I15.8
	Secondary hypertension	I15
Coronary Artery Disease and Hyperlipidemia	Atherosclerotic heart disease of native coronary artery without angina pectoris	I25.10
	Hyperlipidemia	E78.5
Angina and Myocardial Infarction	Angina pectoris	I20
	Angina pectoris with documented spasm	I20.1
	Cardiac tamponade	I31.4
	Coronary atherosclerosis of unspecified bypass graft	I25.810
	Percutaneous transluminal coronary angioplasty status	Z98.61
	ST elevation (STEMI) myocardial infarction of unspecified site	I21.3
	Unstable angina	I20.0
Adjunct Equipment/Devices		

Appendix B	ICD-10 Codes	
Chapter	**Condition/Topic**	**ICD-10 Code**
Peripheral Vascular Disease	Deep vein thrombosis	I82.619
	Occlusive arterial disease	I714.3
	Peripheral vascular disease	I73.9
	Thromboangiitis obliterans (Buerger's disease)	I73.1
	Venous disease	I87.9
Inflammatory Cardiac Diseases	Acute and subacute endocarditis	I33
	Acute pericarditis, unspecific	I30.9
	Chronic pericarditis	I31.1
	Disease of pericardium, unspecified	I31.9
	Endocarditis	I38
Heart Failure	Heart failure, unspecified	I50.9
	Heart failure due to hypertension	I11.0
	Heart failure due to hypertension and chronic kidney disease	I13
	Heart failure following surgery	I97.13
	Rheumatic heart failure	I09.81
Valvular Disease	Disorder of vein, unspecified	I87.9
	Nonrheumatic aortic valve disorder, unspecified	I35.9
	Nonrheumatic aortic valve insufficiency	I35.1
	Nonrheumatic aortic valve stenosis	I35.0
	Nonrheumatic aortic valve stenosis with insufficiency	I35.2
	Nonrheumatic mitral valve insufficiency	I34.0
	Other nonrheumatic aortic valve disorders	I35.8
	Other nonrheumatic mitral valve disorders	I34.8
	Rheumatic mitral stenosis	I05.0
	Unspecified disorder of circulatory system	I99.9
Cardiomyopathy	Dilated cardiomyopathy	I42.0
	Hypertrophy cardiomyopathy	I42.1
	Restrictive cardiomyopathy	I42.5
Arrhythmias	Atrial premature depolarization	I49.1
	Atrioventricular block, complete	I44.2
	Atrioventricular block, first degree	I44.0
	Atrioventricular block, second degree	I44.1
	Bradycardia	R00.1
	Cardiac arrest	I46.9
	Cardiac arrhythmia, unspecified	I49.9
	Other premature depolarization	I49.49
	Other specified cardiac arrhythmias	I49.8
	Other specified conduction disorders	I45.89
	Unspecified atrial fibrillation	I48.91
	Unspecified atrial flutter	I48.92
	Ventricular fibrillation	I49.01
	Ventricular premature depolarization	I49.3
	Ventricular tachycardia	I47.2

Appendix B	ICD-10 Codes	
Chapter	**Condition/Topic**	**ICD-10 Code**
Section 3. Management of Pulmonary Disorders		
Diagnostic Concepts of Oxygenation and Ventilation	Respiratory measurement	4A09
	Respiratory monitoring	4A19
Measures of Oxygen and Ventilation	Respiratory measurement	4A09
	Respiratory monitoring	4A19
The Chest X-Ray	Disease of pericardium, unspecified	I31.9
	Emphysema, unspecified	J43.9
	Heart failure, unspecified	I50.9
	Pericardial effusion	I31.3
	Pneumonia, unspecified organism	J18.9
	Solitary pulmonary nodule	R91.1
Pulmonary Function Testing	Abnormal results of pulmonary function studies	R94.2
Obstructive (Ventilatory) Lung Diseases	Asthma	J45
	Bronchiectasis	J47
	Chronic bronchitis	J42
	Chronic obstructive pulmonary disease	J44.9
	Emphysema	J43.9
	Obstructive airway lesions	J44.9
Restrictive (Inflammatory) Lung Diseases	Acute lung injury	S27.309A
	Acute respiratory distress syndrome	J80
	Cardiogenic pulmonary edema	J81.1
	Congestive heart failure	I50.9
	Idiopathic pulmonary fibrosis	J84.10
	Pneumonia	J18.9
	Pulmonary edema	J81.1
	Restrictive (inflammatory) lung diseases	J98.4
	Sarcoidosis	D86.9
	Tuberculosis	A15.0
Pulmonary Hypertension and Pulmonary Vascular Disorders	Primary pulmonary hypertension	I27.0
	Pulmonary embolism	I26
	Secondary pulmonary hypertension	I27.2
	Wegener granulomatosis without renal involvement	M31.30
Chest Wall and Secondary Pleural Disorders	Chest wall disorders	F45.8
	Pleural condition, unspecified	J94.9
	Pleural effusion	J90
	Pleuritis	R09.1
Respiratory Failure	See Appendix C for respiratory failure ICD codes	
Pneumothorax	Chronic pneumothorax	J93.81
	Pneumothorax and air leak	J93
	Spontaneous pneumothorax	J93.0
	Tension pneumothorax	J93.0
	Traumatic pneumothorax	S27.0
Lower Respiratory Tract Pathogens	See Appendix C for list of lower respiratory tract infections	

Appendix B	ICD-10 Codes	
Chapter	**Condition/Topic**	**ICD-10 Code**
Obstructive Sleep Apnea	Hypoxemia	R09.02
	Obstructive sleep apnea	G47.33
	Sleep apnea	G47.3
Oxygen Supplementation	Dependence on supplemental oxygen	Z99.81
Mechanical Ventilatory Support	Dependence on respiratory ventilator	Z99.11
Section 4. Management of Patients with Gastrointestinal Disorders		
Peptic Ulcer Disease	Gastroesophageal reflux disease	K21.9
	Gastrointestinal mucositis	K92.81
	Peptic ulcer, site unspecified	K27.9
	Personal history of peptic ulcer disease	Z87.11
Liver Disease	Acute hepatitis	B17.9
	Alcoholic liver disease	K70.9
	Biliary cirrhosis	K74.3
	Cholangitis	K83.0
	Hereditary hemochromatosis	E83.110
	Liver disease, unspecified	K76.9
	Wilson disease	E83.01
Biliary Dysfunction	Acute pancreatitis	K85.9
	Cholecystitis	K81.9
Inflammatory Gastrointestinal Disorders	Appendicitis	K37
	Diverticulitis	K57.32
	Peritonitis	K65.9
	Ulcerative colitis	K51.90
Anatomic Intestinal Disorders	Intestinal obstruction	K56.60
	Paralytic ileus and intestinal obstruction	K56.0
	Traumatic ischemia of muscle	T79.6XXS
	Vascular disorder of the intestine, unspecified	K55.9
Gastrointestinal Bleeding	Esophageal varices	I85.00
	Lower gastrointestinal bleeding	K92.2
	Upper gastrointestinal bleeding	K92.2
Section 5. Management of Patients with Genitourinary Disorders		
Urinary Tract Infections	History of urinary tract infections	Z87.440
	Urinary tract calculus	N21
	Urinary tract infection, site not specified	N39.0
Acute Kidney Injury and Chronic Kidney Disease	Acute kidney injury	S37.0
	Chronic kidney disease	N18.9
Benign Prostatic Hyperplasia	Enlarged prostate without lower UTI symptoms	N40.0
	Enlarged prostate with lower UTI symptoms	N40.1
Renal Artery Stenosis	Atherosclerosis of renal artery	I70.1
	Congenital renal artery stenosis	Q27.1
	Fibromuscular dysplasia	I77.3
Nephrolithiasis	Calculus of kidney	N20.0

Appendix B	ICD-10 Codes	
Chapter	**Condition/Topic**	**ICD-10 Code**
Section 6. Management of Patients with Endocrine Disorders		
Diabetes Mellitus	Other specified diabetes mellitus	E13
	Type 1 diabetes mellitus	E10
	Type 2 diabetes mellitus	E11
Diabetes-Related Emergencies	Diabetes mellitus with ketoacidosis	E13.1
	Diabetes mellitus with hyperosmolarity with coma	E11.01
	Hypoglycemia	E16.2
Thyroid Disease	Hyperthyroidism	E05
	Hypothyroidism	E03.9
	Myxedema coma	E03.5
	Thyroid storm (thyrotoxic crisis)	E05.81
Cushing's Syndrome	Cushing's syndrome	E24.9
Primary Adrenocortical Insufficiency (Addison Disease) & Adrenal Crisis	Addison disease	G73.7
	Addisonian crisis	E27.2
	Primary adrenocortical insufficiency	E27.1
Pheochromocytoma	Pheochromocytoma	C74.10
Syndrome of Inappropriate Antidiuretic Hormone	Syndrome of inappropriate antidiuretic hormone	E22.2
Diabetes Insipidus	Diabetes insipidus	E23.2
	Nephrogenic diabetes insipidus	N25.1
Section 7. Management of Musculoskeletal Disorders		
Arthritis	Gout	M10.9
	Osteoarthritis	M19.91
	Rheumatoid arthritis	M06.9
Subluxations and Dislocations	Dislocation of ankle	M24.473
	Dislocation of shoulder	M24.419
	Dislocation of hand	M24.443
	Dislocation and subluxation of hip	S73.0
	Dislocation and subluxation of shoulder joint	S43.0
	Subluxation of unspecified scapula	S43.313A
	Subluxation of wrist and hand	S63.003
Soft Tissue Injury	Disorders of soft tissue	M79.9
	Soft tissue disorder related to use, overuse, and pressure	M70.99
Fractures	Closed fracture	T14.8
	Open fracture	T14.8
	Stress fracture	M84.3
Compartment syndrome	Compartment syndrome	T79.80
	Early complications of trauma, initial encounter	T79.8XXA
Back Pain Syndromes	Herniated disk	M51.9
	Low back pain	M54.5

Appendix xv

Appendix B	ICD-10 Codes	
Chapter	**Condition/Topic**	**ICD-10 Code**
Section 8. Management of Patients with Hematologic Disorders		
Anemias	Anemia of chronic disease (ACD)	D63.8
	Anemias	D64.9
	Folic acid deficiency	D50.9
	Iron deficiency	D50.9
	Pernicious anemia	E61.1
	Thalassemia	D56.9
	Vitamin B12 deficiency	D51.0
Sickle Cell Disease/Crisis	Sickle cell disease/crisis	D57.819
	Sickle cell disease without crisis	D57.1
Coagulopathies	Disseminated intravascular coagulation	D65
	Heparin-induced thrombocytopenia	D75.82
	Idiopathic thrombocytopenic purpura	D69.3
Section 9. Management of Patients with Oncologic Disorders		
Leukemias	Acute lymphocytic leukemia	C91.0
	Acute leukemia of unspecified cell	C95.02
	Acute myeloblastic leukemia	C92.0
	Chronic lymphocytic leukemia	C91.1
	Chronic myelogenous leukemia	C93.11, C93.12
	Refractory anemia with excess of blasts not in transformation	D46.2
Lymphoma	Hodgkin's disease	C81.9
	Lymphoma	C81.90
	Non-Hodgkin's lymphoma	C85.90
Other Common Cancers	Bladder cancer	C67.9
	Breast cancer	C50.919
	Cervical cancer	C53.0
	Colorectal cancer	C19
	Endometrial cancer	C54.1
	Lung cancer	C34.90
	Ovarian cancer	C56.9
	Prostate cancer	C61
Section 10. Management of Patients with Immunologic Disorders		
HIV/AIDS and Opportunistic Infections	Contact with or exposure to viral diseases	Z20.6
	HIV infection	B20-B24
	Immunodeficiency	D84.9
Autoimmune Diseases	Giant cell arteritis	M31.6
	Systemic lupus erythematosus	M32.10
Section 11. Management of Patients with Miscellaneous Health Problems		
Integumentary Disorders	Cellulitis	L03.90
	Dermatitis medicamentosa (drug eruption)	L27.0
	Herpes zoster (shingles)	B02.9
	Integumentary disorders	L98.9
	Skin disorders	C44.90
	Melanoma	C73.9

Appendix B	ICD-10 Codes	
Chapter	**Condition/Topic**	**ICD-10 Code**
Ectopic Pregnancy and STIs	*Chlamydia trachomatis* infection	A74.9
	Ectopic pregnancy	O00.9
	Gonorrhea	A54.00
	Herpes	B00.9
	Pelvic inflammatory disease (PID salpingitis)	N73.9
	Syphilis	A53.9
	Vaginitis	N76.0
Eye, Ear, Nose, and Throat Disorders	See appendix E for ICD-10 codes for common eye, ear, nose, and throat disorders	
Headache	Chronic tension type headache	G44.229
	Cluster headaches syndrome	G44.001
	Episodic cluster headache	G44.019
	Episodic tension-type headache	G44.211
	Headache	R51
	Migraine	G43
Section 12. Common Problems in Acute Care		
Fever	Fever	R50.9
Pain	Acute pain	G89.11
	Chronic pain	G89.29
	Neoplasm related pain	G89.3
	Unspecified pain	R52
Psychosocial Problems in Acute Care	Anxiety	F41.9
	Delirium	F05
	Depression	F32.9
	Psychosis	F06.0
	Substance Use Disorder (Alcohol)	F10.20
	Violence	R45.6
Management of the Patient in Shock	Anaphylactic shock	T78.2XXA
	R57.0	785.51
	Hypovolemic shock	R57.1
	Septic shock	R65.21
	Shock	R57.9
Nutritional Considerations	Encounter for screening for nutritional disorder	Z13.21
	Nutritional deficiency	E63.9

Appendix B	ICD-10 Codes	
Chapter	**Condition/Topic**	**ICD-10 Code**
Fluid, Electrolyte, and Acid-Base Imbalances	Acid-base disorders	E87.4
	Hypercalcemia	E83.52
	Hyperkalemia	E87.5
	Hypermagnesemia	E83.41
	Hypernatremia	E87.0
	Hyperphosphatemia	E83.30
	Hypocalcemia	E83.51
	Hypokalemia	E87.6
	Hypomagnesemia	E83.42
	Hyponatremia	E87.1
	Hypophosphatemia	E83.30
	Metabolic acidosis	E87.3
	Metabolic alkalosis	E87.3
	Respiratory acidosis	E87.2
	Respiratory alkalosis	E87.3
Poisoning and Drug Toxicities	Acetaminophen toxicity	T39.1X2A
	Alcohol (ethanol) toxicity	T51.0X4A
	Antiarrhythmic drug overdose	T46.2X3A
	Anticoagulant overdose	T45.514A
	Antidepressant toxicity	T43.011A
	Antipsychotic toxicity	T433504A
	Barbiturate overdose	T42.3X4A
	Benzodiazepine overdose	T42.4X4A
	Beta-blocker overdose	T46.2X4A
	Calcium channel blocker overdose	T46.2X4A
	Carbon monoxide poisoning	T58.94XA
	Digoxin toxicity	T46.0X4A
	Lithium toxicity	T56.4X4A
	Organophosphate (insecticide) poisoning	T60.0X4A
	Salicylate toxicity	T49.4X4A
	Stimulant toxicity	T50.991A
	Theophylline toxicity	T50.2X1A
Wound Management	Non-pressure chronic ulcer	L98.4
	Pressure ulcer	L89
	Type 1 diabetes mellitus with foot ulcer	E10.621
	Type 2 diabetes mellitus with foot ulcer	E11.621

Appendix B — ICD-10 Codes

Chapter	Condition/Topic	ICD-10 Code
Infections	Cellulitis	L03.90
	Clostridium difficile colitis	A04.7
	Dysentery	A09
	Endocarditis	I38
	Meningitis	G03.9
	Neutropenia	D70
	Nosocomial and ventilator-associated pneumonia	J69.0
	Nosocomial bacteremia	R78.81
	Nosocomial urinary tract infection	J69.0
	Pharyngitis	J02.9
	Pneumonia	J18.9
	Simple diarrhea	R19.7
	Sinusitis	J32.9
	Skin and soft tissue furunculosis	L02.92
	Sepsis	R65.2
	Urinary tract infection	N39.0
Trauma Considerations	Angina	I20.9
	Aortic rupture	I71.8
	Cardiac tamponade	I31.9
	Collapsed lung	J98.11
	Flail chest	S22.5XXA
	Lacerated liver	S36.113A
	Myocardial infarction	I25.2
	Penetrating eye trauma	S05.60XA
	Renal injuries	S37.009A
	Rib fractures	S22.39XA
	Ruptured spleen	D73.3
Solid Organ Transplantation	Complication of transplanted intestine	T86.850
	Complication of transplanted kidney	T86.10
	Complication of transplanted liver	T86.40
	Complication of transplanted lung	T86.819
	Complication of transplanted pancreas	T86.899
	Heart transplantation	V50.0
	Intestinal transplantation	V42.84
	Kidney transplantation	V42.0
	Lung transplantation	V42.6
	Pancreas transplantation	V42.83
Burns	Burns of unspecified body region	T30.0
	First degree burn	T21.10XS
	Second degree burn	T21.20XS
	Third degree burn	T21.30XS
Hospital Admission Considerations		
Managing the Surgical Patient	Pre-operative examination	Z01.818
	Encounter for post procedural aftercare	Z48

Appendix B	ICD-10 Codes	
Chapter	**Condition/Topic**	**ICD-10 Code**
Section 13. Health Promotion		
Guidelines for Health Promotion and Screening	Encounter for general adult medical examination	Z00.0
	Encounter for screening, unspecified	Z13.9
Major Causes of Mortality in the U.S.	Alzheimer's disease	G30.9
	Cerebral atherosclerosis	I67.2
	Chronic ischemic heart disease, unspecified	I25.9
	Influenza due to other identified influenza virus with other respiratory manifestations	J10.1
	Nephritic syndrome	N04.9
	Pneumonia	J18.9
	Respiratory disorder	J98.9
	Systemic inflammatory response syndrome of non-infectious origin without acute organ dysfunction	R65.10
	Type 2 diabetes without complications	E11.9
	Unspecified nephritic syndrome with unspecified morphologic changes	N05.9
Immunization Recommendations	Encounter for immunization	Z23

Note. Appendix B. International Classification of Diseases (2014). ICD10data.com: The Web's free 2015 medical coding reference [Data file]. Retrieved from icd10data.com

Appendix C	ICD-10 Coding, Respiratory Failure (CMS, 2013)
ICD-10 Code	**Disorder**
J96	Respiratory failure not otherwise specified Excludes: acute respiratory distress syndrome (J80) Cardiorespiratory failure (R09.2) Post-procedural respiratory failure (J95.82-) Respiratory arrest (R09.2)
J96	Acute respiratory failure
J96.00	Acute respiratory failure unspecified whether with hypoxia or hypercapnia
J96.01	Acute respiratory failure with hypoxia
J96.02	Acute respiratory failure with hypercapnia
J96.1	Chronic respiratory failure
J96.10	Chronic respiratory failure unspecified whether with hypoxia or hypercapnia
J96.11	Chronic respiratory failure with hypoxia
J96.12	Chronic respiratory failure with hypercapnia
J96.2	Acute and chronic respiratory failure (or acute or chronic respiratory failure)
J96.20	Acute and chronic respiratory failure unspecified whether with hypoxia or hypercapnia
J96.21	Acute and chronic respiratory failure with hypoxia
J96.22	Acute and chronic respiratory failure with hypercapnia
J96.9	Respiratory failure unspecified
J96.90	Respiratory failure unspecified whether with hypoxia or hypercapnia
J96.91	Respiratory failure unspecified with hypoxia
J96.92	Respiratory failure unspecified with hypercapnia

Note. Appendix C. International Classification of Diseases (2014). ICD10data.com: The Web's free 2015 medical coding reference [Data file]. Retrieved from icd10data.com

Appendix D	Former ICD-9 and ICD-10 Coding, Lower Respiratory Tract Infections (see Lower Respiratory Tract Pathogens chapter), for 2014 (CMS, 2013)
Former ICD-9 Coding (2013):	
466.0	Acute tracheobronchitis
496	Chronic obstructive pulmonary disease
486	Pneumonia, community-acquired
ICD-10 Code (2014):	
J09	Influenza due to certain identified influenza viruses
J09.X	Influenza due to identified novel influenza A viruses, including: •Avian influenza •Bird influenza •Influenza A/H5N1 •Influenza of other animal origin, not bird or swine •Swine influenza virus
J09.X1	Influenza due to identified novel influenza A virus with pneumonia
J10	Influenza due to other identified influenza virus
J10.0	Influenza due to other identified influenza virus with pneumonia
J10.00	Influenza due to other identified influenza virus with unspecified type of pneumonia
J10.01	Influenza due to other identified influenza virus with the same other identified influenza virus pneumonia
J10.08	Influenza due to other identified influenza virus with other specified pneumonia
J11	Influenza due to unidentified influenza virus
J11.0	Influenza due to unidentified influenza virus pneumonia
J11.00	Influenza due to unidentified influenza virus with unspecified type of pneumonia
J11.08	Influenza due to unidentified influenza virus with specified pneumonia
J12	Viral pneumonia, not elsewhere classified
J12.0	Adenoviral pneumonia
J12.1	Respiratory syncytial virus pneumonia
J12.2	Parainfluenza virus pneumonia
J12.3	Human metapneumovirus pneumonia
J12.8	Other viral pneumonia
J12.81	Pneumonia due to SAS-associated coronavirus
J12.89	Other viral pneumonia
J12.9	Viral pneumonia, unspecified
J13	Pneumonia due to *Streptococcus pneumoniae*
J14	Pneumonia due to *Hemophilus influenzae*
J15	Bacterial pneumonia, not elsewhere classified
J15.0	Pneumonia due to *Klebsiella pneumoniae*
J15.1	Pneumonia due to *Pseudomonas*
J15.2	Pneumonia due to *Staphylococcus*
J15.20	Pneumonia due to *Staphylococcus*, unspecified
J15.21	Pneumonia due to *Staphylococcus aureus*
J15.211	Pneumonia due to methicillin-susceptible *Staphylococcus aureus*
J15.212	Pneumonia due to methicillin-resistant *Staphylococcus aureus*
J15.3	Pneumonia due to *Streptococcus*, group B
J15.4	Pneumonia due to other streptococci
J15.5	Pneumonia due to *Escherichia coli*
J15.6	Pneumonia due to other Gram-negative bacteria, including *Serratia marcescens*
J15.7	Pneumonia due to *Mycoplasma pneumoniae*
J15.8	Pneumonia due to other specified bacteria

Appendix D	Former ICD-9 and ICD-10 Coding, Lower Respiratory Tract Infections (see Lower Respiratory Tract Pathogens chapter), for 2014 (CMS, 2013)
J15.9	Unspecified bacterial pneumonia due to Gram-positive bacteria
J16	Pneumonia due to other infectious organisms, not elsewhere classified
J16.0	Chlamydial pneumonia
J16.8	Pneumonia due to other specified infectious organisms
J18	Pneumonia, unspecified organism
J18.0	Bronchopneumonia
J18.1	Lobar, pneumonia, unspecified organism
J18.2	Hypostatic pneumonia, unspecified organism
J18.8	Other pneumonia, unspecified organism
J18.9	Pneumonia, unspecified organism
J20	Acute bronchitis
J20.0	Acute bronchitis due to *Mycoplasma pneumoniae*
J20.1	Acute bronchitis due to *Hemophilus influenzae*
J20.2	Acute bronchitis due to *Streptococcus*
J20.3	Acute bronchitis due to Coxsackie virus
J20.4	Acute bronchitis due to parainfluenza virus
J20.5	Acute bronchitis due to respiratory syncytial virus
J20.6	Acute bronchitis due to rhinovirus
J20.7	Acute bronchitis due to echovirus
J20.8	Acute bronchitis due to other specified organisms
J20.9	Acute bronchitis, unspecified
J21	Acute bronchiolitis
J21.0	Acute bronchiolitis due to respiratory syncytial virus
J21.1	Acute bronchiolitis due to human metapneumovirus
J21.8	Acute bronchiolitis due to other specified organisms
J21.0	Acute bronchiolitis, unspecified
J22	Unspecified acute lower respiratory infection

Note. Appendix D. International Classification of Diseases (2014). ICD10data.com: The Web's free 2015 medical coding reference [Data file]. Retrieved from icd10data.com

Appendix E	ICD-9 and ICD-10 Codes for Common Eye, Ear, Nose, and Throat Disorders (see Common Eye, Ear, Nose, and Throat Disorders chapter)
ICD-9 Code (2013) Category	**Disorder**
477.9	Allergic rhinitis
351.0	Bell palsy
362.30	Central and branch retinal artery obstruction
372.30	Conjunctivitis
918.1	Corneal abrasion
362.01	Diabetic retinopathy
464.30	Epiglottitis
784.7	Epistaxis
365.9	Glaucoma
380.10	Otitis externa
382.9	Otitis media
462.0	Pharyngitis
361.9	Retinal detachment
473.9	Sinusitis
524.60	Temporomandibular joint disorder
350.1	Trigeminal neuralgia (tic douloureux)
ICD-10 Code (2014) Category	**Disorder**
Disorders of the eye	
E11 (see also E08)	Type 2 diabetes mellitus (Diabetes mellitus due to underlying conditions)
E11.31	Type 2 diabetes mellitus with unspecified retinopathy
G45	Transient cerebral ischemic attacks and related syndromes
G45.3	Amaurosis fugax
H00.0	Hordeolum (externum) (internum) of eyelid
H00.01	Hordeolum externum (stye)
H00.02	Hordeolum internum (infection of meibomian gland)
H00.1	Chalazion (cyst of meibomian gland)
H01.0	Blepharitis
H01.00	Unspecified blepharitis
H01.1	Noninfectious dermatoses of eyelid
H01.11	Allergic (contact) dermatitis of eyelid
H01.13	Eczematous dermatitis of eyelid
H01.9	Unspecified inflammation of eyelid
H02.0	Entropion and trichiasis of eyelid
H02.00	Unspecified entropion of eyelid
H02.03	Senile entropion of eyelid
H02.1	Ectropion of eyelid
H02.10	Unspecified ectropion of eyelid
H02.13	Senile ectropion of eyelid
H02.4	Ptosis of eyelid
H02.40	Unspecified ptosis of eyelid
H02.6	Xanthelasma of eyelid
H02.60	Xanthelasma of unspecified eye
H04.1	Other disorders of lacrimal gland
H04.12	Dry eye syndrome

Appendix E	ICD-9 and ICD-10 Codes for Common Eye, Ear, Nose, and Throat Disorders (see Common Eye, Ear, Nose, and Throat Disorders chapter)
H04.3	Acute and unspecified inflammation of lacrimal passages
H04.30	Unspecified Dacryocystitis
H04.4	Chronic inflammation of lacrimal passages
H04.41	Chronic dacryocystitis
H05.0	Acute inflammation of orbit
H05.00	Unspecified acute inflammation of orbit
H05.01	Cellulitis (including abscess) of orbit
H05.20	Unspecified exophthalmos
H10.0	Mucopurulent conjunctivitis
H10.01	Acute follicular conjunctivitis
H10.02	Other mucopurulent conjunctivitis
H11.0	Pterygium of eye
H11.00	Unspecified pterygium of eye
H11.3	Conjunctival (subconjunctival) hemorrhage
H11.30	Conjunctival hemorrhage unspecified eye
H25.0	Age-related incipient cataract
H25.01	Cortical age-related cataract
H25.1	Age-related nuclear cataract
H25.10	Age-related nuclear cataract unspecified eye
H33	Retinal detachments and breaks
H33.00	Unspecified retinal detachment with retinal break
H33.8	Other retinal detachment
H34	Retinal vascular occlusions
H34.0	Transient retinal artery occlusion
H34.1	Central retinal artery occlusion
H40.0	Glaucoma suspect
H40.00	Preglaucoma unspecified
S05.0	Injury of conjunctiva and corneal abrasion without foreign body
S05.00	Injury of conjunctiva and corneal abrasion without foreign body unspecified eye
Disorders of the Ear	
H60	Otitis externa
H60.33	Swimmer's ear
H60.50	Unspecified acute noninfective otitis externa
H65	Nonsuppurative otitis media (acute)
H65.0	Acute serous otitis media
H66.0	Suppurative and unspecified otitis media
H66.00	Acute suppurative otitis media without spontaneous rupture of ear drum
H81	Disorders of vestibular function
H81.0	Ménière disease
H81.1	Benign paroxysmal vertigo
R42	Dizziness and giddiness; vertigo, NOS
Disorders of the Face (nerve-related)	
G50	Disorders of trigeminal nerve
G50.0	Trigeminal neuralgia (Tic douloureux)
G51	Facial nerve disorders
G51.0	Bell's palsy

Appendix E	ICD-9 and ICD-10 Codes for Common Eye, Ear, Nose, and Throat Disorders (see Common Eye, Ear, Nose, and Throat Disorders chapter)
Disorders of the Nose and Sinuses	
J01	Acute sinusitis
J01.00	Acute maxillary sinusitis unspecified
J01.10	Acute fontal sinusitis
J30	Vasomotor and allergic rhinitis unspecified
J30.0	Vasomotor rhinitis
J30.1	Allergic rhinitis due to pollen (hay fever)
R04	Hemorrhage from respiratory passages
R04.4	Epistaxis
Disorders of the Temporomandibular Joint	
M26.6	Temporomandibular joint disorders
M26.60	Temporomandibular joint disorder unspecified
M26.62	Arthralgia of temporomandibular joint
Disorders of the Throat and Larynx	
J02	Acute pharyngitis
J02.0	Streptococcal pharyngitis
J02.9	Acute pharyngitis unspecified
J03	Acute tonsillitis
J03.0	Streptococcal tonsillitis
J03.9	Acute tonsillitis unspecified
J04	Acute laryngitis and tracheitis
J04.0	Acute laryngitis
J04.3	Supraglottitis unspecified
J05	Acute obstructive laryngitis [croup] and epiglottitis
J05.0	Acute obstructive laryngitis {croup]
J05.1	Acute epiglottitis
J05.10	Acute epiglottitis without obstruction
J05.11	Acute epiglottitis with obstruction
J06	Acute upper respiratory infections of multiple and unspecified sites
J06.0	Acute laryngopharyngitis
J06.9	Acute upper respiratory infection unspecified

Note. ICD 9 codes (2013) and ICD-10 (2014) codes for disorders of the eye and adnexa (CDC, 2013). Please note that there are 85 pages of coding for these ocular disorders. Codes provided are only for those disorders likely to be encountered in an acute care nurse practitioner role, while caring for elderly patients. Furthermore, there are also codings for right or left eye, which eyelid is involved, and other descriptors. The reader is directed to the following URL for additional information under Chapter 7 of the ICD-10 coding. Additional coding to specify whether the disorder affects the right eye, the left eye, or both is available, especially if the coding below states "unspecified."

Appendix E. International Classification of Diseases (2014). ICD10data.com: The Web's free 2015 medical coding reference [Data file]. Retrieved from icd10data.com

INDEX

A

a-fib, see atrial fibrillation

abciximab (ReoPro), 124

abdomen, (abdominal), 28, 45, 49, 50, 88, 113, 115, 116, 121, 149, 155, 171, 202, 203, 238, 246, 293, 294, 300, 315, 327, 328, 340, 345, 346, 352, 354–355, 359, 360, 362, 363, 365, 366, 369, 370, 371, 372, 373, 375, 378, 379, 387, 396, 399, 400, 421, 429, 441t, 452, 503, 558, 560, 567, 575, 590, 623, 687, 690t, 771, 829, 833, 835, 856t, 862, 876

abdominal trauma, 832

abort, 68, 670t, 671t, 673t

abortion, 4, 330, 629, 860

abscess , 9, 12, 42, 59, 60–61, 73, 164, 356, 359, 360, 362, 363, 366, 386, 506t, 613, 614, 625, 626, 627, 629, 653, 684, 691t, 747, 822, 846, 848

abstinence, 343, 389, 707t, 892t

abuse, 4, 75, 164, 198, 337, 343, 625, 705t, 711–716, 721, 722, 731t, 769, 774, 883, 884t, 892t, 893t, 895, 904

acalculous cholecystitis, 351

accident(s), 3–20, 22, 23, 24, 40, 46, 132, 135, 179, 372, 588, 650, 653, 727, 731t, 835, 857t, 858, 888, 898–903, 905

acebutolol (Sectral), 127, 200, 226, 674t,

ace-I (ACEI), see angiotensin-converting-enzyme inhibitor

acetaminophen, 16, 19, 60, 163, 326, 344, 345, 346, 354, 422, 449, 471, 479t, 485t, 487t, 490, 494, 495, 499, 507, 509, 530, 616, 624, 627, 652, 653, 658, 659, 670t, 675t, 689, 696, 697, 702t, 788, 789, 830

acetaminophen toxicity, 788

acetate, 82, 404, 455, 465, 524, 529, 578, 770, 778, 780, 853

acetazolamide (Diamox),, 781

acetohydroxamic (Lithostat), 422, 423

acetylcholine, 35, 36

acetylcysteine, 251, 345, 394, 789, 846

acetylsalicylic , 251, 345, 394, 449, 696, 748, 857t, 872, 894

ache , 154, 615, 694

acid, 5, 7, 17, 24, 46, 69, 70, 103, 115, 117, 118, 154, 163, 264, 269, 270, 287, 289, 325, 326, 329, 330, 332, 333, 334, 342, 348, 352, 353, 354, 361, 362, 365, 366, 391, 393, 403, 417, 419–423, 443, 449, 458, 473, 474, 482t, 517, 520, 531, 534, 544, 546, 547, 551, 560, 572, 577, 578, 608t, 623, 624, 628, 631, 637, 672t, 673t, 685, 696, 697, 698, 720t, 734, 737, 748, 757, 760, 761, 764, 774, 778, 779, 780, 785, 789, 790, 804, 815, 851, 857t, 891t–894, 896

acid-antisecretory, 329–330

acid-base, 391, 740, 769, 778, 786, 789, 797, 874

acid-fast, 264, 269, 270, 287

acidify, 423, 458, 515, 779

acidity, 330, 335

acidosis, 63, 65, 171, 208, 222, 223, 225, 228, 231, 246, 267, 275, 346, 348, 355, 365, 369, 372, 376, 394, 397, 398, 403, 404, 412, 415, 421, 443, 444, 455, 737–740, 742, 743, 744, 767, 769, 770, 771, 777–783, 789, 791, 793, 794, 796, 802, 804, 805, 829, 830, 831, 846, 848, 852, 853, 854, 868, 872

acidotic, 738, 739

acoustic neuroma, 27

actin-myosin, 170

activated coagulation time (ACT), 137

activated partial thromboplastin time (APTT), 137

active immunity, 905

acute agitation, 732

acute kidney injury, 12, 376, 391–399

acute lung injury, 266–267, 790

acute lymphocytic leukemia, 543–547

acute myelogenous, 544

acute myocardial infarction (AMI), 743

acute pain, 528, 530, 693

acute respiratory distress syndrome (ARDS), 222, 266–267, 309, 314, 316, 319, 355, 597, 738, 847

acute tubulointerstitial nephritis, 394

acyclovir (Zovirax), 62, 597, 616, 635, 636, 651

Addison's disease, 454–456

Addisonian crisis, 249

adefovir (Hepsera), 338

adenocarcinoma, 362, 565, 567, 572, 577

adenoid, 306, 570

adenoidectomy, 166, 306

adenoma, 420, 452, 453, 567

adenosine, 203, 206

adenovirus, 261, 641, 642, 650, 658, 684

adhesion, 368, 370, 601, 622, 625

adjuvant therapy, 571, 621

admission orders, 863

adrenal, 264, 364, 451–459, 462, 479t, 685, 735, 749, 766, 769, 770, 868

adrenal crisis, 455, see Addison disease

adrenal hemorrhage, 454

adrenal medullary, 457

adrenal neoplasms, 452

adrenergic, 103, 105, 109, 202, 248, 251, 252, 274, 332, 373, 459, 649, 698, 749, 750t, 769, 793, 873

adrenoceptor-mediated, 108

adrenocortical, 53, 454, 458, 516

adrenocorticotropic, 50, 452, 454, 735

Adriamycin (doxorubicin), 561

Advair, 248, 253, 254

advance, 444, 521, 548, 560, 564, 566, 567, 570, 574, 575, 581, 588–591, 656, 661, 746, 760, 761, 779, 820, 828, 853, 882

aeromonas, 613, 615

aerosol, 247, 595, 673t, 783, 830

aeruginosa (Pseudomonas), 262, 298, 300, 385, 388, 651, 819, 821, 822, 824, 844t

afebrile, 59, 534, 614, 615

African-American, 102, 255, 430, 603, 648

Aggrenox, 7, 12

aggressive pulmonary toilet, 830

aging, 101, 183, 288, 290, 296, 326, 615, 689, 810

agnosia, 73, 75

agranulocytosis, 202, 472, 482t, 610

AIDS (HIV), 27, 57, 59, 61, 63, 264, 351, 462, 514, 535, 557, 558, 587–593, 595, 596, 597, 615, 616, 627, 631, 633, 639, 665t, 684, 686, 687, 729, 872, 884t, 885, 890t, 892t, 893t, 895, 896, 899t, 900t, 901t, 904, 909t

airborne, 252

albumin, 68, 231, 348, 355, 356, 560, 739, 742, 757, 772, 773, 774, 786, 813, 872

albumin, 68, 75, 231, 347, 348, 355, 356, 361, 376, 560, 739, 742, 757, 772, 773, 774, 786, 813, 864, 872

albuminocytologic, 32

albuterol (Proventil), 248, 253, 749, 769, 771, 772, 783, 830, 874

alcohol, 4, 9, 14, 22, 65, 73, 75, 101, 103, 107, 117, 169, 172, 193, 195, 196, 204, 298, 306, 326, 331, 332, 334, 337, 341, 343, 344, 346, 354, 411, 423, 429, 434, 445, 458, 462, 482t, 498, 517, 520, 521, 522, 634, 652–655, 673t, 678t, 685, 686, 707t, 712, 715, 716, 721, 722, 723t, 729, 731t, 772–777, 779, 780, 788, 789, 790, 803, 845, 858, 884t, 887, 889t, 892t, 893t, 896, 903, 909t

alcohol toxicity, 789

alcoholic ketoacidosis, 779, 780

alcoholism, 354, 903

alcohol-mediated, 343

aldosterone (aldosteronism), 101, 106, 170, 173, 174, 175, 176, 183, 184, 416, 454, 455, 735, 739, 764, 769, 770, 771, 781

aldosterone antagonist, 173, 174, 175, 184

alkaline (phosphate), 340, 341, 342, 344, 345, 347, 352, 355, 404, 529, 551, 570, 789, 848

alkalosis, 171, 223, 225, 228, 278, 329, 368, 369, 376, 393, 398, 647, 735, 739, 740, 770, 776, 778, 780, 781, 783, 784, 796, 829

allergen (subcutaneous), 253, 254, 257, 642, 654–657, 748

allergic reactions, 137, 627, 807

allergic rhinitis, 251, 658

allergist, 254, 655

allergy, 60, 104, 123, 133, 137, 153, 162, 165, 166, 251–254, 257, 280, 299, 331, 361, 365, 388, 397, 476t, 481t, 610, 611, 612, 614, 625, 627, 639, 643, 644, 651, 652, 654–658, 704t, 789, 807, 813, 820, 827

allograft rejection, 838

allopurinol, 395, 423, 474, 544, 547, 551, 608

almotriptan (Axert), 671, 676

aluminum, 330, 404, 410

alveolar diffusion, 222–223

alveolar pattern, 235, 236

alveoli, 221, 222, 226, 235, 236, 243, 290, 316, 610, 735

Alzheimer's, 25, 65, 72, 76, 731t, 882, 898–903

aminotransaminases, 347

amlodipine (Norvasc), 104, 127, 179, 182, 183, 793

ammonia, 63, 371, 721, 737, 759

amnesia, 41, 67, 709t

amoxicillin (Amoxil), 166, 297, 301, 302, 331, 360, 610, 631, 652

amoxicillin-clavulanate (Augmentin), 297, 298, 301, 302, 387, 518, 658, 808

amphotericin (Fungilin), 394, 465, 596, 597, 689, 774, 776, 820, 824

ampicillin, 59, 60, 165, 166, 298, 353, 365, 388, 610, 690t, 823, 826t

amputation, 158, 429, 493, 504, 862

amyotrophic lateral sclerosis, 90–91, 241, 314

anaerobic, 224, 263, 287, 369, 376, 388, 495, 499, 613, 626, 638, 687, 734, 737, 815, 816t, 822

anaesthesia, 140f

analgesia 495, 499, 530, 645, 666t, 696, 697, 699, 700, 707t, 709t, 730, 830, 877, 43, 495, 499, 530, 645, 666t, 696, 697, 699, 700, 707t, 709t, 730, 830, 877

analgesics, 34, 353, 422, 479t, 480t, 481t, 507, 530, 616, 617, 652, 653, 658, 659, 665, 670t, 673t, 678t, 694, 696–702t, 704t, 705t, 807, 813, 814, 815, 874, 877

anaphylactic shock, 748

anaphylaxis, 83, 133, 166, 388, 392, 474, 486t, 487t, 520, 535, 610, 611, 612, 734, 735, 736t, 743, 745, 748, 749, 753t, 800t, 803, 805, 806, 840t

anaplastic large cell lymphoma (ALCL), 555

anastomoses, 325

anastomotic leaks, 847

androgen, 408, 409, 411, 453, 454, 576

anemia(s), anemic, 3, 5, 36, 75, 122, 164, 202, 224, 228, 272, 309, 327, 347, 360, 362, 378, 380, 400, 402, 404, 447, 448, 450, 472, 480t, 481t, 484t, 487t, 513–525, 527–530, 532, 534, 535, 544, 546, 548, 549, 557, 567, 579, 602, 603, 610, 611, 623, 646, 647, 653, 654, 686, 687, 703t, 715, 721, 744, 790, 807, 841, 859, 872, 873, 889t, 891t, 892t, 896

anemia of chronic disease (ACD), 521–523

anesthesia, 19, 49, 232, 313, 319, 320, 466, 614, 710, 786, 865

aneurysm, 13, 15, 16, 17, 21–24, 109, 113, 139, 236, 414, 464, 506t, 601, 602, 645, 666t, 685, 743, 867

angina, 112, 118, 119, 120, 121, 123, 125, 127, 129, 131, 133, 135, 137, 189, 280, 309, 543, 687, 832

angina, 33, 38, 104, 105, 108 (angina-inducing), 109, 112, 118, 119–137, 139, 179, 182, 189, 196, 273, 280, 309, 514, 543, 687, 752t, 801, 805, 832, 867, 868

angioedema, 166, 172, 174, 487t, 610, 611, 612, 748, 749, 806

angiography, 6, 10, 15, 23, 28, 46, 124, 153, 154, 182, 279, 372, 373, 378, 415, 416, 568, 602, 645, 647, 666t, 688, 833, 834, 835, 847 angiomas, 346, 378, 656

angioplasty, 6, 17, 24, 120, 123, 124, 132, 137, 373, 416, 666t, 847

angiotensin receptor blockers (ARBs), 172

angiotensin, 105, 170, 674t, 770

angiotensin-converting-enzyme (ACE), 108, 184, 674t

angiotensin-converting-enzyme inhibitor (ACE-I, ACEI), 101, 102, 106, 172, 173, 175, 252, 354, 392, 415, 417

angiotensin-receptor, 102, 104, 106, 172, 173, 176, 184, 403, 415, 417, 674t, 770

anorectal disease, 379

anorexia, 88, 327, 340, 352, 364, 366, 398, 401, 450, 471, 514, 520, 521, 543, 546, 548, 574, 603, 695, 698, 717t, 718t, 720t, 725t, 760, 779, 795, 801

antacid(s), 108, 325, 326, 328, 330, 334, 404, 775

antiarrhythmic(s), 37, 134, 135, 182, 195, 196, 201, 202, 203, 205, 206, 207, 208, 209, 210, 216, 790

antibacterial, 615

antibiotic(s), 18, 41, 60, 61, 135, 165, 166, 187, 188, 189, 190, 191, 196, 262, 288, 296, 330, 360, 365, 373, 379, 388, 389, 456, 495, 499, 544, 547, 561, 608t, 614, 615, 627, 643, 644, 651, 652, 658, 659, 660, 684, 688, 746, 747, 748, 808, 813–816t, 820, 821, 823–827, 833, 839, 845, 853, 872, 874, 876

antibody(antibodies), 5, 31, 32, 33, 35, 36, 37, 38, 62, 132, 160, 280, 327, 337, 338, 341, 342, 363, 364, 430, 448, 472, 476t, 477t, 478t, 485t, 515, 517, 518, 533–536, 544, 546, 548, 549, 557, 558, 559, 561, 579, 590, 592, 596, 602, 603, 604, 610, 616, 623, 631, 634, 638, 639, 647, 687, 748, 838, 839, 840t, 843, 844, 905

antibody, antinuclear, 5, 36, 67

anticholinergic agents, 248

anticholinergic(s), 77, 86, 88, 248, 250, 251, 325, 332, 362, 409, 641, 642, 799

anticholinesterase, 37

anticoagulant(s), 3, 5, 6, 11, 13, 14, 136, 158, 160, 177, 190, 187, 279, 280, 368, 454, 647, 803, 831, 872

anticoagulant overdose, 803

anticoagulation, 6–7, 9, 11–12, 34, 134, 137, 156, 159, 160, 177, 178, 187, 195, 203, 205, 276, 279, 280, 373, 410, 536, 875

anticonvulsant(s), 28, 45, 60, 62, 63, 66, 68, 69, 70, 404, 507, 509, 611, 697, 708t

antidepressant, 77, 108, 333, 409, 458, 461, 507, 509, 530, 617, 641, 668, 672t, 674t, 685, 698, 708t, 715, 716, 718t, 719t, 725t, 728, 792, 799

antidepressant toxicity, 799

antidysrhythmic drug overdose, 790

antiemetics, 337, 353, 422, 654, 668, 675t, 699

antiepileptic, 16, 68, 69, 610, 672t, 674t

antifibrinolytic, 17, 24

antigen(s), 34, 59, 287, 327, 337, 409, 430, 476t, 477t, 478t, 529, 534, 544, 546, 548, 560, 561, 568, 576, 590, 596, 601, 602, 616, 633, 654, 655, 659, 686, 748, 838, 843, 886, 905

antihistamine, 332, 409, 474, 485t, 487t, 530, 612, 641, 642, 644, 655, 656, 674t, 749, 806

antihypertensive(s), 100, 105, 108, 113, 117, 182, 183, 190, 402, 653, 807, 886

anti-inflammatory, 34, 249, 364, 461, 479t–481t, 530, 578, 603, 652, 670t, 696, 698, 702t, 704t, 830, 839, 872

antimicrobial(s), 63, 165, 250–251 (agents), 261, 262, 263, 288, 296, 297, 365, 370, 387, 389, 518, 597, 627, 633, 652, 659, 685, 689, 746, 814, 815, 816t

antioxidant, 77

antiphospholipid antibodies, 603

antiphospholipid, 3, 5, 603, 647

antiplatelet, 7, 12, 124, 133, 177, 182, 416, 647

antipseudomonal, 299, 300, 388, 615, 821, 823

antipsychotic(s), 77, 409, 641, 716, 720t, 730, 798

antipsychotic toxicity, 798

antiretroviral therapy (ART), 557, 588, 592–595, 598

antiseptics, 387, 389, 815

antispasmodics, 353, 409, 422, 507, 509

antiviral, 63, 337, 338, 345, 616, 651

anxiety, 16, 43, 86, 91, 109, 123, 135, 202, 248, 278, 317, 332, 355, 445, 447, 452, 457, 477t, 669t, 678t, 695, 700, 707t, 709t, 711, 712, 716, 717t, 720t, 722–725t, 727–731t, 741, 748, 772, 782, 783, 784, 798, 806, 860, 874

aorta, 3, 9, 21, 132, 139, 141, 190, 236, 238, 415, 601, 602, 735, 832

aortic regurgitation, 97, 190

aortic rupture, 832

aortic stenosis, 97, 186, 189, 192, 372

aortogram, 602, 832

aphasia, 4, 9, 62, 73, 75, 482t

apnea, 46, 48, 179, 222, 251, 276, 290, 305–307

appendectomy, 366

appendicitis, 363, 366–367, 627, 633

appendix, 366

argatroban (Acova), 279, 536, 803

arrhythmia(s), 3, 4, 50, 98, 105, 135, 179, 199, 202, 203, 205, 207, 210, 211, 216, 273, 459, 514, 603, 653, 718t, 719t, 726t, 729, 737, 738, 743, 744, 748, 753t, 769, 770, 775, 781, 790, 799, 800t, 801, 802, 807, 838t, 847, 867, 868

arterial blood gases (ABGs), 226, 246, 263

arterial blood, 48, 67, 75, 171, 224, 226, 246, 263, 266, 278, 294, 376, 502, 660, 739, 778, 779, 781

arterial ulcers, 813

arteriosclerosis obliterans, 156–157

arteriovenous malformation (AVM), 13

arteriovenous, 14, 24, 25, 76, 136

artery, 4, 6, 9, 10, 13, 21, 52, 120, 122, 131, 132, 133, 134, 141, 152, 187, 190, 224, 229, 236, 238, 276, 291, 371, 377, 414, 415, 416, 450, 490, 591, 601, 602, 646, 647, 653, 665t, 736t, 737, 738, 740, 741, 772, 780, 829, 830, 833, 845, 846, 847, 857t, 863, 871–874, 892t, 894

arthralgia(s), 87, 115, 340, 395, 454, 486t, 487t, 611, 638, 686, 838t, 840t, 860

arthritis, 36, 190, 251, 268, 269, 286, 340, 449, 469, 471, 479t–489, 493, 494, 514, 516, 521, 523, 603, 610, 611, 630, 661, 684, 685, 686, 689, 693, 696, 705t, 860, 882 artificial tears, 650

ascites, 170, 171, 179, 194, 272, 276, 346, 348, 355, 363, 365, 575, 576, 765, 785, 838t, 848

aseptic techniques, 389

aspartate aminotransferase (AST), 376

aspiration pneumonia, 236, 263

aspiration, 18, 33, 51, 263, 300, 310, 318, 328, 370, 387, 473, 494, 495, 560, 565, 570, 577, 623, 683, 687, 690, 761, 780, 797, 820, 822, 845

aspirin, 7, 12, 116, 117, 123, 127, 128, 130, 131, 133, 137, 154, 163, 177, 178, 189, 205, 207, 326, 332, 375, 380, 416, 449, 480t, 518, 608t, 641, 670t, 675t, 696, 702t, 779, 830, 873, 893t, 894

asthma, 105, 174, 241, 242, 243, 246, 248, 249, 252–254, 255, 257, 258, 259, 260, 309, 476t, 480t, 481t, 611, 699, 703t, 749, 783, 858

astrocytoma, 26

asystole, 98, 142, 145, 147, 209, 792, 793

ataxia, 5, 9, 14, 27, 32, 42, 62, 80, 81, 87, 124, 450, 516, 697, 708t, 709t, 720t, 725t, 772, 791, 796, 803, 808

atelectasis, 236, 255, 309, 315, 316, 355, 479t, 564, 695, 702t, 738, 829, 830, 876

atenolol (Tenormin), 103, 126, 176, 196, 202, 674t, 792, 856

atherectomy, 154

atheroembolic, 400

atherosclerosis , 3, 8, 111, 120, 139, 156, 171, 190, 193, 236, 380, 393, 400, 414, 415, 416

atrial fibrillation (a-fib), 3, 4, 6, 8, 11, 96, 105, 134, 135, 137, 171, 172, 173, 177, 179, 186, 187, 188, 189, 194, 195, 196, 201, 203–204, 205, 207, 208, 279, 372, 447, 647, 867

atrioventricular, 82, 95, 142, 147, 178, 199, 790, 792, 793, 795, 796, 799

atrium, 6, 9, 99, 143, 145, 146, 147, 149, 170, 171, 187, 188, 189, 201, 204, 205, 206, 208, 229, 236, 238

atrophy, 72, 75, 81, 90, 414, 508, 515, 564, 608t, 627, 648, 731t

atropine, 36, 50, 199, 212, 645, 748, 790, 794, 798, 847

Augmentin, 301, 658, 814, 825t, 826t

autoimmune, 4, 31, 35, 38, 157, 162, 170, 267, 286, 340, 342, 345, 354, 428, 447, 448, 449, 454, 471, 476t, 477t, 493, 515, 533, 534, 548, 557, 601, 602, 641, 684, 904

automatic internal cardioverter defibrillator (AICD), 149–150, 210

autopsy, 164, 661

axillary adenopathy, 570

azathioprine (Imuran), 34, 37, 269, 271, 281, 341, 354, 361, 362, 363, 364, 484t, 535, 840t

azithromycin (Zithromax), 166, 297, 298, 301, 302, 303, 595, 631, 633, 643, 652, 659

B

Babinski's sign, 59, 62, 81, 516, 730

bacteriuria, 386, 387, 820, 889t

Bactrim, 387, 652, 825t, 843

barbiturate, 65, 345, 608t, 722, 748, 791

barbiturate overdose, 791

Bell's palsy, 650–651

benign prostatic hyperplasia, 105, 395, 396, 408–412

benzodiazepine, 43, 68, 77, 332, 458, 698, 699, 722, 724, 725t, 730, 783, 791, 792, 796, 800, 802, 807, 874

benzodiazepine overdose, 791

benztropine (Cogentin), 86, 88, 799

beta-blocker, see β-blocker

Betaseron, 82

betaxolol, 103, 176, 649

bile, 115, 325, 326, 330, 332, 342, 344, 346, 351, 353, 355, 846

biliary dysfunction, 351–358

bilirubin, 340, 343–347, 352, 355, 376, 524, 529, 738, 739, 789, 838t

biopsy, 6, 28, 62, 90, 195, 255, 269, 270, 294, 327, 333, 341, 344, 345, 360, 396, 400, 409, 515, 519, 534, 544, 548, 557, 558, 560, 564, 565, 568, 569, 570, 572, 573, 577, 579, 581, 597, 602, 612, 618, 619, 620, 626, 637, 687, 688, 821, 838, 845, 887

bipolar, 143, 715, 716, 720t, 731

bismuth, 325, 330, 331

bisoprolol (Zebeta), 103, 176, 184, 674t

bites, 502, 548, 686, 805–808

bladder, 51, 53, 54, 74, 80, 107, 231, 385, 386, 395, 396, 408–411, 421, 439t, 457, 506, 508, 571, 573, 577–581, 747, 819, 820, 834, 844, 847, 848

bladder cancer, 439, 578–580

bleed, 11, 12, 13, 15, 16, 18, 23, 24, 40, 41, 42, 50, 124, 125, 132, 133, 134, 136, 139, 153, 154, 160, 204, 230, 231, 266, 279, 280, 327, 328, 346, 348, 355, 360, 372, 375–381, 398, 421, 479–483, 490, 494, 498, 499, 502, 516, 518, 533, 534, 535, 537, 539, 543, 546, 550, 551, 574, 580, 619, 622, 625, 630, 637, 656, 657, 666, 702t, 703t, 720t, 721, 738, 741, 742, 743, 788, 803, 828, 832, 835, 845–848, 858, 859, 868, 872, 874, 876

blepharitis, 643

blood-borne, 337, 338, 592

blood-brain, 44, 62

blood-neutralizing, 33

bloodstream, 57, 344, 371, 638, 737, 745, 760, 822

blotches, 154

body temperature, 231, 264, 278, 683

bone marrow, 522, 543

bone, 28, 266, 470, 500, 504, 519, 534, 543, 544, 545, 546, 547, 548, 550, 554, 558, 560, 568, 577, 623, 687, 773, 843

bordetella, 297

Bouchard nodes, 470

bowel, 51, 54, 74, 80, 201, 236, 328, 345, 355, 359, 360, 362–365, 368–373, 378, 379, 409, 420, 421, 448, 450, 486, 498, 506, 508, 514, 518, 520, 555, 557, 567, 575, 580, 685, 737, 738, 742, 747, 761, 771, 774, 790, 793, 796, 799, 802, 810, 833, 848, 856t, 860, 862, 887

brachial, 153, 238, 489, 564, 772, 812, 813

brachiocephalic, 236

brachytherapy, 29, 566, 573, 577, 581

bradyarrhythmia, 33, 126, 142, 202, 752t

bradycardia, 16, 32, 42, 50, 53, 76, 82, 98, 104, 105, 129, 132, 145, 149, 174, 178, 196, 198, 199, 202, 203, 212, 271, 272, 403, 450, 649, 709t, 729, 747, 748, 749, 753t, 754t, 790, 792, 793, 798, 801t

bradykinesia, 85, 88

brain, 3–8, 13, 15, 16, 18, 23, 25–28, 40–46, 56, 59–63, 65, 66, 72, 73, 78, 80, 81, 83, 89, 90, 210, 222, 281, 306, 344, 457, 461, 464, 543, 565, 597, 653, 654, 664, 665t, 694, 711, 712, 729, 730, 735, 737, 739, 744, 747, 765, 767, 781, 837, 857t, 868

brainstem, 46

brain tumor, 4, 15, 26–29, 61, 461, 464, 543, 664, 712

breast cancer, 569, 570

breast, 26, 162, 370, 518, 563, 567, 569, 570, 571, 574, 576, 580–582, 773, 856, 862, 886, 887, 891, 892, 893, 894, 895, 897

breathing, 18, 37, 46, 48, 49, 54, 63, 194, 216, 222, 223, 225, 226, 245, 246, 251, 267, 273, 275, 285, 286, 289, 305, 310, 312, 314, 316, 318, 319, 378, 443, 444, 499, 655, 779, 789, 828, 829, 863, 875, 876

Breslow staging, 620

broad-spectrum, 41, 328, 356, 371, 456, 495, 688, 746, 824

Bromocriptine, 87

bronchial provocation testing, 242

bronchiectasis, 60, 255, 298, 461

bronchiolitis, 847

bronchiolitis obliterans syndrome (BOS), 847

bronchitis, 245, 246, 249, 564, 683, 781

bronchoalveolar, 269, 270, 565, 821

bronchoconstriction, 268, 270

bronchodilation, 248

bronchodilator, 240–243, 248–252, 612, 783, 874

bronchogenic carcinoma, 294, 461

bronchopneumonia, 236,

bronchopulmonary, 263

bronchoscopy, 166, 255, 269, 270, 565

bronchospasm, 202, 225, 241, 251, 252, 257, 259, 333, 748, 749, 781, 783, 792, 805, 840t

brown spiders, 806

Brown-Séquard syndrome, 52

bruit, 5, 602, 654, 729, 856t, 861

budesonide (Nasacort, Rhinocort), 243, 363, 364, 656

bumetanide (Bumex), 103, 180, 181, 402

blood urea nitrogen (BUN), 74, 172, 179, 270, 272, 348, 355, 357, 365, 376, 378, 393, 395, 396, 397, 398, 409, 443, 444, 462, 482, 594, 623, 739, 771, 776, 777, 779, 838, 873, 876

BUN-to-creatinine ratio, 393, 395, 396

bupropion (Wellbutrin), 247, 698, 715, 718t, 799

burn, 164, 266, 392, 399, 502, 522, 537, 572, 612, 615, 619, 635, 641, 642, 644, 646, 694, 712, 723t, 741, 742, 764, 767, 776, 851–854

buspirone (BuSpar), 77, 458, 724, 725t

C

coronary artery bypass graft (CABG), 124, 128, 129, 132–135, 871

caffeine, 326, 665, 670t, 675t, 678t, 887, 893t

calcineurin inhibitors, 839, 840

calcitonin (Calcimar, Miacalcin), 774

calcium, 17, 24, 35, 53, 67, 74, 98, 101–105, 107, 108, 112, 120, 126, 127, 135, 155, 157, 179, 182, 183, 191, 198, 200, 201, 203, 206, 211, 216, 270, 273, 277, 330, 332, 356, 357, 397, 398, 402, 403, 404, 416, 417, 419–423, 465, 500, 560, 603, 668, 674t, 697, 742, 771–774, 776, 777, 778, 781, 785, 793, 813, 816t, 839, 843, 864, 873, 887, 893

calcium channel blocker overdose, 793

calories, 112, 117, 403, 429, 444, 760, 762, 763, 775, 785

cancer, 122, 160, 238, 287, 288, 296, 331, 362, 395, 409, 411, 439t, 441t, 448, 452t, 454, 461, 486t, 487t, 506t, 516, 537, 543, 545, 546, 547, 557, 559, 563–582, 596, 610, 617, 618, 636, 637, 665t, 689, 693, 695, 696, 699, 705t, 729, 773, 831, 843, 856t, 858, 872, 882, 884t–891t, 894, 895, 903

candida, 57, 386, 388, 560, 589, 651, 658, 659, 820, 822, 824, 843, 844t, 853

candidiasis, 248, 589, 596, 627, 628, 641, 684

candiduria, 388, 820

cannabis, 716

capillary dynamics, 737

capillary filling time (CFT), 738

captopril (Capoten), 101, 103, 109, 127, 175, 176, 184, 415, 416, 417

Carafate, 325

carbamazepine (Tegretol), 69, 70, 461, 662, 674t, 697, 708t, 720t

carbapenem, 299, 356, 611, 615, 746, 814

carbidopa (Lodosyn), 87, 88

carbidopa-levodopa (Sinemet), 86

carbon monoxide poisoning, 794

carcinoma, 294, 331, 338, 342, 343, 362, 371, 573, 574, 578, 617, 658, 684, 845

cardiac, 3, 4, 6, 9, 10, 16, 17, 32, 44, 49, 50, 73, 76, 95, 98, 111, 120–124, 126–131, 134, 135, 139, 141, 142, 143, 145, 147, 149, 153, 162, 163, 166, 168, 170, 171, 173, 176, 178, 182, 183, 186–190, 193, 194, 195, 198, 201, 209–212, 216, 224, 225, 226, 229, 230, 231, 234, 236, 237, 238, 241, 248, 253, 268, 269, 271, 272, 273, 276, 278, 286, 291, 294, 316, 319, 329, 346, 372, 393, 396, 416, 444, 445, 462, 463, 486t, 487t, 518, 524, 557, 559, 603, 623, 647, 653, 666t, 687, 688, 715, 721, 731t, 735, 736t, 738, 743, 744, 745, 747–751t, 754t, 765, 769, 770, 777, 781, 794, 799, 800t, 801t, 831, 832, 840t, 843, 847, 856t, 857t, 867, 874, 891, 893t, 896, 903

cardiac allograft vasculopathy (CAV), 847

cardiac arrest, 794

cardiac arrhythmias, 32, 33, 87, 101, 104, 123, 189, 194, 195, 198–216, 248, 253, 268, 271, 306, 315, 346, 372, 514, 603, 718, 719, 726, 743, 744, 748, 753, 759, 770, 775, 781, 784, 790, 799, 800, 801, 802, 807, 838, 847, 867, 868

cardiac catheterization, 182, 187, 188, 190, 195, 276

cardiac conditions, 166

cardiac cycle, 95

cardiac failure, 445, 524, 738

cardiac markers, 128, 129
cardiac tamponade, 135, 163, 557, 559, 745, 832, 867
cardioembolic, 6, 12
cardiogenic, 134, 135, 139, 230, 231, 237, 271, 290, 393, 734, 736t, 740, 743, 744, 750t, 751t, 792, 867
cardiogenic pulmonary edema, 237, 271–274, 738
cardiologist, 11, 198–201, 204, 206, 208, 209, 211, 212, 873
cardiomegaly, 9, 101, 172, 194, 195, 272, 401, 529, 729
cardiomyopathy, 3, 96, 97, 149, 170, 173, 178, 187, 193–196, 200, 209, 210, 248, 271, 559, 561, 735, 743, 744, 847
cardiopulmonary bypass, 135, 266
cardiovascular, 35, 49, 51, 68, 77, 97, 98, 103, 104, 107, 113, 154, 169, 172, 174, 176, 179, 183, 248, 251, 278, 401, 404, 427, 429, 440t, 443, 445, 471, 480t, 481t, 638, 684, 687, 703t, 704t, 742, 745, 748, 765, 768, 782, 784, 790, 799, 839, 847, 856t, 859, 873, 885, 886, 894, 903
cardiovascular assessment, 95–99
cardioversion, 122, 149, 187, 204, 205, 206, 207, 208, 209, 216
Cardizem, 126, 135, 195, 203
carotid, 3–6, 10, 12, 13, 21, 25, 95, 97, 113, 140, 190, 222, 647, 654, 729, 735, 856t
carotid bruits, 654, 729
carotid TIAs, 6
catabolic, 396, 399, 403, 767
Catapres, 104, 109, 403, 698, 722
cataract, 251, 430, 641, 644, 646, 648, 859
catecholamine, 51, 101, 105, 201, 204, 205, 274, 393, 457, 458, 459, 744, 750, 769
catheter, 18, 23, 44, 51, 132, 134, 141, 143, 160, 164, 166, 205, 207, 224, 227, 229, 230, 231, 237, 238, 273, 291, 311, 318, 370, 373, 376, 380, 386, 388, 389, 395, 396, 399, 410, 411, 443, 445, 525, 580, 684, 687, 688, 699, 740, 744, 746, 798, 819, 820, 822, 823, 826, 829, 832–835, 845, 856t, 863, 869, 874, 875, 876
Cauda equina syndrome, 506
causative organisms, 164, 262, 624
cauter, 378, 657
carcinoembryonic antigen (CEA), 6, 13, 568, 570
cefaclor (Ceclor), 387
cefazolin (Kefzol), 165, 166, 353, 366, 388, 495, 499, 614, 691, 813, 823, 824, 825t
cefepime (Maxipime), 60, 360, 367, 373, 388, 615, 690t, 691t, 747, 814, 820, 822, 823, 826t, 833
cefoperazone (Cefobid), 300
cefotaxime (Claforan), 59, 60, 165, 360, 365, 366, 388, 615, 626, 660, 690t, 691t
cefotetan (Cefotan), 366, 370, 626, 691t
cefoxitin (Mefoxin), 366, 370, 624, 626, 825
cefpodoxime (Vantin), 387, 653
ceftazidime (Tazicef), 299, 300, 367, 373, 388, 820, 822, 823, 826t, 833
ceftriaxone (Rocephin), 59, 60, 165, 166, 353, 360, 365, 366, 379, 387, 388, 615, 626, 633, 643, 660, 826t
celecoxib (Celebrex), 470

cellulitis, 613, 684, 691, 812, 815, 822, 825
central nervous system (CNS), 65, 684
cephalexin, 166, 388, 389, 495, 614, 659, 813, 814, 825t
cephalosporin, 59, 60, 166, 297, 298, 299, 353, 360, 365, 388, 389, 394, 499, 611, 626, 633, 660, 825
cerebellar, 14, 19, 25, 26, 27, 80, 81, 653
cerebellar hemangioblastoma, 27
cerebral, 3, 6, 8–19, 21, 23–28, 40, 42, 43, 44, 46, 60, 61, 62, 65, 67, 72, 75, 81, 109, 136, 171, 222, 306, 345, 443, 444, 445, 462, 465, 558, 646, 664, 665, 666t, 730, 735, 737, 739, 768
cerebral abscess, 60–61,
cerebral cortex, 222
cerebrospinal, 15, 24, 32, 40, 56, 58, 81, 687
cerebrospinal fluid (CSF), 15, 40, 81
cerebrovascular, 3, 4, 8, 128, 132, 135, 179, 650, 653, 731t, 857t, 858, 888, 898–903
cerebrovascular accidents, 3–20, 22–24, 132, 179, 650, 653, 731, 857, 858, i
cerebrovascular diseases, 898, 899, 900, 901, 902
certolizumab (Cimzia), 363, 364, 486t
cervical, 35, 36, 41, 45, 47, 48, 49, 52, 53, 90, 270, 340, 395, 472, 498, 507, 548, 560, 564, 571, 572, 573, 581, 596, 623, 625, 626, 628, 630, 633, 636, 637, 651, 659, 661, 665, 672t, 828, 829, 885, 886, 889t, 891, 895, 903
cervical cancer, 571, 582, 583, 596, 889
cervical spine, 47, 491, 498
cervical spondylosis, 665
cervical, 35, 36, 41, 45, 47, 49, 52, 53, 54, 90, 270, 340, 395, 472, 507, 560, 564, 571, 581, 582, 583, 623, 625, 626, 630, 633, 636, 637, 651, 659, 672, 828, 829, 885, 886, 891, 895, 903
cetirizine (Zyrtec), 655
CHAD score, 177, 204, 205, 207
charcoal, 789, 790, 802
chemoreceptor, 222, 289, 735
chemotherapy, 26, 27, 28, 256, 262, 268, 420, 535, 544, 545, 547, 549, 551, 558, 559, 561, 565, 566, 568, 571, 573, 574, 575, 577, 578, 580, 581, 621, 770, 777, 843
chest wall, 96, 145, 222, 226, 236, 238, 243, 245, 285–286, 288, 290, 293, 315
chest trauma, 829
chest x-ray, 6, 15, 28, 135, 194, 195, 239, 247, 252, 255, 263, 265, 266, 270, 272, 276, 279, 287, 294, 352, 365, 531, 560, 564, 568, 575, 592, 660, 730, 746, 821, 829, 830, 831, 832
chlamydia, 77, 79, 261, 297, 298, 299, 302, 387, 622, 626, 629, 631, 633, 642, 643, 659, 684, 891t, 895
chlorine, 268
chlorothiazide (Diuril), 103, 177, 179, 180, 181, 402,
chlorpropamide (Diabinese), 466
cholecystectomy, 353
cholecystitis, 351, 352, 353, 363
cholelithiasis, 351, 857t
cholesterol, 7, 78, 112–115, 117, 118, 120, 131, 351, 353, 356, 415, 416, 647, 760, 843, 885, 886, 889t, 891t, 892t, 903

cholinergic, 36, 37, 72, 76
cholinesterase, 35, 36, 76
cholinesterase inhibitors, 36
chronic kidney disease, 102, 106, 290, 399–405, 414, 514, 521, 603, 882
chronic lower respiratory disease, 898, 899, 900, 901, 902, 903
chronic lymphocytic leukemia, 533, 547, 554, 555, 556, 558
chronic myelogenous leukemia, 550
chronic obstructive pulmonary disease (COPD), 105, 245–252, 254, 255, 261, 263, 264, 273, 275, 276, 279, 290, 296, 297, 298, 309, 310, 782
chronic venous insufficiency (CVI), 152
cigarette, 22, 101, 107t, 113, 119, 245, 267, 271, 326, 578, 622, 655, 884t
cilostazol (Pletal), 153
cimetidine (Tagamet), 34, 108, 251, 329, 334, 354, 534, 678t
ciprofloxacin (Cipro), 299, 300, 302, 360, 363, 366, 367, 379, 387, 388, 652, 820, 822, 823, 826t
circumcision, 386, 591
cirrhosis, 286, 338, 339, 342, 343, 344, 363, 372, 375, 377, 378, 379, 463, 685, 764, 783, 898t–901t
citalopram hydrobromide (Celexa), 77, 715, 717t
clarithromycin (Biaxin), 166, 297, 301, 302, 303, 331, 595, 659
claudication, 124, 152, 153, 157, 506, 514, 601, 665t, 810, 859
claustrophobic, 312
clavicle, 49, 235, 236, 602
clavulanate, 297, 298, 301, 302, 360, 387, 518, 643, 658, 808
clindamycin (Cleocin), 166, 298, 299, 300, 499, 614, 615, 626, 628, 629, 659, 660, 691t, 813, 814, 822, 825
clindamycin hydrochloride (Cleocin), 626
clinging, 287
clinical perfusion, 229–230
clonal stem cell disorder, 550
clonazepam (Klonopin), 77, 674t, 698, 725t, 791
clonidine (Catapres), 104, 105, 108, 109, 403, 459, 674t, 698, 700, 722
clopidogrel (Plavix), 7, 12, 123, 127, 130, 133, 136, 154, 177, 178
closed-angle glaucoma, 649
Clostridium difficile colitis, 824
clozapine (Clozaril), 685
cluster headache, 664, 669, 679
coagulopathies, 533–537
cocaine, 4, 7, 14, 108, 128, 193, 200, 337, 678, 685, 801, 805
coccidioidomycosis, 267, 268, 270, 596
cognitive, 17, 73, 74, 80, 81, 83, 307, 525, 603, 695, 700, 709t, 724, 727, 730
colchicine, 163, 420, 474
colestipol (Colestid), 115, 348
colic, 352, 369, 421, 422, 774

colitis, 342, 360–363, 379, 380, 684, 685, 824, 826, 848
colloid, 134, 231, 232, 325, 348, 376, 570, 666t, 737, 742, 786, 852
colloid solutions, 231
colloidal bismuth suspension, 325
colon, 287, 359, 360, 362, 364, 369, 370, 379, 380, 478t, 563, 567, 568, 569, 573, 574, 576, 684, 689, 771, 819, 825, 887
colon cancer and, 887
colonoscopy, 166, 360, 380, 568, 886, 887, 889t, 892t
colorectal cancer, 567, 582, 889
coma, 14, 41, 62, 63, 300, 427, 430, 443, 444, 445, 449, 450, 528, 765, 766, 767, 773, 779, 781, 782, 788–793, 796, 797, 798, 804, 807, 828, 854, 867, 868
comatose, 42, 44, 62
community-acquired, 261, 262, 296–299, 302, 353, 683, 825, 826t
community-acquired infection, 825
community-resistance, 389
comorbidities, 33, 38, 89, 154, 158, 173, 179, 187, 188, 192, 248, 253, 254, 257, 261, 290, 296, 298, 392, 420, 431, 433, 448, 459, 591, 593, 596, 614, 647, 686, 689, 760, 868, 896
compartment syndrome, 502, 504
complete blood count (CBC), 5, 263
concussion, 41
congenital, 21, 24, 25, 56, 60, 97, 164, 166, 170, 189, 190, 275, 285, 469, 488, 489, 498, 588, 620, 622, 847, 900t
congestion, 172, 173, 179, 652, 655, 657, 668, 669t, 743
congestive, 3, 4, 49, 73, 75, 83, 100, 118, 125, 181, 191, 194, 237, 276, 278, 286, 372, 393, 402, 445, 486t, 516, 735, 743, 757, 764, 783, 867, 873
congestive heart failure, 764
conjunctiva, 58, 401, 518, 641, 642, 644, 667, 669t
conjunctivitis, 603, 630, 641–644, 655, 777
continuous positive airway pressure (CPAP), 316
contraceptive, 3, 7, 101, 111, 113, 372, 428, 521, 531, 574, 608t, 622, 625, 629, 647, 678t, 728, 872
contrast-induced, 394, 407, 415, 416
contusion, 41, 52, 122, 490, 492, 743, 829, 831
Cooling blankets, 689
core needle biopsy, 570
cornea, 46, 344, 641–644, 648, 649, 650, 777, 791
corneal abrasion, 641, 643, 644–645
coronary, 98, 100, 109–113, 119, 120, 122–127, 129–137, 139, 140, 141, 149, 152, 156, 169, 171, 173, 179, 182, 187, 190, 191, 207, 248, 271, 378, 416, 450, 591, 668, 735, 737, 738, 744, 847, 856t, 857t, 871, 872, 873, 891t–894
coronary artery, 119, 131, 133, 196, 207, 271, 873
coronary artery disease, 100, 110, 111–118, 119, 129, 131, 134, 149, 152, 156, 169, 173, 187, 190, 191, 207, 248, 271, 348, 416, 450, 591, 847, 857, 872, 873, 892, 894

corticosteroids, 12, 28, 33, 44, 53, 163, 196, 248–254, 257–260, 269, 271, 298, 326, 354, 361–364, 400, 465, 471, 474, 479t, 485t, 498, 545, 597, 603, 608t, 612, 616, 644, 648, 652, 655, 656, 658, 698, 746, 747, 749, 806, 838, 839, 841t, 843, 847, 872

cortisol, 264, 453, 454, 455, 765, 766

Cortisporin otic, 652, 653

costochondral junctions, 286

costochondritis, 286

costophrenic, 236, 237, 287

costosternal, 285, 286

costovertebral, 386, 421

cough, 37, 57, 82, 104, 164, 171, 172, 174, 179, 201, 240, 242, 243, 245, 247, 248, 249, 252, 255, 261, 262, 264, 268, 270, 272, 280, 305, 318, 333, 508, 564, 597, 611, 655, 656, 821, 829, 830, 838t, 841t, 847, 859, 876

coumadin (Warfarin), 6, 160, 205, 279, 604, 674t

Coxiella, 164, 906

coxsackie, 162, 650

crackles, 171, 263, 268, 270, 329, 355, 765, 856t

cramp, 37, 115, 121, 154, 360, 369, 372, 380, 402, 415, 462, 551, 625, 694, 748, 760, 762, 769, 783, 797

craniectomy, 27, 45

craniofacial, 86

craniopharyngioma, 27

c-reactive, 123, 355, 359, 478t, 602, 626, 746

creatine, 122, 129, 131, 372, 392, 398, 401, 503, 614, 739, 777, 797

creatinine, 9, 11, 74, 76, 101, 172, 174, 175, 179, 270, 272, 296, 346, 348, 357, 369, 376, 378, 392–399, 401, 402, 405, 409, 411, 428, 438t, 444, 446, 458, 465, 529, 536, 594t, 598t, 623, 666t, 739, 740, 771, 776, 777, 779, 787, 808, 838t, 844, 845, 873, 876

cremasteric, 49

crisis intervention, 727, 895

critical care monitoring, 443, 445

Crohn's disease, 326, 360, 362, 364, 368, 369, 516, 685, 688, 848

cryoprecipitate, 538

cryotherapy, 572, 577, 646

cryptococcus, 57, 613, 844t

cryptosporidium, 351, 589, 844t

crystalloid solutions, 231

Cushing's syndrome, 63, 101, 427, 452, 769, 780

cyanosis, 156, 210, 226, 318, 538, 564, 782, 793, 796, 804, 830, 831

cyanotic, 68, 166, 738, 742

cyclobenzaprine (Flexeril), 490, 494, 507, 509

cyclophosphamide (Cytoxan), 83, 269, 271, 280, 281, 400, 462, 535, 545, 549, 558, 560, 561, 571

cyclosporine, 108, 361–364, 394, 472, 483t, 770, 839, 840t, 842t, 843

cyst, 470, 570, 574

cystic, 268, 351, 352, 428, 846

cystic fibrosis, 274, 428

cystine calculi, 421, 422

cytokines, 683, 838

cytologic smears, 581

cytology, 558, 565, 579, 865, 889

cytomegalovirus, 31, 57, 59, 61, 326, 344, 351, 354, 394, 592, 597, 650, 684, 843, 844t

D

dabigatran (Pradaxa), 11, 160, 177, 205, 279, 803

dalteparin (Fragmin), 159, 803

d-dimer, 159, 538, 546

deafness, 56, 396

death, 7, 14, 18, 32, 40, 46, 48, 53, 80, 83, 111, 114, 119, 120, 128, 129, 131, 149, 169, 196, 203, 209, 210, 262, 278, 291, 306, 343, 356, 414, 465, 479, 485–487, 543, 557, 559, 563, 569, 571, 573, 619, 620, 667, 702, 714, 716, 727, 734, 739, 745, 793, 807, 843, 847, 848, 851, 854, 858, 886, 898–904

debridement, 61, 471, 473, 499, 811, 813, 814, 815, 816, 826, 853

decongestants, 396, 409, 656, 825

defibrillator, 149, 178, 196, 238

dehydration, 44, 175, 190, 221, 263, 278, 353, 355, 362, 365, 368, 369, 402, 412, 419, 428, 429, 442–444, 462, 465, 477, 507, 514, 530, 531, 627, 641, 653, 796

delirium, 72, 75, 171, 449, 687, 716, 723, 726, 729–731, 788, 790, 792, 796, 800, 808, 874

dementia, 25, 26, 72–78, 86, 136, 251, 290, 296, 514, 516, 597, 711, 726, 729–731, 796, 808, 882, 894

demyelination, 32, 33, 79, 462

denervation, 847

depression, 36, 51, 68, 74, 75, 77, 82, 86, 88, 105, 120, 121, 122, 124, 126, 130, 131, 133, 174, 195, 248, 290, 310, 314, 450, 452, 490, 516, 525, 529, 603, 668, 670, 678, 695, 698, 712–719, 724, 727, 728, 772, 773, 860, 889, 892–896

dermatitis medicamentosa (drug eruption), 453, 463, 470, 476, 608, 610–612

desmopressin, 465

dexamethasone (Decadron), 28, 60, 101, 453, 545, 656, 675

dexlansoprazole (Dexilant), 330, 335, 659

dextran, 348, 520, 748

dextrose, 60, 231, 345, 353, 443, 763, 768, 780, 785, 786, 789, 790, 820, 875

diabetes mellitus, 4 6, 9, 13, 43, 102, 106, 111–116, 119, 128, 131, 135, 152, 153, 154, 156, 157, 169, 173, 174, 179, 204, 251, 262, 263, 271, 296, 300, 341, 342, 386, 392, 402, 416, 419, 427–447, 449, 464–466, 521, 580, 591, 596, 613, 641, 645–647, 650, 653, 686, 687, 711, 715, 720, 729, 731, 741, 746, 767, 768, 773, 796, 810, 826, 839, 844, 847, 856–858, 873, 882, 885, 889, 891, 894, 898–904

diabetes insipidus, 43, 392, 464–466, 720, 741, 767, 768, 773, 796

diabetic retinopathy, 645–646

diabetic ulcers, 814

diagnostic criteria for PID, 625

diarrhea, 37, 82, 83, 88, 105, 115, 116, 175, 202, 203, 231, 330, 340, 346, 359, 360, 364, 366, 369, 380, 392, 421, 422, 441, 445, 454, 482, 483, 487, 551, 589, 597, 623, 708, 709, 714, 720, 724, 741, 748, 759, 762, 764, 767, 769, 774, 779, 790, 792, 794, 795, 797, 824, 826, 840, 841, 859

diastolic dysfunction, 193, 316

diazepam (Valium), 67, 84, 86, 87, 92, 490, 494, 507, 509, 654, 698, 721, 725, 791, 800, 802, 805

differential diagnosis, 86, 453, 592, 623, 749, 862

digital plethysmography, 812

digitalis toxicity, 199, 771

digoxin (Lanoxin), 108, 176, 177, 196, 201, 203, 211, 373, 769, 794, 795, 847

digoxin toxicity, 795

dilated cardiomyopathy, 194, 195

dilaudid, 353, 356, 367, 373, 499, 530, 696, 706, 830, 831

diltiazem, 104, 126, 127, 135, 179, 191, 195, 200, 225, 201, 203, 206, 277, 793

diphenhydramine (Benadryl), 403, 520, 612, 655, 749, 806

diphtheria, 906

dipyridamole, 7, 12, 126, 872

discharge summary, 865

disequilibrium, 653

dislocations, 488, 489, 491

disorientation, 74, 444, 731

disseminated intravascular coagulation (DIC), 537–539, 546, 614, 739

diuretics, 28, 43, 101–108, 172, 173, 174, 177, 179–183, 190, 195, 196, 277, 348, 354, 387, 392–396, 402, 409, 412, 416, 421, 423, 428, 459, 462, 504, 641, 654, 741, 744, 764–766, 769, 770, 772, 773, 774, 776, 780, 781, 796, 839

diverticulitis, 359, 360, 363, 370, 371, 684

dizziness, 7, 41, 87, 88, 105, 116, 124, 126, 189, 198, 202, 203, 409, 445, 479–483, 486, 487, 514, 519, 550, 623, 697, 702, 704, 707–709, 717–720, 725, 752, 790, 794–796, 859

dobutamine (Dobutrex), 126, 134, 181, 273, 356, 373, 744, 747, 749–751, 847

dopamine, 18, 50, 85, 86, 87, 134, 199, 212, 356, 458, 666, 744, 747–750, 753, 791, 793, 801

Doppler echocardiogram, 126, 187, 188

Doppler pressure studies, 812

doxycycline (Vibramycin), 297, 298, 302, 303, 614, 615, 626, 631, 633, 635, 643, 658, 690, 814

drainage, 20, 43, 53, 56, 247, 255, 288, 294, 357, 396, 494, 495, 568, 652, 655, 657, 658, 691, 747, 767, 779, 811, 812, 814, 816, 819, 825, 831, 844, 846, 848, 865, 875, 876

drowsiness, 14, 42, 61, 63, 88, 105, 415, 443, 482, 707, 709, 717–720, 725, 739, 782, 791, 797, 798, 803

drug interactions with, 105, 108, 593

drug-induced, 394, 485, 520, 535, 602, 610

drug-resistant, 264, 592, 595, 746

dual-chamber, 143, 144, 196

duodenal ulcers, 326, 329, 331

duodenum, 238, 325, 326, 377, 761

dysfunctional grief, 727, 728

dysgerminoma, 574

dyspareunia, 625

dyspepsia, 115, 327, 352, 481, 574, 704

dysplasia, 3, 362, 414, 415, 469, 480, 481, 545, 572, 636, 637, 703

dyspnea, 121, 124, 163, 164, 171, 179, 186, 188, 189, 191, 194, 196, 203, 226, 240, 245, 247, 251, 252, 255, 261, 268, 270, 272, 276, 278, 280, 286, 294, 347, 364, 365, 401, 447, 458, 514, 519, 543, 551, 564, 597, 660, 748, 782, 838, 840, 847, 854, 856, 859

dyspnea on exertion (DOE), 859

dysuria, 359, 386, 408, 421, 630, 632, 634, 860

E

echocardiogram, 101, 126, 135, 163, 164, 172, 178, 186, 187, 188, 190, 194, 195, 208, 211, 212, 276, 740, 743, 744

ectopic pregnancy, 200, 201, 622–639, 777

ectopic tissue calcification, 777

ectopy, 98, 135, 172, 203, 856

edema, 5, 12, 16, 18, 19, 28, 41–44, 48, 49, 61, 62, 82, 109, 128, 129, 135, 153–155, 159, 160, 170, 171, 179, 181, 183, 194, 202, 203, 225, 230, 236, 237, 252, 271–274, 276, 290, 306, 314, 328, 329, 345, 346, 348, 372, 398, 401, 415, 443, 445, 455, 462, 465, 480, 481, 487, 514, 537, 570, 576, 580, 608, 610–614, 630, 632, 633, 642, 645, 646, 651, 652, 658, 659, 665, 702, 704, 708, 709, 726, 737, 738, 742, 743, 744, 748, 749, 757, 765, 768, 783, 785, 806, 811, 812, 823, 838, 840, 841, 845, 847, 852, 853, 856, 859, 875

Ehlers-Danlos syndrome, 189, 488

electrocardiogram, 9, 36, 75, 76, 83, 98, 101, 129, 141, 216, 276, 352, 616, 715, 769, 829, 832, 863, 871

electroencephalogram, 62

electroencephalography, 6, 28, 46, 75, 712, 730

electrolytes, 5, 15, 34, 44, 59, 63, 67, 74, 101, 133, 163, 177, 209, 211, 272, 346, 353, 368, 378, 421, 445, 499, 503, 654, 666, 712, 721, 744, 763, 778, 781, 785, 790, 796, 875

electromyelography (EMG), 508

electrophoresis, 515, 524, 529, 647

eletriptan (Relpax), 668, 671

embolism, 31, 32, 35, 157, 249, 276, 299, 301, 302, 303, 396, 440, 460, 647, 685, 688, 783

emesis, 769

emphysema, 237, 241, 245, 246, 249, 275, 276, 294, 318, 781

enalapril (Vasotec), 103, 175, 176, 182, 184, 417

encephalitis, 61–63, 73, 636, 653, 664, 665, 684

encephalopathy, 10, 63 109, 337, 344, 345–347, 363, 377, 399, 464, 597, 721, 752, 770, 788, 846

end-diastolic filling pressure, 230

endobronchial lesions, 255

endobronchial, 846

endocarditis, 5, 6, 9, 60, 97, 163–166, 186–191, 647, 684, 688, 822, 823, 826

endocrine, 27, 32, 46, 63, 101, 170, 195, 522, 731, 856, 860, 868

endocrinopathies, 685

endodermal sinus tumor, 574
endometrial biopsy (EMB), 581
endometrial cancer, 567, 569, 574, 576, 582
endoscopic retrograde cholangiopancreatography (ERCP), 352
endoscopic third ventriculostomy, 26
endoscopy, 327–329, 331, 333, 376–378, 517, 519, 688
enema, 347, 359, 360, 361, 364, 371, 398, 568, 575, 688, 863, 886
enoxaparin (Lovenox), 124, 159, 279, 280, 803
enteral nutrition, 357, 760, 763
enteral therapy, 768
eosinophilia, 395, 400, 610
ependymoma, 26
epigastric, 66, 326–328, 352, 354, 355, 415
epigastric pain, 326, 328
epigastric tenderness, 326, 355
epiglottitis, 660–663
epilepsy, 65, 67, 528,
epinephrine, 18, 40, 41, 170, 210, 212, 378, 457, 458, 520, 611, 612, 744, 747–750, 753, 769, 793, 800, 806
epistaxis, 101, 109, 401, 641, 656, 657
epithelial cell, 572
eplerenone (Inspra), 103, 175, 176, 184, 770, 781
epoprostenol (Flolan), 277
eprosartan (Teveten), 104, 176, 417
Epstein-Barre, 57, 59, 79, 162, 344, 471, 557, 559, 650, 684, 843, 844
eradication therapy, 330
erection, 49, 411
Erysipelothrix rhusiopathiae, 613
erythema, 378, 483–486, 494, 608, 610, 611, 613, 615, 618, 628, 630, 632–634, 651, 659, 705, 748, 806, 811, 812, 823, 838, 875
erythromycin, 300–303, 354, 614, 631, 643, 813, 825
erythropoietin, 404, 531
Escherichia coli, 57, 299, 380, 385, 559, 613, 745, 819, 826
esmolol (Brevibloc), 18, 135, 202
esomeprazole (Nexium), 330, 335, 659
esophageal varices, 375–377, 378, 846
esophagitis, 121, 327, 329, 332–335
esophagostomy, 761
ethambutol (Myambutol), 59, 265
ethanolamine, 376
ethylene glycol toxicity, 804
eustachian tube dysfunction, 652
euvolemia, 17, 19, 400, 740, 765
euvolemic hyponatremia, 764
expiratory flow rates, 246
extended-release, 7, 12, 116, 301, 302, 387, 437, 441, 696, 700, 706, 770
extubation, 319
eyes, 9, 14, 41, 46, 62, 66, 86, 442, 450, 516, 617, 619, 636, 641, 655, 686, 836, 856, 859, 861

F

famciclovir (Famvir), 616, 636
famotidine (Pepcid), 329
fascia, 502
fatigue, 35, 48, 80, 82, 83, 105, 115, 124, 154, 164, 171, 179, 186, 188, 189, 191, 194, 198, 200–206, 208, 245, 267, 276, 309, 340, 345, 401, 430, 433, 443, 447, 450, 454, 471, 482, 483, 485, 514, 519–522, 524, 528, 543, 546, 548–550, 567, 589, 615, 634, 650, 687, 695, 697, 698, 708, 713, 717, 720, 725, 795, 838, 840, 856, 858, 903
fecal occult blood testing (FOBT), 567
fecaliths, 366
feces, 368, 370
felodipine (Plendil), 104, 108, 127, 793
fenoldopam (Corlopam), 110
fentanyl, 43, 356, 530, 696, 699, 700, 701, 706
ferritin, 343, 380, 472, 515, 517, 522, 523, 525
fever, 17, 45, 57, 60–62, 135, 158, 159, 162–164, 186, 190, 200, 224, 249, 252, 262–264, 287, 328, 340, 351, 352, 355, 356, 359, 360, 362–364, 366, 386, 394, 395, 400, 412, 447, 449, 455, 465, 473, 476, 485, 487, 506, 528–530, 543, 546, 548, 550, 557, 559, 564, 588, 589, 592, 596, 597, 601–603, 611, 613–615, 625, 627, 632, 634, 635, 638, 651, 657–660, 665, 683–691, 729, 783, 796, 806, 807, 819, 821–826, 838, 840, 841, 843, 858, 876, 898, 906
fexofenadine (Allegra), 655
fibrates, 115, 117, 118
fibrillation, 3, 4, 6, 8, 11, 96, 105, 132, 134, 135, 137, 147, 171–173, 177–179, 186, 187, 188, 189, 194–196, 201, 203–205, 207–210, 214, 279, 372, 447, 647, 805, 867
fibrinogen, 266, 376, 537, 538, 539, 546, 647
fibrinogen consumption, 537
fibrinolytic therapy, 120, 124, 127–133, 136, 137, 280, 537
fibromuscular dysplasia, 414, 415, 418
fibrosis, 157, 186, 194, 202, 212, 235, 267–270, 294, 341, 342, 368, 428, 472, 559, 561, 846, 847
finasteride, 409, 576
fish tapeworm, 517
Flagyl, 331, 360, 363
flail chest, 309, 315, 782, 830
flank pain, 386, 473, 804
flecainide, 202, 207, 790
Flomax, 409, 422
fluconazole (Diflucan), 388, 471, 596, 597, 628, 659, 689, 820, 824, 843
fludarabine (Fludara), 549
fluid resuscitation, 49, 136, 231, 262, 267, 345, 365, 376, 378, 443, 499, 739, 744, 747, 786, 832–834, 852
flumazenil (Romazicon), 783
fluoroquinolone, 35, 297–299, 360, 365, 387, 388, 658
fluoxetine (Prozac), 685, 715
fluticasone (Flonase), 656
folate, 73, 75, 361, 364, 515, 517, 518, 520, 521, 571, 715
folic acid deficiency, 520–521
fondaparinux (Arixtra), 159, 160, 279, 536, 803

fracture, 40, 41, 46, 47, 52, 54, 60, 236, 278, 286, 330, 461, 469, 488–490, 494, 497–500, 502, 504, 524, 543, 656, 699, 712, 741, 743, 829–832, 834, 835, 890

Framingham score, 101, 886

friction rub, 97

frovatriptan (Frova), 671, 676

fungal, 56, 57, 60, 61, 135, 164, 267–270, 287, 386, 484, 522, 613, 651, 657, 658, 684, 745, 826, 843, 844

furosemide (Lasix), 103, 108, 180, 181, 348, 354, 396, 402, 462, 463, 504, 641, 766, 769, 771, 774

G

gabapentin (Neurontin), 34, 69, 70, 507, 674, 697, 708

galantamine hydrobromide (Razadyne), 76

gallbladder, 351–353, 747

gallstones, 115, 351–357, 524

gangrene, 153, 352, 366, 429, 430, 537, 812, 815, 816

gardasil, 573

gastrectomy, 51

gastric atony, 51

gastric lavage, 792, 796

gastric outlet obstruction, 328

gastric ulcers, 326

gastritis, 121, 327, 335, 364, 378, 515

gastroepiploic artery, 134

gastroesophageal, 251, 329, 332–335, 500

gastroesophageal reflux disease (GERD), 332, 333, 334, 335

gastrointestinal, 26, 50, 53, 62, 121, 163, 166, 237, 266, 269, 325–381, 392, 396, 398, 401, 417, 422, 449, 480, 481, 482, 484, 487, 518, 519, 521, 522, 537, 592, 694, 696, 721, 722, 760, 764, 768, 773, 774, 826, 848, 859, 868

gastrointestinal bleeding, 348, 375–381, 398, 537, 721, 848, 868

gastrostomy, 761

gemfibrozil (Lopid), 139, 141

generalized seizures, 66

genetic, 80, 85, 101, 116, 157, 170, 189, 252, 278, 326, 340, 342, 343, 419, 428, 430, 458, 469, 471, 477, 523, 524, 531, 544, 545, 558, 569, 574, 578, 602, 607, 716, 728, 838, 845, 881, 882, 885, 893

genital lesions, 638, 862

genitourinary, 26, 51, 164, 385–426, 518, 537, 632, 746, 835, 856, 860, 862

gentamicin (Garamycin), 165, 299, 365, 388, 495, 499, 626, 643, 645, 747, 820, 822, 823, 826, 827

germ cell tumors, 574, 575

giant cell arteritis, 5, 6, 601–602, 647, 664, 665, 684

glaucoma, 430

glioblastoma multiforme, 26

Global Institute for Chronic Obstructive Lung Disease (GOLD), 256

glucagon, 434, 441, 446, 793, 794

glucocorticoid, 106, 271, 280, 326, 427, 452–455, 487, 659, 735, 749

glucose, 58, 62, 67, 74, 287, 347, 365, 441, 443, 446, 592, 695, 785, 794

glycosuria, 428, 443, 453, 458

gonorrhea, 642, 643

gout, 420, 422, 473, 474, 494, 685, 860

graft thrombosis, 844

gram-negative, 60, 165, 261, 298, 299, 362, 363, 365, 388, 389, 468, 495, 537, 559, 561, 613, 624, 632, 745, 746, 815, 816, 821, 823, 825, 826, 844, 853

gram-positive, 388, 389, 495, 499, 613, 745, 814–816, 821, 823, 825, 826, 853

grief, 727, 728

guaifenesin (Mucinex), 251

Guillain-Barré, 31–43, 290, 314, 458, 461, 781

gynecomastia, 329, 411

H

H&P, 855, 865, 869

Haemophilus influenzae, 262

hallucinations, 62, 66, 87t, 88t, 667, 709t, 714, 716, 723t, 731(t), 782, 795, 799

haloperidol (Haldol), 77, 404, 685, 713, 719t, 726t, 730, 798

head trauma, 12, 40–46, 57, 60, 65, 300, 461, 684, 690, 731, 783

headache, 7, 14, 16, 22, 23, 25–28, 41, 42, 51, 57, 59–63, 67, 82, 87t, 88t, 101, 104, 105, 109, 116, 126, 164, 202t, 203t, 249, 262, 415, 442, 452, 454, 457, 462, 479t–483t, 485t–487t, 516, 519, 546, 596, 601, 615, 634, 638, 648, 655, 657, 661, 662, 664, 665(t), 666(t), 667–668, 669t–676t, 702t, 704t, 707t–709t, 717t–720t, 723t, 724, 725t, 749, 752t, 765, 781, 782, 793–797, 804, 806–807, 842t, 854, vi, xvi

Healthy People 2020, 882, 883, 896

heart failure (HF), 49, 73, 75, 77, 83, 88, 96, 100, 118, 123, 125, 126, 130, 134, 135, 136, 153, 158, 168–184, 186, 188, 191, 193–196, 202, 204, 207, 216, 236, 237, 252, 262, 263, 268, 271–273, 276, 287, 290, 296, 306, 329, 372, 393, 394, 402, 412, 415, 438, 439, 443, 445, 480, 481, 486, 487, 514, 516, 597, 603, 649, 687, 702, 725, 735, 743, 744, 750, 752, 757, 764, 783, 794, 816, 847, 867, 873

heart transplant, 108t, 173f, 241, 847

heartburn, 326, 333, 334

heatstroke, 685

HEENT (head, ears, eyes, nose, and throat), 859

hematemesis, 327, 375, 378, 859

hematochezia, 327, 375, 859

hematocrit, 17, 43, 50, 133, 231, 247, 276, 277, 328, 355, 357, 361t, 362, 365, 369, 371, 375, 378, 443, 513, 520, 529, 544, 561, 623, 624, 654, 739, 742, 758, 833–4, 873–4, 876

hematology, 526, 531, 532, 536, 538, 539, 544, 547, 548, 551, 558, 560, 859

hematoma, 4, 12, 15, 19, 22, 41, 42, 47, 52, 54, 73, 75, 133, 368, 490, 493, 665(t), 685, 711–2, 730, 876

hematuria, 101, 164, 366, 386, 397t, 400f, 409, 421, 472, 537, 576, 578–9, 603, 819, 834, 844–5, 848, 860

hemiparesis, 14, 41, 42, 60, 62, 482t

hemodialysis, 164, 262, 340, 398, 403–405, 500, 504, 517, 771, 774, 776, 778, 781, 789, 796–7, 804–5

hemodynamic monitoring, 740, 744, 755, 833, 834
hemodynamic support, 280, 747, 791
hemophilia, 364, 469, 539
hemorrhage, 4, 5, 9–12, 14, 15, 17, 19, 22, 23, 24, 45, 52, 75, 109, 125t, 127, 132, 136t, 164, 221, 230, 231, 236, 333, 345, 346, 355, 362, 372, 375–379, 392, 416, 454, 459, 464, 502, 518, 528, 535, 537–8, 603, 623, 645–7, 653, 664–5(t), 666t, 684–5, 735, 737, 740, 803, 828, 833, 835, 867, 889t, x, xxiii, xxiv
hemorrhagic stroke, 7, 11, 13–19, 136
hemorrhoids, 379, 862
hemothorax, 237, 286, 831
heparin, 6, 7, 10, 11, 13, 34, 45, 50, 124, 130f, 137t, 156, 159, 160, 187, 227, 279, 280, 373, 533–6, 538, 647, 666t, 770, 803, v, xv
heparin-induced thrombocytopenia (HIT), 159, 279, 535–536
hepatic, 63, 69t, 76, 108t, 115, 190, 247, 251, 329, 337, 341–345, 347, 353, 363, 377, 393, 437t–8t, 479t–82t, 536, 568, 612, 623, 685, 701t–2t, 708t, 715, 721, 730, 757, 759, 764, 766, 770, 783, 788, 833, 845–6, 868, iii
hepatic artery thrombosis (HAT), 845
hepatic artery, 845, 846
hepatic encephalopathy, 344, 347
hepatitis, 31, 162, 202t, 336–341, 343–346, 348, 473, 486t–7t, 531, 557–8, 573, 592, 596, 610, 631, 636, 684, 685, 844t, 845, 858, 889t, 893t, 896, 901t, 906, 908t–9t, iii, ix, xiii
hepatitis A virus (HAV), 336
hepatitis B vaccine (Hep B), 338
hepatitis B virus (HBV), 337
hepatitis D virus (delta agent), 339
hepatitis G virus (HGV), 339
hepatomegaly, 170, 171, 179, 340, 516, 529, 550, 557, 564, 578
hepatosplenomegaly, 514, 524, 544, 546, 548, 872
hepatotoxic, 115t, 116t, 117, 202t, 337, 343, 348, 364t, 788
hernia, 10, 15, 23, 25, 42, 43, 44, 52, 237, 332, 335, 368, 369, 371, 856b
herniated disk, 52, 506, 508
herpes, 57, 59, 61, 62, 79, 344, 589, 597, 615–7, 627, 634–6, 641–2, 644, 650, 684, 844t, 906, v, vi, xv, xvi
herpes simplex virus (HSV), 61
herpes zoster, 616, 617, 650
histamine, 242, 329, 503, 515, 611, 693, 749
Histoplasmosis, 267, 268, 270, 597, 684
Hodgkin's lymphoma, 558, 616, 647, 843, v, xv
holosystolic, 96, 67, 188
Home Access Express Test, 590
homeostasis, 375, 428, 518
homosexuality, 386
hordeolum, xxii
hormone, 22, 32, 42, 43, 50, 62, 101, 158, 170, 272, 391, 393, 403, 408, 409, 414, 420, 433, 447, 449–50, 452, 454, 458, 461–2, 464, 570, 654, 735, 764, 773–4, 843, 860, 892t, 894, 896, iv, xiv

hospital-acquired, 262, 299t, 300t, 388, 683, 819–20, 822
hospital-acquired infection, 819
hospital-associated, 393
human papillomavirus (HPV), 571, 618, 636–637, 903, 906
Huntington's disease, 72, 731t
hydralazine (Apresoline), 16, 103t, 110, 173f, 174, 175, 183, 403, 602, 608t
hydrobromide, 76
hydrocephalus, 15, 16, 18, 23–27, 29, 73, 75, 666t, i, x
hydrochloride, 108t, 109, 389, 403, 404, 439t, 441t, 466, 615, 626
hydrocodone, 163, 422, 490, 495, 499, 507, 509, 652, 696, 701t, 706t, 797
hydrocortisone (Solu-Cortef), 361, 364t, 449, 451, 455–6, 479t, 612, 675t, 747, 749
hydromorphone (Dilaudid), 353, 356, 367, 373, 422, 499, 530, 696, 699, 700, 701t, 706t, 806, 830–1
hydroxychloroquine, 603
hymenoptera, 805
hyperactivity, 712
hyperaldosteronism, 780
hyperbilirubinemia, 342
hypercalcemia, 63, 75, 98, 104, 270, 354, 420, 444, 448, 455, 458, 465, 570, 773–4, 868, vii, xvii
hypercalciuria, 441, 444, 446, 447
hypocalciuric, 420
hypercalciuric calcium nephrolithiasis, 420
hypercarbia, 246
hypercatabolic, 403
hypercellular, 544
hyperchloremic, 231, 770
hypercholesterolemia, 131t, 443, 450
hypercoagulability, 158, 278, 695,
hypercoagulopathy, 5
hyperextension, 46, 52
hyperflexion, 46
hyperglycemia, 5, 28, 104, 116t, 249, 269, 271, 355, 357, 376, 427, 442, 444, 449, 453, 458, 479t, 645, 695, 726t, 739, 753t, 762–3, 766–8, 770, 793, 796, 800t, 802, 838t, 840t–1t, 872
hyperkalemia, 98, 104, 105, 108t, 174, 175, 355, 396, 398, 403, 412, 443, 455, 466, 480t–1t, 703t, 770, 792–3, 795, 852, 868, vii, xvii
hyperlipidemia, 4–8, 111, 119, 152, 154, 156, 416, 591, 764, 766, 839, 840t, 856b–7b, 889t, 890t–1t, i, x
hypermagnesemia, 98, 330, 398, 404, 775, 868, vii, xvii
hypermetabolic, 309, 448
hypernatremia, 43, 346, 394, 398, 412, 453, 465–6, 767–8, 771, 785, 868, vii, xvii
hyperosmolar, 44, 427, 430, 444–5, 786, 868, iv
hyperosmolar hyperglycemic nonketosis (HHNK), 430, 434, 444–445, 868
hyperoxaluric calcium nephrolithiasis, 420
hyperparathyroidism, 63, 404, 419, 420, 522, 773–4, 776
hyperphosphatemia, 398, 403, 404, 777, vii, xvii

hyperpigmented, 154

hypersensitivity, 263

hypertension (HTN), 8, 100

hypertension, 4, 6, 8, 10, 16, 17, 23, 24, 33, 42, 43, 96, 98, 100, 102t–107t, 109, 111, 112, 113, 117, 118, 119, 131t, 132, 134, 135, 136t, 154, 169, 173f, 176t, 179, 181, 182, 186–191, 193, 200, 204, 207t, 237, 271, 273, 275, 276, 277, 281, 345, 346, 364t, 372, 375, 377, 378, 393, 399–402, 414, 415, 416, 430, 433, 452, 455, 457–9, 480t–1t, 483t, 486t–7t, 523, 551, 603, 645, 647, 650, 656, 664, 665t–6t, 695, 702t, 704t, 712, 717t, 721, 724, 725t, 729, 745, 754, 769, 774, 785, 802, 804–7, 839, 840t–1t, 844, 846, 858, 876, 884t, 885–86, 891t–2t, 894, 898t, 899t, 902t, 903, i, iii, x, xi, xii

hyperthermia, 224, 228, 309, 410, 411, 451, 685, 689, 796, 799, 802, 805, 868

hyperthyroidism, 73, 75, 170, 204, 205, 271, 309, 427, 447–50, 685, 773, iv, xiv

hypertonic, 12, 16, 18, 44, 345, 403, 462–3, 764, 766–7, 780

hypertonic hyponatremia, 764, 766

hypertrophy, 96, 101, 168, 169, 170, 173f, 188, 190, 193, 194, 195, 207t, 248, 252, 275, 411, 414, 543–4, 546, iv, xi

hyperuricemia, 422, 544

hyperventilation, 43, 345, 347

hypocalcemia, 65, 98, 355, 398, 404, 464, 772, 775, 777, vii, xvii

hypofibrinogenemia, 538

hypogammaglobulinemia, 548

hypoglycemia, 4, 5, 63, 65, 75, 108t, 174, 346, 347, 429, 431–3, 437t–8t, 440t–1t, 443, 445–6, 450–1, 455, 458, 466, 653, 678t, 721, 789–90, 792, iv, xiv

hypokalemia, 5, 98, 104, 177, 329, 346, 348, 355, 360, 368, 369, 443, 453, 455, 464–5, 517, 744, 751t, 766, 768–9, 802, 852, 868, vii, xvii

hypomagnesemia, 98, 104, 744, 769, 772, 774–5, 868, vii, xvii

hyponatremia, 5, 17, 42, 63, 65, 104, 172, 181, 346, 347, 348, 393, 398, 412, 450–1, 455, 462–3, 465, 764–6, 785, 868, vii, xvii

hypoparathyroidism, 516, 772

hypophosphatemia, 330, 420, 444, 776–7, 840t, 868, vii, xvii

hypotension, 4, 8, 33, 43, 44, 49, 50, 53, 76, 86, 87t, 88t, 98, 105, 109, 110, 123, 128t, 129t, 134, 174, 177, 179, 181, 182, 198, 200–207t, 211, 212, 216f, 225, 231, 249, 267, 273, 278, 280, 291, 296, 328, 345, 347, 353, 355, 364t, 365, 369, 372, 376, 378, 380, 393, 409, 443–4, 451, 454–5, 459, 465, 484t, 487t, 520–1, 537–8, 611, 613, 623, 654, 705t, 709t, 717t–9t, 729, 741–2, 747–9, 750t–4t, 766–7, 774, 776, 779, 781, 784, 788–93, 795, 799, 800(t), 801t, 803–4, 806, 823, 831, 839, 840t, 868, 876

hypotensive, 68, 124, 181, 332, 445, 746, 750t

hypothalamic activity, 687

hypothalamus, 50, 464, 683

hypothermia, 45, 50, 134, 223, 224, 228, 231, 443, 450, 462, 748, 788, 791, 797, 799, 829, 868

hypothyroidism, 73, 75, 271, 447, 449–50, 513, 522, 654, 715, 765–6, iv, xiv

hypotonic hyponatremia, 764, 765

hypoventilation, 450

hypovolemia, 17, 40, 49, 135, 190, 200, 232, 309, 328, 348, 356, 369, 373, 375, 376, 455, 735, 738, 743–5, 765

hypovolemic hyponatremia, 764

hypovolemic shock, 834

hypoxemia, 43, 73, 222, 225, 227, 246, 247, 253, 254, 266, 267, 268, 270, 275, 276, 278, 290, 291, 294, 306, 309, 318, 347, 355, 538, 738–40, 829, 838t, 847, xiii

I

ibuprofen (Motrin), 163, 480t, 661, 670t, 675t, 689, 696, 703t, 830

ibutilide (Corvert), 202

idiopathic pulmonary fibrosis (IPF), 235, 267–269, 846

idiopathic thrombocytopenic purpura (ITP), 533–535

ileum, 325, 369, 516–7

imipenem (Primaxin), 300t, 353, 356, 360, 367, 373, 388, 615, 747, 814, 833

imipramine (Tofranil), 77, 608t, 698, 719t, 799

immunization, 296, 596, 645, 882, 891t–3t, 894–5, 905, 907, 908t–9t, ix, xix

immunocompromised, 57, 58, 164, 264, 265, 298t, 360, 367, 495, 615–6, 635, 637, 826t, 906

immunodeficient, 27, 57, 905

immunoglobulin, 5, 32, 33, 59, 336, 342, 477t, 515, 548, 595, 602, 610, 654, 805, 905

immunosuppressant, 34, 36, 37, 53, 57, 83, 249, 265, 268, 269, 271, 280, 299t, 363, 399, 603, 838

immunosuppressive medications, 840, 841, 843

immunotherapy, 253, 254, 257f, 549, 558, 580

indomethacin (Indocin), 158, 163, 466, 474, 608t, 703t

infarction, 3, 5, 7, 9, 10, 13, 16, 73, 75, 96, 97, 109, 112, 118–122, 125t, 127, 129t–132, 136t, 137t, 139, 149, 154, 169, 172, 173f, 176t, 178, 208, 211, 212, 271, 272, 273, 278, 280, 306, 352, 372, 373, 393, 458, 480t–1t, 468t, 522, 685, 702t, 731t, 735, 737, 743–4, 856b, 858, 867, 873, 903, i, viii, x, xviii

infection, 819–825

inflammation, 17, 31, 32, 34, 53, 56, 58, 61, 79, 97, 135, 157, 159, 162, 163, 241, 249, 242, 255, 261, 266, 269, 270, 285, 286, 332, 333, 336, 340, 341, 342, 351, 352, 353, 354, 356, 357, 359, 360, 362, 363, 364t, 366, 368, 376, 379, 385, 420, 421, 470–3, 476t–8t, 494, 507, 521–2, 569, 572, 592, 620, 624, 628, 641, 646, 650–1, 657–8, 660, 664, 696, 739, 745, 749, 757, 838, 861, xxii, xxiii

inflammatory bowel disease, 379, 420, 514, 567, 685

inflammatory cardiac disease, 135, 162–166, 187–191

infliximab (Remicade), 361, 363, 364t, 485t

influenza, 56, 57, 59, 60t, 61, 82, 162, 261, 262, 263, 269, 296, 298t, 299t, 301t, 531, 550, 596, 650, 658, 684, 844, 858–9, 891t–3t, 898, 899t–902t, 904, 906, 908t–9t, ix, xix, xx

ingestion, 326, 345, 420, 673, 721, 765, 769, 780, 788, 789, 795, 796, 799, 802, 804, 868, 887

inguinal lymphadenopathy, 635

inhalation injury, 263, 851

inhaler, 248, 250–254, 257f, 874

insecticide, 797–8, vii, xvii

insomnia, 88t, 105, 115t, 202t, 203t, 411, 479t, 481t, 702t, 704t, 707t–8t, 717t–20t, 722, 725t, 801

inspiratory rhonchi, 255

insulin, 108t, 116, 326, 357, 398, 403, 427, 429–34, 436t–9t, 441t, 442–6, 695, 762, 769–72, 775, 779–80, 794, 814, 839, 856b, 873

intercostal nerve blocks, 830

intermittent mandatory ventilation (IMV), 317

international normalized ratio (INR), 137

interstitial pattern, 235

interstitial, 29, 171, 194, 222, 231, 235, 236, 268, 269, 270, 274, 275, 395, 397, 410, 503, 737, 738, 742, 784

intestinal transplantation, 848

intestine, 328, 364t, 368, 369, 370, 379, 380, 516, 838t, 847, viii, xiii, xviii

intra-aortic balloon pump, 139–142, 238, 744, 793

intracerebral hemorrhage (ICH), 4

intrauterine device (IUD), 622

intravenous urography, 579

intubation, 18, 33, 48, 225, 291, 820, 853

ipratropium bromide (Atrovent), 248

ipsilateral, 4, 5, 9, 14, 27t, 41, 52, 647, 650, 668, 772

iritis, 269

iron, 108t, 196, 330, 342, 343, 380, 404, 472, 515–6, 518–20, 522–25, 531, 757–8, 762, 889t, x, xv

iron deficiency, 380, 515, 516, 518–520, 522–524, 889

iron dextran (Imferon), 520

ischemia, 3, 5, 7, 10, 17, 24, 43, 53, 109, 119, 120, 121, 123–126, 128t, 129t, 130f, 132, 139, 141, 154, 156, 171, 172, 174, 207t, 209, 212, 271, 272, 273, 291, 306, 351, 368, 369, 371, 372, 373, 378, 393, 400f, 414, 502–3, 528, 537, 645, 647–8, 666t, 670t, 685, 735, 737–9, 744, 751t, 753t–4t, 770, 800t–1t, 810, 813, 845–6, 872, iii, xiii

ischemic colitis, 380

ischemic stroke, 7, 8–13, 136

islet cell transplantation, 847

isoniazid, 59, 264, 265, 354, 521, 595, 602, 608t, 685

isoproterenol, 199, 212, 458, 790–1, 793

isotonic hyponatremia, 764, 766

J

jaundice, 336, 340, 342, 345, 346, 352, 355, 401, 514, 524, 529, 567, 738, 788, 838t

jaw, 48, 601, 661

jejunum, 325, 357, 380, 420, 761, 846

joint, 8, 102, 105, 107, 108, 110, 473, 494, 495, 500, 504, 603, 632, 684, 685, 699, 836, 839, 860, 862, 885, 897

K

ketoacidosis, 179, 427, 430, 433, 442, 444, 769, 775, 779–80, 868, iv, xiv

ketonuria, 428

ketorolac (Toradol)163, 422, 644, 670t, 675t, 696, 703t, 830, 877

kidney, 12, 21, 22, 73, 102t, 106f, 170, 266, 281, 289, 290, 291, 344, 370, 371, 376, 385, 387, 391–394, 396, 399, 401, 403, 405, 411, 414, 415, 416, 419, 422, 423t, 466, 514, 521, 596, 603, 611, 616, 720t, 740, 765–6, 770, 778–9, 834, 837, 838t, 839, 842t, 844–5, 847, 872, 882, 909t, viii, xi, xiii, xviii

kidney transplantation, 844

kyphoscoliosis, 782

L

labetalol (Trandate), 11, 16, 18, 103t, 109, 176t, 458, 792

labialis, 634

labyrinthine hydrops, 653

Lactated Ringer's solution, 49, 231, 785

lactic acidosis, 372, 779, 780

lactulose, 63, 347, 377, 771

lamivudine (Epivir), 338, 594t, 598t

lamotrigine (Lamictal), 69t, 70t, 662, 674t, 708t, 716, 720t

lansoprazole (Prevacid), 330, 331, 335, 659

lanthanum, 404, 776, 778

laparoscopic diskectomy, 509

laparoscopy, 158, 353, 370, 422, 560, 623

large bowel obstruction, 370–371

laryngeal edema, 853

laryngitis, xxiv

laryngopharyngitis, xxiv

larynx, 296, xxiv

lasix (Furosemide), 103t, 348, 354, 396, 402

lateral films, 234

laxatives, 16, 360, 404, 863

left ventricular ejection fraction(LVEF), 172, 174, 176, 177, 178, 179, 181, 182

leg ulcers, 529

lepirudin (Refludan), 803

lesions, 24, 25, 26, 27, 28, 46, 48, 52, 61, 65, 67, 81, 133, 152, 153, 164, 187, 237, 242, 263, 269, 430, 458, 492, 498, 564, 565, 570, 572, 579, 592, 603, 607, 608, 609, 610, 615, 616, 617, 618, 619, 620, 630, 634, 635, 638, 650, 729, 741, 814, 861

leukemias, 543, 545, 547, 549, 551, 553

leukocyte esterase dipstick test, 387

leukocytosis, 163, 261, 262, 327, 328, 355, 359, 360, 365, 369, 372, 443, 453, 473, 499, 522, 626, 687, 746, 770, 796, 821

levamisole HCl (Ergamisol), 568

lidocaine, 40, 202, 210, 617, 675, 790

ligamentous laxity, 488, 489

linear salpingostomy, 623

lipoprotein, 112, 113, 115, 116, 127, 433, 886, 891, 893

Liquiprin, 788

lithium toxicity, 795

liver, 59, 67, 82, 88, 116, 170, 177, 179, 202, 203, 204, 232, 236, 262, 266, 291, 294, 336, 337, 338, 339, 340, 341, 342, 343, 344, 345, 346, 347, 349, 350, 360, 375, 376, 377, 378, 400, 401, 439, 462, 464, 473, 479, 480, 481, 482, 483, 485, 486, 487, 516, 538, 551, 560, 567, 590, 592, 596, 597, 617, 662, 666, 684, 694, 702, 703, 704, 709, 715, 721, 722, 725, 735, 738, 739, 740, 741, 757, 759, 763, 785, 788, 808, 830, 832, 833, 838, 840, 843, 844, 845, 846, 848, 849, 850, 862, 872, 887, 898, 899, 900, 901, 909

liver disease, 336–348, 376–378, 393, 401, 483, 522, 537, 538, 596, 666, 757, 788, 845, 898–901

liver transplantation, 845

loop diuretics, 177, 180, 181

lorazepam (Ativan), 43, 68, 77, 713, 721, 722, 725t, 730, 800, 802

low back pain, 505–507, 509, 576, 666, 708

lower respiratory tract pathogens, 251, 263, 296–303, 597

lumbar nerve root findings, 508

lumbar puncture (LP), 10, 58

lumbar spine, 47

lumbar vertebrae, 52

Lund and Browder chart, 852

lung, 26, 75, 222, 223, 225, 233, 234, 235, 236, 237, 238, 239, 240, 241, 242, 243, 244, 246, 247, 248, 249, 251, 255, 260, 261, 262, 266, 267, 268, 269, 270, 272, 275, 276, 277, 279, 288, 290, 292, 293, 294, 300, 315, 452, 461, 563, 564, 565, 566, 569, 582, 583, 596, 603, 740, 759, 773, 778, 783, 820, 830, 831, 838, 843, 844, 846, 849, 850, 856, 871, 873, 875, 876, 887, 909

lung cancer, 238, 288, 452, 563–566, 569, 831

lung parenchyma, 268, 269, 270, 272

lung transplantation, 846

LV systolic dysfunction, 174, 175, 176, 177, 178, 183, 191

lymph node, 577, 613, 686, 687, 859

lymphadenopathy, 557, 564

lymphedema, 578, 614

lymphocele, 845

lymphocyte depletion (LD), 555

lymphocyte, 555, 559, 560, 758

lymphoma, 326, 485, 486, 554, 555, 557, 558, 559, 561, 597, 684

lymphomatoid granulomatosis, 281

lysis syndrome, 487, 770, 777

M

maalox, 121, 334, 775

macrocyte, 516

macrocytosis, 37, 515

macrolide, 35, 297t–299t, 301t–303t, 643, 658, 690t

maculopapular rash, 638

magnesium (Mg), 36, 67, 74, 98, 103, 107t, 134, 179, 203, 209, 210, 272, 330, 419, 421, 423t, 721, 763, 769, 772, 774–776, 780, 781, 785, 805, 864

magnetic resonance angiography (MRA), 6, 153

magnetic resonance, 23, 55, 78, 153, 155, 182, 342, 356, 372, 396, 415

malabsorption, 115t, 364t, 419, 498, 517, 520, 772, 774, 776

malaise, 61, 164, 340, 386, 471, 482t, 528, 548, 549, 560, 601, 603, 611, 613, 615, 625, 638, 657, 659, 687, 698, 765, 807, 838t, 840t

malaria, 684

malformation, 13, 24, 25, 56, 97, 136t, 377, 506t, 666t, 900t

malignancy, 158, 268, 278, 286–288, 409, 461, 470, 485t, 486t, 514, 520–522, 543, 545, 557, 560, 561, 569, 571, 573, 576, 579, 641, 684, 686, 689, 773, 774, 837, 843

malignant, 10, 27t, 28, 80, 136t, 238, 288, 315, 327, 379, 415, 457, 461, 485t, 487t, 523, 537, 558, 559, 561, 564–566, 617, 619, 620, 652, 656, 685, 720t, 726t, 799, 898, 898t–902t, 903

malnourished, 329, 763, 861

malnutrition, 291, 346, 360, 521, 522, 729, 746, 757, 762, 772, 775

malodorous, 386, 628, 632

mammogram, 28, 581, 892t, 893t, 896

mammography/mammographic, 569, 570, 886, 887

mannitol (Osmitrol), 12, 16, 18, 28, 43, 44, 345, 764, 766, 767, 769

Marcus Gunn pupil, 646

mass lesion, 665

mastoiditis, 56

McCoy cell culture, 630

measles, 57, 61, 79, 893t, 906, 908t, 909t

mechanical ventilatory support, 314–319

mediastinal, 134, 234, 236, 270, 294, 555, 560, 561, 565, 831, 876

mediastinum, 36, 135, 236, 286, 293, 832

medicaid, 149

MedicAlert bracelet, 455

medicare, 149, 169, 399

medulloblastoma, 26t

Mefoxin, 366, 370, 624, 626

megacolon, 362

megaloblastic, 122t, 515–517, 520

meglitinides, 434, 438

melanoma, 485t, 487t, 619–621

melena, 327, 375, 378, 859

memantine (Namenda), 76, 697

ménière, 641, 653, 654

meninges, 746

meningioma, 26, 27t

meningismus, 57, 665t

meningitides, 57

meningitidis, 56, 59, 60t, 690t

meningitis, 42, 56–59, 58t, 60t, 63, 73, 75, 461, 464, 530, 596, 597, 636, 641, 653, 664, 665t, 684, 825t, 867

meningococcal, 56, 58, 59, 858, 891t, 908t, 909t

meningococcus, 745, 906

meningoencephalitis, 25

menopause, 90, 569, 580, 860, 894

menses, 136t, 622, 625, 635

mental health, 883, 884, 895, 896

meperidine (Demerol), 87t, 356, 675t, 696, 701t, 797
mercaptopropionylglycine, 422
mercaptopurine, 361–363, 364t, 545
meropenem, 353, 367, 373, 615, 747, 814, 833
mesalamine, 361–363, 364t
mesenteric ischemia, 371, 372, 373, 374, 685
mesylate, 86, 104t, 403, 417t, 531, 552, 670t, 673t, 799
metabolic, 6, 32, 43, 45, 63, 65, 108t, 113, 116, 117, 119, 120, 123, 133, 163, 164, 168, 169t, 171, 172, 173f, 198, 200, 212, 227, 248, 289, 307, 329, 344, 346, 365, 368–370, 376, 392, 398, 412, 415, 420, 427, 433, 443–445, 455, 469, 498, 546, 665, 666t, 712, 734, 737, 739, 740, 747, 761–763, 769, 770, 777–781, 783, 789, 793, 794, 796, 802, 804, 805, 848, 852, 867, 885
metabolic acidosis, 739, 778
metabolic alkalosis, 368, 780, 781, 786
metabolism, 224, 251, 290, 329, 376, 391, 405, 449, 473, 522, 689, 701t, 737, 738, 740, 805
metaxalone (Skelaxin), 490, 494, 507, 509
metformin (Glucophage), 394, 437t–441t, 517
methacholine, 242
methadone (Dolophine), 87t, 675t, 696, 701t, 706t, 797
methanol, 779, 780
methanol toxicity, 803
methemoglobinemia, 202t, 228
methicillin, 165, 299t, 300t, 465, 821–823, 825t, 826t
methicillin-resistant, 300t, 821–823, 825t, 826t
methicillin-sensitive, 299t, 821
methicillin-susceptible, 165
methionine, 423t
methotrexate (Trexall), 37, 83, 271, 280, 281, 362, 363, 364t, 472, 473, 482t, 483t, 485t–487t, 520, 545, 547, 623, 624
methyldopa (Clonidine), 104t, 105, 108t, 354, 434, 458, 602, 608t, 685
methylene, 228
methylprednisolone (Medrol), 28, 82, 249, 280, 361, 362, 364t, 487t, 602, 603, 617, 651, 749
metolazone, 103t, 177, 179, 180t, 181t, 402
metoprolol (Lopressor), 103t, 124, 126, 127, 176t, 184t, 195, 196, 202t, 448, 672t, 674t, 792
metronidazole (Flagyl), 298t, 331, 353, 354, 356, 360, 363, 365–367, 373, 518, 626, 628, 629, 690t, 747, 814, 824, 826, 833
microaneurysms, 645
microaspiration, 298t
microcrystalline arthritis, 685
microcytic anemia, 518
microcytic, 472, 521, 522, 523, 524
microscopic, 164, 339, 578, 631
microscopy, 386, 396, 544, 557, 626
microvascular, 120, 400f, 645
midazolam, 68
midbrain, 27t, 85
midclavicular, 95, 188, 294, 832, 857b

migraine, 4, 104, 641, 647, 664, 667, 668, 699t–672t, 674t, 675t, 678t, 707t
military antishock trousers (MAST), 743
milrinone (Primacor), 134
mineralocorticoid, 174, 445, 769
mineralocorticoid excess, 769
mini-mental status exam, 74, 730
minipress (Prazosin), 104t, 403, 409
misoprostol (Cytotec), 325, 330
mitral regurgitation, 97, 187, 189
mitral stenosis, 8, 11, 97, 186, 187, 192
mitral valve prolapse, 9, 166, 189
mixed cellularity (MC), 555
model for end-stage liver disease (MELD), 346
Mobitz type I, 211, 215
Moraxella, 297t–299t, 642, 652, 657, 825t
morbidity, 8, 43, 44, 104, 174, 204, 241, 337, 345, 357, 410, 504, 514, 525, 528, 624, 625, 689, 843, 854, 886, 896, 903, 905
morphine, 43, 123, 124, 130f, 132, 274, 353, 356, 367, 373, 461, 499, 530, 624, 666t, 696, 697, 699, 700, 701t, 705t, 706t, 797, 830, 831, 853, 877
morphine sulfate, 356, 367, 831
motor assessment, 48
mouth-to-mouth ventilation, 310
moxifloxacin, 298t, 301t, 302t, 303t, 366, 658, 814
mucinex (guaifenesin), 251
mucolytics, 255
mucopurulent, 625–627, 629, 630, 632, 633
mucosa, 166, 312, 318, 325, 326, 332, 334, 359, 377, 378, 410, 454, 470, 507, 515, 555, 557, 610, 659, 696, 761
mucosal barrier, 325
mucosal, 306, 330, 360, 362, 533, 534, 741
mucous, 58, 252, 311, 330, 369, 444, 477t, 514, 610, 617, 620, 655, 657, 660, 686, 758, 861
multidrug-resistant, 264
multiple sclerosis, 79–83, 386, 641, 653, 662, 698
mumps, 57, 61, 162, 354, 560, 893t, 906, 908t, 909t
murmur, 96, 97, 129t, 163, 164, 186, 188–191, 194, 514, 519, 743, 782, 823, 856b, 859, 862
Murphy's sign, 352
musculoskeletal, 51, 62, 170, 243, 467, 492, 499, 698, 705t, 773, 829, 840t, 856b, 860, 862
myalgia, 57, 82, 340, 487t, 634, 659, 665t, 686, 838t
myambutol (Ethambutol), 265
myasthenia gravis, 35–38, 170, 290, 314, 447, 781
myasthenic, 35–37
mycobacterium, 57, 261, 264, 354, 595, 597, 844t
mylanta, 121, 334
myocardial biopsy, 195
myocardial infarction (MI), 3, 73, 96, 97, 109, 112, 118, 119–137, 139, 149, 154, 169, 172, 173, 176, 208, 211, 273, 280, 352, 393, 458, 480, 481, 486, 522, 685, 702, 735, 743, 744, 832, 856, 858, 867, 873, 903
myocardial ischemia, 212, 271, 306, 738, 754

myocarditis, 122t, 271, 472, 603, 743

myopathy, 4, 115t, 843

myositis, 115t, 117

mysoline, 69t

myxedema, 449, 450, 516, 868, see also hypothyroidism

N

n-acetylcysteine (Mucomyst), 345, 394, 789, 846

nadolol, 103t, 126, 176t, 377, 674t, 792

nafcillin, 165, 614, 823, 826t

naloxone (Narcan), 697, 783

naproxen (Aleve), 163, 474, 481t, 661, 670t, 675t, 704t

naratriptan (Amerge), 671, 676

narcotic, 123, 422, 489, 490, 509, 653, 658, 722, 748

narrow-spectrum, 297

nasal prongs, 311

nasogastric (NGT), 17, 41, 51, 53, 134, 238t, 311, 328, 329, 345, 347, 353, 356, 360, 364, 365, 369–371, 373, 376, 378, 380, 392, 657, 688, 689, 741, 761, 764, 769, 780, 790, 794, 821, 830, 833–835, 863, 874, 875

nasojejunal, 357, 761, 762

nasopharyngeal, 59, 311, 603, 656

nasopharynx, 56, 62, 311, 656

nasotracheal, 52, 172

natalizumab, 83

National Cancer Institute, 547, 552, 561, 886

National Comprehensive Cancer Network, 561, 567

nausea, 5, 22, 26, 37, 41, 58, 60, 62, 66, 67, 76, 83, 87t, 88t, 105, 116t, 121, 126, 202t, 203t, 327, 328, 337, 340, 345, 346, 352, 355, 359, 363, 364t, 366, 370, 386, 398, 401, 415, 421, 441t, 442, 454, 457, 466, 479t–482t, 484t–487t, 516, 528, 530, 567, 611, 623, 627, 632, 648, 652–654, 666t, 667, 669t, 670t, 698, 699, 702t, 703t, 705t, 707t–709t, 717t–720t, 723t, 725t, 737, 748, 759, 760, 765, 767, 769, 773, 776, 779, 788–790, 792, 794–797, 804, 806, 838t, 840t, 841t, 854, 856b, 859

necrosis, 34, 53, 61, 82, 119, 122t, 212, 342, 347, 355, 356, 363, 364t, 368, 369, 387, 393, 397t, 399, 400f, 410, 471, 486t, 487t, 499, 503, 527, 530, 535, 537, 614, 635, 646, 683, 685, 734, 737, 739, 754t, 771, 800t, 804, 806, 807, 812, 838, 841t, 844–846

Neisseria, 56, 164, 387, 622, 658, 825t

neoplasm, 9, 26, 67, 75, 136t, 351, 377, 379, 452, 453, 537, 554–556, 559, 579, 652, 657, 662, 893t, 898, 898t–902t, 903

nephritis, 394, 395, 397t, 399, 400f, 604, 610, 898, 899t–902t, 904

nephrolithiasis, 419, 421, 423, 424

nephrology, 500

nephron, 108t, 180t, 181t, 392, 399

nephropathy, 153, 399, 414–416, 427, 430, 770, 839, 845

nephropathy, 427, 430

nephrosclerosis, 414

nephrosis, 397t, 898, 899t–902t, 904

nephrostomy, 396, 845

nephrotic, 397t, 486t, 764, 899t–902t

nephrotoxic, 393, 394, 824, 839

nephrotoxicity, 394, 405, 412, 472, 824, 839

nervousness, 88t, 445 ,447, 707t, 725t

nesiritide, 181

neuralgia, 23, 81, 615–617, 661, 693, 694, 698, 708t

neurofibromatosis, 22, 27t, 458

neurogenic, 53, 231, 386, 395, 464, 506, 664, 734, 736t, 745, 747, 748

neurogenic shock, 747

neurologic, 1, 3, 7, 9, 14, 17, 18, 22, 23, 28, 40, 42, 48, 49, 53, 56, 58–63, 74, 80, 132, 135, 198, 344, 347, 402, 404, 444, 445, 462, 469, 498, 505, 509t, 510, 514, 517, 521, 528, 564, 662, 665t, 667, 709t, 730, 735, 748, 765, 767, 773, 775, 796, 828, 829, 854, 856b, 860, 862, 867

neurologic examination, 42, 74

neurological, 3, 10, 16–18, 27, 41, 43, 45, 79–81, 189, 590, 709t, 783

neurologist, 10, 11, 36, 43, 86

neurology, 11, 33, 82, 89

neuromuscular blocking agents, 35, 43

neuromuscular, 35, 36, 38, 43, 226, 241, 242, 263, 320, 398, 489, 498, 867

neuropathy, 31, 32, 121, 176t, 265, 266, 395, 402, 427, 430, 433, 469, 487t, 559, 602, 603, 648, 693, 694, 698, 810, 811, 840t

neurosurgeon, 15, 16, 43, 52

neurosyphilis, 75, 638, 639

neutropenia, 455, 480t, 481t, 487t, 549, 613

neutrophil, 56, 249, 472, 473, 487t, 517, 551

New York Heart Association (NYHA), 168, 272

niacin, 116t, 117

nicardipine, 11, 16, 18, 104t, 108t, 109, 188, 459, 666t, 674t, 793, 802, 805

nicotine, 247, 333, 462

nifedipine (Procardia), 104t, 108t, 277, 422, 674t, 793

nimodipine, 24

nipride, 109, 134, 802, 832

nissen fundoplication procedure, 335

nitrates, 120, 126, 127, 128t, 132, 174, 175, 182, 190, 195, 196, 273, 333, 376, 387, 665, 678t, 873

nitrofurantoin, 268, 354, 387, 389

nitrogen, 9, 101, 245, 328, 357, 369, 392, 397t, 398

nitroglycerin, 109, 120, 121, 123, 124, 126, 130f, 132, 135, 181, 273, 376, 678t, 744, 752t, 805, 856b, 857b

nitroprusside (Nitropress), 109, 134, 181, 188, 191, 428, 459, 666t, 744, 752t, 802, 805, 832

nizatidine (Axid), 329

n-methyl-d-aspartate (NMDA) 76, 694, 696, 697, 700

nodular sclerosis (NS), 555

non-adherence, 251, 444, 592

non-Hodgkin's lymphoma, 554, 557, 558, 597, 843

nonopioid analgesics, 616, 696

non-rebreather masks, 312

nonrenal potassium loss, 769

non-small cell carcinoma (NSCC), 565

non-ST segment elevation MI (NSTEMI), 121, 123, 124, 127, 130f, 131t, 136

nonsteroidal anti-inflammatory drugs (NSAIDs) 16, 34, 77, 101, 108t, 158, 163, 175t, 182, 286, 325, 326, 330, 333, 353, 375, 380, 393, 395, 397t, 422, 449, 461, 470, 471, 474, 480t, 481t, 489, 490, 494, 507, 509, 530, 578, 603, 644, 652, 653, 658, 659, 661, 670t, 673t, 696, 697, 700, 702t–704t, 770, 830, 839, 872

norepinephrine, 18, 134, 170, 345, 457, 458, 666t, 674t, 694, 697, 698, 715, 717t, 735, 744, 747–749, 750b, 751t, 753t, 754t, 791, 793, 799, 800t, 801t

norfloxacin, 363, 379, 518

normochromic, 164, 450, 521, 522, 602

normocytic, 164, 450, 515

normocytosis, 521, 522, 602

normotensive, 15, 188

Norvasc, 104t

nosocomial bacteremia, 822

nosocomial urinary tract infection, 819, 827

nosocomial, 158, 330, 388, 819, 820, 821, 822, 824, 825, 826

numbness, 27t, 47, 80, 153, 156, 157, 490, 506, 508, 509t, 516, 667, 723t, 811, 835

nutrition, 19, 34, 73, 76, 89, 91, 170, 267, 291, 297, 318, 329, 343, 357, 362, 370, 376, 396, 444, 498, 517, 520, 525, 670t, 731t, 740, 741, 757, 758, 760–763, 776, 779, 780, 785, 810, 815, 822, 871, 874, 883, 884t, 892t, 893t, 903

nystagmus, 62, 81, 654, 789

O

obesity, 4, 6, 101, 111, 116, 117, 119, 135, 153, 158, 169, 169t, 173f, 241, 271, 278, 305, 306, 332, 341, 343, 351, 388, 419, 433, 452, 469, 493, 505, 508, 580, 591, 782, 837, 872, 873, 884t, 885, 890t, 892t, 894, 895, 903

obstipation, 369

obstructive airway lesions, 255–256

obstructive sleep apnea, 314, 317, 699

occlusive arterial disease, 156

occlusive disease, 372

occupational therapy, 52, 490

octreotide (Sandostatin), 328, 376

ocular, 35, 62, 447, 645, 649, 662

ofloxacin (Floxin), 302t, 631, 643

olanzapine (Zyprexa), 77, 685, 713, 720t, 726t, 730–732, 798

oligodendroglioma, 26

oliguria, 135, 347, 369, 393, 395, 421, 742, 743

olsalazine, 361, 364t

omalizumab, 254, 257t

omeprazole (Prilosec), 325, 330, 331, 335, 659

oncological emergencies, 558, 560, 565, 621

oncologist, 28, 551

oncology, 281, 544, 547, 548, 551, 556, 557

ondansetron, 422, 654

open-angle glaucoma, 663

ophthalmic corticosteroids, 644

ophthalmic zoster, 616

ophthalmologic, 22, 271, 472, 616, 649

ophthalmologic examination, 22, 271

ophthalmologist, 616, 643–647, 649

ophthalmopathy, 448

ophthamology, 429, 836

opiates, 16, 353, 354, 409, 479t, 700, 702t, 716, 781

opioids, 34, 41, 43, 290, 306, 314, 333, 362, 373, 422, 470, 490, 494, 499, 507, 509, 530, 611, 616, 617, 652, 653, 673t, 694, 696–700, 701t, 705t–707t, 722, 783, 797, 830

opioid toxicity, 797

opportunistic infections, 589, 596, 600, 684

oral contraceptive, 3, 428, 521, 531, 574

oral diuretics, 180

organ rejection, 838

organophosphate (insecticide) poisoning, 797

oromandibular dysfunction, 661

oropharyngeal, 32, 35, 310, 311, 659

oropharynx, 32, 305, 311, 632, 656

orthopnea, 171, 179, 186, 194, 272, 856b, 859

orthostatic, 33, 50, 86, 87t, 88t, 105, 179, 198, 369, 378, 443, 455, 521, 717t–719t, 741

orthostatic, 33, 88, 105, 179, 198, 443, 455, 717, 718, 719

osmolality, 12, 16, 18, 393, 395, 402, 442, 443, 461, 462, 465, 740, 764, 765, 768, 784, 785

osmolarity, 44, 397, 402, 444, 465, 762

osteoarthritis, 469, 484t, 505, 506, 705t

osteopenia, 472

osteoporosis, 47, 251, 285, 364t, 453, 479t, 498–500, 524, 592, 843, 882, 887, 890t, 894, 896

otitis externa, 651–652

otitis media, 60, 651–652

otorrhea, 41, 651, 652

outpatient management, 127, 830

outpatient, 36, 127, 211, 271, 335, 360, 410, 614, 623, 626, 627, 715, 766, 830

ovarian cancer, 567, 569, 574, 582, 583

ovarian, 287, 560, 573, 574, 575, 580, 582, 625, 626, 627, 629, 887, 893, 895

overdose, 73, 290, 449, 608, 697, 706, 707, 714, 715, 722, 783, 789, 790, 791, 792, 795, 797, 802, 803, 808, 868

over-the-counter, 334, 335, 518, 587, 591, 607, 627, 643, 659, 686, 858, 871

oxacillin, 165, 614, 691t

oxcarbazepine, 69t, 70t, 674t, 697, 708t

oximetry, 123, 216f, 228, 229, 246, 247, 263, 268, 270, 272, 318, 740

oxycodone (Oxycontin), 490, 494, 499, 507, 509, 617, 624, 696, 701, 797

oxygen supplementation, 251, 308–312, 450, 531

oxygenation, 3, 45, 50, 221, 225–229, 246, 247, 272, 309, 317, 319, 735, 810, 821, 847

oxyhemoglobin, 223

P

pacemakers, 141–143, 144f, 145–147, 146t, 147t, 148f, 149, 178, 199, 201, 206, 208, 211, 212, 238t, 684, 867

pain, 430, 442, 454, 458, 462, 469, 470, 471, 473, 477, 480–485, 487–490, 493, 495, 498, 499, 503, 505–509, 516, 519–521, 528–531, 543, 546, 548, 550, 557, 559, 560, 564, 569–571, 574, 576, 577, 580, 601, 603, 615–617, 622–627, 630, 632, 634, 638, 641, 644, 646–648, 650–652, 657–659, 661, 662, 664, 666, 667, 669, 693–710

palliative, 91, 166, 269, 558, 566, 570, 591, 635

pallor, 66, 81, 152, 156, 157, 164, 327, 376, 378, 380, 401, 445, 503, 514, 518, 521, 524, 623, 741

palpitations, 128t, 186, 188, 189, 191, 200, 201, 202t, 204–206, 208, 209, 276, 445, 447, 449, 457, 516, 519, 724, 752t, 769, 859

panadol, 788

pancreas, 326, 327, 354, 434, 694, 738, 838, 838t, 844, 847, 848

pancreas transplantation, 847

pancreatic, 352, 354–357, 428, 461, 506t, 517, 738, 739, 772, 779, 848

pancreatitis, 117, 266, 352, 354–357, 363, 364t, 372, 373, 428, 441t, 444, 685, 721, 741, 763, 772, 848, 868

pancytopenia, 544, 546

panel reactive antibody (PRA), 838

pantoprazole, 163, 330, 331, 335, 379, 380, 659

Papanicolaou (Pap) smear, 572

papaverine, 373

papilledema, 15, 26, 58, 665t, 729, 782

parainfluenza, 684, 906

paralysis, 32, 34, 43, 49–52, 62, 65, 152, 156, 503, 564, 650, 769, 771, 773, 776, 782, 794, 798, 807, 831, 860

paralytic ileus, 769

paralytics, 44, 45, 54

paraplegia, 47, 49

parasitic infestation, 642

parathion, 797

parenchyma, 13, 24, 237, 240, 241, 247, 268–270, 272, 385, 833, 834

paresthesias, 4, 5, 32, 47, 65, 66, 86, 152, 156, 202t, 445, 450, 486t, 490, 503, 516, 519, 667, 776, 783

Parkinson's disease, 72, 85, 86, 87t, 88t, 731t, 902t

paroxysmal sweats, 723

past medical history (PMH), 858

past surgical history (PSH), 858

pathogens, 59, 60t, 61, 165, 251, 261, 263, 287, 296, 297t, 298t, 363, 385, 386, 389, 592, 597, 614, 651, 659, 690t, 691t, 746, 747, 813, 814, 819–825, 825t, 826t, 844, 905

peginterferon, 338, 339

penetrating eye trauma, 835

penicillin, 59, 60t, 165, 166t, 298t–301t, 331, 365, 388, 394, 499, 608t, 610, 614, 615, 639, 643, 652, 658, 659, 691t, 813, 825, 857

penicillin-allergic, 165, 166t, 299t, 331, 365, 813

penicillin-resistant, 298t, 301t, 660

penicillin-sensitive, 298t, 388, 611

penicillin-susceptible, 59, 165

pentoxifylline (Trental), 153

peptic ulcer disease (PUD), 325, 377

percutaneous coronary intervention (PCI), 123, 124, 125, 132–133, 136

percutaneous transluminal coronary angioplasty (PTCA), 124, 132–133, 134, 137, 857

perforation, 133, 142, 156, 166, 236, 293, 327, 328, 352, 357, 359, 360, 362, 363, 366, 368, 370, 371, 487t, 643, 653, 836, 848, 868

pericardial, 135, 163, 237, 401, 486t, 564, 667

pericardial effusion, 237

pericardiocentesis, 135

pericarditis, 97, 122t, 135, 162, 163, 170, 195, 275, 398, 399, 401, 472, 486t, 603, 745

pericardium, 162, 195

pericholecystic, 352

perihepatitis, 632

perineal flora, 819

peripheral arterial disease (PAD), 152

peripheral pulse amplitude, 98

peripheral smear, 519

peripheral vascular disease, 118, 152–160, 161, 174, 228, 416, 427, 872, 895

peritoneal dialysis, 399, 405, 778

peritonitis, 359, 360, 363, 365, 373, 603, 742, 848

periumbilical, 366, 369, 372

pernicious anemia, 447

pH, 50, 222, 224, 227, 228, 287, 315, 319, 327, 328, 332, 334, 346, 348, 357, 398, 420, 421, 422, 423, 442, 443, 444, 628, 734, 740, 777, 778, 779, 780, 781, 782, 783, 784, 789, 796, 800, 865

pharyngitis, 340, 632, 634, 658, 825t

phenobarbital, 68, 69t, 70t, 108t, 404, 666t, 722, 791, 802

phenylephrine, 18, 666t, 744, 747–749, 750t, 754t, 801t

phenytoin (Dilantin), 16, 19, 28, 45, 68, 69t, 70t, 329, 395, 404, 428, 498, 520, 662, 666t, 772

pheochromocytoma, 101, 170, 427, 457–459, 685

phlebectomy, 155

phlebitis, 278, 520, 684, 822

phlegm, 247

photocoagulation, 646

photophobia, 57, 644, 648, 667

physical restraints, 713

phytotherapy, 409

Pickwickian syndrome, 315

pineal tumor, 27

piperacillin, 388, 820, 821, 823

piperacillin-tazobactam, 299t, 353, 360, 367, 373, 388, 615, 660, 690t, 691t, 747, 814, 822, 825, 826t, 833

pituitary failure, 454

placebo, 165, 377

plasmapheresis, 33, 34, 37, 38, 400f

plasmin, 132

plasminogen, 4, 5, 132, 137t, 156, 280

Plasmodium falciparum, 523, 528
Plavix, 7, 12, 127, 154
pleural disorders, 286–288
pleural effusion, 237, 272, 286, 357, 401, 472, 575, 821
pleuritis, 286
pneumococcal, 56, 174, 264, 269, 296, 531, 535, 550, 561, 596, 856b, 858, 893t, 908t, 909t
pneumococcus, 164, 296, 363, 906
pneumocystis, 268, 589, 595, 597, 843, 844t
pneumomediastinum, 267
pneumonia, 48, 56, 77, 179, 222, 225, 236, 237, 250, 251, 255, 261–263, 268, 291, 293, 296, 297, 298t–300t, 302t, 309, 314, 318, 330, 333, 352, 461, 472, 564, 595, 597, 603, 610, 630, 683, 695, 746, 783. 820, 822, 823, 825, 825t, 830, 844, 856b, 859, 876, 898, 899t–902t, 904
pneumoniae, 56, 59, 60t, 77, 261, 262, 264, 296, 297t–299t, 301t–303t, 385, 528, 642, 652, 657, 658, 660, 690t, 745, 819, 825t
pneumothorax, 225, 237, 267, 291, 293, 294, 310, 315, 316, 745, 782, 828–832
Pneumovax, 264
poikilothermy, 50
point of maximal impulse (PMI), 861
poisoning, 46, 109, 228, 291, 525, 779, 780, 788, 794, 797, 851, 854
polio, 893t
polioviruses, 61, 906
pollen, 410, 642
polycythemia, 3
polymyalgia, 601, 689
polymyalgia rheumatica, 601
polynephritis, 388
polyneuropathy, 31, 33
polysomnography (PSG), 306
polyurethane, 141, 815
polyuria, 395, 412, 428, 430, 433, 442, 444, 452, 458, 464, 465, 767, 769, 773, 860
portal vein thrombosis, 846
positional hypotension, 654
positive end-expiratory pressure (PEEP), 316
postencephalitic syndrome, 73
posterior cord syndrome, 52
postmenopausal, 22, 111, 113, 523, 571, 580, 892t, 894
postoperative, 134, 135, 410, 459, 580, 696, 697, 699, 700, 763, 771, 825, 838, 839, 844, 847, 863, 868, 874–876
postremission therapy, 545
postrenal, 395, 397
potassium-sparing, 103t, 108t, 180t, 412, 770
P-Q-R-S-T, 120
PR interval, 790
prazosin (Minipress), 104t, 108t, 403, 409, 459
prednisone (Deltasone), 163, 249
preeclampsia, 170, 345, 464

pregnancy, 96, 101, 104, 105, 109, 136t, 332, 345, 351, 386, 388, 449, 464, 483t, 518, 520, 531, 560, 569, 574, 591, 622–625, 627, 629, 631–633, 635, 639, 783, 829, 889t, 892t, 893t, 894–896
pregnant, 330, 339, 388, 389, 448, 484t, 616, 617, 623, 627, 629, 794, 889t, 891t, 894, 896, 900t, 909t
prehypertension, 100, 885, 886
premenopausal, 22, 111, 523
preoperative lymphatic mapping, 620
preoperative, 190, 217, 269, 371, 459, 700, 873, 874
pressure control ventilation, 317
pressure ulcers, 51, 812, 815, 817, 818
Prevacid, 330, 335, 659
priapism, 49, 528, 531, 551
Prilosec, 325, 330, 335, 659
primary aldosteronism, 780
primary adrenocortical insufficiency, see Addison disease
primary cerebral lymphoma, 27
Prinzmetal's, 120
procainamide, 35, 202t, 208, 216f, 354, 608t, 685, 790
procalcitonin, 263, 359, 746
procarbazine, 28, 561
procedure note, 864
prodromal phase, 340
progress note, 864
propafenone, 202, 207
prophylactic, 41, 45, 165, 166, 178, 255, 330, 356, 377, 389, 561, 655, 808
prophylaxis, 8, 16, 18, 44, 45, 50, 165, 166, 187–191, 195, 196, 265, 280, 338, 363, 365, 379, 389, 417, 422, 474, 535, 545, 589, 591, 593–597, 619, 666t, 672t–674t, 807, 821, 824, 825, 840t, 841t, 843, 875, 892t
propofol, 43, 68
propranolol, 103t, 108t, 126, 176t, 196, 202t, 211, 403, 448, 459, 672t, 674t, 676t, 677t, 792
prostacyclins, 277
prostaglandin, 157, 326, 330, 333, 373, 470, 507, 649, 683, 693, 846
prostate, 28, 248, 385, 395, 397t, 408–411, 506t, 563, 567, 576–578, 687, 835, 862, 886, 887, 892t
prostate cancer, 576, 887
prostate-specific antigen (PSA), 409, 576, 886
prostatic, 105, 386, 395, 396, 408, 410, 461, 577
protease inhibitors, 339, 593
proteinuria, 164, 340, 387, 395, 397t, 400f, 402, 472, 480t, 481t, 603, 703t
prothrombin, 5, 12, 15, 123, 137t, 160, 260, 340, 343, 345, 347, 348, 371, 372, 375, 376, 378, 538, 546, 647, 666t, 865b, 740, 788, 803, 813, 833, 857t, 864, 872
prothrombotic, 117, 375
proton pump inhibitors (PPIs), 327
pruritic, 806
pruritus, 116t, 342, 346, 348, 364t, 401, 433, 448, 479t–482t, 484t, 560, 616, 699, 702t, 703t, 705t, 706t, 748, 777, 838t, 846
pseudocysts, 356

pseudohyperkalemia, 770
pseudomonas, 262, 298t, 300t, 385, 387, 559, 561, 642, 651, 745, 819, 826t, 844t
pseudotumor cerebri, 665
psoas, 366
psychiatric, 75, 685, 686, 709t, 713, 716, 728, 730–732, 805, 860
psychiatrist, 713, 715, 716, 729,
psychiatry, 51
psychomotor agitation, 714
psychosis, 86, 364t, 449, 458, 479t, 603, 709t, 711, 726t, 728–731, 790, 794
pulmonary angiography, 279
pulmonary blood flow, 221, 735
pulmonary edema, 128, 129, 135, 194, 225, 290, 314, 783
pulmonary function testing, 240–243, 246, 249, 268, 269, 270, 271, 276, 871
pulmonary hypertension, 274, 281, 282, 283, 284
pulmonary nodules, 237, 472
pulmonary perfusion, 5, 10, 17, 18, 20, 25, 42, 43, 53, 54, 125, 126, 139, 140, 141, 142, 171, 181, 182, 190, 198, 200, 201, 204, 205, 206, 210, 212, 226, 227, 231, 268, 270, 276, 279, 290, 309, 333, 373, 376, 380, 392, 396, 414, 416, 465, 503, 648, 688, 734, 735, 737, 738, 739, 740, 743, 744, 745, 748, 750, 754, 758, 780, 801, 810, 813, 845
pulmonary vascular disorders, 275–281
pulmonary vasculitis, 280
pulmonic ejection click, 97
pulse oximetry, 123, 228, 246, 263, 268, 270, 272, 318, 740
pulsus paradoxus, 135
pyelonephritis, 386–389, 394, 464, 683
pyrazinamide, 59, 265
Pyridium, 389
pyridostigmine, 36, 37
pyridoxine, 59, 265, 266, 344, 595, 805
pyuria, 366, 387, 409, 578

Q

QRS complex, 98, 122, 143, 145, 148, 198, 199, 200, 203, 205, 211, 403, 771, 790, 792, 793, 799
QT intervals, 98, 551
quadriparesis, 35
quadriplegia, 14, 47–49, 458
quantiferon, 265
quinapril (Accupril), 103t, 176t, 184t, 417t
quinidine, 35, 108t, 202t, 602, 608t, 685, 790
quinolones, 356, 363, 379, 387, 388

R

radiation, 26–28, 96, 120, 153, 162, 235, 256, 268, 356, 368–370, 380, 414, 415, 421, 545–547, 549, 550, 559, 561, 563, 565, 566, 568, 569, 571, 573, 575–578, 580, 581, 602, 615, 619, 641, 843, 848, 851, 857, 872, 885, 890t
radical prostatectomy, 577
radioablation, 416
radioactive iodine, 448
radioallergosorbent Test (RAST), 476
radiography, 9, 242, 328, 369, 371, 372, 688, 777
radiology, 8
radionuclide bone scan, 577
Ramsay Hunt syndrome, 650
ranitidine (Zantac), 28, 34, 50, 108t, 329, 331, 334, 354, 612, 749
ranolazine, 127
reabsorption, 393, 464, 465, 720, 735
rebleeding, 17, 24
rebreathing, 784
receptor antagonist, 76, 174, 277, 282, 329, 462, 466, 644, 696, 697, 700
Recombivax, 338, 596
red blood cell (RBC), 3
reflex, 9, 32, 34, 35, 46, 49, 50, 58, 59, 62, 81, 85, 90, 105, 110, 127, 156, 201, 221, 243, 311, 447, 450, 462, 508, 509, 516, 650, 747, 754t, 774, 776, 782, 783, 791, 801t, 804, 862
rehabilitation, 8, 13, 34, 53, 54, 127
renal artery differential pressure (RADP), 416
renal artery stenosis (RAS), 414–417
renal biopsy, 396
renal calculi nephrolithiasis, 419–423
renal disease, 101, 464, 873
renal failure, 44, 98, 100, 105, 153, 292, 300, 345, 355, 379, 392, 393, 394, 396, 397, 398, 402, 405, 415, 416, 421, 463, 480, 481, 482, 486, 504, 529, 696, 703, 737, 746, 759, 771, 772, 777, 778, 779, 835, 841, 847
renal function, 272, 413, 623
renal hypercalciuria, 422
renal injuries, 834
renal osmotic diuresis, 767
renal osteodystrophy, 404
renal potassium loss, 768
renal replacement, 401
renal tubule defects, 776
renal vascular hypertension, 414
renal vascular, 839
renin-angiotensin, 101, 770
renin-angiotensin-aldosterone, 170, 184t, 416
renin-secreting tumor, 769
replacement fluid, 786
reserpine, 105, 459
respiratory, 31–33, 35, 36, 38, 42, 48, 49, 51, 53, 57, 59, 62, 68, 90, 91, 166, 171, 222, 223, 225, 228, 229, 240, 241, 246, 250, 251, 261, 263, 266, 272, 274, 278, 280, 281, 285, 286, 288–291, 296–299t, 305, 306, 309, 314, 316–319, 340, 347, 348, 355, 365, 376, 462, 479t, 487t, 537, 550, 592, 597, 636, 652, 657, 658, 660, 699, 702t, 705t, 707t, 735, 738–740, 746, 748, 749, 759, 776–778, 780–784, 789–792, 794, 796–798, 806, 807, 820, 825t, 829–831, 847, 851, 856t, 859, 863, 867, 868, 883, 895, 898–903, 907
respiratory acidosis, 225, 740, 780, 791

respiratory alkalosis, 171, 225, 278, 376, 735, 739, 740, 776, 778, 783, 796, 829

respiratory failure, 738, 867

respiratory rate, 246, 319

respiratory tract, 57, 166, 280, 281, 296, 297, 298, 537, 746, 749, 820, 825

resuscitation, 43, 46, 47, 49, 122t, 125t, 129t–131t, 136, 150, 216f, 229, 231, 232, 267, 345, 346, 362, 365, 371, 375, 376, 378–380, 396, 443, 449, 503, 520, 737, 740, 742, 744, 746, 747, 753t, 762, 767, 785, 800, 832–834, 852

retinal artery obstruction, 646–647

retinal detachment, 641, 646, 835

retinopathy, 100, 427, 429, 529, 645

retroperitoneal lymph node sampling, 581

revascularization, 6, 25, 131t, 134, 153, 154, 156, 157, 173f, 182, 209, 373, 416, 744, 847

rhabdomyolysis, 115t, 117, 394, 397t, 614, 770, 777, 802

rheumatic fever, 162, 190, 192

rheumatoid arthritis (RA), 471

rhinitis, 251, 252, 654, 656, 658

rhinorrhea, 41, 655, 668, 669t

rhinovirus, 261

ribavirin, 298t, 339

rifampin, 59, 78, 108t, 264, 265, 300t, 395

rifaximin, 347, 518

Ringer's solution, 49, 60, 231, 356, 371, 376, 380, 499, 624, 742, 746, 749, 785, 807, 830, 832, 834, 875

risk assessment, 903

risperidone (Risperdal), 77, 713, 720t, 726t, 730, 798

Rivaroxaban, 11, 160, 280, 803

rivastigmine (Exelon), 76

rizatriptan (Maxalt), 671, 677

Robitussin, 251

rocephin, 59, 365, 379, 633, 660

Rocky Mountain spotted fever, 61, 394, 684

rosiglitazone, 341, 438t–440t

rosuvastatin, 114t, 115t, 127

R-wave, 141

S

salicylate poisoning, 779, 780 797

salicylate, 470, 484, 705, 779, 783, 796

Salmonella septicemia, 597

salpingitis, 622, 624

Sandostatin, 328, 376

sarcoidosis, 170, 194, 196, 269–271, 276, 294, 295, 420, 650, 684, 689, 773, 774, 846

schizophrenia, 731

scintillating scotoma, 667

sclerosis, 79, 90, 97, 241, 314, 386, 414, 555, 641, 653, 662, 698, 838, 845

scoliosis, 895

sedative, 43, 290, 306, 314, 404, 653, 697, 698, 722, 730, 781, 783, 874

seizure, 4, 6, 12, 16, 23, 24, 27, 28, 41, 44, 45, 57, 58, 60, 62, 63, 65–68, 70t, 73, 76, 80, 83, 202t, 210, 309, 402, 444, 445, 462, 463, 479t, 482, 485, 486, 523, 603, 666t, 684, 696, 698, 702t, 711, 712, 716, 718t, 720t, 721, 725t, 726t, 765, 766, 772, 773, 775, 781, 783, 789, 790, 792, 793, 796, 798–800, 802, 804, 805, 807, 854, 859, 860, 868

selective serotonin reuptake inhibitors (SSRIs), 715

selegiline, 77, 86, 87t

sepsis syndrome, 291

septic shock, 743, 745, 751, 755, 868

sequential nephron blockade, 180, 181

Seroquel, 77, 720t, 726t, 730, 732

serotonin, 77, 87t, 536, 674t, 693, 694, 697, 698, 715, 717t, 718t, 724, 725t

sertraline, 77, 698, 715, 717t, 725t, 799

sexual assessment, 728

sexual dysfunction, 83, 86

sexual intercourse, 386

sexual orientation, 686, 860

sexuality, 729

sexually active, 625, 634, 636, 637, 890, 891, 892, 893

shingles, 589, 592, 615, 650, 908t, 909t, see herpes zoster

shock, 49, 51, 53, 134–136, 139, 146t, 149t, 200, 201, 206, 209, 210, 212, 216f, 228, 231, 266, 278, 280, 291, 309, 314, 315, 327, 356, 372, 375, 378, 380, 393, 421, 422, 530, 610, 612, 613, 623, 694, 707t, 734, 736t–751t, 753t, 779t, 792t, 800t, 807, 833, 834, 854, 867, 868

sickle cell anemia (SS), 528

sildenafil, 157, 277

silhouette sign, 235

simvastatin, 114t, 115t, 593

sinemet, 86, 87t

sinusitis, 56, 60, 251, 485t, 656–658, 664, 683, 825t

skin cancer, 567, 610, 618, 843, 890, 895

skin testing, 264, 612

small bowel feces sign, 370

small bowel obstruction, 368–370

small cell carcinoma (SCC), 564

smoking, 4, 6–8, 22, 101, 103, 107t, 111, 113, 119, 120, 131t, 152, 154, 156–158, 170, 172, 182, 238, 245, 247, 252, 266, 267, 271, 273, 326, 332, 334, 340, 354, 416, 429, 563, 571, 578, 604, 622, 625, 645, 646, 670t, 858, 871, 874, 885, 887, 892t–894, 903

socioeconomic status, 881

soft tissue injury, 492

solid organ transplantation, 837

Solu-Medrol, 28, 249, 362, 364t, 597, 749, 841t

somatic efferent, 687

space-occupying lesions, 26–29, 65

speculum examination, 628, 630

spermicide, 386, 389

S-phase fraction (SPF), 570

spinal cord, 46–54, 55, 158, 314, 395, 868

spinal cord trauma, 46–54

spinal stenosis, 505, 506

spine, 54, 285, 488, 510

spirometry, 240–242, 252, 254, 259t, 821, 830, 838t, 863, 875, 876

spironolactone, 103t, 175t, 176t, 180t, 184t, 348, 770, 781

spleen, 171, 534

splenomegaly, 164, 171, 340, 472, 516, 527, 529, 550, 557

sputum, 245, 250, 252, 262, 264, 266, 564, 565, 687, 821, 859, 876

ST segment, 120, 121, 124, 125, 126, 127, 128, 129, 130, 131, 133, 163, 194, 195, 206

ST-segment elevation myocardial infarction (STEMI), 120, 121, 123, 124, 125t, 127, 130f, 131t, 136t

Staphylococcus, 57, 158, 164, 165, 262, 298t–300t, 385, 387, 613, 642, 651, 652, 691t, 745, 819, 823–826t

statin, 78, 113–117, 127, 130f, 173f, 328, 333, 353, 356, 367, 373, 376, 388, 401, 416

steatorrhea, 355, 421, 422

stenosis, 4, 6, 7, 97, 131, 133, 155, 156, 188, 189, 192, 275, 372, 373, 399, 414, 415, 417, 418, 507, 581, 735, 744, 780, 846, 848

steroid, 18, 28, 35, 44, 82, 108t, 241, 250, 300t, 344, 361–363, 364t, 403, 420, 507, 509, 535, 603, 644, 648, 651, 652, 699, 758, 806, 810

stimulant, 109, 189, 242, 716, 801t, 805

stimulant toxicity, 801

stings, 805–808

stomach, 115, 238, 311, 325, 326, 328, 329, 375, 377, 378, 437, 516, 548, 557, 761, 792

stool cultures, 360

streptococci, 57, 165, 613, 624, 691, 745

Streptococcus pneumoniae, 262

stress, 16, 46, 50, 55, 111, 112, 120, 124, 125, 126, 127, 140, 172, 182, 195, 376, 419, 420, 424, 442, 444, 449, 454, 458, 462, 489, 490, 499, 615, 635, 650, 673, 687, 714, 716, 724, 728, 731, 740, 758, 759, 821, 872, 874, 876, 893, 894, 896

stretta procedure, 335

stroke, 4, 6–14, 73, 75, 100, 113, 114, 132, 136, 141, 154, 168, 177, 192, 203–205, 263, 306, 309, 344, 386, 528–531, 603, 641, 647, 711, 738, 740, 748, 867, 882, 894, 903

stromal tumors, 574

struvite calculi, 421, 422

subclavian steal syndrome, 4

subluxation, 472, 488, 489, 505

submaximal tests, 125

substance use disorder, 716–723

sucralfate, 325, 330, 331, 821

suctioning, 43, 50, 657, 821

sufentanil, 43

suicidal risk, 714

sulfapyridine, 364t

sulfasalazine, 354, 361, 362, 364t, 472, 482t

sulfonamide, 354, 387–389, 395, 434, 533, 592, 608t, 611

sulfonylureas, 108t, 434, 437t, 441t, 608t

sulfur dioxide, 268

Sulindac, 354, 474, 481t, 704t

sumatriptan (Imitrex), 671, 673

surgical biopsy, 620

surgical wound infections, 824

surgical wound, 824

sympathomimetics, 108, 458

symptomatic bacteriuria, 820

symptomatic candiduria, 820

syndrome of inappropriate antidiuretic hormone (SIADH), 461–463

synovial fluid, 470, 472

syphilis, 57, 73, 464, 592, 603, 631, 633, 638, 639, 647, 653, 730

systemic circulation, 737

systemic disease, 638, 642, 729, 810

systemic lupus erythematosus (SLE), 188, 193, 286, 395, 448, 449, 461, 493, 533, 534, 602–604, 608, 684

systemic panarteritis, 601

systolic BP (SBP), 10

systolic dysfunction, 174, 175, 176, 182

T

tachyarrhythmia, 33, 98, 142, 143, 145, 146t, 189, 195, 202t, 203t, 208, 216f, 750t, 752t, 753t, 784, 800t

tachycardia, 32, 53, 88t, 98, 105, 110, 127, 129t, 130f, 132, 135, 147, 149t, 171, 178, 189, 191, 193, 194, 199–203t, 205–207t, 209, 214f, 216f, 231, 248, 249, 251, 263, 271, 272, 278, 279, 328, 353, 355, 365, 369, 378, 380, 386, 443–445, 447, 449, 455, 457, 465, 514, 516, 519, 529, 537, 623, 687, 695, 712, 720t, 721, 725t, 729, 738, 741, 742, 748, 750t, 753t, 767, 781, 784, 789, 794, 795, 798, 799, 801t, 802, 804–807, 823, 830, 831, 854, 867, 876

tachypnea, 355

tacrolimus, 37, 364t, 840t, 842t, 843

tadalafil, 277, 752t

Tagamet, 329

Tamiflu, 298t

tamoxifen, 571

tamponade, 135, 163, 377, 379, 557, 559, 564, 743, 745, 832, 834, 867

tamsulosin, 409, 422

tazobactam, 299t, 353, 360, 367, 373, 388, 615, 660, 690t, 691t, 747, 814, 822, 825, 826t, 833

T-cell, 34, 473, 544, 545, 555, 556

telithromycin, 297t, 301t–303t

temporomandibular joint disorder, 661

tenecteplase (TNKase), 132, 137

tenofovir, 338, 591, 594t, 598t

Tenormin, 103t, 126, 202t

tension-type headache, 679

terazosin, 104t, 409, 459

tertiary prevention, 887

testosterone, 409, 411

tetanus, 41, 499, 645, 807, 826t, 858, 893t, 894, 906, 908t, 909t tetracycline, 78, 297t, 303t, 331, 354, 403, 608, 626, 643, 845

tetracyn, 331

thalassemia, 515, 516, 523–525, 527–529

thallium stress test, 125

the six Ps, 503

theophylline, 108, 199, 203, 250, 251, 257f, 329, 333

theophylline toxicity, 802

therapeutic coagulation values, 137

thiamine, 63, 170, 721, 780, 790, 805

thiazide, 43, 102t–107t, 108t, 177, 179–181t, 354, 412, 421–423t, 533, 608t, 765, 769, 773, 774

thiazolidinediones, 182, 434

thoracentesis, 287, 294

thoracic spine, 47

thoracic vertebrae, 52

thoracotomy, 832

thorax, 852

thromboangiitis obliterans (Buerger's disease), 157, 161

thrombocytopenia, 3, 5, 7, 159, 202t, 230, 279, 400f, 472, 480t–482t, 484t, 485t, 487, 514, 525, 533–536, 538, 546, 548, 549, 603, 610, 623, 703, 746, 751, 790, 840t, 872

thrombocytosis, 3, 522, 529, 551, 602, 770

thromboembolectomy, 157

thromboembolism, 11, 34, 276, 277, 279, 414, 537, 894

thrombolytic therapy, 12, 124, 127, 136, 160, 846

thrombophlebitis, 685

thrombosis, 8, 25, 50, 137t, 155, 157–160, 276, 278–280, 372, 416, 535–538, 551, 613, 614, 647, 653, 685, 688, 844–846, 872, 875, 876

thyroid, 36, 74, 271, 272, 403, 447, 448, 449, 451, 458, 462, 642, 653, 654, 715, 774, 868, 895, 896

thyroid storm, 448–449, 868

thyroidectomy, 450

thyroid-stimulating hormone (TSH), 447, 774

thyrotoxicosis, 38, 170, 447, 665t, 685, see also hyperthyroidism

thyroxine, 272, 447, 448, 450, 451

timolol, 103, 176t, 649, 674t, 792

tinnitus, 25, 27, 81, 396, 480t, 481t, 484t, 514, 516, 653, 665t, 702t, 705t, 790, 796, 859

TMP-SMX 389, 595, 597, 614

TobraDex, 652

tobramycin, 299, 388, 495, 690t, 691t, 747, 822, 823, 826, 827

tonic-clonic, 67, 70t

tonsillitis, 658

topiramate, 70, 672t–674t, 697

total parenteral nutrition (TPN), 370

toxic, 5, 6, 57, 73, 88t, 98, 163, 177, 199, 202t, 203, 224, 251, 271, 309, 315, 330, 336, 341, 345, 362, 364t, 368, 398, 404, 447, 470, 472, 477t, 479t, 481t–484t, 486t, 487t, 499, 525, 551, 561, 577, 592, 611, 612, 614, 626, 641, 649, 686, 690t, 691t, 702t, 704, 715, 720, 729, 747, 752, 771, 774, 776, 780, 783, 788, 789, 792, 794–799, 801–805, 808, 826t, 827, 840t, 854, 867

toxic megacolon, 362

toxin, 36, 193, 249, 251, 275, 344, 398, 400f, 477t, 731, 745, 824, 826t, 851, 903, 905

toxoplasmosis, 27t, 61, 592, 595, 597, 684

tracheobronchitis, 297t

tracheostomy, 307, 320

trandolapril, 103t, 176t, 184t, 417t

transesophageal echocardiography (TEE), 6

transient ischemic attack, 3–7, 177, 179, 204, 528, 653, 858

transurethral incision of the prostate (TUIP), 410

transurethral laser-induced prostatectomy (TULIP), 410

transurethral microwave therapy (TUMT), 410

transurethral needle ablation of the prostate (TUNA), 410

transurethral resection of the prostate (TURP), 410

transvaginal ultrasound, 623

transvaginal, 575, 626

traumatic pneumothorax, 294

tremor, 81, 445, 723, 782, 795, 840

Treponema pallidum, 638

treponemal antibody absorption test, 639

triamterene, 180t, 420

trigeminal neuralgia (Tic disorders), 23, 81, 661–662, 694, 708

tuberculosis, 57, 59, 162, 255, 261, 264, 267, 287, 294, 364t, 454, 461, 464, 473, 498, 506t, 592, 595, 597, 683, 686, 689, 844t, 885, 893t

tumor, 4, 9, 12, 15, 25–28, 34, 52, 61, 65, 75, 236, 252, 255, 263, 268, 276, 278, 326, 363, 364t, 366, 368, 372, 376, 386, 387, 395, 447, 449, 453, 457, 459, 461, 464, 471, 486t, 487t, 498, 505, 506t, 543, 546, 558, 561, 564–568, 570–576, 579, 615, 617–619, 622, 638, 641, 648, 650, 653, 656, 657, 664, 665, 683, 687, 688, 694, 712, 731t, 734, 740, 744, 745, 769, 770, 777, 847

Tums, 334, 404

Tylenol, 19, 495, 499, 507, 627, 658, 659, 696, 788

type 1 diabetes, 430–433, 438

type 2 diabetes, 433–434, 441

U

U.S. Public Health Service disease prevention and health promotion model, 882

ulcer, 34, 50, 51, 87t, 116t, 121, 136t, 153–158, 325–331, 333, 335, 342, 357, 360–363, 376, 377, 379, 429, 470, 480t, 481t, 506t, 507, 529, 531, 557, 572, 603, 608t, 609f, 612–614, 617–619, 623, 630, 635, 637, 638, 656, 659, 684, 691, 703, 704t, 737, 806, 810–816t, 821, 841t, 857t, 858

ulcerative colitis, 342, 360, 367, 685

ultrasonography, 6, 10, 126, 153, 159, 287, 356, 369, 415, 529, 531, 570, 575, 577, 579, 581, 623, 688, 812, 838t, 845, 846

ultrasound, 6, 17, 155, 341, 352, 353, 356, 365, 366, 370, 372, 387, 396, 397t, 399, 409, 410, 415, 421, 474, 490, 623, 833, 844, 845, 889t

ultrasound-guided needle aspiration, 845

unstable angina, 109, 867

ureteral obstruction, 845

Index xlix

urethral stents, 411
urethritis, 386, 387, 625, 630, 848
urinalysis, 67, 101, 266, 271, 340, 366, 371, 386, 389, 395, 409, 421, 428, 499, 503, 579, 687, 730, 807, 819, 834, 863, 871, 891t
urinary output, 852
urinary sediment, 393, 396, 397
urinary tract infection, 51, 385–389, 409, 420, 421, 683, 687, 819, 822, 823, 825, 844, 845, 896
urine, 290, 386, 392, 393, 395, 397, 402, 409, 420, 421, 445, 453, 465, 529, 579, 590, 687, 737, 740, 741, 746, 765, 768, 779, 781, 819, 844
urticaria, 166t, 364t, 486t, 608t, 610–612, 706t, 748, 749, 805, 806, 840t
uveitis, 642, 646, 648
uvulopalatopharyngoplasty (UPPP), 306

V

vaccine, 56, 57, 174, 251, 263–265, 269, 296, 337–339, 478t, 486t, 487t, 531, 535, 550, 561, 573, 596, 608t, 616, 617, 637, 748, 844, 856t, 858, 884t, 891t, 893t, 904–909t
vagina, 337, 380, 386, 389, 571–574, 580, 581, 588, 589, 622–630, 632–635, 712, 829, 835, 886
vaginal discharge, 628, 635
vaginitis, 627–629
valacyclovir (Valtrex), 616, 636
valproic, 69t, 70t, 354, 672t, 673t, 697, 720t
valsartan, 104t, 176t, 184t, 417t
valvular disease, 3, 164, 169, 186–192, 193, 275, 372, 740, 744
vancomycin, 60t, 165, 300t, 388, 499, 611, 614, 615, 660, 690t, 691t, 747, 814, 822–827
varicella-zoster, 57, 59, 61, 162, 592, 596, 615–617, 684, 844t, 885, 891t, 893t, 906, 908t, 909t
vascular ectasias, 379
vasculitis, 3, 5, 8, 75, 275, 280, 286, 414, 485t, 603, 610, 647, 684, 685
vasoconstriction, 43, 51, 105, 108t, 134, 170, 221, 275, 393, 735, 737, 738, 744, 839
vasodilation, 104, 105, 153, 157, 181, 183, 664, 750t, 751t
vasomotor center depression, 747
vasopressin, 210, 328, 376, 379, 380, 462, 464, 465, 744, 747–750t, 754t, 768, 799, 800t
vasospasm, 15–17, 23, 24, 98, 111, 666t, 868, 876
vasovagal reflex, 50
venous disease, 158
venous stasis, 278, 876
venous thrombosis, 50, 551, 844
venous ulcers, 812, 813
ventilation, 221–225
ventilator adjustments, 225
ventilatory failure, 290
verapamil (Calan), 104, 108t, 127, 179, 191, 196, 200, 201, 203t, 206, 211, 666t, 673t, 674t, 793
vertebrobasilar, 5
vertigo, 5, 9, 14, 27t, 58, 80, 482t, 623, 652, 653, 709t, 859

Vibramycin, 302t, 303t
violence, 46, 712, 713, 881, 883, 884, 890, 892, 893, 895
viral infections, 528, 843
visual disturbances, 41, 445
vitamin B, 36, 73, 75, 516, 526, 551, 715
vitamin B12 deficiency, 73, 515–517, 521, 641
vitamin, 36, 73, 75, 77, 341, 343, 348, 349, 404, 420, 516, 526, 551, 592, 715, 759, 772, 773, 774, 777, 889
vomit, 5, 14, 26, 37, 41, 51, 58, 60, 62, 83, 87t, 116t, 121, 202t, 203t, 327, 328, 329, 337, 340, 345, 346, 352, 355, 356, 359, 363, 364t, 366, 368–371, 378, 386, 392, 398, 401, 415, 421, 441t, 442t, 445, 454, 462, 479t–482t, 484t, 487t, 528, 530, 611, 623, 627, 632, 648, 653, 654, 666t, 667, 669t, 670t, 697, 702t, 703t, 705t, 707t, 709t, 717t–720t, 723t–725t, 741, 748, 759, 760, 773, 779–781, 788–790, 792, 794–797, 802, 804, 806, 838, 841, 854, 856t, 859

W

Wagner Ulcer Grade Classification System of Staging, 811, 812
warfarin (Coumadin), 6, 7, 11, 160, 177, 178, 187, 204, 207t, 279, 329, 434, 536, 604, 803
Western blot test, 590
wheezing, 246, 252, 564, 611, 612, 748, 782, 830
whiplash, 46
widow spiders, 806
work of breathing (WOB), 222
World Health Organization (WHO), 275, 556

X

Xigris, 756
x-ray, 6, 15, 26t–28, 52, 53, 75, 101, 130f, 135, 146, 147, 187, 188, 190, 191, 194, 195, 229, 234–238, 247, 252, 255, 261–263, 265–268, 270, 272, 276, 279, 287, 294, 318, 328, 352, 360, 362, 365, 369, 370, 387, 396, 399, 404, 455, 470, 490, 494, 499, 506, 508, 525, 530, 531, 560, 564, 568, 575, 592, 660, 661, 712, 730, 744, 746, 807, 821, 825, 829–832, 834, 835, 857t, 863
x-ray film, 499

Y

yeasts, 823

Z

zanamivir, 298t
ziprasidone, 77, 713, 720t, 798
Zithromax, 301t–303t, 595, 631, 633, 652
zolmitriptan (Zomig), 671, 677
Zyloprim, 422
Zyprexa, 77, 685, 713, 720t, 726t, 730

ß

ß-blocker, 35, 106f, 108t, 120, 123, 124, 126, 127, 130f, 132, 135, 172, 174–177, 179, 182–184t, 188, 195, 196, 200, 201, 203, 206, 209, 211, 216f, 273, 377, 459, 610, 611, 672t, 674t, 750t, 751t